ADAPTIVE RADIOGRAPHY

WITH TRAUMA, IMAGE CRITIQUE AND CRITICAL THINKING

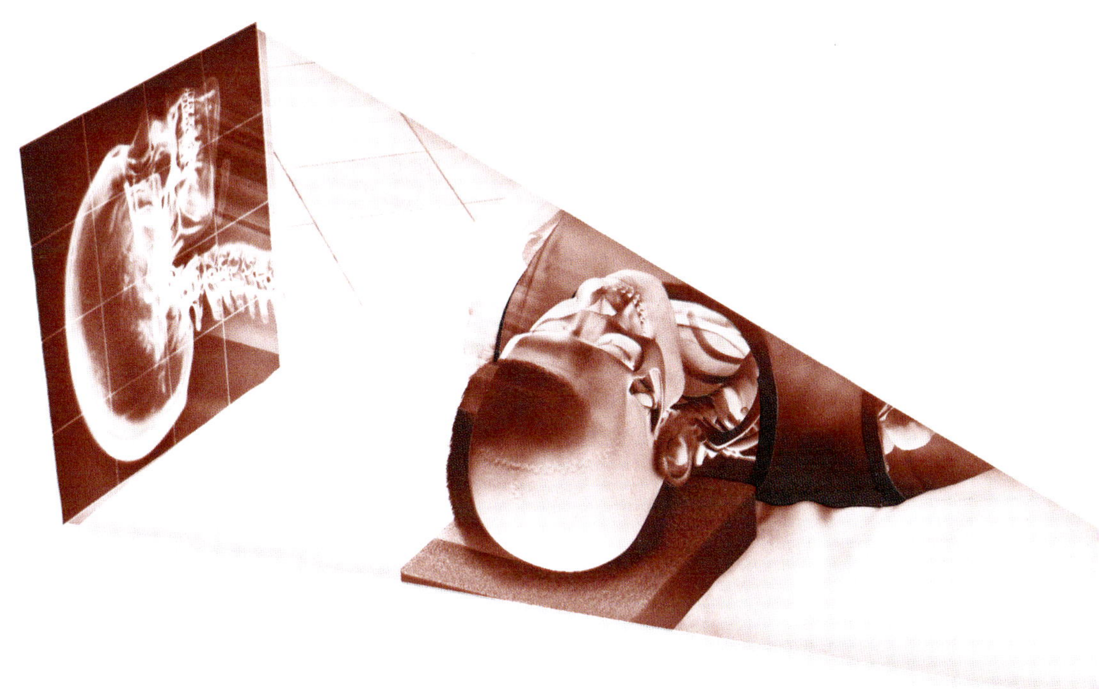

ADAPTIVE RADIOGRAPHY WITH TRAUMA, IMAGE CRITIQUE AND CRITICAL THINKING

First Edition

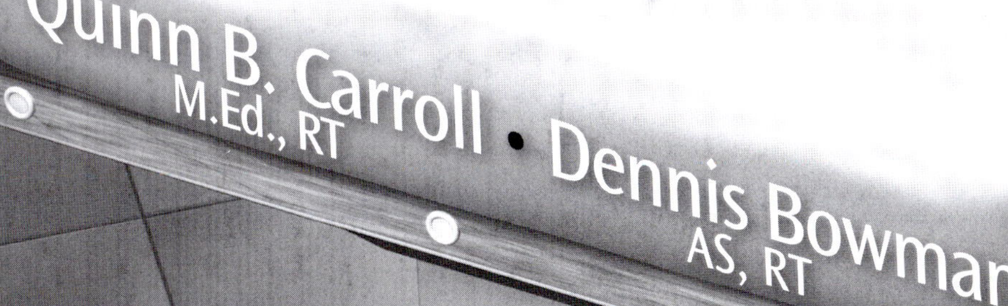

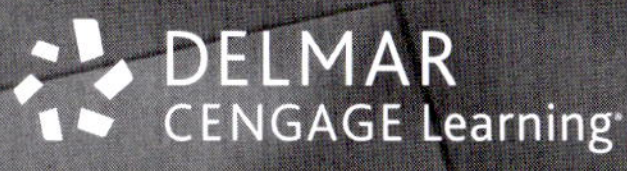

Australia • Brazil • Japan • Korea • Mexico • Singapore • Spain • United Kingdom • United States

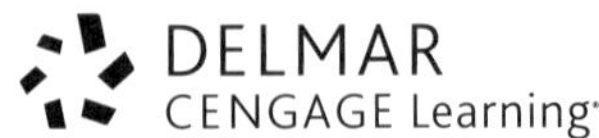

Adaptive Radiography with Trauma, Image Critique, and Critical Thinking, First Edition International Edition
Quinn B. Carroll, M.Ed., RT and Dennis Bowman, AS, RT

Vice President, Careers & Computing: Dave Garza

Publisher: Stephen Helba

Associate Acquisitions Editor: Christina Gifford

Director, Development- Careers & Computing: Marah Bellegarde

Product Development Manager: Juliet Steiner

Senior Product Manager: Laura J. Stewart

Editorial Assistant: Cassie Cloutier

Executive Brand Manager: Wendy E. Mapstone

Associate Market Development Manager: Jonathan Sheehan

Senior Production Director: Wendy A. Troeger

Production Manager: Andrew Crouth

Senior Content Project Manager: Kara A. DiCaterino

Senior Art Director: David Arsenault

Media Editor: William Overocker

Interior Design Images: Courtesy of Sharon and Joel Harris/Deborah Wolfe Ltd.

Cover Image: © CLIPAREA | Custom media/ www.Shutterstock.com

International Edition:
ISBN-13: 978-1-285-19783-8
ISBN-10: 1-285-19783-6

Cengage Learning International Offices

Asia
www.cengageasia.com
tel: (65) 6410 1200

Australia/New Zealand
www.cengage.com.au
tel: (61) 3 9685 4111

Brazil
www.cengage.com.br
tel: (55) 11 3665 9900

India
www.cengage.co.in
tel: (91) 11 4364 1111

Latin America
www.cengage.com.mx
tel: (52) 55 1500 6000

UK/Europe/Middle East/Africa
www.cengage.co.uk
tel: (44) 0 1264 332 424

Represented in Canada by Nelson Education, Ltd.
www.nelson.com
tel: (416) 752 9100/(800) 668 0671

Cengage Learning is a leading provider of customized learning solutions with office locations around the globe, including Singapore, the United Kingdom, Australia, Mexico, Brazil, and Japan. Locate your local office at: **international.cengage.com/region**

Cengage Learning products are represented in Canada by Nelson Education, Ltd.

To learn more about Delmar, visit **www.cengage.com/delmar**

Purchase any of our products at your local college store or at our preferred online store **www.cengagebrain.com**

Printed in the United States of America
1 2 3 4 5 6 7 17 16 15 14 13

DEDICATIONS

I have received ongoing support and love from a wonderful family, and especially from my wife, Margaret, who has never faltered in sustaining me. Since I have acknowledged my children in other publications, I wish to dedicate this work to a growing list of ***grandkids,*** namely, Lauren, Emily, Zachary, Colbie, Kade, Maira, Paxton, Rowan, Dylan, Ethan, Aiden, Lyndin, Caleb, Ashlyn, and Peyton. All my love.

Quinn B. Carroll

I want to thank my family, especially my remarkable wife Kristi. The endless hours I've spent on the computer these past 2 years can never be made up but she filled me with confidence and supported me through it all. I also want to thank my two wonderful stepsons Cris and Daniel and Cris's lovely wife Katie, our cherished daughter-in-law, and Daniel's fiance Nicole, our soon to be treasured daughter-in-law #2. I love you all.

Dennis M. Bowman

Brief Table of Contents

Table of Contents

Preface

Introduction and Conceptual Approach

Through the development of analytical and critical thinking, this textbook is designed to raise radiographic positioning skills and image critique skills to the "next level," from rote learning to generic understanding. It will be of great interest to the *practicing clinical radiographer* as well as to educational programs with a curricular emphasis on challenging radiography students to excel.

Students are generally taken chapter by chapter through positioning textbooks, simply *memorizing* the various body positions, beam angles, and centering points. The conceptual approach used here is truly foundational, and leads to an understanding of *why* those particular positions, angles, and centering points are used, and in the process, empower the radiographer and student to *adapt* positions for difficult patients and situations including mobile and trauma procedures.

Some educational programs will prefer to use this book in their advanced courses on trauma positioning, mobile procedures, and image critique, or in their *capstone* course targeted at integrating all that has been learned throughout the program. Others will integrate it throughout their curriculum, using it over several semesters as a supplement to each positioning course.

Organization and Features

Chapters 1 through 5 present spatial relations principles that no other text in the field has addressed in any thorough or logical progression, yet these are foundational, essential skills that underpin the radiographer's generic ability to adapt to the great variety of patients and clinical situations encountered in daily practice.

Unique to this textbook is the effort to *quantify* the degree and manner in which anatomy shifts with various positioning movements of the patient's body (rotation, flexion, extension, tilt, abduction, and adduction), with various angles of the x-ray beam, and with various degrees of off-centering from the central ray, and also *quantify* the expansion of the x-ray beam as it passes through the body. Corrections in centering for all these variables are not only specified, but again *quantified*. All of this information is presented in the form of concise rules of thumb that can be immediately applied in daily practice.

Chapter 6 presents several positioning adaptations necessitated by DR equipment and other new imaging units that have limited movement in the x-ray tube or table, as well as new positions made possible by *increased* flexibility of movement in some upright units.

Chapter 7 gets to the heart of trauma positioning, presenting *generic* skills in working around the trauma patient. This is immediately followed by specific tips for trauma and mobile positions in Chapter 8, including a step-by-step approach to mobile chest and abdomen positions.

Chapter 9 provides a comprehensive treatment of adaptive head positions, for both routine and trauma situations. The *quantification* of head tilt, rotation, flexion, and extension that leads to specific CR angle corrections is a unique feature here. Positions that have certainly become rarer but are still encountered on occasion (the Townes, SMV, and TMJ projections) are included for two reasons: The classroom instructor may leave out whichever specific positions she chooses, whereas eliminating these positions from the textbook leaves the instructor no option. More important is the fact that these positions provide excellent material for reinforcing the generic positioning and visualization skills that are desired for adaptive radiography.

Finally, Chapter 10 progresses through the typical list of routine positions covered by positioning atlases, but with an eye to simplified centering and positioning tips that apply the foundational rules and paradigms presented in Chapter 1.

Chapter 11 presents essential skills for image critique including the *quantification* of positioning errors apparent in the image; then these are followed by specific corrections from image evaluation in Chapter 12.

Chapter 13 is a short review of clinically useful technique adjustments. The capstone Chapter 14 is uniquely dedicated to critical thinking skills. Essential intellectual traits identified by the *Foundation for Critical Thinking* are discussed in detail, then the application of these principles to *clinical evaluation of radiography students* is demonstrated along with suggested forms for grading clinical challenge cases or case studies. This material is supported by several exercises on sequencing clinical exams.

Reinforcement of essential concepts for the reader is prominent throughout the book by the use of highlighted *Best Practice Tips*, numerous *Case Studies* sprinkled throughout each chapter, and *Critical Thinking Challenges* presented at the end of each chapter (with answers in the appendix).

The entire work revolves around 22 *basic paradigms* for adaptive positioning skills, which are presented in Chapter 1. These paradigms were developed with an eye to *simplifying* radiographic positioning, while at the same time improving accuracy.

Ideas for the ongoing improvement of this textbook are actively solicited from all of our colleagues in radiography, and much appreciated.

The authors' intent and hope is that this will be a truly innovative and valuable contribution to the clinical practice of radiography and the improvement of quality patient care.

Quinn B. Carroll
Dennis M. Bowman

Also Available

Instructor Companion Website
ISBN-13: 978-1-111-54121-7

The instructor companion website contains instructor support materials designed to accompany the textbook. Included on the companion website are the following materials:

- Customizable instructor support slide presentations in **PowerPoint**® format focus on key points for each chapter. Use during class lectures, as handouts for student note taking and review. Over 550 slides are available with one presentation for each chapter.
- The **Instructor's Manual** contains a list of suggested course materials, chapter learning objectives, chapter summary, and lesson plans for each chapter that include additional activities. A sample syllabus for a 16-week course is also provided for you to modify and adapt to your course.
- A **test bank** created using ExamView® software contains over 200 additional questions related to each chapter's content. Available formats include true/false, multiple choice, multiple response, short answer, and essay. Use the test banks to create exams and customize to add or edit questions.

To access these materials, log on to login.cengage.com and sign up for a faculty account or contact your sales representative for more information.

ACKNOWLEDGMENTS

A number of good friends and colleagues in clinical practice have assisted with the production of this work. We wish to extend heartfelt thanks to them.

Mr. Carroll wishes to thank Lisa Moore, RT, Dendra Whisman, RT, and Elise Fielder, RT for their assistance in modeling for radiographic positions.

ReeDunna Young, clinical instructor and supervisor at Midland Memorial Hospital in Texas, was not only instrumental in photographing and modeling for a number of illustrations in this book, but she also contributed several positioning tips and ideas in this book. Combining extensive clinical experience with an open mind, she provides a professional role model for students. Special gratitude is extended to ReeDunna for her assistance, teaching, and personal support over many years.

Mr. Bowman wishes to express special gratitude to Lito Lopez, RT for all the positioning work over the past few years—thanks for taking many for the team. Thanks to Carter Doupnik RT for all the incredible "magic" he has done with Excel and the charts he's created. In addition, thanks to both Ramiro Villanueva RT(R)(CV), CIIP, CPSA and Frank Gin CIIP, CPSA for the endless PACS images work you've done for me.

Many thanks to Laura Stewart, Christina Gifford, and Sherry Dickinson, editors at Cengage, for their extensive assistance and counsel, and to all the copy editors and artists at Cengage who contributed to this important work.

Cengage Learning would also like to acknowledge the reviewers who took the time to provide invaluable feedback on the content during development of this project. Those reviewers include:

Brenda Cliff, MRT(R), BTech
Medical Radiation Technology, Program Coordinator
Cambrian College of Applied Arts and Technology
Sudbury Ontario, Canada

Terri Crutcher, RTR(C), BA
Instructor, Clinical Coordinator
Volunteer State Community College
Gallatin, TN

Donna Endicott, MEd, RT(R)
Program Director
Xavier University
Cincinnati, Ohio

Ismael Garcia, BAAS, RT (R)
Associate Professor
Del Mar College
Corpus Christi, TX

Warren Hejny, BS, RT(R)(CT)
Professor
Truckee Meadows Community College
Reno, Nevada

Sandra J. Nauman, MS, RT(R)(M)
Radiography Program Director
Riverland Community College
Austin, Minnesota

Jera Roberts, RT(R)(M), EdS
Radiologic Technology Program Director
Washburn University
Topeka, Kansas

Shellie Son, BSRT(R)(MR)
Clinical Coordinator/Faculty
North Idaho College
Coeur d'Alene, Idaho

Karen Steinhoff, BS, Ed RT(R)
Clinical Coordinator & Assistant Professor
MassBay Community College
Framingham, MA

William Sykes, MBA, RT(R)(M)(CT)(MR)(QM)
Professor and Chair, Radiologic Technology Program
Shawnee State University
Portsmouth, OH

ABOUT THE AUTHORS

After 33 years as a radiography program director, Quinn B. Carroll recently took his retirement from Midland College in Texas as an assistant professor to write full time. Quinn has published three textbooks, workbooks, and a number of journal articles. His newest publication is *Radiography in the Digital Age*, released in 2011 along with several instructional ancillaries. Quinn has presented over 120 seminars in Canada and the USA, and many dozens of presentations for state societies and the ASRT. Quinn received his Master of Education degree from the University of Wyoming and his BS degree from the University of Utah, where he also obtained his radiography training at the University Medical Center.

Dennis Bowman RT(R) has been an active radiographer for over 30 years. He has been employed as a Staff Technologist at Community Hospital of the Monterey Peninsula (CHOMP) in Monterey, California since 1990. He has also been the Clinical Instructor (CI) for the Cabrillo College Radiology Program since 1991. In addition to the weekly classes he gives his students, Dennis has travelled internationally lecturing on how best to use and critique digital radiography. Because Dennis still is a "shooting tech" and CI, he truly understands all the problems techs run into and has figured out a fun and lighthearted way to explain it.

Both authors have extensive speaking experience, having presented hundreds of seminars for practicing radiographers throughout the United States and Canada, and have benefited from being able to glean from these radiographers their experiences and tips for better practice over the years.

As a team, the authors combine years of real clinical experience with innovative teaching experience. This has produced a "chemistry" that we believe has resulted in the best possible approach to this critical subject of adapting radiographic positions to all circumstances and learning to "think out of the box."

How to Use This Text *Adaptive Radiography with Trauma, Image Critique and Critical Thinking*

OBJECTIVES

Upon completion of this chapter, you should be able to:

1. As a universal rule for all projections and distances, state the *minimum* amount of expansion for each edge of the projected x-ray field, from the upside surface of the typical adult patient to the image receptor.
2. In both AP and lateral projections for average adult head and torso procedures, and for very large patients, state the typical expansion for each edge of the x-ray field, from the upside surface of the anatomy to the image receptor.
3. Apply this understanding by trusting the collimator readout and by never using a field size exceeding the size of the image receptor.
4. Adapt these rules in practice for various angled x-ray beams.
5. Appreciate and apply long-SID technique anytime there is concern for fitting all of the anatomy of interest on the IR.

Adaptive Radiography with Trauma, Image Critique, and Critical Thinking offers numerous features to facilitate understanding of the content being discussed.

OBJECTIVES

Chapter objectives highlight the critical concepts you should understand upon completion of each chapter.

BEST PRACTICE TIP

For average and small patients, chests, ribs, AP and lateral T-spines, all C-spines, skulls, shoulders, knees, and femurs can all be radiographed in trauma situations without a grid by using one-third (or one-quarter) the usual technique.

BEST PRACTICE TIPS

Best Practice Tips offer recommended practice guidelines for various positioning techniques and situations.

CASE STUDIES

Case Studies appear throughout the textbook and provide in-depth discussions of specific techniques and recommendations for optimal positioning. In many instances, figures are used to illustrate key points.

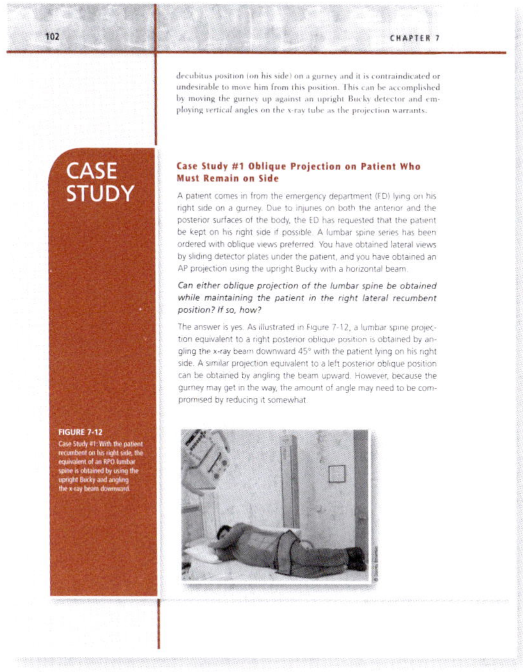
102 CHAPTER 7

decubitus position (on his side) on a gurney and it is contraindicated or undesirable to move him from this position. This can be accomplished by moving the gurney up against an upright Bucky detector and employing *vertical* angles on the x-ray tube as the projection warrants.

CASE STUDY

Case Study #1 Oblique Projection on Patient Who Must Remain on Side

A patient comes in from the emergency department (ED) lying on his right side on a gurney. Due to injuries on both the anterior and the posterior surfaces of the body, the ED has requested that the patient be kept on his right side if possible. A lumbar spine series has been ordered with oblique views preferred. You have obtained lateral views by sliding detector plates under the patient, and you have obtained an AP projection using the upright Bucky with a horizontal beam.

Can either oblique projection of the lumbar spine be obtained while maintaining the patient in the right lateral recumbent position? If so, how?

The answer is yes. As illustrated in Figure 7-12, a lumbar spine projection equivalent to a right posterior oblique position is obtained by angling the x-ray beam downward 45° with the patient lying on his right side. A similar projection equivalent to a left posterior oblique position can be obtained by angling the beam upward. However, because the gurney may get in the way, the amount of angle may need to be compromised by reducing it somewhat.

FIGURE 7-12
Case Study #1: With the patient recumbent on his right side, the equivalent of an RPO lumbar spine is obtained by using the upright Bucky and angling the x-ray beam downward.

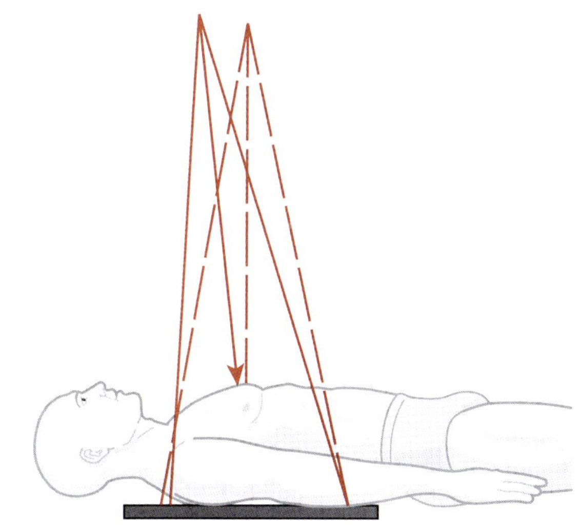

PHOTOGRAPHS, RADIOGRAPHS, AND ILLUSTRATIONS

Photographs, radiographs, and illustrations are used to demonstrate every positioning technique discussed in the textbook. Conceptual illustrations help you visualize core principles related to adaptive techniques.

CRITICAL THINKING CHALLENGES

Critical Thinking Challenges appear at the end of each chapter and prompt you to review and apply key principles you have learned.

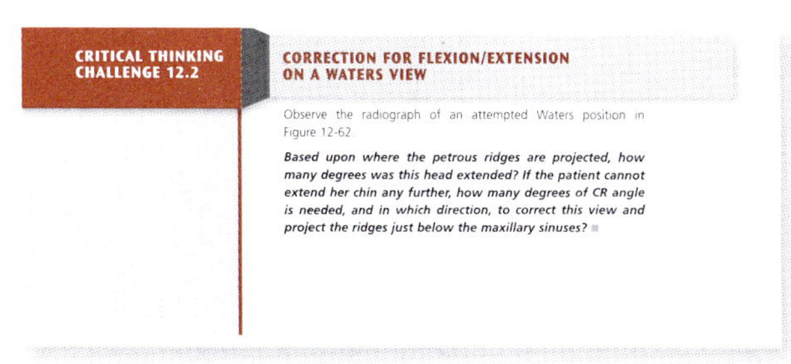
CRITICAL THINKING CHALLENGE 12.2

CORRECTION FOR FLEXION/EXTENSION ON A WATERS VIEW

Observe the radiograph of an attempted Waters position in Figure 12-62.

Based upon where the petrous ridges are projected, how many degrees was this head extended? If the patient cannot extend her chin any further, how many degrees of CR angle is needed, and in which direction, to correct this view and project the ridges just below the maxillary sinuses?

ADAPTIVE RADIOGRAPHY

WITH TRAUMA, IMAGE CRITIQUE AND CRITICAL THINKING

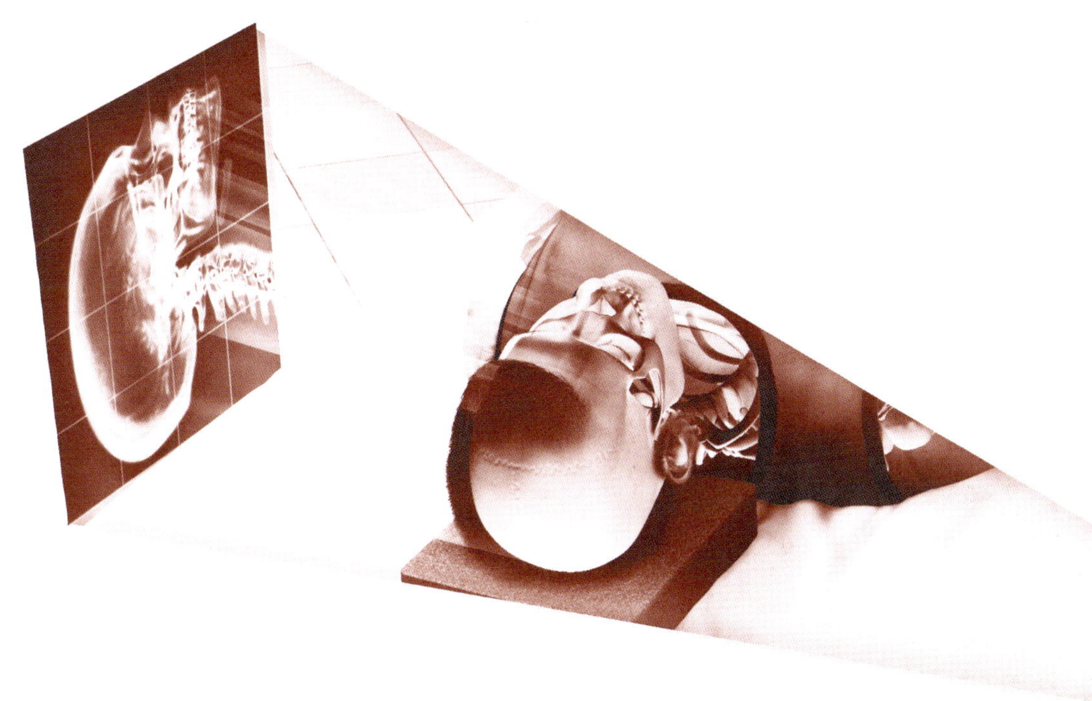

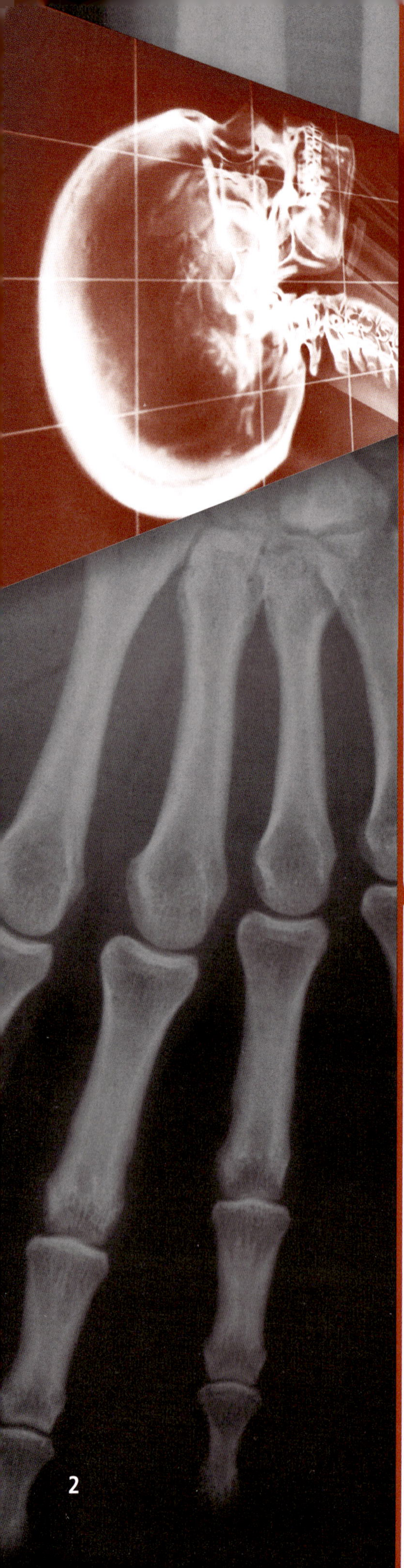

CHAPTER 1
Foundational Principles

OUTLINE

OBJECTIVES

Upon completion of this chapter, you should be able to:

1. Appreciate the need for applying basic, universal principles to the clinical practice of radiography.
2. State the fundamental paradigms that will be used throughout this book.
3. Understand the importance of palpation in locating body landmarks.
4. Avoid the use of "blanket rules" that are not strictly based upon actual anatomy.
5. Describe the relationship of the shift of upside and downside anatomy to body part thickness, and to rotation, tilt, flexion, and extension of the body part.
6. Explain the primary method of identifying upside versus downside anatomy.
7. State how parts of the human hand can be used to estimate distances in inches and centimeters.

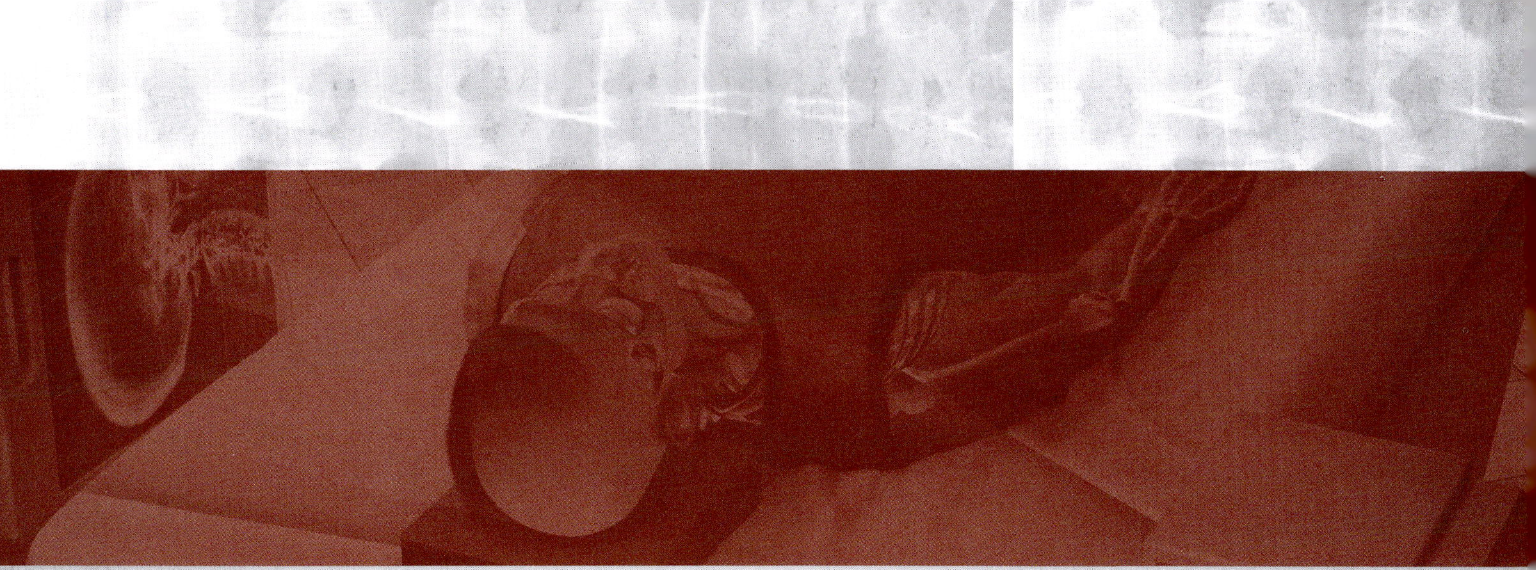

INTRODUCTION

The capacity to *adapt* to different patients, circumstances, and challenges that arise in the daily practice of clinical radiography is what sets apart the professional radiographer from a "technician." The radiographer in possession of these skills is frequently approached by other members of the clinical staff seeking assistance or advice. Critical thinking skills are important to daily practice and include many aspects of radiography. A radiographer may be very adept at critiquing radiographs, yet this does not automatically translate into the ability to accurately recenter an x-ray beam in order to adjust for an angle that was required by the presence of traction devices.

Although we tend to think of *adaptive skills* in terms of a radiographer's ability to be inventive, in reality, the secret of truly capable radiographers is a full understanding and *appreciation* for basic principles. Skull positioning provides a wonderful example: The difference between radiographers who find it frustrating and those who embrace it is not that there are esoteric "tricks" or particularly difficult details in skull positioning. Rather, those in the positive group have learned to position *themselves* where they can site down the planes of the skull end-on, keeping their eyes level with the anatomy, maintaining their viewpoint perpendicular to the body movements they are adjusting, and using two anatomical points to define each positioning line they use. Those who master these basics often find skull positioning stimulating rather than frustrating.

In our society, "common" sense is becoming increasingly uncommon. The reason time must be taken in our education to ensure that the *basics* are fully understood is because these basics have *wide and often universal application*. They broadly affect many of the daily procedures performed, preventing repeats and saving many patients from unnecessary radiation exposure. Students are generally capable of recognizing those important patterns or concepts immediately, *once they have heard them*. But, sometimes it is assumed that students will (or should) pick up these basics on their own. Often they are simply neglected in lessons or textbooks, or worse yet, they are contradicted.

For example, look up centering for the oblique hand projection in many textbooks, and you will find that the centering point is listed as the third metacarpophalangeal joint, *the same centering point as for the posteroanterior (PA) hand.* Perform this actual procedure with the hand properly positioned at 45° and with a well-collimated field, and following this centering rule, you will see that it tends to clip off the thumb. Now, look up the oblique position for an intravenous urogram and you will find instructions to shift centering *upside* from the midline because of the rotation of the body part. Why is this concept of shifting the centering point to the upside applied to urography but not to the oblique hand? Perhaps because it is assumed that the hand is not thick enough for it to matter. But simple application shows that it *does* matter. This demonstrates that we can, at times, superficially grasp a universal concept but fail to see all of its applications.

Care must be taken to provide students (and practicing radiographers) with these basic tools. For this reason, the first five chapters of this book are devoted to laying a foundation in the spatial relations of projection geometry. The next four chapters *apply* these concepts to trauma situations, pediatrics, and other cases in which we must adapt and work around the patient, as well as improve routine positioning skills. The last two chapters are dedicated to applying the same concepts to image critique and corrective positioning.

One of the main themes of this book is that there *are* common patterns that can be followed, generic rules that can be learned, and *basic* principles that, if appreciated and applied, will result in the ability to innovate and to adapt in systematic ways that produce much more consistent results, whatever the situation.

THE BASIC PARADIGMS

In keeping with this spirit, we will lay out, as follows, the 22 paradigms or "foundational principles" upon which the format of this entire book is based. (Note that each principle will be fully explained in subsequent chapters. The concepts are listed here in summary format to provide an overview.) They are:

1. The use of anatomical landmarks for centering and collimating the x-ray beam is always more reliable than "blanket rules" based on gender or other unscientific notions.
2. Stable bony landmarks are generally more reliable than soft-tissue landmarks.
3. For most landmarks, physical palpation (feeling) of the landmark is more reliable than visually estimating its location.
4. The best landmarks are those directly related to or directly adjacent to the anatomy of interest being radiographed.
5. Certain landmark methods *automatically adjust* for differing patient habitus: They cause you to center higher on a tall patient

or lower on a short patient automatically, without additional "rules." These methods are more reliable and should be adopted over those that do not automatically compensate for body habitus.

6. With the exception of specific joints or foramina that must be "opened up," the ideal collimation and centering for most radiographic projections is determined by what anatomy is *included within the view* rather than by the specific location of the central ray. For example, on a skull series or a hand series, where the *edges of the collimated field* fall is actually more critical than the exact centering point for the central ray (CR).
7. *All* body part movements are equivalent to some type of angulation of the x-ray beam: In frontal positions, flexion is equivalent to a cephalic beam angle and extension is equivalent to a caudal angle. In lateral positions, tilt, abduction, and adduction are equivalent to cephalic or caudal angles. In any position, rotation is equivalent to a transverse angle. Thus, the following rules of shift for centering (#8, #9, and #10) have broad, universal application for positioning, and can be applied to body part movement as well as angles.
8. Angulation of the x-ray beam affects the centering point for deep anatomy. For all projections of skull, thoracic, and abdominal anatomy, centering of the CR must be shifted by 1 inch for every 10° of tube angle (or ½ inch for every 5°).
9. Rule #8 also applies to body part rotation, flexion, extension, tilt, abduction, or adduction. For all positions of skull, thoracic, and abdominal anatomy, centering of the CR must be shifted by 1 inch for every 10° (or ½ inch for every 5°).
10. To adjust Rule #8 and Rule #9 for large patients, add an additional 1 inch of shift for every added 5 centimeters (2 inches) of body thickness.
11. Each edge of the collimated field as observed on the surface of the patient's torso can be expected to expand by 2 inches by the time it reaches the image receptor. In *all* circumstances, each edge of the field will expand by *at least* 1 inch.
12. X-ray beam divergence for a 40-inch source-to-image receptor distance (SID) is 2° per inch in any direction from the CR. Anatomy that is off-centered from the CR will be projected by an *angled ray* equivalent to this amount. This is critical to understand when considering the correction needed when an initial projection fails to properly "open" a joint space of interest.
13. For *accurate* positioning, each of the following is essential:
    A. Two points must always be used to define a positioning line.
    B. Positioning planes must be evaluated from a true end-on viewpoint. The radiographer must do what it takes to align *herself* with the patient in order to achieve this viewpoint.

C. The radiographer must view positioning lines and planes from the same *vertical* level that the patient or the anatomy is on.

D. At least two different viewpoints, perpendicular to each other, are required for the radiographer to assess all positioning planes.

14. When adapting a position for trauma or other circumstances, correct alignment of the CR *with the anatomy* always takes precedence over perpendicularity of the CR with the cassette or image receptor (IR).

15. In trauma positioning, *alignment* of the x-ray beam and the anatomy generally takes precedence over the need to minimize the object-to-image receptor distance (OID).

16. In trauma positioning of long bones, when the part cannot be placed parallel to the IR, angle the CR to half of the angle formed between the part and the cassette or IR.

17. In trauma positioning (especially for the cross-table lateral cervical spine), cut-off or superimposition problems caused by beam divergence can be minimized by:

    A. using the maximum feasible SID.

    B. recentering (usually lower) such that the cut-off anatomy is closer to the CR.

18. Good centering rules are those that:

    A. make good *anatomical* sense and use reliable bony landmarks;

    B. *automatically compensate* for larger or smaller patients, *self-correcting* for normal variations in anatomy;

    C. are *independent* of the radiographer's own body size;

    D. are *simple*, and able to be applied *easily* without special equipment;

    E. are easy on the *patient* and quick to use; and

    F. *consistently* produce the desired results in the image, so that *repeat rates are actually reduced*.

19. The degree of off-angling, off-rotation, tilt, abduction, adduction, or improper flexion or extension can be quantified, and universal rules for what constitutes *repeatable* error in all of these criteria can be established.

20. Generally, the amount of off-angle, off-rotation, incorrect tilt, flexion, or extension that is considered to warrant a repeated exposure is *more* than 3°.

21. When critiquing torso or skull images, to accurately correct an improper position, note that every 1 inch of shift observed between landmarks represents 10° of beam angulation, body rotation, tilt, flexion, or extension. For spines or extremities, cut

this rule in half (½ inch = 10°). For the lateral chest, double this rule (2 inches = 10°).

22. For critiquing a position on a radiograph, the best criteria to observe will always be a pair of stable, bony anatomical parts that:
    A. are distant from each other *and* from the midline of the body;
    B. have a long axis perpendicular to the expected direction of shift; and
    C. are close to the central ray in the direction of expected shift.

The chapters that follow provide the details on how each of these principles should be applied, and provide numerous case studies as examples. The specific positioning guidelines provided in Chapters 11 and 12 for each radiographic projection are completely grounded in these concepts. In addition, Chapter 13 presents guidelines for adjusting the technical factors of mA, exposure time, and kVp for several common circumstances that challenge our ability to adapt.

ANATOMICAL LANDMARKS AND SILLY RULES

Whenever possible, use *bony* anatomy as a landmark for centering the x-ray beam. A centering rule that uses a soft-tissue landmark, such as "center to the belly button," is subject to obvious limitations: On an obese patient the belly button may fall higher or lower, or to the side, as adipose tissue shifts around when the body is rolled into oblique and other positions. Even with thin patients, the navel will be found lower on some people than on others as a normal variation. It is true that bony landmarks may also be subject to change from surgery or disease, and some may be shifted by movement, such as those in the jaw or shoulder blades. However, bony landmarks are generally much more consistent than soft tissue landmarks.

Identifying landmarks by *palpation* (location by feel) is more reliable than locating them by visual identification alone. There are many examples. The anterior superior iliac spine (ASIS) may be easily visible on very thin patients, but must be palpated on large patients and even on many average patients for confirmation of what one sees. Likewise, in order to count down the spinous processes, physically palpate them on most patients. Even the iliac crest, one of the most prominent landmarks used, must be located by feel on larger patients and on many average patients.

For some landmarks, it can help to have the patient *move* the anatomy while palpating for it. Examples are having the patient swallow while feeling for the thyroid cartilage, or having the patient open and close the jaw while feeling for the temporomandibular joint (TMJ).

Palpation of bony anatomy is *strongly* recommended in determining appropriate beam angles for radiography of the spine and other anatomy where the joint spaces may lie in variable planes. The lateral L5–S1 projection is particularly vulnerable to this problem. It can and often does lie at a wide range of angles depending on patient habitus, condition, and position. It can even change on the same patient performing the same projection from one time to the next, because of changes in the particular way the patient lies or shifts his or her weight. Palpation is the scientific, logical approach. Palpation *does not lie*, but it must be done *correctly* to properly locate the landmarks as instructed. Properly used, there is no more reliable way to determine centering and angles for the x-ray beam.

The very worst thing a radiographer can do in determining beam angles is to adopt a "blanket" rule for all patients, for all males, or for all females that does not allow for any automatic adjustment according to actual body conditions and variations. Using the lateral L5–S1 projection as an example, many radiographers follow the maxim to "angle caudal on all female patients, and use a vertical beam on all male patients." It may be true that 65%–70% of all female patients require a caudal angle on this projection, but then, is a 30%–35% repeat rate acceptable? Palpation can bring this repeat rate down to 5%–10% for this difficult projection. The following true story is an experience the author had early in his career, before the AP view was immediately available to check on an LCD screen. With film-based radiography, one would generally expose all of the projections in a series before being able to see the results. It illustrates the concept of not making assumptions or using "blanket rules" in a most convincing way that still applies in digital radiography practice:

> I was performing a lateral L5–S1 "spot" projection on a very thin, fragile female patient. With her lying on her side, I noticed that her waist was substantially thinner than her pelvis, and the expected "sagging" of the lumbar spine area was unmistakable. Visually, there seemed to be no question that a significant caudal angle would be needed to open this lowest of the lumbar joints. I decided to palpate the spinous process of L5 and the tip of the sacrum anyway to confirm this impression. I could not find L5 either in the apparent midline of the back or even below the midline.
>
> Finally, I palpated higher up vertically and found it, lying above the midline. The slope between my fingers, one on L5 and one on the tip of the sacrum, indicated that the slant of the joint would be opposite to the usual, and a cephalic angle would be needed. Against all visual intuition, I angled the beam 7° cephalic as palpation indicated and made the exposure. The joint was beautifully opened on the first exposure. The patient had severe scoliosis.

Physical palpation is always safer than visual assessment, and far more reliable than "blanket" rules. An angle should be determined (and a centering point) by where the anatomy actually lies when this can be determined, not by the gender of the patient.

Another common example of a "blanket" rule based on gender is cassette placement on the PA chest. The slogan, "Place the cassette (or IR plate) crosswise on all male patients, and lengthwise on all female patients," would better read, "Place the cassette (or IR plate) crosswise on broad-shouldered patients, and lengthwise on narrow-shouldered patients." After all, broad-shouldered females, as well as thin males, are not uncommon. Radiographers and students should be suspicious of any "blanket" rule that is not strictly based upon the actual anatomy of the patient.

Physical palpation of landmarks is the most reliable way to determine centering points and angles. Visual identification of clear landmarks is also helpful, but do not solely rely upon this.

Chapter 10 begins with a list of criteria for judging what makes a good centering rule. This is followed by recommended centering rules and angles for each of the routine projections.

BEST PRACTICE TIP

Physical palpation of landmarks is the most reliable way to determine centering points and angles. Visual identification of clear landmarks is also helpful, but do not solely rely upon this.

RELATIVE SHIFT OF ANATOMY

The following discussion applies to both the expected shifting of anatomy while positioning the body and the apparent shift of the same anatomy on the finished radiographic image. It is equally applicable to positioning and to film critique.

When the torso is rotated into an oblique position, organs close to the front or anterior surface of the body, such as the bladder, will naturally be expected to shift in the direction of rotation. When turning the patient to the right, the bladder will shift to the right. Adjust centering to the bladder with this in mind. This adjustment is fairly simple. However, shifting will be *negligible* for midline anatomy, and actually *reversed* for downside anatomy. This is much more difficult to visualize, yet it is a critical skill for proper centering. To further complicate things, the reversal of shift for downside anatomy is true not only when rotating the torso or skull, but also when tilting, flexing, or extending the body part.

Figure 1-1 illustrates this concept. When the patient's torso is rotated to the right, the kidneys, lying posteriorly on the downside, will shift to the *left*. The amount of shift is a direct function of the distance of the anatomy from the exact midline of the body. If, for example, the sternum lies 4 inches *anterior* to the midline, and the spinous processes of the thoracic spine lie an equidistant 4 inches *posterior* to the midline, the sternum and the spinous processes will shift by the same amount, only in opposite directions from the midline structures. Structures closer to the midline, however, will shift less.

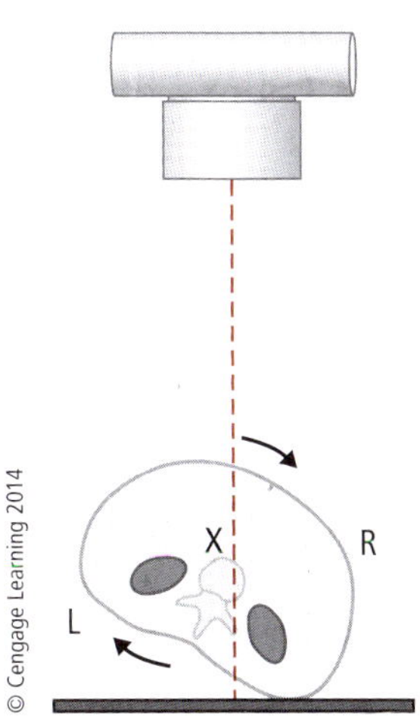

FIGURE 1-1

Rotation of the torso toward the patient's right shifts downside anatomy such as the kidneys (shaded) to the left. The farther the anatomy from the midline axis of the body, the greater the shift. For most oblique positions, the central ray as observed on the patient's surface must be recentered by shifting it toward the upside, even if the anatomy of interest is midline, marked by the X.

Anatomy very close to the midline of the body, marked as **X** in Figure 1-1, will not technically shift much with body rotation. However, side-to-side centering of the x-ray beam *will* still need adjusting, because in most cases, the centering landmarks used are also on the upside, observable surface of the body, as is the observed light field. These landmarks shift to the right as the body is rotated to the right, so one must recenter the beam toward the *left* in order for the central ray to pass through the midline structures of interest.

Thus, almost all oblique positions require some kind of recentering side to side in order to adjust for either the shift of the anatomy of interest or the shift of the landmarks used. This is just as true for procedures involving the skull as for those involving the torso. Even the extremities generally require this *upside* shift adjustment in centering for oblique positions. As was described with the oblique hand position at the beginning of this chapter, even though the degree of shift is less for the smaller diameter extremities, failure to adapt the centering for an oblique position, combined with tight collimation, can result in clipping one side of the anatomy.

Particularly for skull positions, the radiographer must fully appreciate the effects of flexion, extension, or tilt upon vertical (up-and-down) shift. As shown in Figure 1-2, for all *frontal* projections of skull anatomy (including the PA, AP, Caldwell, Waters, and Townes projections), extension of the chin will cause posterior anatomy to shift *downward* as the anterior anatomy moves up, and vice versa. For example, raising the chin will *lower* the petrous pyramids, which lie posterior. On all *lateral* projections of skull anatomy, tilting of the head will cause anatomy *of that side* to shift downward, while anatomy on the opposite side will shift upward. As demonstrated in Figure 1-3, tilting the head to the right brings the *right* orbital plate of the frontal bone downward, while the *left* plate moves upward by an equal amount.

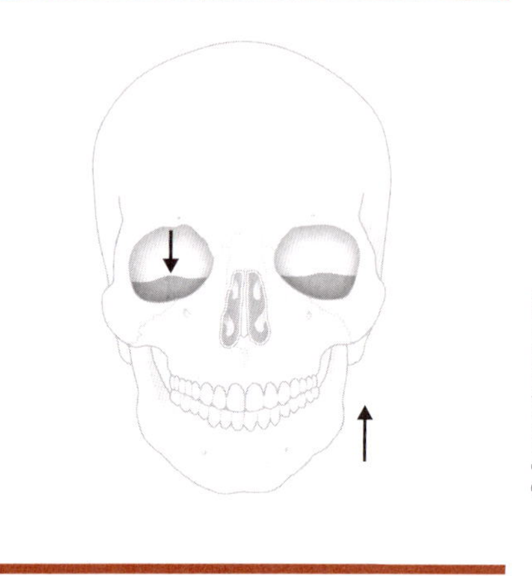

FIGURE 1-2

For frontal skull projections, extending the chin upward will lower posterior anatomy such as the petrous ridges (small arrow), relative to the anterior anatomy.

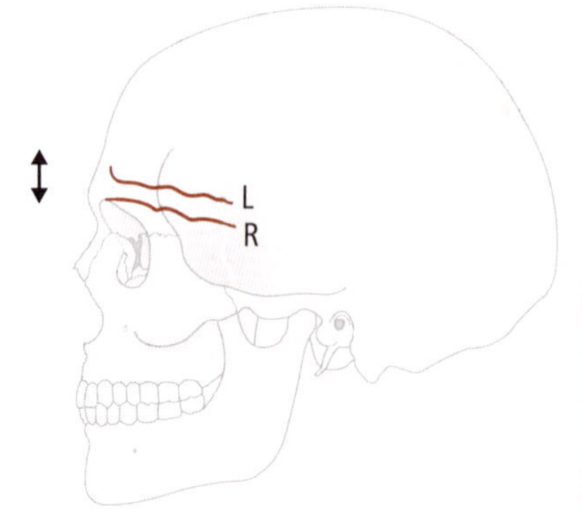

FIGURE 1-3

For lateral skull projections, tilting the head toward the patient's right will shift right-side anatomy downward. In this diagram, the right orbital plate is projected below the left orbital plate, indicating tilt to the right.

When *axial* projections are performed, such as an axial patella or a submentovertex projection of the skull, side-to-side shift will no longer be due to rotation, but rather due to *tilt* of the body part, shown in Figure 1-4. Vertical (up-and-down) shift on axial projections will be due to flexion or extension of the body part, just as on frontal projections.

Finally, the radiographer must consider that the amount of expected shift increases for thicker body parts and for larger patients. Shift decreases for thinner parts or thinner patients. Figure 1-5 illustrates that the farther two anatomical parts are away from each other, the more they will shift when rotating the body. When centering side to side for an oblique position (to include both kidneys during a urinary study, for example), the CR must be recentered *more to the upside* on thick patients than on average patients, as shown in Figure 1-6. This difference is substantial for hypersthenic patients, and if the positioner does not keep this in mind it may very well result in repeated exposures due to clipping off the upside kidney.

Chapter 5 further explains positioning shift and gives formulas for actually *quantifying* it so that the amount of shift as well as the direction of shift can be predicted, used to advantage in positioning, and evaluated on the final image.

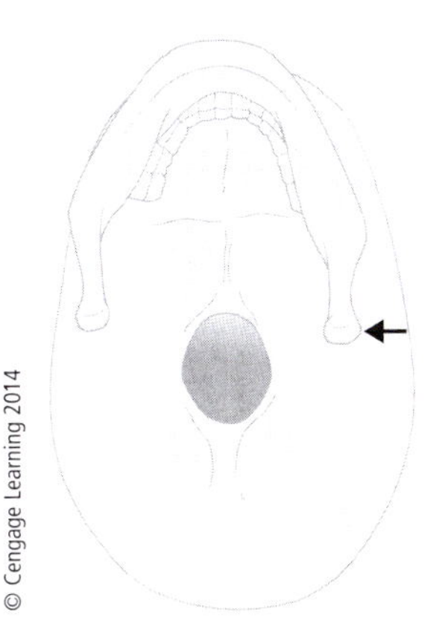

FIGURE 1-4
For axial (SMV) projections of the skull, side-to-side shift is caused by *tilt,* not by rotation. In this diagram, tilting the head toward the patient's *left* caused the jaw to shift to the patient's *right* (arrow).

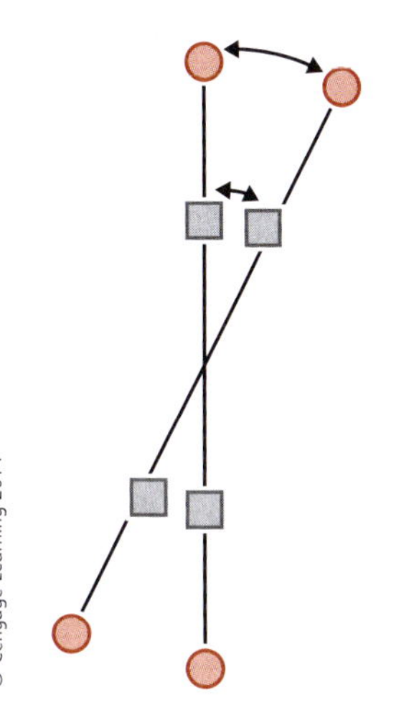

FIGURE 1-5
The farther two objects lie from the fulcrum or center of rotation, the more they shift. In this diagram, the circular objects shift much more than the squares. Therefore, on larger patients, anatomy will shift more with rotation of the body part.

> Upside anatomy always shifts *with* the rotation of the body part. Downside anatomy always shifts *against* the rotation of the body part.

These principles can be generally applied to all radiographs. To apply them, however, the radiographer must also be able to determine which anatomical landmark is more posterior, or downside. This is addressed in the next section.

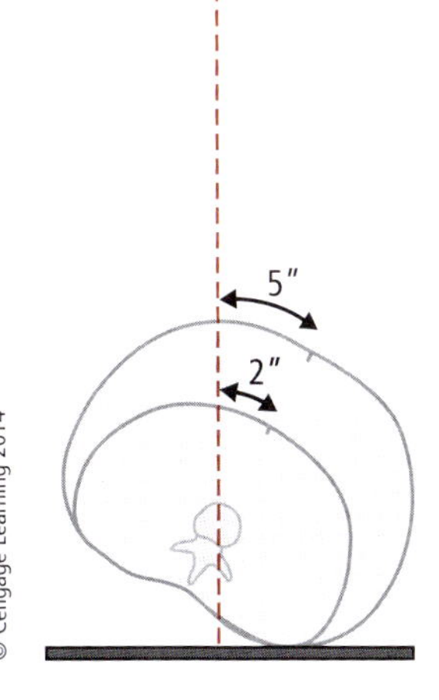

FIGURE 1-6
The larger the patient, the more upside shift is necessary for the CR. In this example, the objective is for the CR to pass through the midspine. Note that for the obese patient, the CR had to be shifted 5 inches upside from the midline as observed on the patient's upper surface, whereas for the thinner patient, it only had to be shifted 2 inches upside.

IDENTIFYING UPSIDE AND DOWNSIDE ANATOMY ON RADIOGRAPHS

It would seem at first glance that one could identify on a radiographic image which set of ribs, which TMJ, or which condyle is the *upside* and which is the *downside* by the appearance of magnification and blur. We know that, in principle, the upside anatomy, farthest from the image receptor, will always demonstrate more blur and be larger in size. In practice, however, at least three problems complicate this observation.

First, some anatomical parts are of such small thickness that the *degree* of difference between the upside and downside is just not obvious on the radiograph. Second, differences in size can be *anatomical* rather than geometrical: Some diseases result in the bones on one side of the body to be physically larger than the opposite side. Further, even *normal* anatomical differences can be misinterpreted as magnification. An example is the left lung being naturally longer than the right lung. In the case of the lateral chest view, the resulting higher anatomical position of the right hemidiaphragm actually cancels out the geometrical projection of the right diaphragm downward by the diverging x-ray beam, enough so that the two diaphragms often cross over each other in the image. This renders it impossible to simply "pick the lower diaphragm as the left diaphragm." Rather, one must learn the anatomy, that is, the shape of each hemidiaphragm, more intimately.

Finally, some anatomy has very low inherent radiographic contrast, such as the ribs. Visually, this low contrast can be easily misinterpreted as blur. High-contrast bones subjectively seem to have sharp edges, and low contrast bones, whose edges are less apparent, mimic blur that is in fact not present.

Figure 1-7 demonstrates the use of obvious magnification and blur in evaluating a radiograph of the temporomandibular joint. In practical application, there are many positions where the differences in magnification and blur are obvious on the image, and these will be used. But, given the preceding limitations, it is often necessary to also use other anatomical clues to confirm one's assessment of the image. Chapter 9 details all of these aids to image evaluation.

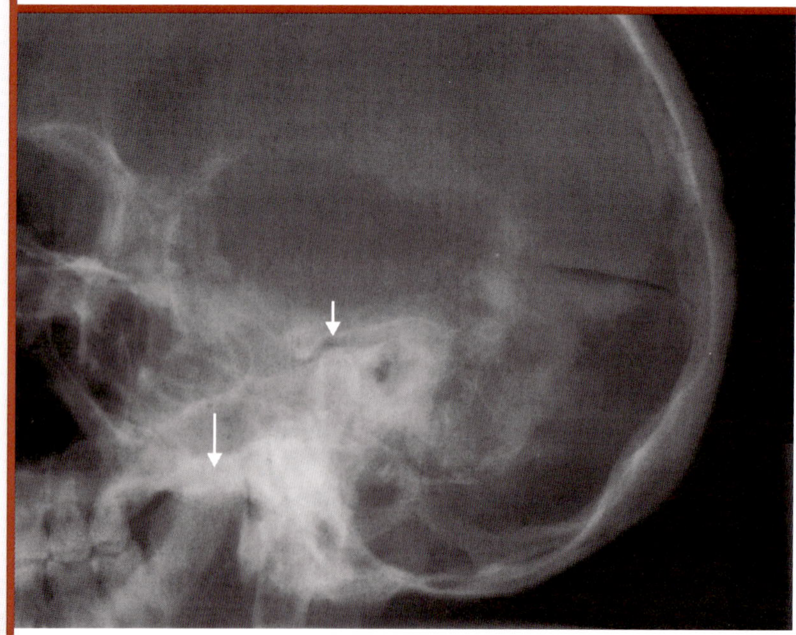

FIGURE 1-7

For this TMJ projection, the upside TMJ (large arrow) can be distinguished from the downside TMJ (small arrow) by its comparative magnification and blurriness. However, on many radiographs there is an insufficient difference between the two to make this distinction.

Carroll, Q. Evaluating Radiographs, 1993. Courtesy of Charles C Thomas Publisher, Ltd., Springfield, Illinois.

RELATIVE SIZING OF IMAGES IN THIS TEXT

Illustrations in this text are smaller than original radiographs from which they are reproduced. The reader must take references to all distances, "one inch of shift," and so on in the context of the typical sizes of conventional radiographs, i.e., the size of the image receptor plate or *cassette* used in producing the image. This is a particular problem for CR or DR images, which are presented on an LCD (TV screen) rather than on "hard-copy" film, frequently smaller in size than the cassette originally used. For radiographs presented on these pages, the reader can use his or her imagination to visualize the actual distances in the context of the original cassette or IR plate size. It may help to use as a reference that 1 inch is typically about two fingerbreadths for a female, somewhat less on a male—about the *width* of the average male thumb. When evaluating a radiograph, the radiographer must visualize these relationships relative to the *patient* in the image (not to the radiographer's own hand).

PRACTICAL RULES OF THUMB VERSUS "INCHES" AND "CENTIMETERS"

Many radiographic positioning textbooks include centering rules designating distances from a selected landmark, such as centering "2 inches above the symphysis pubis" or "4 centimeters below the iliac crest." Realistically, most radiographers never go to the trouble of actually measuring such distances, but mentally estimate or "eyeball" them. People do "see" distances differently. For many, it takes some practice to become reasonably accurate at estimating these distances.

In this text, *practical centering rules of thumb* shall be used in every instance. These will be handy references for comparison, such as the positioner's own fingerbreadths. While specific distances will be referred to, some method will always be added whereby the positioner may make a good estimate of that distance using the tools at hand (no pun intended).

Generally, it may be said that for the average female radiographer, 2 fingerbreadths will approximate 1 inch. For the average male radiographer, 1 inch will be somewhat less, slightly more than the *width* of the thumb. Either gender can use the width of the smallest fingernail to estimate 1 centimeter. For the highest degree of accuracy, you should take actual measurements of your own thumb width, and fingerbreadth in centimeters or inches. Find which fingernail has a width closest to 1 centimeter. Measure the width of these digits at the most distal joint. This simple exercise, performed once, can reap perpetual benefits for you in daily practice throughout your career.

Much of the remainder of this textbook is devoted to application of the 22 paradigms listed in this chapter. These, and the other guidelines

BEST PRACTICE TIP

Generally, it may be said that for the average female radiographer, 2 fingerbreadths will approximate 1 inch. For the average male radiographer, 1 inch will be somewhat less, slightly more than the *width* of the thumb. Either gender can use the width of the smallest fingernail to estimate 1 centimeter.

For the highest degree of accuracy, you should take actual measurements of your own thumb width, and fingerbreadth in centimeters or inches. Find which fingernail has a width closest to 1 centimeter. Measure the width of these digits at the most distal joint. This simple exercise, performed once, can reap perpetual benefits for you in daily practice throughout your career.

presented here, will facilitate the daily practice of radiography and result in more accurate positioning.

SIZING OF PATIENTS

Throughout this book, references will be made to "small, average, and large" patients. We define a *small* patient as a person who weighs 120–160 pounds (54–73 kg), and normally measures in the abdomen from 15–18 centimeters in AP measurement, about ¾ average thickness. We define an *average* patient as a person who weighs 160–200 pounds (73–91 kg), and measures 19–23 centimeters for the AP abdomen. A *large* patient will be defined as a person who weighs 200–240 pounds (91–109 kg), and measures 24–27 centimeters (about 1¼ times average). A *very large* patient weighs over 240 pounds (110 kg) and exceeds 28 centimeters in abdominal thickness (more than 1½ times average).

CRITICAL THINKING CHALLENGES

At the end of each chapter a *Critical Thinking Challenge* is presented. These do not always correlate strictly with the material in the same chapter, but are designed to progressively stimulate analytical thinking about problems specific to radiography. It is *strongly* recommended that the student engage in these challenges to get the full benefit out of this textbook. Unlike the case studies in each chapter, the answers are not given in the text, but may be found in the Appendix. The first three challenges follow the summary for this chapter.

SUMMARY

1. Palpation (feeling) for landmarks is more reliable than visual identification alone. Stable bony landmarks are generally more reliable than soft-tissue landmarks.
2. Generalized "blanket" rules based on the patient's gender, race, and so on are *not* consistent and are not recommended.
3. Downside anatomy shifts *opposite* to the direction the patient is being rotated. Even midline anatomy shifts opposite to the observed light field on the surface of the patient, requiring recentering of the CR toward the *upside* when rotating the body part.

4. The larger the patient, the *greater* the shift of anatomy from rotation, tilt, flexion, and so on.
5. Generally, *upside* anatomy can be identified on radiographs by its increased magnification and blur relative to the downside anatomy. However, this is not always reliable without additional confirmation.
6. Rules of thumb for measuring are that, on average:
   - For a female radiographer, 2 fingerbreadths equal 1 inch.
   - For a male radiographer, the width of the thumb equals 1 inch.
   - The width of the smallest fingernail equals 1 centimeter, on average.
7. The 22 paradigms listed at the beginning of this chapter form the basis for the entire format of this book. They represent principles and fundamental skills that are critical for the radiographer to be able to adapt radiographic positions.

CRITICAL THINKING CHALLENGE 1.1

CENTERING A PORTABLE CHEST

A radiographer and a student are performing a mobile (portable) chest exam with the patient sitting up in a bed. The student has just placed the gridded image receptor behind the patient and is still standing next to the head of the bed. The radiographer has pointed the tube at the patient's chest and is asking the student if the x-ray tube is parallel with the gridded IR (or if the central ray is perpendicular).

From the student's position, can the student assess whether the tube face is parallel, or the CR perpendicular, to the IR?

CRITICAL THINKING CHALLENGE 1.2

ROUTINE CHEST EXAM ON A KYPHOTIC PATIENT

A routine chest x-ray has been ordered on a very old patient with severe kyphosis. She is able to stand at the upright Bucky, so you set the SID at 72 inches (180 centimeters). You notice that in standard PA position, because she cannot lift her chin out of the way, a substantial OID gap of about 6 inches (15 centimeters) is created.

How can magnification of the heart and other mediastinal structures be kept at a minimum? ■

CRITICAL THINKING CHALLENGE 1.3

HEAD POSITION FOR THE OBLIQUE CERVICAL SPINE

Some textbooks recommend that, for the oblique projection of the cervical spine, the head must be kept in line with the obliquity of the body, so that the midsagittal planes of both the body and the head lie at 45° from the tabletop.

Explain how this might prevent the proper visualization of all cervical vertebrae. ■

(Answers to Critical Thinking Challenges are found in the Appendix.)

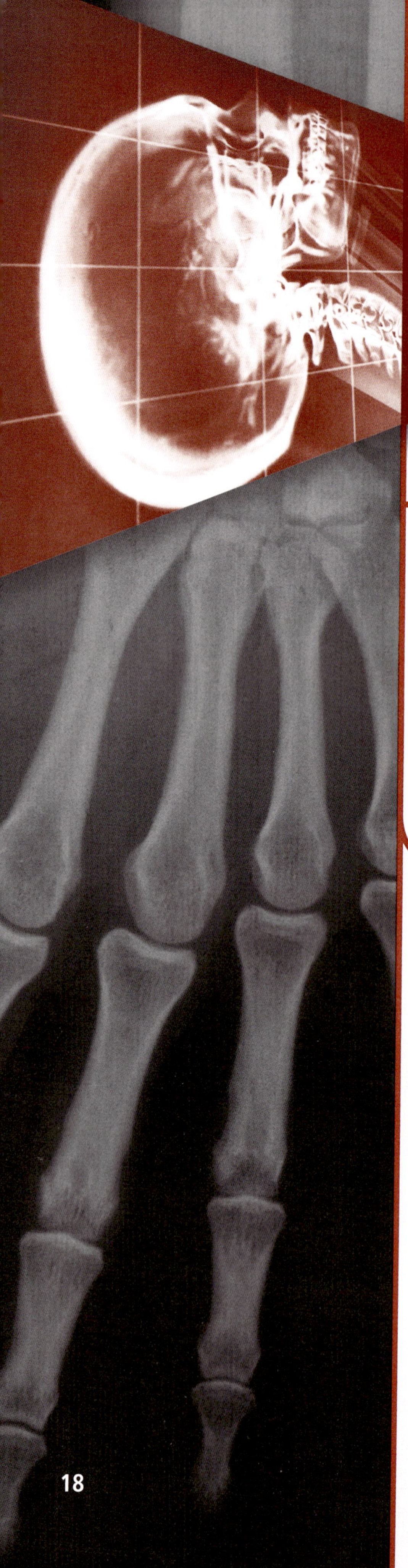

CHAPTER 2

Adapting Centering for Beam Angles

OUTLINE

OBJECTIVES

Upon completion of this chapter, you should be able to:

1. State the direction, and specify the distance, by which the central ray must be shifted to compensate for various angles of the x-ray beam in order to always project the anatomy of interest that lies deep in the body part to the center of the view.
2. State the direction (upside, downside, cephalic, caudal, distal, or proximal) and specify the distance by which the central ray must be shifted to compensate for various degrees of body part obliquity or rotation, tilt, flexion, or extension in order to always project the anatomy of interest that lies deep in the body part to the center of the view.

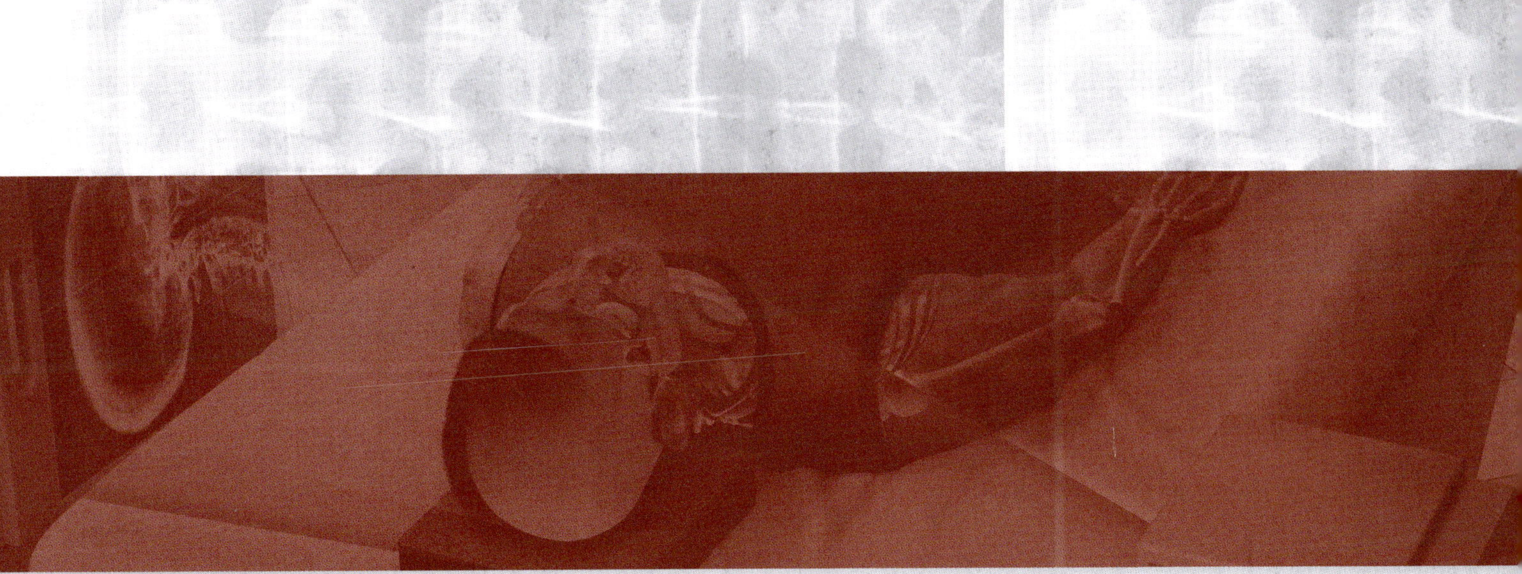

ADAPTING FOR TYPICAL ANGLES

For anatomy of interest that lies near the surface of the body facing up toward the x-ray tube, the x-ray beam centering does not need to be adjusted in any way when the x-ray beam is angled. Likewise, for anatomy of interest that lies near the back surface of a patient lying supine, centering to *exit* points needs no adjustment. However, these two instances represent only a small percentage of common radiographic positions for torso and skull anatomy. Most centering rules for torso and skull anatomy are designed to demonstrate organs, vertebrae, and other structures *deep* within the body rather than at the surface.

Clearly, when the anatomy of interest is deep within the torso or head as the x-ray beam traverses through it, the radiographer must compensate for any angle placed on the x-ray beam by recentering the beam. Failure to do so not only places the anatomy of interest off-centered on the resulting image, but can also result in closed-off joint spaces and overlapping of anatomical parts. This defeats the purpose of radiographic positioning—the *desuperimposition* of overlying structures. Thus, understanding this concept is not just an important and essential positioning skill, but it cuts to the very heart of positioning. A general rule may be stated as follows:

> For deep anatomy, any caudally-angled beam must be re-centered in a cephalic direction; any cephalic angle must be adjusted for by re-centering more caudal.

This is demonstrated in Figure 2-1. No matter what "normal" centering rule the radiographer uses to locate the anatomy for a vertical x-ray beam, if the beam is then angled caudally without recentering it, the central ray will pass below the desired point in the actual anatomy of interest. The greater the angle, the more critical it becomes to recenter.

For radiography of extremities, with their smaller thicknesses, this is a nonissue. However, for radiography of the skull and torso, it is worthwhile to go as far as to quantify this rule for adult patients.

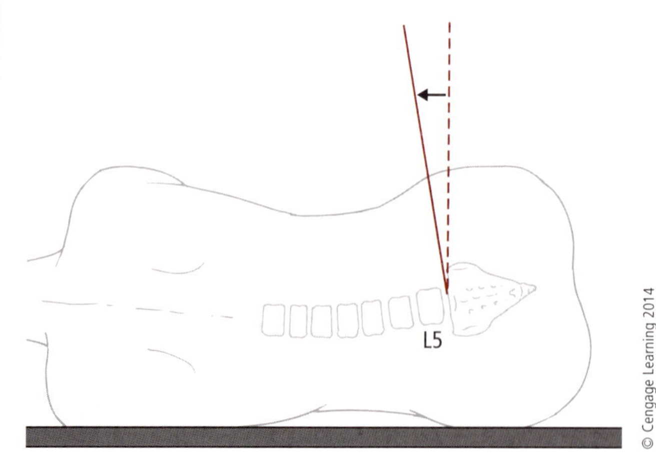

FIGURE 2-1

Here, the centering is to the L5–S1 joint space in lateral projection. Note that if a caudal angle is placed on the x-ray beam, the centering point observed on the upside surface of the patient must be shifted toward the head (arrow) in order to pass through the joint at L5–S1.

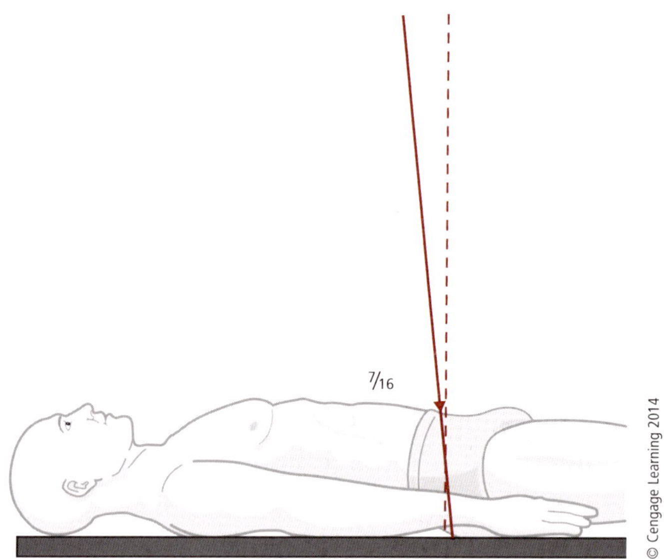

FIGURE 2-2

For a 5° angle with the patient supine, the amount of shift required to recenter the x-ray beam on the anterior surface of the average patient is about 7/16 inch, just under ½ inch. This can be rounded to the very useful rule of thumb: *Recenter ½ inch for every 5° of angle.*

In doing so, the *middle axis* of the body may be considered as the average depth for internal organs or structures of interest.

Theoretically we should develop two rules of thumb: one for frontal (AP or PA) projections of the average chest, abdomen, pelvis, or skull, with a thickness range of 19–25 centimeters; and one for lateral projections of the average chest, spines, or pelvis, with thicknesses from 28–32 centimeters. As it turns out for a 40-inch SID, illustrated in Figures 2-2 and 2-3, these two experiments produce results so close that, luckily, a single rule of thumb can be derived for all torso and head positioning.

The recentering shift required for a 5° CR angle to the AP spine, located 9 centimeters above the table on a 21-centimeter patient, is 7/16 inch. For the same angle on a lateral spine in the midline of a 31-centimeter patient, the recentering shift required is 9/16 inch. Both measurements can be reasonably rounded to ½ inch, (being within 1/16 inch of it). The derived rule of thumb is that *on* all *positions within*

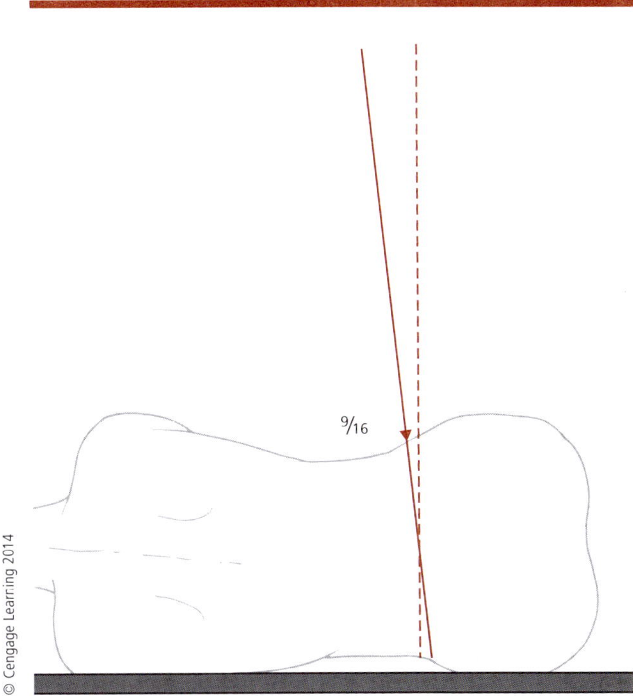

FIGURE 2-3

For a 5° angle with the patient in the lateral position, the amount of shift required to recenter the x-ray beam on the upper surface of the average patient is about 9/16 inch, just over ½ inch. This is so close to the measurement in Figure 2-2 that the ½-inch shift rule of thumb can be used for *all* positions—AP, oblique, or lateral.

the skull, chest, abdomen, and pelvis, shift the CR centering by ½ inch for every 5° of beam angle. For caudal angles, shift in the cephalic direction; for cephalic angles, shift caudally.

This rule is based only upon body thickness and typical anatomical geometry. Therefore, it need not be modified for the use of a 72-inch SID. It is generally applicable regardless of the distance used. By doubling all amounts, a corollary rule can be obtained, which might be easier to remember. This rule is: *Shift the CR centering by 1 inch for every 10° of beam angle.*

On ALL positions within the skull, chest, abdomen, and pelvis, shift the CR centering by ½ inch for every 5° of beam angle. Shift the CR centering by 1 inch for every 10° of beam angle. For caudal angles, shift in the cephalic direction; for cephalic angles, shift caudally.

Using the metric system, unfortunately, one cannot derive any nicely rounded numbers for any of these measurements, but the rule of thumb will be translated to the following:

For a 1-meter SID, shift the CR centering by about 1.3 centimeters for every 5° of beam angle.

BEST PRACTICE TIP

On ALL positions within the skull, chest, abdomen, and pelvis, shift the CR centering by ½ inch for every 5° of beam angle.

Shift the CR centering by 1 inch for every 10° of beam angle.

For caudal angles, shift in the cephalic direction; for cephalic angles, shift caudally.

Practical Application Examples

Figures 2-4 and 2-5 demonstrate the practical application of this rule of thumb for lateral positioning of the L5–S1 joint space, a position that poses several challenges for radiographers. There are, of course, many approaches used by different radiographers to locate the centering point for the lateral L5–S1 projection. *Most of these centering rules assume a vertical x-ray beam (zero angle).* Some may be based on an

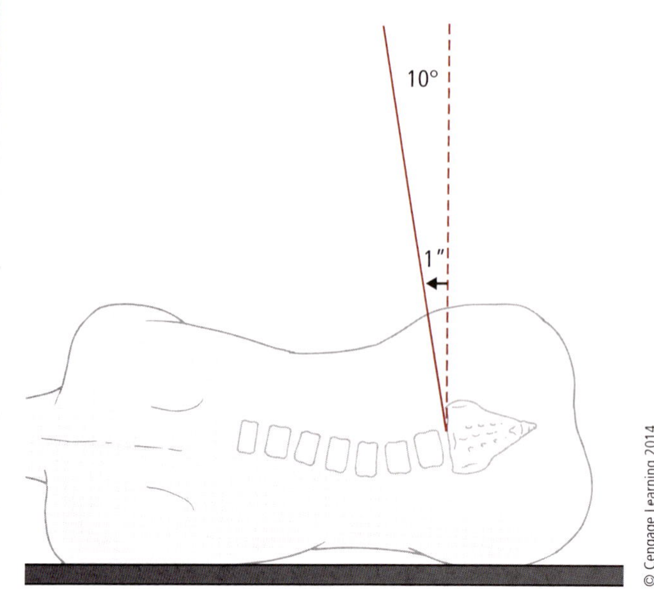

FIGURE 2-4

Application of the rule, 1 inch for every 10°, for a lateral projection of a tilted L5–S1 joint due to severe lumbar levoscoliosis. With a caudal angle of 10°, recenter the x-ray beam 1 inch more cephalic.

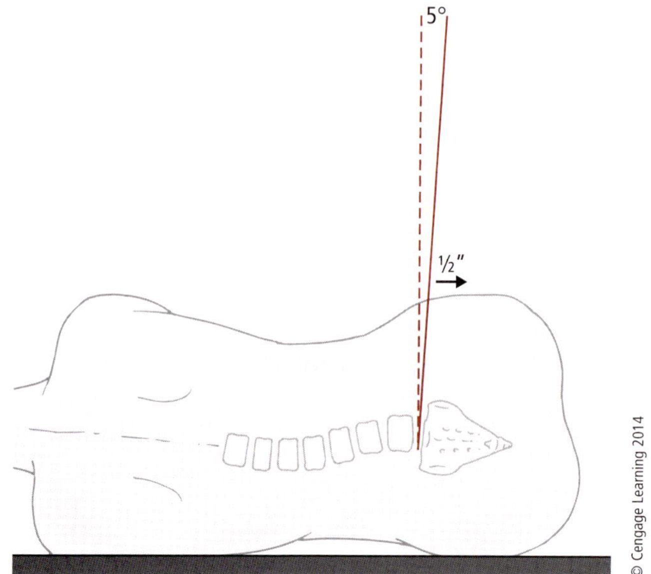

FIGURE 2-5

Further application of the shift rule: With a cephalic angle of 5° for a patient with lumbar dextroscoliosis, recenter the x-ray beam ½ inch more caudally.

already existing 5° caudal angle, and this should be clarified if this is the case.

It is essential to understand that the adjustments for angulation discussed here can be used universally, *regardless of which initial centering rule is applied*. No matter which method one uses to center to the anatomy, the principles here still apply when any change in the CR angle is made. For example, if the centering method used is already based on a 5° angle, these rules still apply for an *additional* 5° or for a *reduction* of 5° *from that point*.

The following case studies provide some practice in applying this rule.

CASE STUDY

Case Study #1: Lateral L5–S1 "Spot"—Levoscoliosis

Let us assume that the superior-to-inferior centering rule you normally use for the lateral L5–S1 projection is "Center 3 fingerbreadths (or 1½ inches) below the iliac crest." Upon palpating the bony anatomy of a patient with lumbar levoscoliosis, you estimate that the joint of interest is tilted roughly 10°, and you decide to angle the x-ray beam 10° caudally. How much and in which direction must you shift the CR centering point to compensate for this angle?

ANSWER: *As shown in Figure 2-4, starting from the "3 finger-breadth or 1½ inch" rule, you will need to recenter the CR 1 inch more superior (i.e., 1 inch of shift for every 10°). This will place the CR less than ½ inch, or roughly 1 fingerbreadth, below the iliac crest after adjusting. This is the proper centering for this angled view.*

Case Study #2: Lateral L5–S1 "Spot"—Dextroscoliosis

Let us assume that the superior-to-inferior centering rule you normally use for the lateral L5–S1 projection is "Place your index finger on the ASIS and your thumb at a right angle on the iliac crest, making an 'L,' and center at the junction of the thumb and finger." You find that the patient has lumbar dextroscoliosis, such that the lateral "S" curvature of the lumbar spine actually slants the L5–S1 joint space opposite to the usual, as shown in Figure 2-5. You estimate that you will need a 5° *cephalic* angle. How much and in which direction must you shift the CR centering point to compensate for this angle?

ANSWER: *From the original "junction of the L" centering point, you should recenter the beam an additional ½ inch (roughly 1 fingerbreadth) lower, as shown in Figure 2-5.*

Transverse Angles and Equivalent Positioning

The same rule of thumb certainly applies for transverse angles (across the table). While transverse angles cannot be used on "Bucky" procedures, there are many instances, especially in trauma and mobile positioning, where transverse angles may be used to effectively obtain oblique projections without moving the patient. These must all be done either nongrid or with a grid/cassette rotated to a crosswise orientation (see Chapter 7). Angling toward the patient's left side, the CR should be recentered to the *right* ½ inch for every 5° of angulation, and vice versa.

As discussed in Chapter 1, tilt, flexion, or extension of a part of the body is equivalent to cephalic or caudal angling of the CR, and rotation is equivalent to a transverse angle of the x-ray beam toward the right or the left of the patient. This same rule of thumb can therefore be applied also to a number of positioning situations. As an example, for an oblique projection of the lumbar spine, the patient is typically rolled up 45° from the supine position. If the patient is of average thickness, the *1 inch of shift for every 10°of angle* rule would indicate a transverse centering point 4½ inches upside from the midline. Thirty degrees of rotation would require 3 inches of upside shift, and so on. This application of the rule for body part position is further discussed in Chapter 5.

The example of a Laws projection for the TMJ, given in Case Study #4, provides a beautiful example of the utility of this rule of thumb, wherein it compensates for *both* the rotation of the head and the beam angle employed in that position.

SHIFT OF CENTERING FOR DOWNSIDE "SURFACE" ANATOMY

The centering shift was recalculated for downside "surface" anatomy situated 2 inches above the tabletop in AP position (since the actual anatomy is not literally at the exit surface, and this exit surface is frequently raised an inch off the table, such as is caused by the lordotic curvature of the lumbar spine in the lower back). The measured shift comes to about 9⁄16 inch, and so does not significantly deviate from the previous rule of thumb for midline anatomy.

Repeating the experiment for lateral torso positions with a thickness of 31 centimeters, it may be worth noting that the rule of thumb almost precisely doubles to 1 inch of shift for every 5° of angle. However, angled projections using a lateral position to demonstrate downside surface anatomy are rare in practice.

Thus, *for most situations involving angled beams to demonstrate downside anatomy, the same rule of thumb as is used for midline structures may be generally used:* ***1 inch of shift for every 10° of angle.***

CASE STUDY

Practical Application Examples

Case Study #3: Modified PA Oblique Sternum

A trauma patient is sitting with her legs off the side of a stretcher, having just completed a PA chest at the chest board. The radiographer needs to obtain a diagnostic projection of the sternum, and opts to use a transverse angle rather than twist the patient precariously on the edge of the stretcher. The patient "hugs" the cassette to her chest, or a holding device is used in *front* of the chest board, to allow for a 20° tube angle toward the patient's right. If the patient is of average thickness, how far should the radiographer center the 20° angled CR to the left of the spine?

ANSWER: *The radiographer should center the CR about 2 inches to the left of the spine (1 inch for every 10°). This is illustrated in Figure 2-6.*

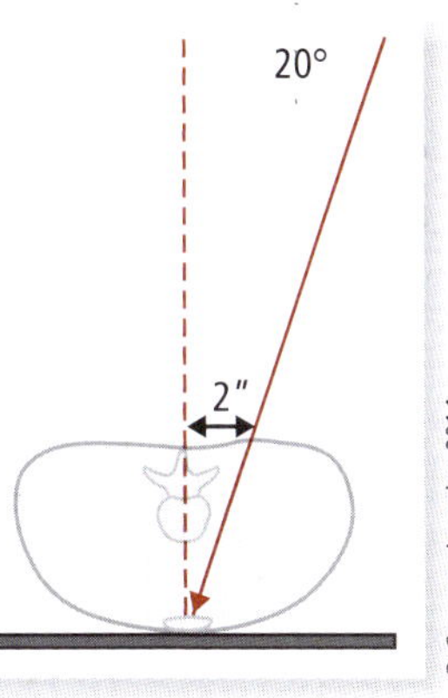

FIGURE 2-6

Adapting a trauma PA-oblique position for the sternum, a 20° left-to-right *transverse* angle is used. The x-ray beam must be recentered 2 inches to the left of the spine. (This diagram is looking down from above the patient's head, so the patient's *left* is to the viewer's *right*.)

Case Study #4: Laws Projection for TMJ

A tightly collimated field is used to obtain a Law's view of the right TMJ. The patient's face is rotated downward toward the tabletop 15°, and the x-ray tube is angled 15° caudally. From the easily visible upside TMJ (just anterior to the tragus of the ear), how should the CR centering be located for this projection?

ANSWER: *From the upside TMJ, center the crosshairs of the light field 1½ inches superior, and then also 1½ inches posterior to this upside TMJ, as shown in Figure 2-7. This will place it just at the upper back "corner" of the ear. This centering will project the downside TMJ right in the middle of a tightly collimated field as shown in Figure 2-8.*

(continues)

CASE STUDY

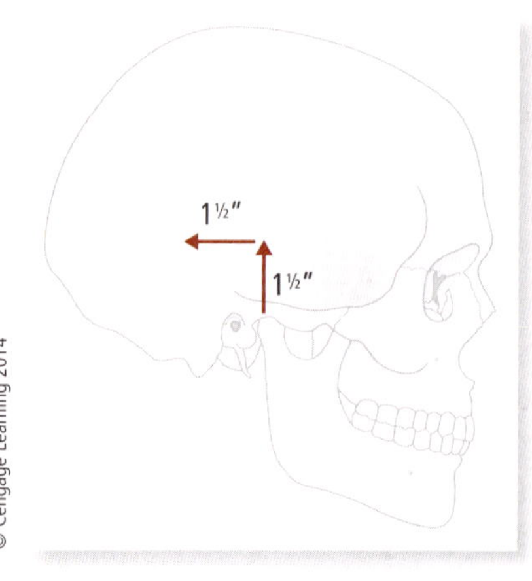

FIGURE 2-7

Lateral oblique projection for the downside TMJ. Due to the 15° caudal angle, centering must be shifted 1½ inches upward from the upside TMJ. Due to the 15° rotation of the head, centering must *also* be shifted more *posterior* by 1½ inches.

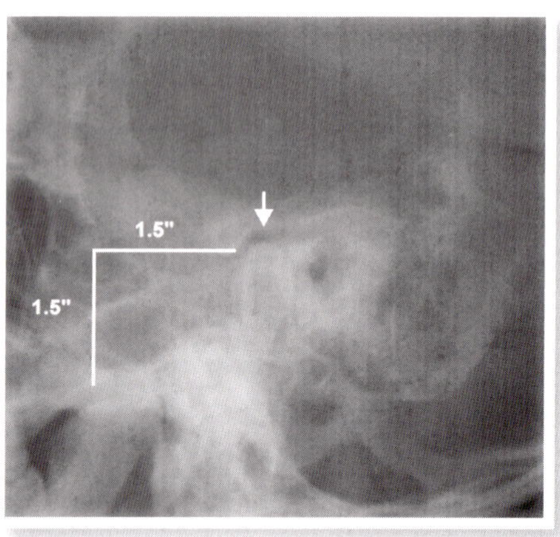

FIGURE 2-8

Radiograph using the recentering shift rule described in Figure 2-7. Note that the downside TMJ (arrow) is precisely centered within the field.

Carroll, Q. Evaluating Radiographs, 1993, Figure 199, Courtesy of Charles C Thomas, Publisher, Ltd., Springfield, Illinois.

Source-To-Image Receptor Distance

The rule of thumb for recentering an angled x-ray beam derives only from the thickness of the body and average anatomical geometry. No adjustment in this rule is necessary for a 72-inch (180-cm) SID as opposed to a 40-inch (100-cm) SID. The rule may be applied just as written at all distances.

Other Applications

Beside CR angles, the same shift rule can be applied for recentering according to changes in body part position: for obliques, for rotation, tilt, flexion, or extension. These are discussed in Chapter 5.

SUMMARY

1. On ALL positions within the skull, chest, abdomen, and pelvis, shift the CR centering by ½ inch for every 5° of beam angle. Shift the CR centering by 1 inch (2.5 cm) for every 10° of beam angle. This rule of thumb may be used with any SID.
2. For caudal angles, shift the CR centering in the cephalic direction, for cephalic angles, shift caudally. For angles toward the patient's right, shift centering to the left, and vice versa.
3. The same rule of thumb can be applied for recentering according to body part obliquity, tilt, flexion, or extension (see Chapter 5).

CENTERING FOR DIFFERENT CERVICAL SPINE VIEWS

CRITICAL THINKING CHALLENGE 2.1

A textbook recommends the following CR centering points for cervical spine projections: For the AP and the AP oblique (posterior oblique) projections, center at the *bottom of the thyroid cartilage* entering at the level of C5. For the lateral (and PA oblique) projection, center at the *top of the thyroid cartilage* entering at the level of C4.

Why are these different? At what vertebral level should the CR always exit? How do these recommendations relate to the rule taught in this chapter: "For every 10° of CR angle, shift the centering of the CR by 1 inch?"

CENTERING FOR THE PA OBLIQUE CERVICAL SPINE

CRITICAL THINKING CHALLENGE 2.2

As discussed in the preceding Critical Thinking Challenge 2.1, the two projections of the C-spine that use a 15° cephalic angle require the centering point to be shifted 1½ inches lower, all in agreement with the shift rule taught in this chapter. Yet, the projection requiring a 15° *caudal* angle (the PA oblique) lists the same centering point as the lateral projection that has no angle.

With a 15° caudal angle, why is the centering point for the PA oblique not shifted 1½ inches upward, placing it higher than the top of the thyroid cartilage? Does this contradict the shift rule? ■

CRITICAL THINKING CHALLENGE 2.3

CENTERING FOR A TRAUMA AP OBLIQUE CERVICAL SPINE

Imagine performing a trauma oblique C-spine with the patient still strapped on the backboard and in full precautions. You have a mobile unit and the x-ray tube is easily angled in any direction. You decide to use both the 45° side angle and the 15° cephalad angle.

With these angles, where would the proper centering point be from the starting point of midline at the level of C4? ■

(Answers to Critical Thinking Challenges are found in the Appendix.)

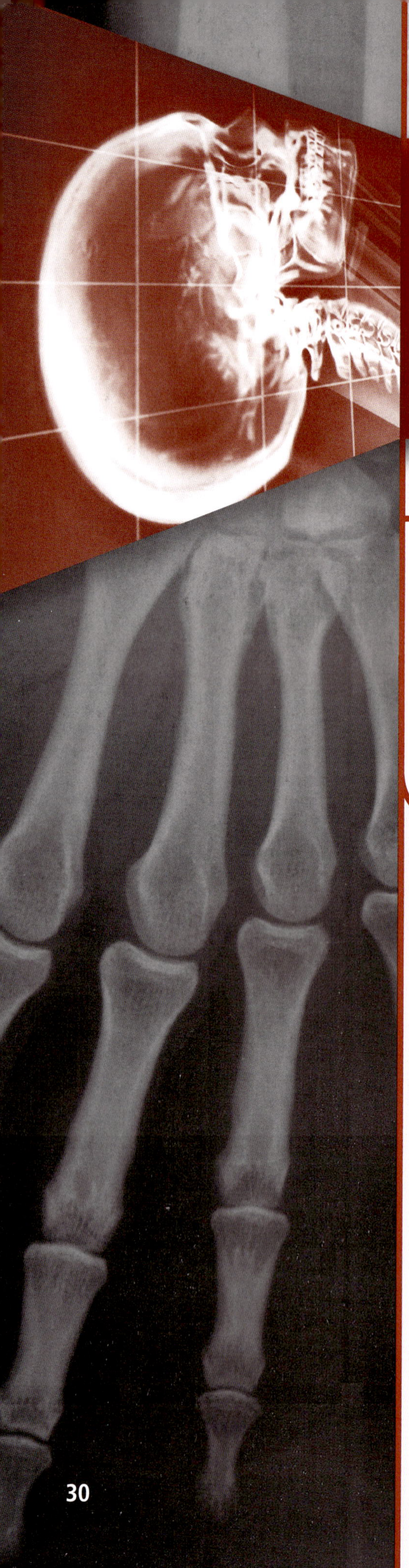

CHAPTER 3

Adapting for Light Field Expansion and Magnification

OUTLINE

OBJECTIVES

Upon completion of this chapter, you should be able to:

1. As a universal rule for all projections and distances, state the *minimum* amount of expansion for each edge of the projected x-ray field, from the upside surface of the typical adult patient to the image receptor.
2. In both AP and lateral projections for average adult head and torso procedures, and for very large patients, state the typical expansion for each edge of the x-ray field, from the upside surface of the anatomy to the image receptor.
3. Apply this understanding by trusting the collimator readout and by never using a field size exceeding the size of the image receptor.
4. Adapt these rules in practice for various angled x-ray beams.
5. Appreciate and apply long-SID technique anytime there is concern for fitting all of the anatomy of interest on the IR.

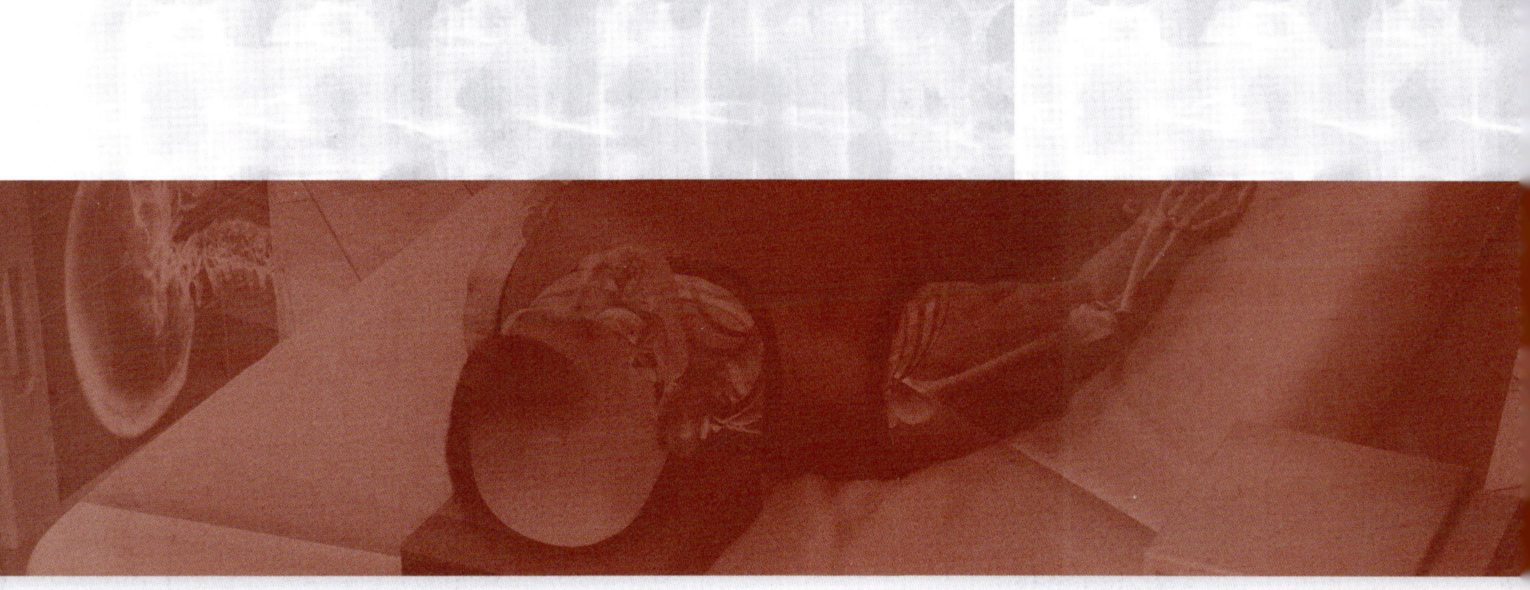

REGULATIONS AND X-RAY BEAM GEOMETRY

By law, the collimated light field should not be larger than the size of the image receptor being used. Yet when doing torso or head procedures, radiographers are often tempted to override the automatically collimated field or reset a "manually" collimated field because the light field projected onto the surface of the patient appears too small to include all of the anatomy of interest. Subjectively, it looks as though anatomy may be clipped off on the final radiograph. This is especially true for very large patients and for any lateral projection, such as the lateral lumbar spine illustrated in Figure 3-1. Here, the observed light field on the patient's upper surface is only 8 inches long. The radiographer must *not* overreact by opening the field larger than the receptor size, but should rather trust the collimation indicator. By the time the actual x-ray beam reaches the image receptor, it will have expanded by *2 inches on every side*, making it 12 inches long just as indicated by the collimator setting.

This effect is nothing more than the normal expansion geometry of a projected beam. It may be appreciated by setting the collimator at a 6-inch by 8-inch field, placing a piece of paper or stiff white card stock on the table and moving the paper or card up vertically while observing the light field as it shrinks. Students are always impressed with how small the field appears when holding the paper about 30 centimeters above the tabletop, yet this is the normal thickness of the adult abdomen in lateral projection. When performing a cross-table (horizontal beam) projection of the lumbar spine for a myelogram, the properly collimated light field always appears subjectively very small on the patient's side, yet it will invariably fill the length of the film cassette as indicated by the collimator settings.

Regulations require that each edge of the projected light field be accurate to within about ½ inch (or 1 cm) of the actual edge of the x-ray field when exposure is made, and it is rare for the light field to be outside this range. All seasoned radiographers have had the experience of finding one edge of the field on a radiograph clipped off by about ½ inch when they had set the collimator exactly to the receptor

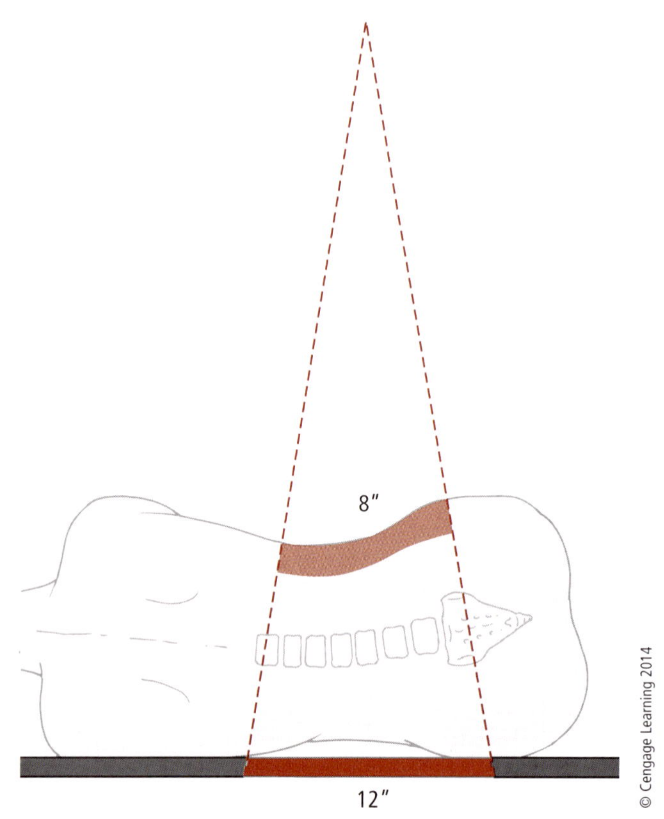

FIGURE 3-1

Here, the observed light field on the patient's surface, only 8 inches long, may appear too small to include all of the anatomy. The radiographer must not open the field, but rather trust the collimator setting. When the actual x-ray beam reaches the image receptor, it has expanded by 2 inches on each side. It is 12 inches long, just as indicated by the collimator.

size. On a very large patient, this can mean clipping off the costophrenic angles of the lungs and result in a repeated exposure. As a practical matter, the technologist may override the preset collimation by ½ inch or so to make sure this does not happen. It cannot be overstressed, however, that going beyond this compensation (i.e., intentionally setting the actual collimated *x-ray* field to a size larger than the receptor), is an unethical practice and illegal in many areas.

Generally, the field size indicators on collimators may be trusted implicitly. Regardless of how small the light field may appear on top of the patient, one may be assured that by the time the field *exits* the patient it is indeed the size indicated by the machine, give or take ½ inch on every side. Therefore, as long as the accepted rules for *centering* that field are correctly followed, one may be assured that the anatomy of interest will nearly always be included in its entirety on the finished radiograph.

A rule of thumb may be stated for mentally picturing the geometrical expansion of the light field as it progresses through the torso or skull: "For AP (or PA) projections, as you examine the light field projected onto the average patient's surface, you may expect more than 1 inch to be added to *each edge* of the field by the time it exits the patient's back." By picturing in your mind's eye the light field an inch larger on every side, it gives you confidence that you will indeed not clip off the anatomy of interest. This reduces the temptation to override

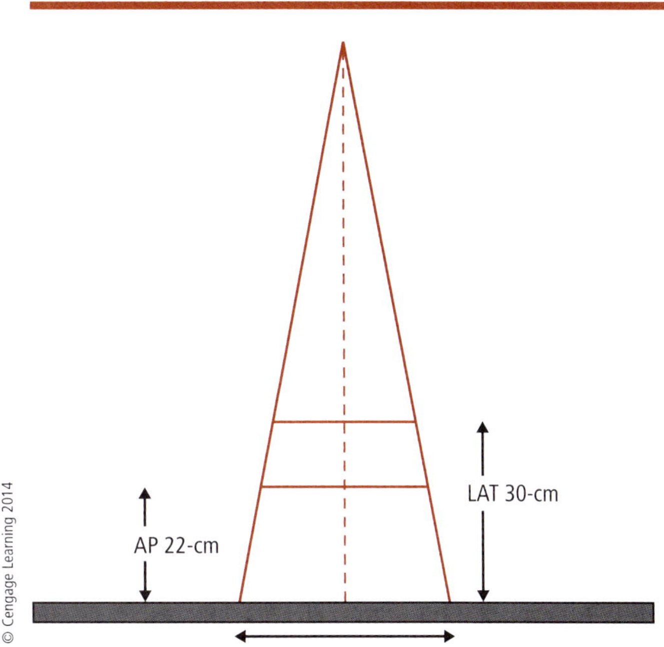

FIGURE 3-2
Diagram of an experiment from which the measurements in Table 3-1 were acquired. The expansion of the x-ray field can be measured at the image receptor, and at the patient's surface in both AP and lateral positions. Measurements were taken for a 40-inch (100-cm) SID, and then repeated for a 72-inch (180-cm) SID.

preset collimation or manually open the field size beyond recommended limits. As it turns out, this simple rule of thumb is an understatement, demonstrated by the following geometrical experiment.

One may plot the divergence of a 40-inch (100-cm) x-ray beam on paper and simply measure the width of the expanding field at the simulated lateral surface of the patient (average, 30 cm), the AP surface of the patient (average, 22 cm), and at the receptor (see Figure 3-2). The results vary according to the field size, and are presented with some precision (plus or minus 1/16 inch) in Table 3-1. This table also lists the measured expansion of the field edges using a 72-inch (180-cm) SID. The conclusions from this table are presented in the next section. Note that even with the smallest fields, smallest patient sizes, and longest

TABLE 3-1

EXPANSION OF EACH EDGE OF PROJECTED X-RAY BEAM FROM PATIENT SURFACE TO RECEPTOR
Assumed Average Patient Torso Thicknesses: AP = 21 cm, LAT = 31 cm

	8-INCH FIELD (20 CM)	12-INCH FIELD (30 CM)	17-INCH FIELD (43 CM)
AP / PA @ 40″ SID	1 1/8 inches	1 11/16 inches	2 1/4 inches
LAT @ 40″ SID	1 1/2 inches	2 1/4 inches	3 1/8 inches
AP / PA @ 72″ SID	11/16 inch	1 inch	1 5/16 inches
LAT @ 72″ SID	15/16 inch	1 5/16 inches	1 13/16 inches

distances, each edge of the field still expands by *at least* 1 inch in *all* circumstances.

PRACTICAL RULES OF THUMB FOR LIGHT FIELD EXPANSION

The data from Table 3-1 may be reduced to these helpful rules of thumb for memorization and practical application:

1. For most common torso and head projections done with a 40-inch (100-cm) SID, EACH EDGE of the light field observed on the patient's surface expands **2 inches** (5 cm) by the time it exits the patient's back. This is true for most AP **and** lateral projections.
2. With very large patients in AP projection, or with large fields in lateral projections, this amount increases to **3 inches** (7 cm).
3. Using a 72-inch (180-cm) SID, this amount decreases to about **1 inch** (2.5 cm) for **all** projections. With very small fields, such as a "cone-down" over a single vertebra, even at 40-inch (100-cm) SID, each edge still expands about **1 inch (2.5 cm)**.

BEST PRACTICE TIP

Each edge of the light field (and x-ray field), in all situations, expands outward by *at least 1 inch (2.5 cm)* prior to reaching the image receptor. For most torso and head projections, it expands by 2 inches.

As an overall conclusion, it may be stated that each edge of the field, in all situations, expands outward by at least 1 inch (2.5 cm) prior to reaching the image receptor.

Each edge of the light field (and x-ray field), in all situations, expands outward by at *least 1 inch (2.5 cm)* prior to reaching the image receptor. For most torso and head projections, it expands by 2 inches.

Practical Application Examples

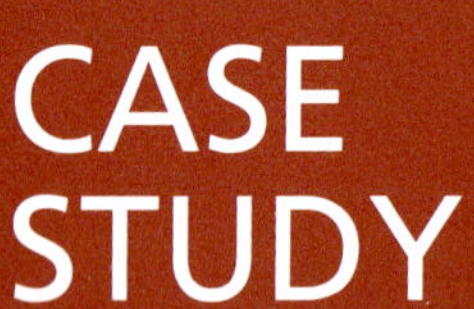

Case Study #1: Waters or Caldwell Projection of Sinuses

The collimated field projected onto the back of the patient's head appears to the radiographer to be about 5 inches in width. Because there is no light on the table off any side of the patient's head, the radiographer is concerned that sinuses may be clipped off. Should the field be opened up more?

ANSWER: *No. By imagining an added 1 inch to every side of the apparent field, the radiographer may be confident that the resulting actual field exiting the patient's face in PA position is at least 7 inches in diameter and that all of the sinuses will be included.*

CASE STUDY

Case Study #2: Collimated AP Lumbar Spine on Large Patient

The radiographer prefers side-to-side collimation to an 8-inch wide field on AP projections for the lumbar spine. Upon collimating in this way on a large patient, the light field at the patient's surface appears to be just 5 inches wide and 10 inches lengthwise. Subjectively, the field certainly looks as though the entire lumbar spine might not fit within it. Should the field be opened more?

ANSWER: *No. By picturing in one's mind each edge of this field expanding by an average of 2 inches (somewhat less for the side-to-side collimation and somewhat more for the lengthwise collimation), the radiographer can be confident of getting all anatomy of interest, including the SI joints, within this field, which will have expanded to about 8 inches wide and a full 14 inches lengthwise by the time it exits the patient's back.* ■

NOTE: This scenario is not for an extremely large patient. In that case, one may count on each edge of the field expanding by *3 inches.*

Case Study #3: PA Chest, 72-inch SID, on Large Patient

Performing an upright PA chest at 72 inches (180 cm) on a large patient, the radiographer notices that, having centered as usual, the upper edge of the light field is about ½ inch below the patient's shoulder line, so that there is no light at all on the chest board above the shoulders. Nor is there any light to either side of the patient's large upper chest: Both lateral edges of the light field fall about 1 inch inside the tissue. Even the lower edge of the field appears that it might clip off the bases of the lung fields. Should the field be opened up more?

ANSWER: *No. The radiographer may be confident that this anatomy will be included all the way around. The field will gain an inch on every side by the time it exits the patient, even when using a 72-inch distance.* ■

Figure 3-3 demonstrates what the light field should look like when centering chest radiographs on very large patients. In Figure 3-3*A*, the patient represents an average male with fairly level shoulders. With proper centering of the field, there will typically be ½ inch to 1½ inches of light on the table above the shoulder shadows. Compare this with the patient in Figure 3-3*B*, a large and muscular male whose overgrown trapezius muscles cause a distinct *slope* to the shoulders from the neck. On this patient, proper centering will result in only a bit of light on the board at the outermost corners of the shoulders. The student will worry about clipping off the apices of the lungs, because close to the neck the top of the light field falls well below the shoulder line (arrow). Do not yield to the temptation to pull the board and field up higher! It will result in clipping off the costophrenic angles at the bases of the lungs. Remember that *this top edge of the light field will be another inch higher by the time it exits the patient, even at 72-inch SID*. Figure 3-3*B* is the correct centering and will not clip the upper lungs.

In Figure 3-3C, the patient represents an obese, hypersthenic patient. Proper centering of the crosswise field is as shown, with the upper edge of the light field somewhat below the shoulder line. (This can actually range all the way from ½ inch below the shoulders to as much as 2 inches below the shoulders on very large patients.) Again, do not yield

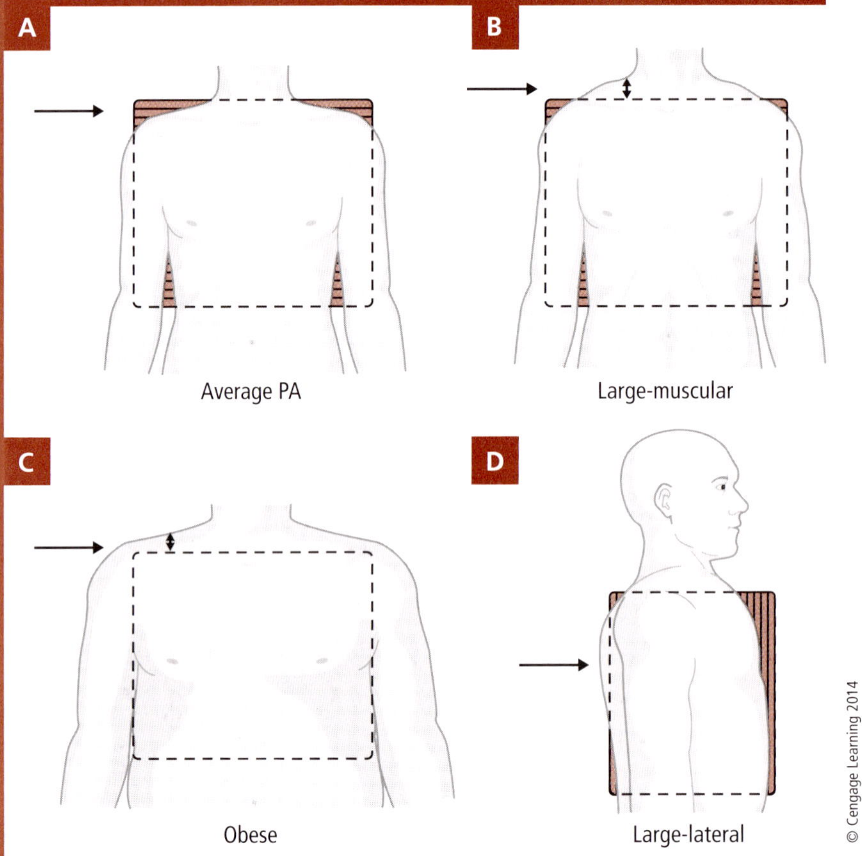

FIGURE 3-3

Application of field size rules of thumb to chest centering and collimation on large patients. **A**. PA chest on an average male for comparison: Typically, ½ inch to 1½ inches of light field extend above the shoulder shadows (arrow); **B**. Recommended centering for a large, muscular male: The top edge of the flight field will expand at least 1 more inch upward to include the apices of the lungs; **C**. Recommended centering for an obese patient: The top and side edges of the field will expand at least 1 inch on every side to include the entire lung field; **D**. Recommended centering for the lateral chest projection on a large patient: The back edge of the light field will expand at least 1 inch to include the posterior lungs.

to the temptation to raise the film and field, or the costophrenic angles at the bases of the lungs will be clipped. Remember that *each edge* of this light field will grow by 1 to 2 inches before it exits the patient. Also, recall that while fat grows primarily outside the bony thorax, the lungs are contained within the bony rib cage and are not much larger than average on these patients (in fact, their internal fat tends to compress the lung fields somewhat *smaller* than average). The centering as shown in Figure 3-3*C* is correct and will include all of the lung fields.

Figure 3-3*D* illustrates proper centering for a *lateral* chest position on any large patient (whether large boned and muscular or of the hypersthenic body habitus). Fat grows more thickly on the back of the chest than on the front. Although a small amount of surface tissue may be clipped by the field anteriorly, take care not to clip the *anterior* costophrenic angles. But, you should intentionally position the patient so that most cut-off occurs at the *upper back* as shown in Figure 3-3*D*. Remember, in doing this, that this edge of the light field will grow by at least another inch before exiting the patient, even with 72-inch SID.

Angled Beams

When the x-ray beam is angled substantially, more than 15°, elongation of the light field becomes obvious, along with a change in shape from rectangular to trapezoid, shown in Figure 3-4. This is normal elongation distortion, but can result in an x-ray field longer than the image receptor (cassette) in the direction of the angle. Some radiation is thus "wasted" at the ends of the field, exposing additional tissues and organs unnecessarily and generating additional scatter radiation. One can collimate the field prior to angling the beam, observe the length of that light field, and then with a little practice, learn how much to *reduce* the collimator setting for field length to bring it back to the size of the cassette or image receptor.

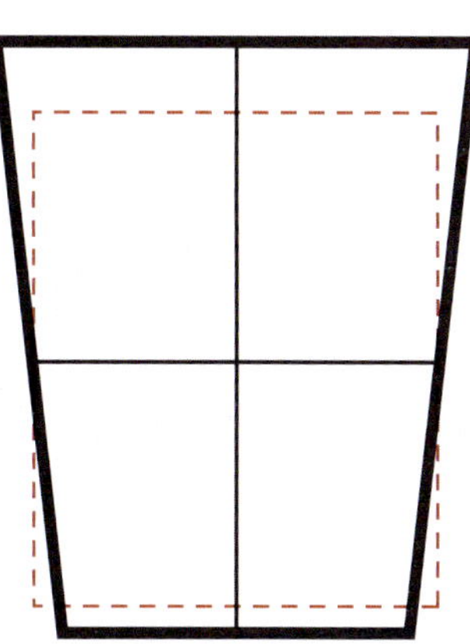

FIGURE 3-4

With substantial angles, the field distorts into an elongated trapezoid. The lengthwise setting may be collimated a little more than usual to avoid wasted exposure at the ends of the field.

USING LONG SID TO FIT MORE ANATOMY ON THE IR

For rib series, spines, and abdominal procedures, many imaging departments now use a 72-inch (180-cm) SID rather than 40 inches (100 cm) because more anatomy is demonstrated on any given projection due to reduced magnification effects. To demonstrate how effective this can be, Figure 3-5 illustrates an SID experiment using an abdomen phantom in AP position. As this series progresses from 40 inches (**A**) to 50 inches (**B**), 60 inches (**C**), and finally 72 inches (**D**), note the marked difference in the position of the top of the first lumbar vertebra relative to the top of the image receptor. At 72-inch SID, approximately

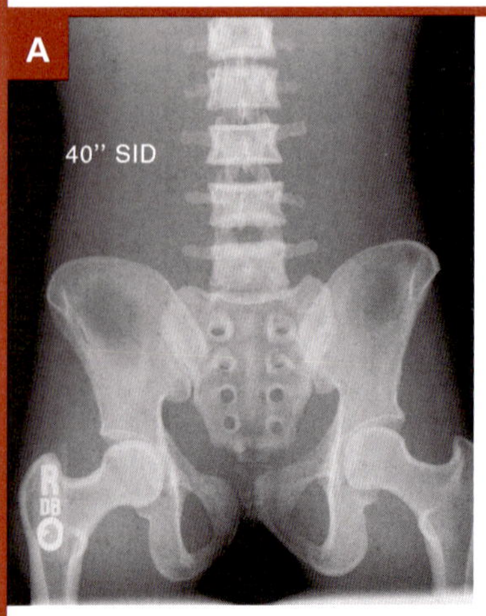

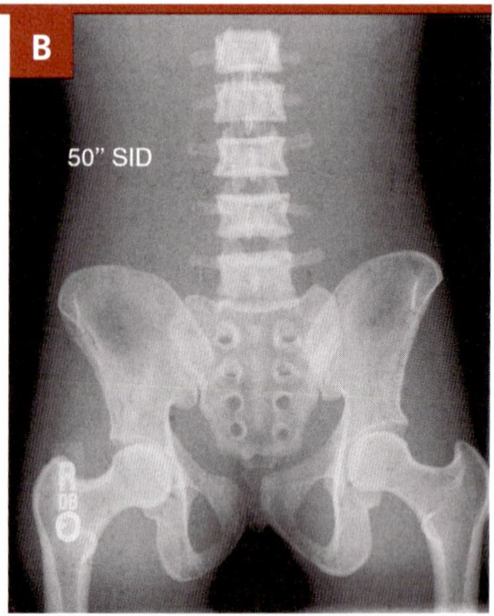

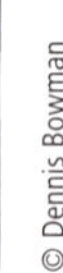

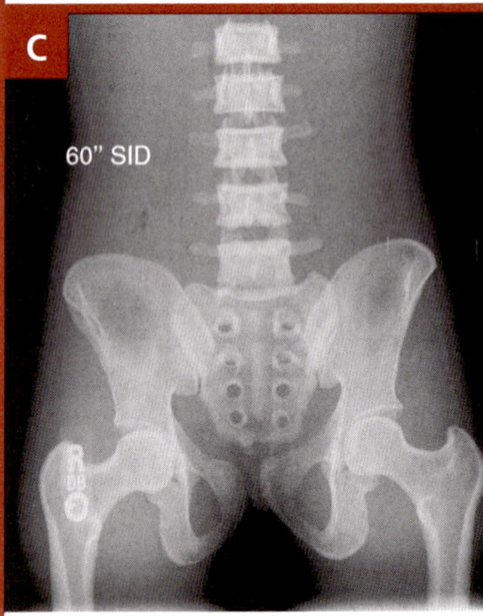

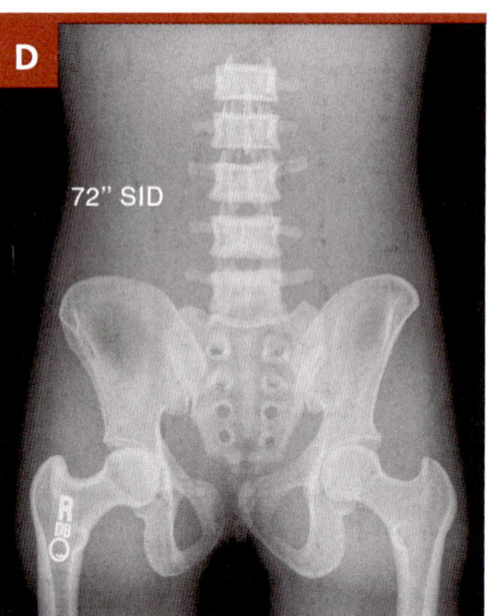

FIGURE 3-5

Effectiveness of increasing SID to fit more anatomy within the length of the image receptor: *An additional 1 inch (2.5 cm) of anatomy is demonstrated for every 10-inch (25 cm) increase in SID.* Image **A** was taken at 40-inch (100-cm) SID. In **B**, taken at 50 inches, ½ inch is gained at each end of the IR, particularly notable at the top where the upper edge of L1 now lies ½-inch below the upper edge of the IR. In **C**, taken at 60 inches, about 1 inch is now visible above L1. Finally, in image **D**, taken at 72 inches (180 cm), more than 1½ inches is visible above L1. The same geometrical compression of the anatomy is occurring at the bottom of the image, so that at 72 inches there is a total of 3 more inches of anatomy included in the view.

1½ inches of additional anatomy above L1 will be included when compared to a 40-inch SID (A). The same amount is also gained at the bottom of the image, for a total of 3 inches more anatomy included lengthwise at 72 inches.

The use of a 72-inch (180-cm) SID can be beneficial when a patient is unusually large or for *any* circumstance in which you are concerned about being able to fit all of the anatomy of interest within the area of the CR cassette or DR detector. To adjust the radiographic technique from the factors you would use at 40-inch SID, simply *triple* the 40-inch technique (triple the mAs or increase kVp by 22%). This will precisely cancel the effect of increased distance and does *not* result in increased patient exposure. This method is especially helpful with rib series, spines, abdominal procedures, humerus, leg, and femur.

BEST PRACTICE TIP

Any time there is concern for fitting all of the anatomy of interest within the area of the image receptor (IR), use a 72-inch SID to minimize magnification. This is especially helpful with ribs, spines, abdominal procedures, and long bones.

Any time there is concern for fitting all of the anatomy of interest within the area of the image receptor (IR), use a 72-inch SID to minimize magnification. This is especially helpful with ribs, spines, abdominal procedures, and long bones.

SUMMARY

1. For torso and head procedures, even when using a 72-inch SID or a very small field, *each edge* of the projected x-ray field expands by *at least 1 inch* (2.5 cm) as it progresses from the patient's upside surface to the image receptor.
2. For most torso and head procedures done with a 40-inch SID, each edge of the field expands by *2 inches* (5 cm); on large patients, it expands even more. With large fields in lateral projection, each edge of the field expands by *3 inches* (7.5 cm).
3. You should implicitly trust the field size reading indicated by the collimator. Actual field size must never exceed the size of the image receptor.
4. Any time there is concern for fitting all of the anatomy of interest within the area of the image receptor (IR), use a 72-inch SID.

CRITICAL THINKING CHALLENGE 3.1

PLACEMENT OF A LEAD MARKER ON A PATIENT

A particular radiographer has become very adept at estimating field size visually without checking the collimator setting. He is performing an AP abdomen on a 23-centimeter patient, and opens the light field to 14 × 17 inches (35 × 42 cm) *as he sees the field on the patient's surface*. He places a lead marker on top of the patient in the lower corner of the light field.

Why might this lead marker not appear on the final image?

CRITICAL THINKING CHALLENGE 3.2

ROTATION ON A LATERAL CHEST POSITION

If the lateral projection of the chest is performed with the patient's back surface *perfectly perpendicular* to the chest board or IR, the view will *always* turn out rotated as judged by the superimposition of the right and left posterior ribs or the posterior costophrenic angles.

Why is this so?

CRITICAL THINKING CHALLENGE 3.3

PROBLEMS WITH THE TUBE ON A GROIN LATERAL HIP

You are attempting to perform a "groin" (cross-table) lateral hip projection with the patient on the x-ray table. It is a *left* hip projection, and the patient is in the usual supine position with her head to your left. You angle the x-ray tube to the *right* into horizontal position. You then swivel the entire tube assembly counterclockwise 135° so that it is pointed horizontally with the proper 45° cephalic angle relative to the patient. When you then vertically lower the tube, you find that the handles of the tube bracket run into the tabletop before you can get the CR all the way down to the midlevel of the patient's thigh.

By trial and error, you discover that both "fixes" for getting the handles off of the table present their own problems: If you simply pull the tube laterally off the table, you have to swivel it back clockwise to recenter to the hip, placing the cephalic angle only 30° or so, too transverse across the table, and an improper angle for the neck of the femur. If you slide the tube toward the foot-end of the table, you can get the proper 45° angle *and* maintain centering through the hip, but now your SID is over 50 inches. This then raises the problem of how to adjust the technique.

Starting over again,* all *of these problems with distance, angles, and the handles could have been prevented in the first place. How would you do this?

As a secondary solution, which of the two preceding options would be better, and why?

(Answers to Critical Thinking Challenges are found in the Appendix.)

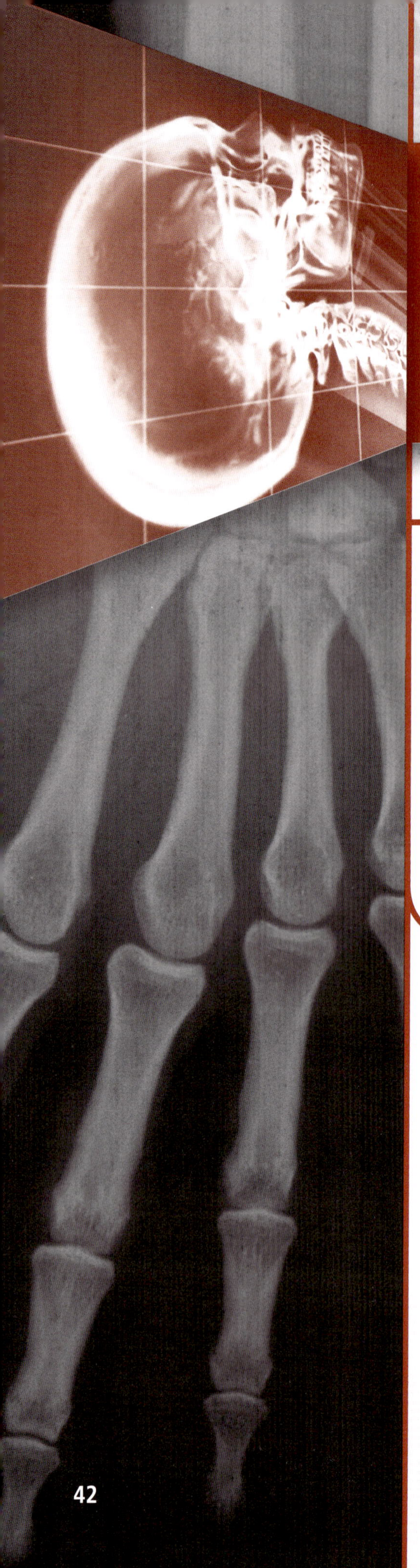

CHAPTER 4

Adapting for Beam Divergence

OUTLINE

OBJECTIVES

Upon completion of this chapter, you should be able to:

1. Take advantage of normal x-ray beam divergence, when it can be applied to the positioning of body parts with multiple joints.
2. Illustrate why reducing the SID, such as for the AP chest projection, requires any compensating angle to be *increased*.
3. Explain why off-centering of anatomy within the x-ray beam is equivalent to angling the beam to that anatomy. Apply this understanding by translating off-centering in either direction to the required angle for an x-ray beam that is recentered to that specific anatomy.

Continues

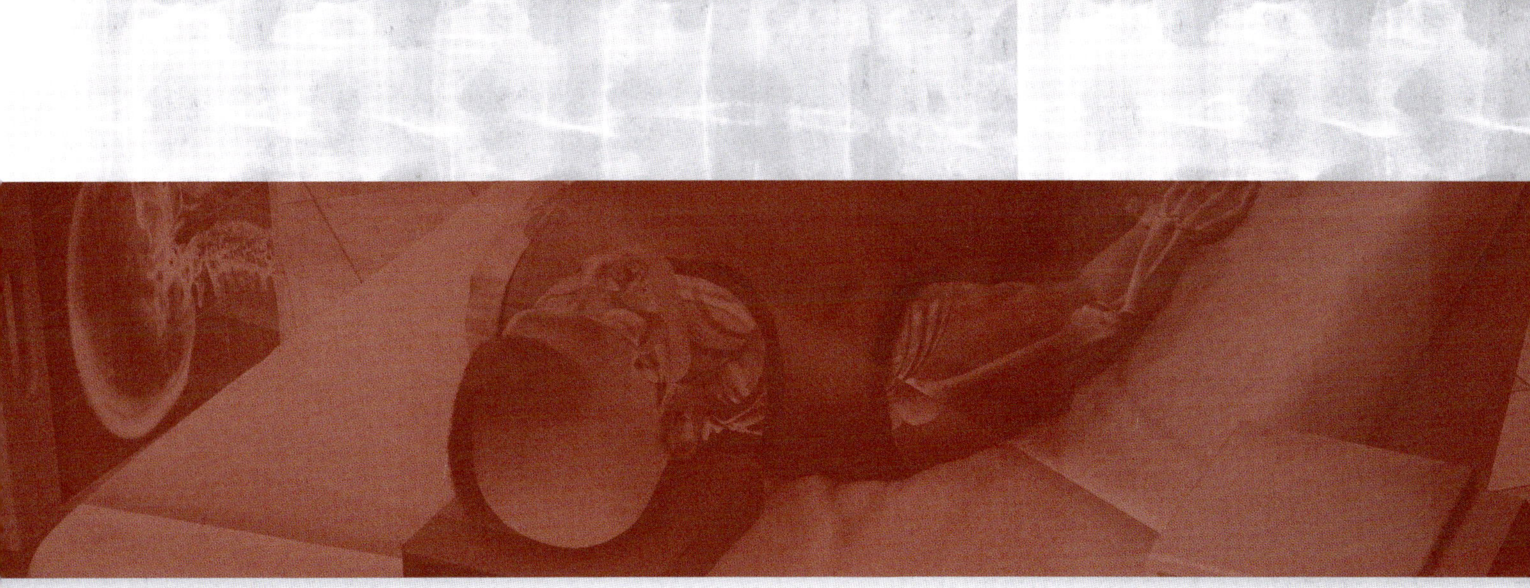

OBJECTIVES *continued*

4. Memorize the degrees of x-ray beam divergence for every inch (or cm) of off-centering, for both 40-inch (100-cm) and 72-inch (180-cm) SID receptor distances.
5. Describe how changes in SID affect beam divergence. Explain and give examples of how short-SID techniques can be used to advantage for some projections.

BEAM DIVERGENCE

The normal divergence and fanning, triangular shape of the projected x-ray beam have many important implications both for routine radiography and for adaptive trauma positioning. Indeed, one of the most valuable skills a radiographer can have is the ability to visualize the spatial relations of a fanning beam as it is projected to, through, and beyond the body to the image receptor.

Surprisingly, any serious discussion of beam divergence has been completely absent from most radiography texts through the years, which has contributed to the misinterpretation of several positioning concepts.

Using the lateral lumbar spine projection as an example, many positioning textbooks have strongly recommended that the waist portion of the patient's body be built up with sponges or sheets until the spine is *parallel* to the tabletop, thus eliminating any and all "sagging" of the lumbar spine. The diagram in Figure 4-1 demonstrates how this practice actually results in blocking the upper and lower rays of a diverging x-ray beam from making it through their respective disk spaces. There will be a poor radiographic demonstration of all but perhaps the two or three most central lumbar disk spaces, as illustrated in radiograph A in Figure 4-2. If the x-ray beam consisted of a "sheet" of rays all projected perfectly vertical and parallel to each other from a very wide area, the recommendation might make sense. But the x-ray beam is fan shaped, none of the rays are parallel to each other, and the only ray that is projected vertically is the central ray.

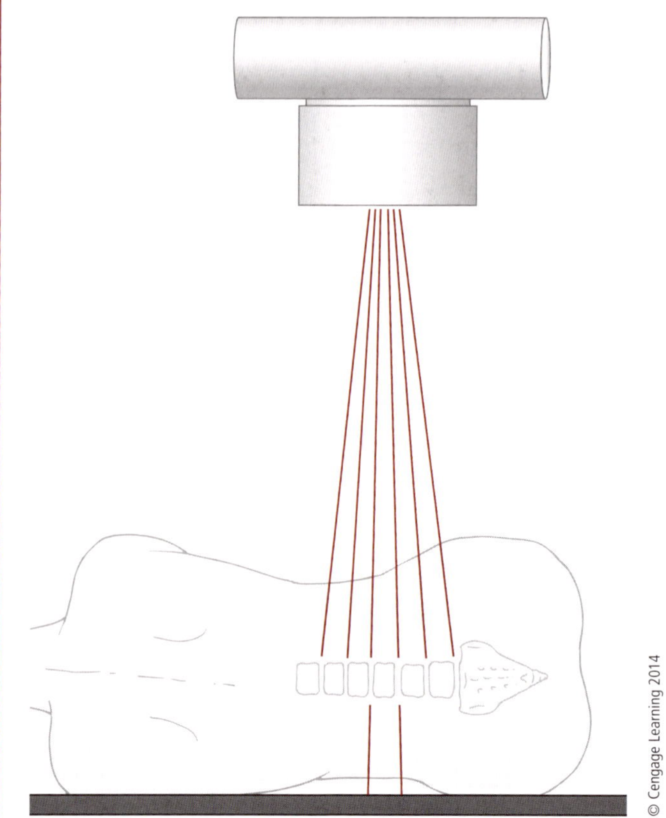

FIGURE 4-1

The common recommendation to build up the lateral L-spine until it is *parallel* to the tabletop actually results in closing off of the upper and lower spinal joint spaces. This is a failure to properly visualize the fanning shape of the x-ray beam's divergence.

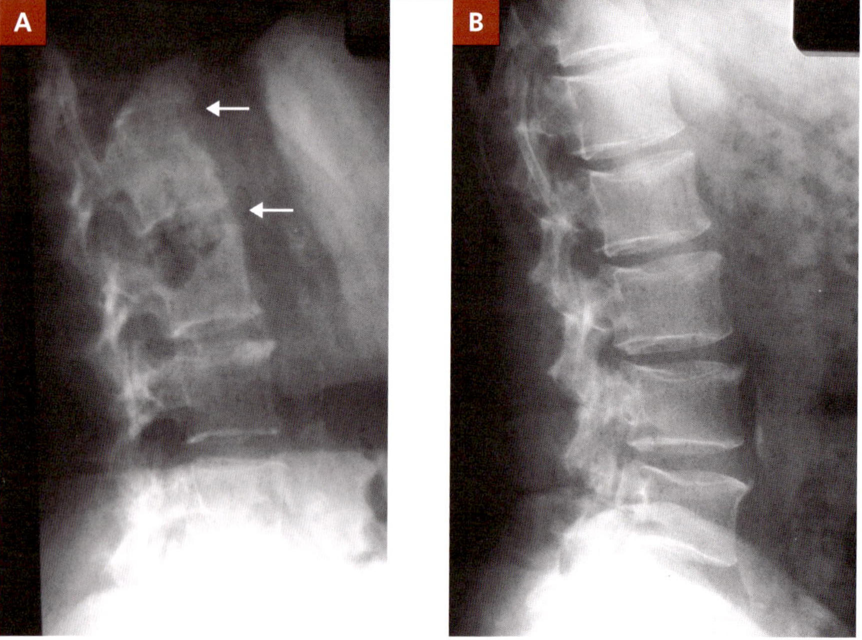

FIGURE 4-2

Radiograph **A** shows how building up the lateral L-spine until it is *parallel* to the tabletop actually results in closing off of the upper and lower spinal joint spaces (arrows). In radiograph **B**, slight sag was allowed in positioning the lumbar spine, aligning the joint spaces with the divergence of the x-ray beams. All of the joints spaces are open.

The closing off of the upper and lower disk spaces from normal beam divergence, as shown in Figure 4-3, is more than just a matter of demonstrating the spaces themselves. Any time a joint space is closed, it means that the two adjacent vertebrae or other bones are projected to overlap each other to some degree. If a small lesion or fracture is

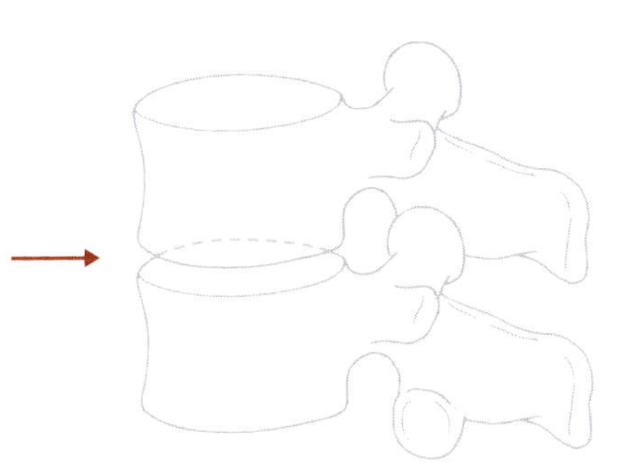

FIGURE 4-3

Diagram showing how when a joint space between two vertebrae is "closed" by beam divergence, the actual bones overlap, making it impossible to be sure if a lesion or object (arrow) is lodged, in this case, in the lower plate of the upper vertebra or in the upper plate of the vertebra below.

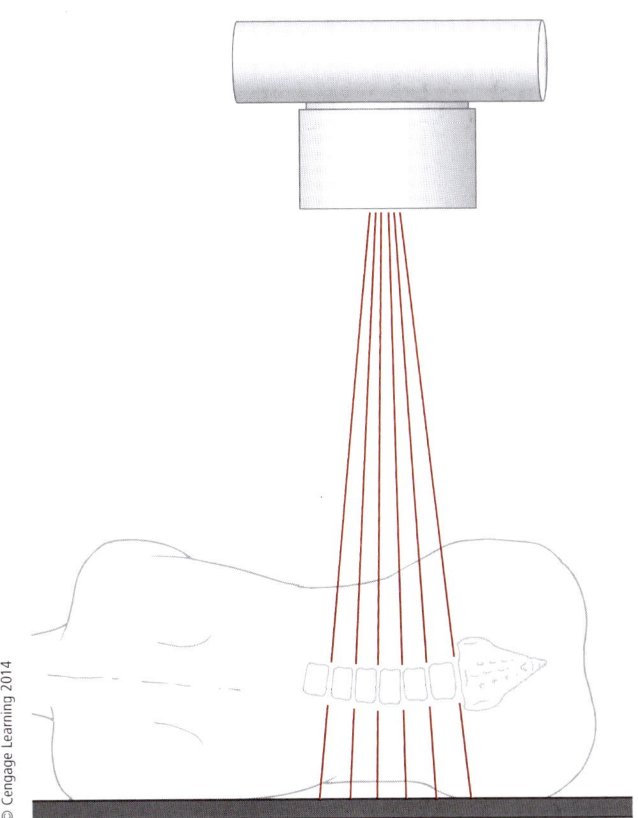

FIGURE 4-4

Allowing a moderate amount of "sagging" on the lateral L-spine serves to line up the joint spaces with the normal divergence of the x-rays in the beam for the best demonstration of this anatomy. See radiograph B in Figure 4-2.

present in this area of overlap or superimposition, it is difficult for the radiologist to discriminate which of the two bones is in fact fractured or pathological. Desuperimposition of overlying anatomy from the anatomy of interest is the central purpose of radiographic positioning. Successful desuperimposition always leaves adjacent joint spaces as open as possible. In fact, the openness of these joint spaces becomes the *gauge* by which you may evaluate the position.

In the case of the lateral lumbar spine projection, a moderate amount of "sagging" of the spine is actually desirable, as illustrated in Figure 4-4. It can result in lining up nearly all of the joints in the area with the diverging x-rays, maximizing the radiographic demonstration of the entire lumbar spine. This is shown in radiograph B, Figure 4-2.

There are several other applications for this concept, and further examples of exploiting normal beam divergence are given in the next section. The important point here is that *the radiography student must develop an ability to mentally visualize the fan shape of the x-ray beam in relation to the anatomy through which it passes.* This will save a good deal of mistakes and dose to the patient.

Practical Examples of Exploiting Normal Beam Divergence

CASE STUDY

Case Study #1: Hand and Digit Survey with Fingers Bent

Most students learn about the Norgaard or "ball-catcher" position for arthritic hands, in which the fingers remain flexed and an AP projection is performed rather than the usual PA projection. This type of position exploits normal beam divergence to advantage, and should not be limited to arthritis patients only. Often, trauma patients cannot fully straighten their fingers. In all such cases, reverse the position to AP to maximize the opening of the joints and desuperimposition of the phalanges, as shown in Figure 4-5. (A further recommendation for a full survey of severely flexed fingers is to take three projections in AP position with increasing *distal* angulation of the beam, the first at 15° shown in Figure 4-5, the second at 25°, and the third at 35°.)

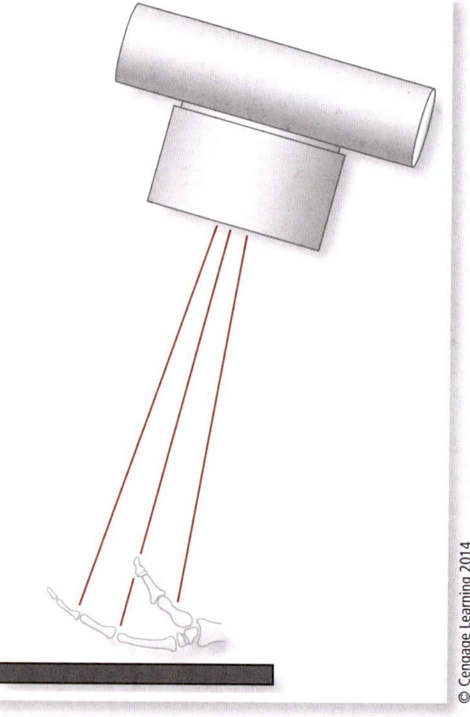

FIGURE 4-5

Modified AP projection of the hand with semiflexed digits, using a 15° angle and taking advantage of normal beam divergence.

CASE STUDY

Case Study #2: Frontal Projection of Lumbar Spine

Radiology departments may want to consider using the PA projection rather than the AP projection as a part of their lumbar spine routine. The PA can also be used as a valuable optional position. Figure 4-6 demonstrates the advantage of the PA projection, in that it closely aligns the lumbar intervertebral disk spaces with the diverging x-rays in the beam. This opens the disk spaces and optimizes the demonstration of the vertebral bodies, as shown in Figure 4-7. (It also reduces female gonadal dose by distancing the ovaries under increased tissue filtration.) Note that although the PA position places the spine slightly farther away from the image receptor, the loss of sharpness on the average patient is negligible.

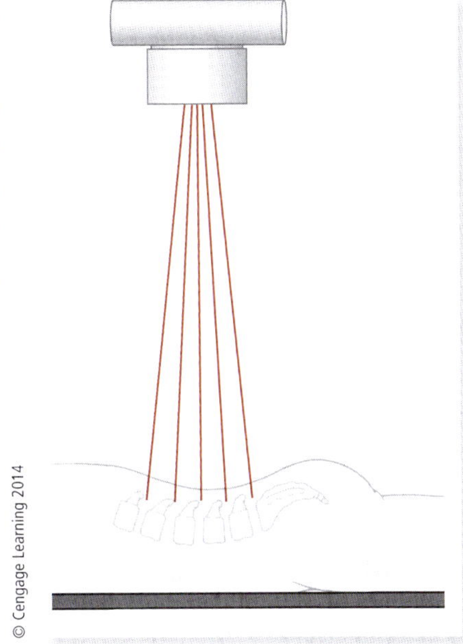

FIGURE 4-6 The PA projection of the lumbar spine takes advantage of normal beam divergence with only a slight increase in object-image receptor distance (OID), achieving far better desuperimposition and opening of the joints than the AP projection.

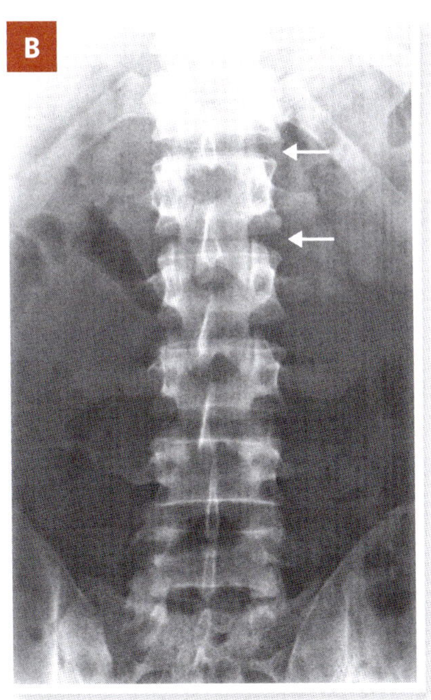

FIGURE 4-7 Lumbar spine radiographs comparing the AP projection and the PA projection. In radiograph **A**, only one intervertebral joint space (L2–L3) is open. Note the closing of T12–L1 and L1–L2 (arrows). In **B**, the PA projection aligns the joints better with the divergence of the x-ray beam, opening T12–L1 and L1–L2 (arrows).

SID and Beam Divergence: Compensating Angles for the AP Chest

Any reduction in the SID causes beam divergence at all points away from the CR to increase, as shown in Figure 4-8. In the very last section of this chapter, we describe how such increased divergence can be turned to advantage in certain projections because of its effects in *de-superimposing* anatomical structures. For most radiographic positions, however, x-ray beam divergence is generally considered deleterious to the image because of its impact on magnification and distortion. In most cases, then, we wish to minimize beam divergence by maximizing the SID.

The AP chest projection adds a unique consideration to this rule, because the normal kyphotic curvature of the thoracic spine and chest cavity is *combined* with the effects of beam divergence, such that a *compensating angle* is often recommended. Many positioning atlases recommend that a *caudal angle* of 5°–7° be placed on the central ray. For a perpendicular x-ray beam, with normal beam divergence the apical portions of the lungs and upper bony thorax fall within beams that are effectively "angled" cephalic, as shown in Figure 4-9. This results in a *lordotic* distortion of the upper lungs, rib cage, and clavicles. There is also a projected lordotic "straightening" of the normal (kyphotic) curvature of the spine and rib cage throughout. A caudal angle reduces

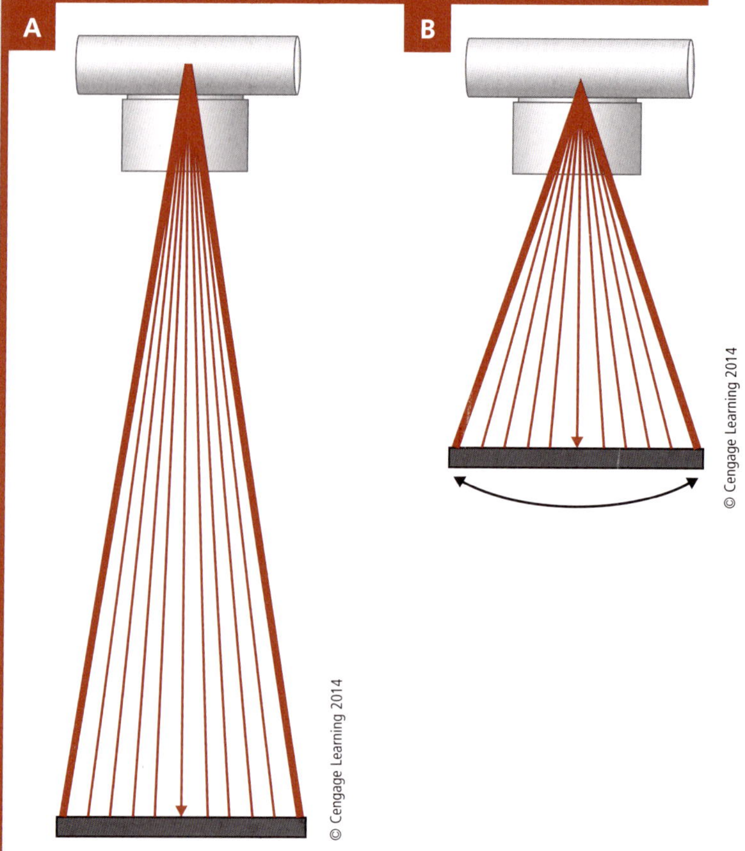

FIGURE 4-8

Any reduction in the SID increases beam divergence, **B**, at all points away from the CR. Compared to **A**, beams that diverge in a *cephalic* direction will be angled more cephalic. Beams that diverge caudally will be projected *more caudally*.

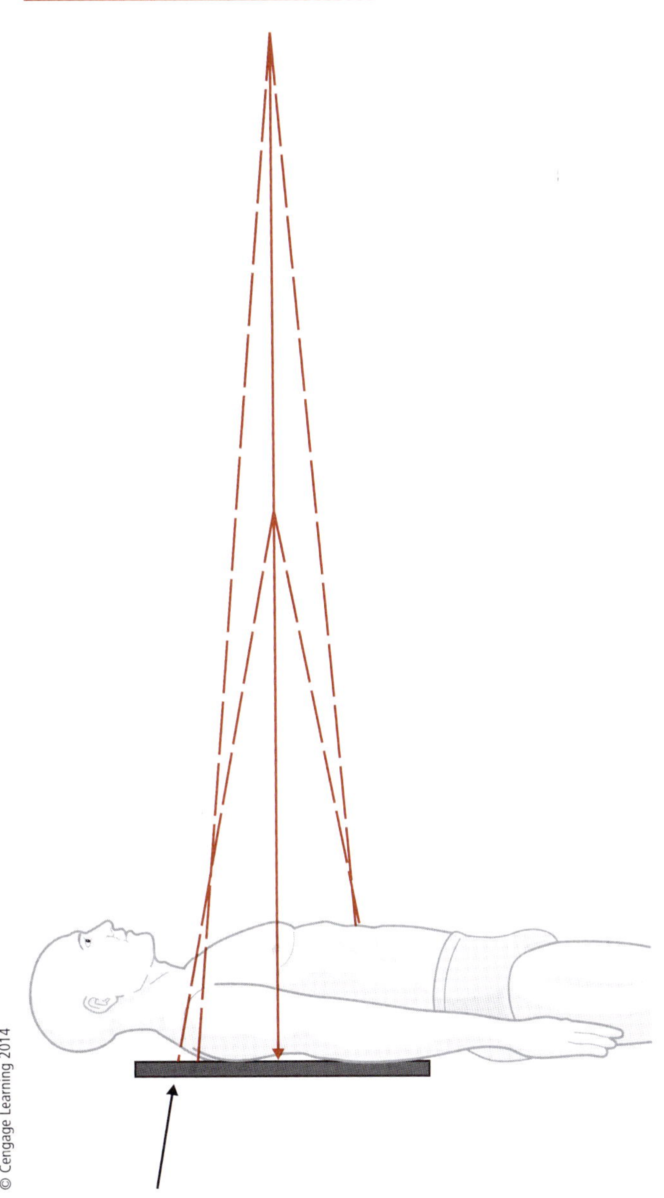

FIGURE 4-9

For an AP chest projection, with the CR perpendicular to the IR, *lordotic distortion* of the upper chest is caused by *cephalic* divergence of the x-ray beam in this area. Reduced SID *increases* this upward divergence and lordotic distortion.

these effects, and also better demonstrates the posterior bases and costophrenic angles of the lungs where small amounts of fluid will first accumulate. As shown in Figure 4-10, these effects on the mid- and upper chest are reduced by using the caudal angle.

The shorter the SID, the more extreme the x-ray beam divergence. Thus, when performing mobile or trauma chests at 40-inch (100-cm) SID (as opposed to 72 inches or 180 cm), these effects are all worsened. At the shorter 40-inch (100-cm) SID, it is more critical to use the caudal angle, *and more caudal angle is needed.*

For the AP chest projection, the shorter the SID, the more caudal angle is needed. When changing from 72-inch (180-cm) SID to 40 inches (100 cm), add about 3° of angulation (in most cases, from 4°–5°at 72 inches to 7°–8°at 40 inches). This is done to counter the effects of beam divergence.

BEST PRACTICE TIP

For the AP chest projection, the shorter the SID, the more caudal angle is needed. When changing from 72-inch (180-cm) SID to 40 inches (100 cm), add about 3° of angulation (in most cases, from 4°–5°at 72 inches to 7°–8°at 40 inches). This is done to counter the effects of beam divergence.

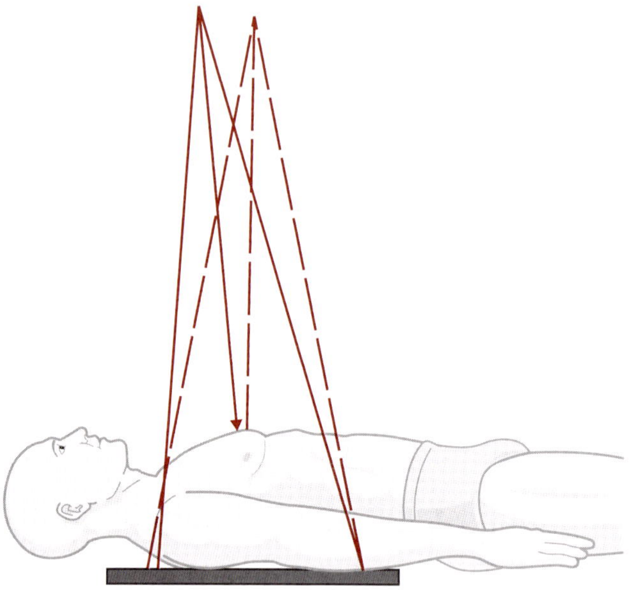

FIGURE 4-10

Slight caudal angulation of the x-ray beam (solid lines) reduces lordotic projection of the upper chest and better demonstrates the posterior costophrenic angles of the lungs. At shorter distances, more caudal angulation is indicated.

EQUIVALENCE OF OFF-CENTERING TO ANGLING

As one considers the fanning shape of the x-ray beam as illustrated in Figure 4-11, it becomes apparent that *any* object that does not fall directly within the central ray is being projected by a ray that is diverging to one degree or another. In effect, *all objects outside the central ray are projected by an angled beam*. This covers most of the objects in view!

The critical point is that when the central ray is off-centered from the anatomy of interest, the projection of that anatomy is also angled. The farther the central ray is off-centered, the greater is its angulation. If this effect can be quantified, it would be extremely valuable in both avoiding positioning errors and in correcting positioning errors. On a radiograph, for example, if a joint that lies 4 inches (10 cm) away from the central ray is seen well opened, then a subsequent projection centered directly to that joint should be taken with an 8° angled beam. Without this knowledge, one can only guess at corrections. The divergence effects of off-centering certainly *can* be quantified. The following discussion presents these very helpful rules and their application.

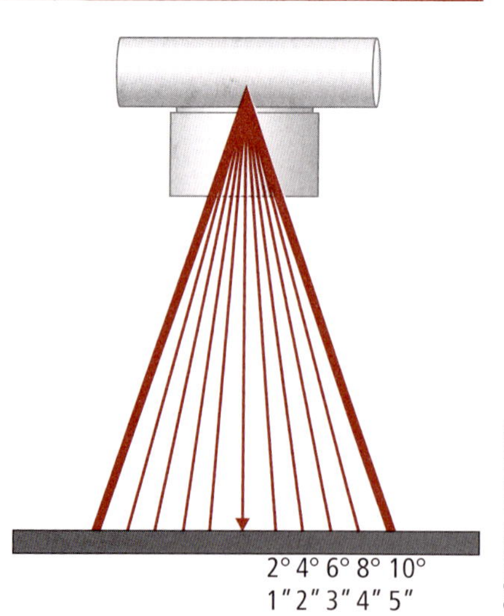

FIGURE 4-11

Careful measurements with a 40-inch SID show that for each inch in any direction away from the central ray, beam divergence increases by 2°. Thus, each inch of off-centering is equivalent to 2° of angle.

Rule for Quantifying Beam Divergence

An experiment can be done to measure the actual amount of divergence for 40-inch (100-cm) and 72-inch (180-cm) x-ray beams, as a function of distance from the CR location (see Figure 4-11). Because x-rays spread out *isotropically* in the beam (i.e., equally in all directions), the resulting rules can be applied no matter which direction one moves outward from the CR as located by the crosshairs in the light field—lengthwise, crosswise, or diagonally.

Accurate measurements show that at a 40-inch SID, each inch away from the central ray at the tabletop corresponds to about 1.7° of divergent angle. At a SID of 72 inches, the measurement comes to about 0.9° per inch. These numbers can be rounded up to formulate very workable rules of thumb. These may be stated as follows:

> At 40-inch (100-cm) SID, moving away from the CR in any direction results in approximately 2° of beam divergence per inch at the tabletop. This divergence is equivalent to 2° for those x-rays passing through joints that lie 1 inch away from the CR, 4° for anatomy lying 2 inches away, and so on. At 72-inch (180-cm) SID, moving away from the CR in any direction results in approximately 1° of beam divergence per inch at the tabletop. Note, for easy memorization, that this is one-half of the rule for 40 inches (100 cm).

BEST PRACTICE TIP

At 40-inch (100-cm) SID, moving away from the CR in any direction results in approximately 2° of beam divergence per inch at the tabletop.

This divergence is equivalent to 2° for those x-rays passing through joints that lie 1 inch away from the CR, 4° for anatomy lying 2 inches away, and so on.

At 72-inches (180-cm) SID, moving away from the CR in any direction results in approximately 1° of beam divergence per inch at the tabletop. Note, for easy memorization, that this is one-half of the rule for 40 inches (100 cm).

Metric Equivalents

Using the metric system, the measured divergence comes out to about 0.7° per centimeter using a 100-cm SID, and 0.4° per centimeter using a 180-cm SID. Although it requires a little more stretch of the imagination to round these values up, one may derive a functional and helpful rule: *At 100-cm SID, beam divergence is very roughly 1° per centimeter from the CR. At 180-cm SID, beam divergence is about 1° for every 2 centimeters.*

Practical Applications of the Divergence Rule

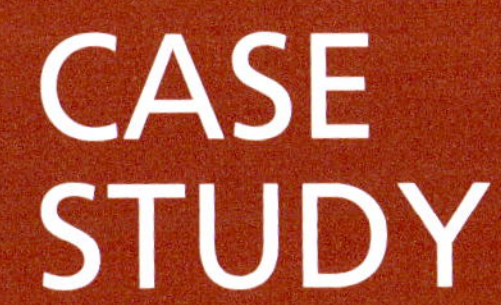

Case Study #3: Predicting the Required Angle for a Lateral L5–S1 Projection

A useful "trick of the trade" gives some guidance for angulation of the beam on the lateral L5–S1 "spot" view, by observing the routine lateral view of the lumbar spine. It states, "On the routine lateral view, if the L5–S1 joint is nicely opened, angle caudally for the 'spot' projection. If L5–S1 is closed off on the routine lateral, the L5–S1 spot view should

(*continues*)

CASE STUDY

be taken with a vertical beam (with no angle)." This rule is based on beam divergence, and works well. Yet, those who use it frequently *underestimate* the amount of angle required. Using the *beam divergence rule* mentioned earlier, you can quantify the actual *amount* of caudal angle with confidence.

Centering for the routine lateral L-spine is to the midbody of L–3, about 1 inch above the iliac crest. On average, the L5–S1 joint lies about 3½ inches below this level. The amount of normal x-ray beam divergence at this point on the routine lateral view can be found by multiplying this distance by 2° per inch. This comes to $2 \times 3.5 = 7°$ of caudal divergence. That is to say, on the *routine lateral L-spine view,* the angle of those beams passing through L5–S1 is about 7°, as shown in Figure 4-12. If that joint space is nicely opened on this view, the indicated angle to use for the "spot" lateral that will be centered directly at L5–S1 is 7° caudal.

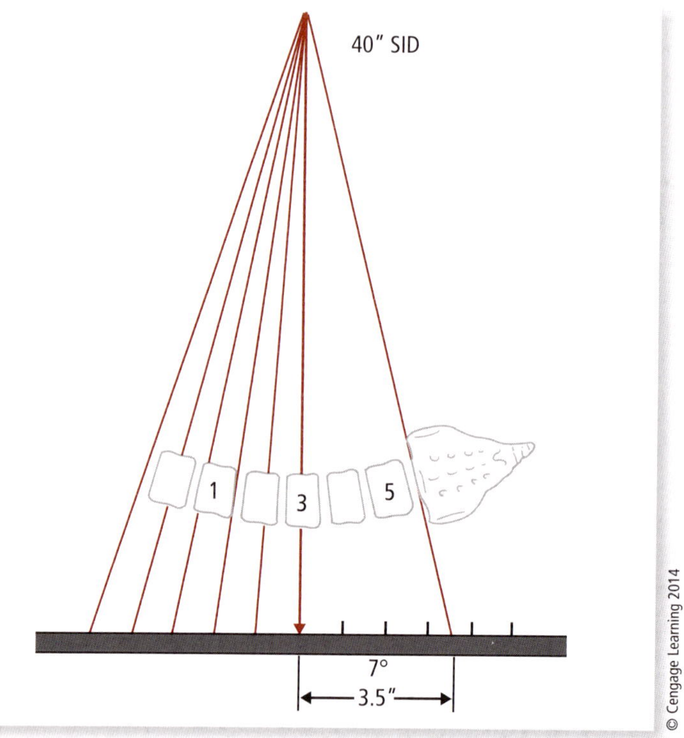

FIGURE 4-12
Using the beam divergence rule of thumb, one can predict that for a routine lateral projection of the lumbar spine, those rays passing through the L5–S1 joint space are angled about 7°. If the joint space is nicely opened, a 7° caudal angle is indicated for the "spot" lateral projection of L5–S1.

Radiographers often underestimate the amount of angle required for lateral L5–S1 projection. Many are hesitant to angle more than 5°. When all variations in the degree of "sagging" and conditions such as scoliosis are taken into consideration, the caudal angle required for different patients can range from 0° up to more than 15°. It is not uncommon for the angle needed to be significantly more than 5°.

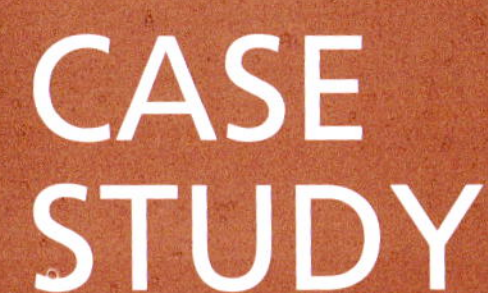

Case Study #4: Predicting the Required Angle for an AP "Coned-Down" Spot of T1

Suppose, upon examining an AP view of the thoracic spine, the radiologist asks for an AP "coned-down spot" view over T1. It is observed that on the full AP view, the joint space just below this vertebra is well opened. What beam angle, if any, would best demonstrate this vertebra for a tightly collimated projection centered directly on it? On the full AP view, T1 is located about 2 ½ inches (6 cm) below the top of the cassette or IR plate. For a 17-inch (42-cm) long cassette or IR plate, this places T1 about 6 inches (15 cm) above the location of the CR. Using the beam divergence rule, the divergence at this distance is about $2 \times 6 = 12°$ cephalic. For the spot projection of T1, angle the tube 12° cephalic.

By both quantifying and more fully appreciating the effects of beam divergence, positioning skills can be improved.

THE LOST ART OF SHORT-DISTANCE RADIOGRAPHY

Traditionally, a shortened SID of 30 inches (75 cm) has been recommended for several projections. For the PA oblique sternum or for the SC joints, beam divergence at 30 inches caused magnification and blurring of the spine and posterior ribs that otherwise get in the way. On the resulting view, visibility of the sternum or SC joints was enhanced as one "saw through" these obstructing bones. The method is extremely effective because of the substantial distance from these posterior bones to the image receptor plate (OID). In the prone position, the sternum lies right against the IR plate, nullifying any magnification and blurring effects of the reduced SID for the sternum itself.

The concept can be applied to any other anatomy where there is a marked difference in OID between the anatomy of interest and the obscuring anatomy. For TMJs and mastoid series, it has been used to better see the specific downside anatomy through the magnified and blurred upside skull anatomy.

For the angled sigmoid projection during a barium enema, the increased beam divergence from a 30-inch SID has been used to "uncoil" the loops of bowel, better opening the rectosigmoid flexure and the flexure between the sigmoid and descending portions of the colon.

During a cervical spine series, for the open-mouth projection of the odontoid, the use of a 30-inch (75-cm) SID magnifies the open mouth, with the upward diverging beams projecting the upper teeth higher, and the lower diverging beams projecting the lower teeth more

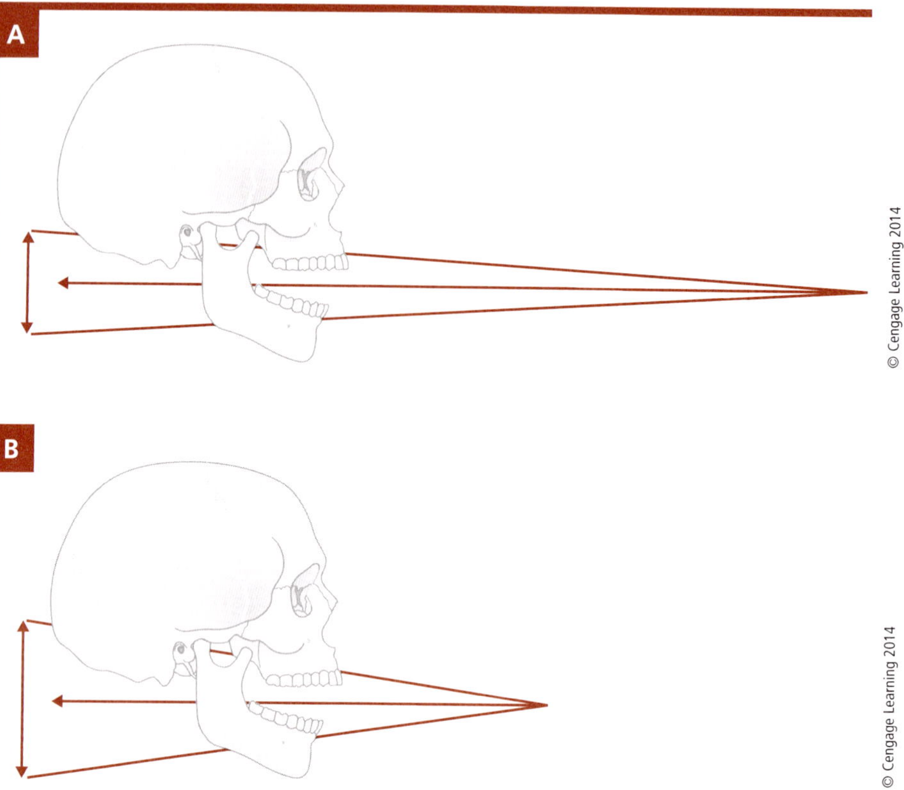

FIGURE 4-13

For the open-mouth projection of the odontoid, note that reducing the SID from **A** to **B** results in increased projected divergence of the upper and lower teeth, effectively opening the mouth wider.

downward (see Figure 4-13). In effect, this "opens" the mouth wider, such that more of C1 and C2 are visible.

Truly, there are instances where one can use a short-distance approach to diagnostic advantage, so one might ask why its use has declined. Two explanations come to mind: concerns over radiation exposure to the patient, and discomfort with how to adjust the technique (kVp and mAs). When changing from 40-inch to 30-inch (100-cm to 75-cm) SID, the inverse square law allows us to reduce the mAs to about one-half. This should cancel out the effects of moving the x-ray tube closer to the patient, so that the actual patient exposure is approximately the same.

Empirically, at least one experimental study has been done that indeed demonstrated an increase in the entrance skin exposure of approximately 10% *even with the proper technique adjustments* employed according to the inverse square law. This result then became the rationale behind a trend to stop using shortened SID methods. It is asserted here, rather, that a 10% increase is so minor as to be easily justified by the improvement in the image. (Bear in mind, by comparison, that the use of CR systems, widely embraced by the entire imaging community in the 1990s and early 2000s, resulted in a widespread *doubling* of mAs. This is over a *100%* increase in patient exposure, and was widely accepted.) Weighing risks against benefits, a significant improvement in the visibility of the anatomy of interest for diagnosis can render such a small change in patient exposure as 10% to be negligible. The reader must judge.

The rule for adjusting technique for a 30-inch SID may not be widely familiar, but it is quite simple: If a 30-inch (75-cm) SID is elected, simply cut the typical mAs used for a 40-inch (100-cm) technique *in half*. We can state that this restores patient exposure to very nearly the original (within 10%).

SUMMARY

1. Where multiple joints are concerned, such as in the spine or hands, positioning the part so as to allow for slight *concavity* in relation to the x-ray beam, rather than aligning it precisely parallel to the table, opens joints and improves desuperimposition.
2. At 40-inch (100-cm) SID, there are 2° of beam divergence for every inch (or roughly 1° per cm), of increased distance from the CR. Thus, every inch of off-centering results in the equivalent of 2°. An example is allowing slight "sagging" of the lumbar spine for the routine lateral projection.
3. At 72-inch (180-cm) SID, there is 1° of beam divergence for every inch of deviation from the central ray (or roughly 1° for every 2 cm).
4. These rules are extremely valuable in both avoiding and correcting positioning errors. A joint that lies 4 inches (10 cm) away from the central ray is being projected with an 8° angled beam. One can only guess at corrections without this knowledge.
5. Use of a shorter 30-inch (75-cm) SID can be diagnostically advantageous in several instances, and, if applied with correct adjustments in technique, it is safe for the patient.

CRITICAL THINKING CHALLENGE 4.1

IDENTIFYING THE UPSIDE ILIAC CREST

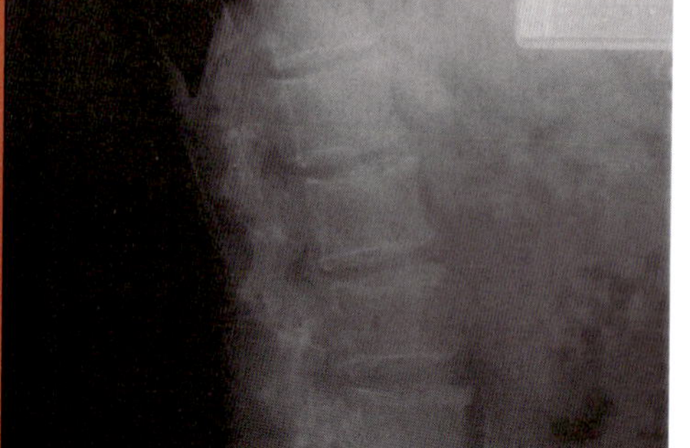

FIGURE 4-14

Identification of the upside iliac crest on a lateral lumbar spine projection.

Carroll, Q. Evaluating Radiographs, 1993, Courtesy of Charles C Thomas, Publisher, Ltd., Springfield, Illinois.

Observe the radiograph in Figure 4-14 of a lateral view of the lumbar spine. The two iliac crests are marked **A** and **B**.

Assuming the patient is lying in a left lateral position, which of the two iliac crests, **A** ***or*** **B**, ***is the*** **right** ***iliac crest? Explain how this can be proven, by referring to x-ray beam geometry.***

CRITICAL THINKING CHALLENGE 4.2

SPATIAL RELATIONS APPLIED TO A LATERAL KNEE VIEW

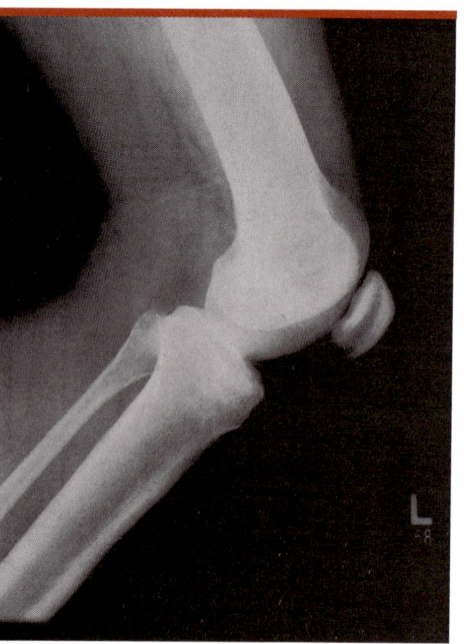

FIGURE 4-15

Spatial relations analysis of a lateral knee view.

Carroll, Q. Evaluating Radiographs, 1993, Courtesy of Charles C Thomas, Publisher, Ltd., Springfield, Illinois.

Observe the radiograph in Figure 4-15 of a lateral knee.

Describe why the two condyles of the femur are not projected directly on top of each other. Is the position rotated? Explain your answer.

SAG ON THE LATERAL LUMBAR SPINE

CRITICAL THINKING CHALLENGE 4.3

To best open all of the joint spaces for the lateral view of the lumbar spine, some textbooks recommend that you completely eliminate any sag by "building up the patient's waist with sponges until the entire lumbar spine is parallel to the tabletop."

What geometrical flaws are there in this reasoning, if any? ■

(Answers to Critical Thinking Challenges are found in the Appendix.)

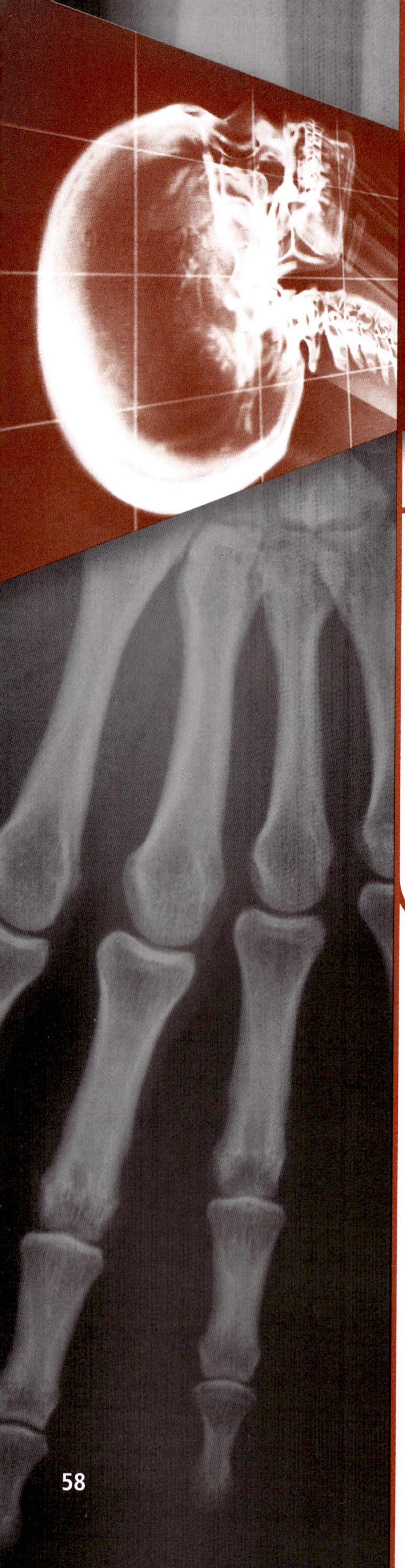

CHAPTER 5

Spatial Relations In Positioning

OUTLINE

OBJECTIVES

Upon completion of this chapter, you should be able to:

1. Always apply two points of reference in defining a positioning landmark line, and always identify positioning lines and planes *end-on* and from a straight viewpoint.
2. Evaluate a radiographic position by always positioning *yourself* square to and centered to the patient.
3. Always evaluate radiographic positions from a viewpoint at the same *vertical level* in which the patient or anatomy of interest lies.
4. Always employ at least two different viewpoints, perpendicular to each other, in evaluating a radiographic position.
5. State the direction and specify the *amount* by which the CR must be recentered to adjust for body part obliquity, tilt, flexion, or extension.

Continues

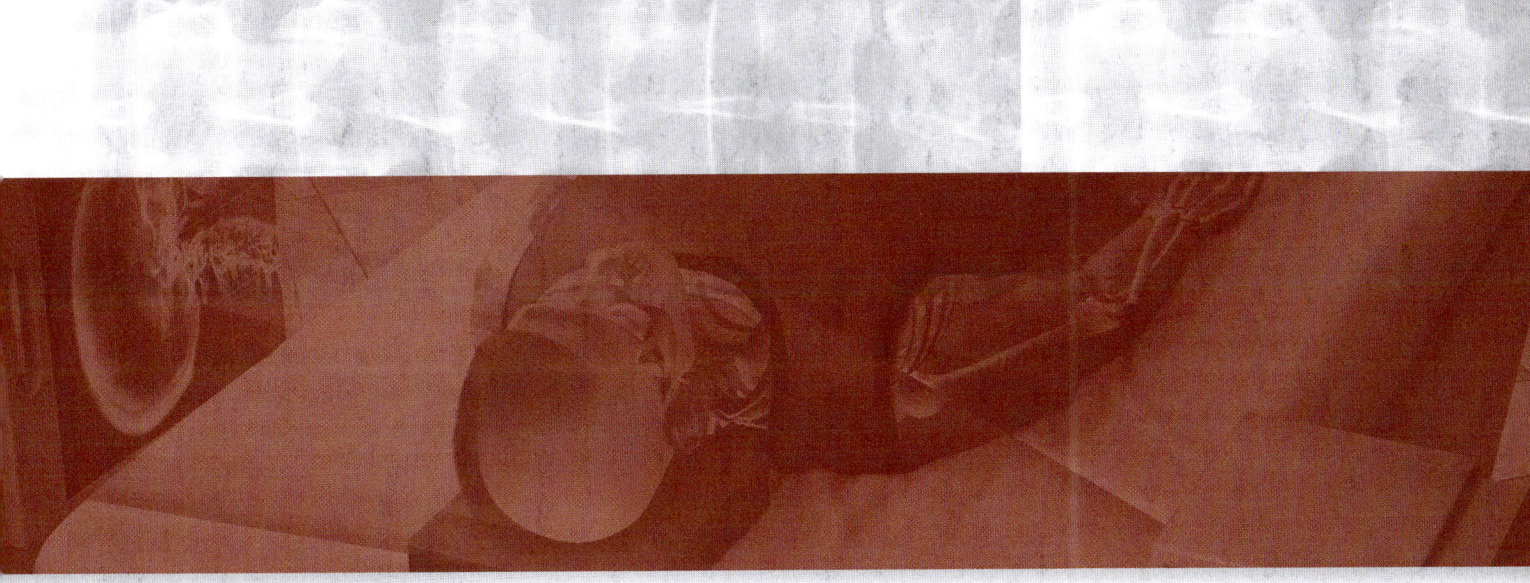

OBJECTIVES *continued*

6. Specify the amount by which the CR recentering rule must be adjusted for very thick patients.
7. Explain how the CR recentering rule must be adapted for organs that lie more anterior or posterior (from the midline of the torso).
8. Accurately sketch the major organs of the torso in cross section from a viewpoint above the head.

THE CRITICAL POSITION OF THE POSITIONER

Several years of observing students learning how to position a lateral chest without rotation, led to the identification of an essential behavioral pattern, a single element that differentiated between those who struggled with rotation and those who just seemed to "have the knack" for getting the position straight every time: It is how the radiographer positions *himself* or *herself* in order to sight along the body. Some would step to their left slightly in order to sight directly down the patient's back surface; others might step to their right in order to better see the light field, then tilt their head into the field to sight along the patient. Examples are shown in Figure 5-1. The best positioners would stand straight with their own midsagittal plane perfectly aligned to the patient's midcoronal plane, even though this meant that they would be blocking out the light field. They would keep themselves centered and their head erect, mentally focused on the single question of body rotation. They knew that the light field could be checked later on, and from a much better vantage point behind the x-ray tube.

In a twist of irony, it turns out that the most ideal position for the lateral chest projection is a slightly rotated position with the patient's upside shoulder rotated forward. As demonstrated in Figure 5-2, this takes into account normal x-ray beam divergence and corrects for it. It aligns the patient's back (and posterior ribs) with those diverging

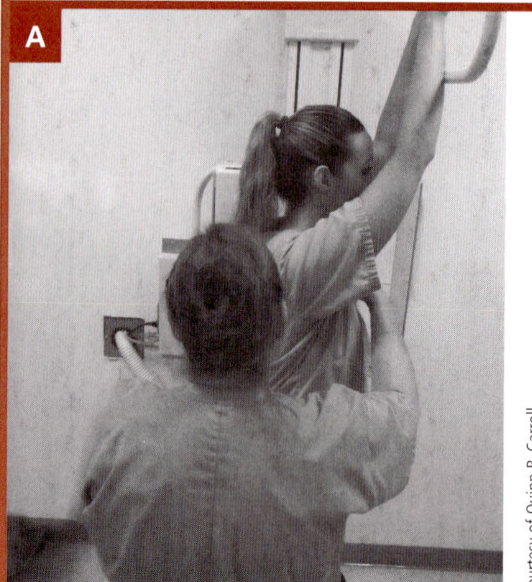

Courtesy of Quinn B. Carroll

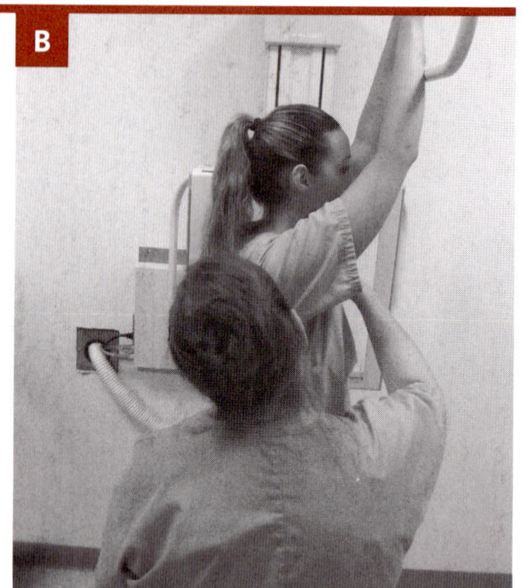

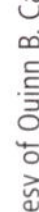

Courtesy of Quinn B. Carroll

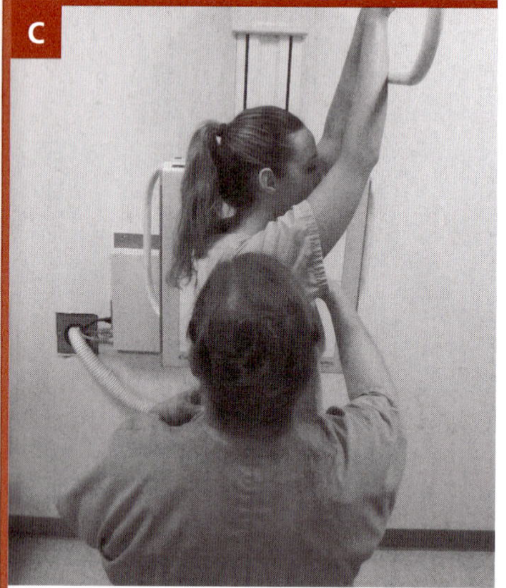

Courtesy of Quinn B. Carroll

FIGURE 5-1

When positioning a lateral chest, do not stand to the left **A** nor tilt your head to the left **B** to sight down the patient's back. Your midsagittal plane should be in line with the patient's midcoronal plane as in **C**.

rays that are angled posteriorly as they skim across the back. On a lateral chest view, rotation is evaluated by superimposition of *posterior anatomy* (the posterior ribs or posterior costophrenic angles). It is therefore this part of the body that must be aligned with the x-ray beams passing through it. These beams are *not* perpendicular to the chest board or tabletop. As with so many other adaptations discussed in this book, accurate positioning is achieved only when the radiographer can adequately *visualize* and fully *appreciate* normal divergence, that is, the *fanning shape*, of the x-ray beam.

Figure 5-2 also shows that when radiographers stand correctly centered to the midcoronal plane of the patient, as in Figure 5-1**C**, their viewpoint *matches* that of the diverging x-ray beam. There will be a natural tendency to bring the upside shoulder slightly forward in order to sight along the patient's back surface, and this is precisely what is required to perfect the position.

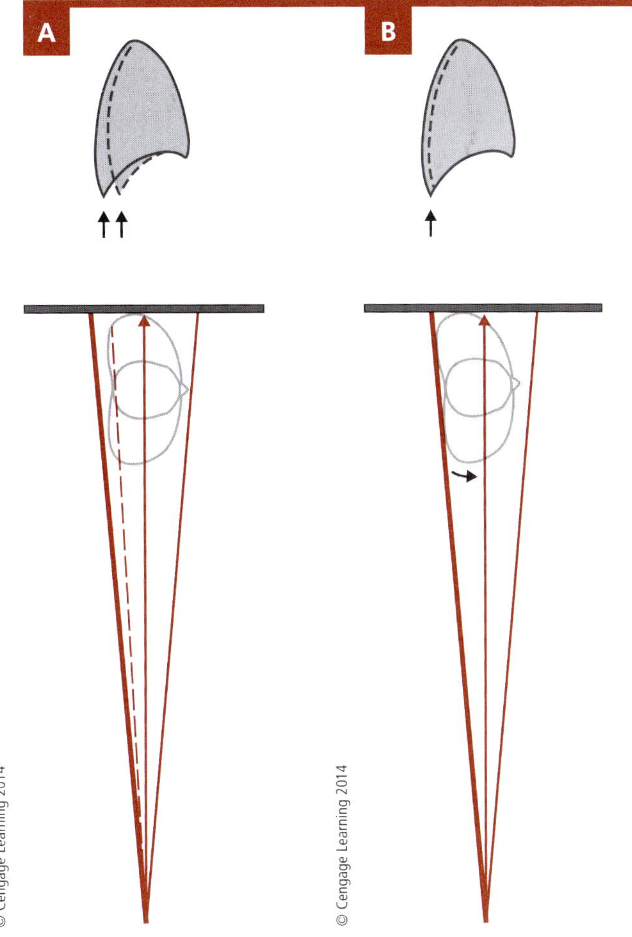

FIGURE 5-2

On a lateral chest projection, note that the beam skimming the patient's back (solid line) is not perpendicular but diverging at an angle. With the patient's back perpendicular to the IR **A**, the upside posterior lung is projected behind the downside lung (dotted line) in a rotated view. To prevent a rotated view **B**, the patient's upside shoulder must be rotated slightly forward (arrow) to align the back with this beam.

While the proper alignment for our own viewpoint may come about intuitively for some, they may not apply the concept consistently for all procedures (such as skull positions). It is, therefore, worth discussing at some length the underlying principles for positioner alignment. An attempt to fully appreciate these concepts should ultimately result in fewer repeated exposures. The key points might be enumerated as follows, and will each be extensively discussed.

1. Two points must always be used to define a positioning line.
2. Positioning planes must be evaluated from a true end-on viewpoint. The radiographer must be willing to do whatever it takes to position himself or herself such that this viewpoint can be achieved.
3. Positioning planes and lines must be viewed by the radiographer from the same vertical level that the patient or anatomy is on.
4. At least two different viewpoints, perpendicular to each other, are required in order to properly evaluate all positioning planes necessary for a position.

BEST PRACTICE TIP

1. Two points must always be used to define a positioning line.
2. Positioning planes must be evaluated from a true end-on viewpoint. The radiographer must be willing to do whatever it takes to position himself or herself such that this viewpoint can be achieved.
3. Positioning planes and lines must be viewed by the radiographer from the same vertical level that the patient or anatomy is on.
4. At least two different viewpoints, perpendicular to each other, are required in order to properly evaluate all positioning planes necessary for a position.

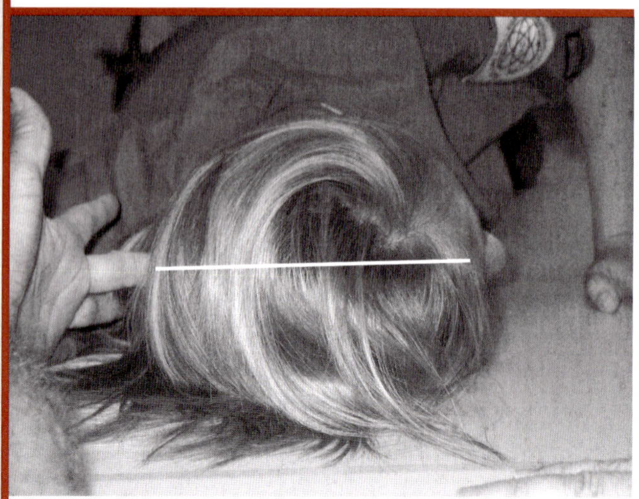

Courtesy of Quinn B. Carroll

FIGURE 5-3
Always use two points to define a line. For the lateral skull, extending your finger from the external occipital protuberance (EOP) allows you to visualize a line from it through the glabella to accurately define the midsagittal plane.

1. Always use two points to define a positioning line.

This concept is well demonstrated in skull and sinus positioning, where the tip of the nose is often used to determine rotation without really defining a positioning line. As shown in Figure 5-3, the midsagittal plane of the skull is easy to locate on a lateral position because a finger can be placed on the external occipital protuberance (EOP), and an imaginary line mentally drawn from that finger through the glabella as a second point of reference. However, on an AP trauma projection or Townes projection of the skull, with the patient on his or her back, the EOP cannot be felt without moving the patient's head out of position. One way to determine a "midpoint" for the back portion of the head is to place your palms squarely against each parietal eminence on the sides of the skull, then carefully draw the thumbs together such that they are perfectly symmetrical in their angle. An imaginary line can then be drawn from the junction of your thumbs through the glabella as a second point of reference. For PA projections, you may place your fingers on each mastoid tip and determine if they are equidistant from the tabletop. In any case, *two* points of reference must always be used to avoid "guessing" at these positions.

In most body parts, pairs of landmarks can be identified in order to visualize true lines for rotation. Examples of pairs of landmarks in the torso include the two ASISs, or the heads of the two humeri (Figure 5-4), which are recommended for visualizing upper and lower torso rotation.

2. Evaluate positioning planes from a true end-on viewpoint. You must be willing to do whatever it takes to position yourself such that you can achieve this viewpoint.

Rotation of the skull or any other body part can only be seen from an *axial* viewpoint, looking down from above the patient's head or looking up from his or her feet. Tilt of the skull can be seen only from a face-on viewpoint. Flexion or extension of the skull can be seen only

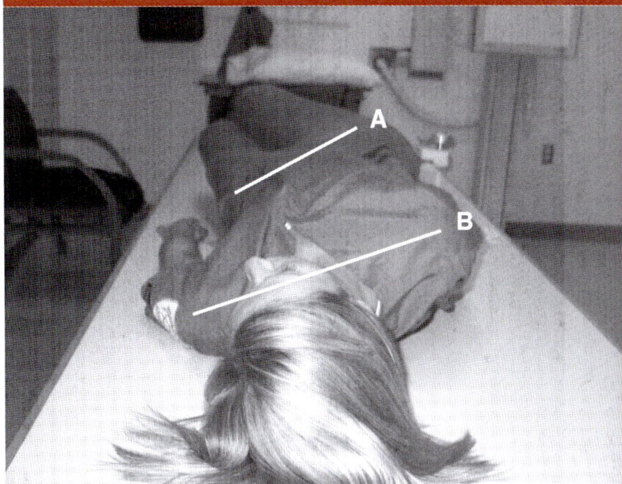

Courtesy of Quinn B. Carroll

FIGURE 5-4

Use a line **A** through the two anterior superior iliac spines (ASISs), which can be palpated, to determine obliquity of the pelvis. Use a line through the heads of the humeri, **B** to determine obliquity of the shoulders. A common error in positioning obliques is to place the shoulder line shallower than the ASIS line, as shown here.

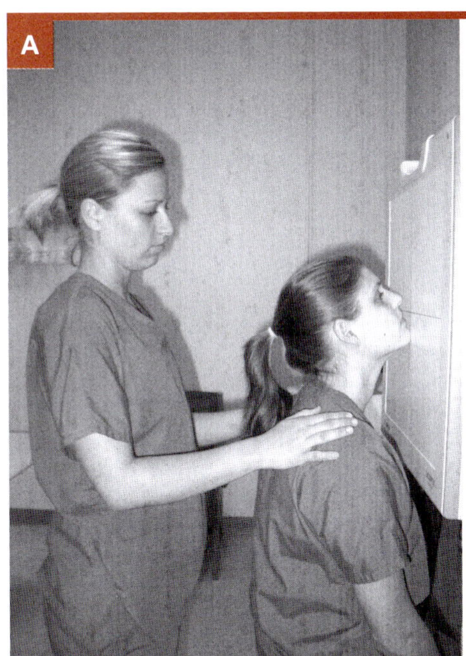

Courtesy of Quinn B. Carroll

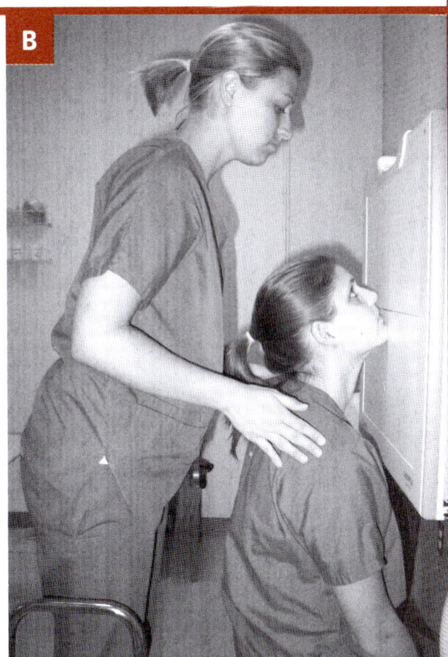

Courtesy of Quinn B. Carroll

FIGURE 5-5

Waters projections for the sinuses. In **A**, the radiographer cannot properly evaluate rotation of the patient's head. If necessary, use a stool to see down over the top of the patient's head to determine rotation **B**. See Figure 5-6.

from the side or lateral viewpoint. Any obliquity to one's viewpoint will likely result in crooked alignment of the anatomy; that is, the planes must be viewed from *straight* above the head, from *straight* in front of the face, and from *straight* to the side. Investing a little time and effort to do this will save much more time and effort in the form of repeated exposures, and is always well worth the trouble.

Figure 5-5*A* shows a radiographer positioning an upright Water's projection for the sinuses. Even with this patient seated, the radiographer is unable to see directly down over the top of the head in order to properly evaluate rotation or tilt of the head. To continue is to effectively "guess" at the position, assuming that rotation and tilt are correct without really knowing by observation. A repeated exposure is likely. It is well worth the effort to obtain a stool (Figure 5-5*B*), and even to remove any

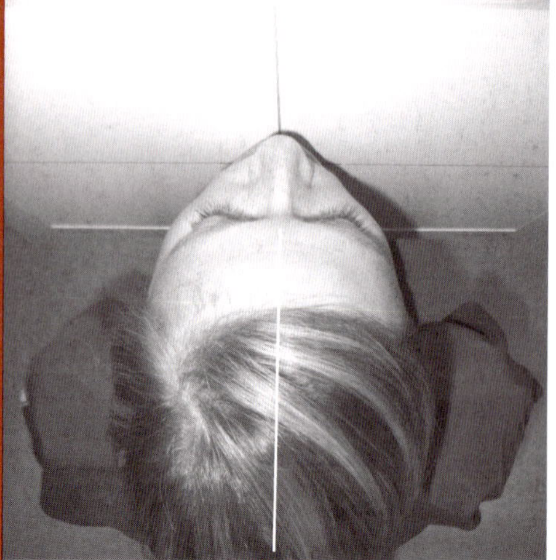

Courtesy of Quinn B. Carroll

FIGURE 5-6

Only from a true axial viewpoint can you evaluate the Waters position for head rotation and side-to-side centering.

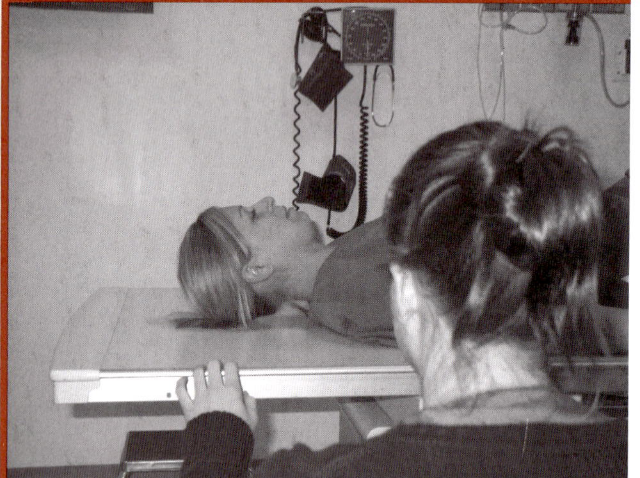

Courtesy of Quinn B. Carroll

FIGURE 5-7

In order to see skull positioning lines properly, you must kneel, squat, or bend to place your own viewpoint at the same vertical level as the patient.

cylinder or "cone" from the x-ray tube or move the tube back temporarily (while center-locked). This allows the radiographer to properly sight down over the patient's head as shown in Figure 5-6. *Only* from this viewpoint can the radiographer accurately evaluate the Waters position for rotation and for side-to-side centering.

3. **View positioning planes and lines from the same vertical level that the patient or anatomy is on.**

This is a direct outgrowth of Rule #2, because it is absolutely necessary in order to see any plane from a true end-on viewpoint. When evaluating a patient who is lying on the x-ray table for rotation, tilt, flexion/extension, or other body movements, the radiographer must *squat, kneel, bend over,* or *sit on a stool* as needed in order to observe the anatomy at the patient's level (Figure 5-7). When the patient is standing at the chest board for a cervical spine or sinus projection, a shorter radiographer may need to use a stool while centering the beam in order to see the top of the image receptor, the central ray, and related anatomical landmarks *from a level viewpoint*. When the patient is

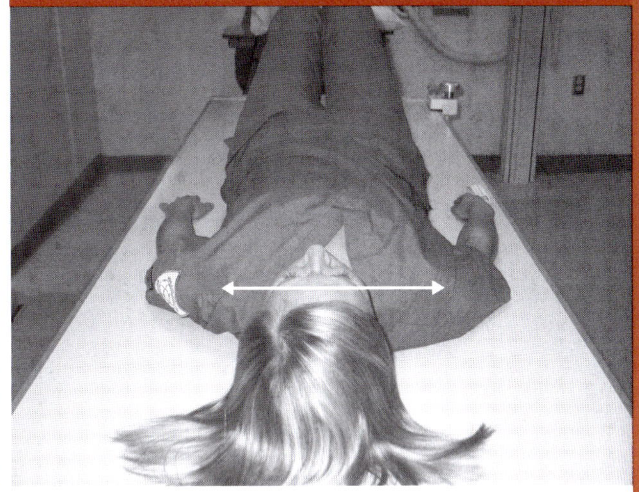
Courtesy of Quinn B. Carroll

FIGURE 5-8

You can properly see side-to-side centering only from the head of the table.

seated at the chest board, you will often need to squat, kneel, or bend over to see positioning lines at the level of the patient's head or neck.

4. **At least two different viewpoints, perpendicular to each other, are required in order to properly evaluate all positioning planes necessary for a position.**

As described under Rule #2, rotation can only be properly seen from an *axial* viewpoint; tilt, abduction, and adduction from a *frontal* viewpoint; and flexion/extension from a *lateral* viewpoint. *All* radiographic positions require at least *two* of these criteria to be evaluated. This is done not only for the part position, but also for centering: Side-to-side centering can be properly evaluated only from the head or foot of the table (Figure 5-8). Superior-to-inferior centering can be properly seen only from the side of the table (Figure 5-7). When one performs an entire position from the side of the table, one can only make a rough estimate of side-to-side centering or part rotation. A good rule to adopt is that, *for every position, it will be necessary at some point to go to the head of the table.* When performing skull or sinus positions at the chest board, it will always be necessary at some point to look down over the patient's head from above.

The small investment of time and effort required to stay cognizant of these four rules and apply them in daily practice will pay big dividends. When performing mobile and trauma positions, it is to the benefit of both the patient and radiographer to "get it right the first time." A key to avoiding many repeats is to remain mindful of the importance of the *position of the positioner*.

ADAPTING CENTERING FOR CHANGES IN PART POSITION

Almost every radiographic body position can be achieved using beam angles and working around the patient in the place of part rotation, tilt, flexion, or extension. This is the essence of the trauma positioning skills discussed in Chapter 7. We can surmise, then, that the rule presented in Chapter 2 for recentering the x-ray beam to compensate for various beam angles would also work for various degrees of rotation, tilt, and so forth. This is true for the average body habitus in the torso, and for the head. We might restate this "shift rule" as:

> In torso or head positioning, for every 10° of rotation, tilt, flexion, or extension, adjust the centering of the CR by 1 inch. Shift the centering towards the *upside*.
>
> Restated, for every 5° of rotation, and so on, shift the CR centering by ½ inch.

Practical Application Examples for Rotation

CASE STUDY

Case Study #1: AP Oblique for IVP

Full abdominal survey views are being taken during an IVP series using 14-inch × 17-inch (35-cm × 43-cm) cassettes. The patient is supine and rotated 25° into a left posterior oblique (left AP oblique) position. Assuming the patient is of average thickness (20–24 cm), how far *upside* from the midline should you center the field?

ANSWER: *Using the preceding rule of thumb, the lengthwise crosshair in the light field should fall about 2½ inches upside from the midline of the patient's stomach. (Palpation of the xiphoid process is recommended when there is any question as to where the midline lies.) As illustrated in Figure 5-9, this 2½-inch upside shift will project the central ray to exit right out the spine posteriorly, close to the midline between the two kidneys (which lie posterior in the body.)*

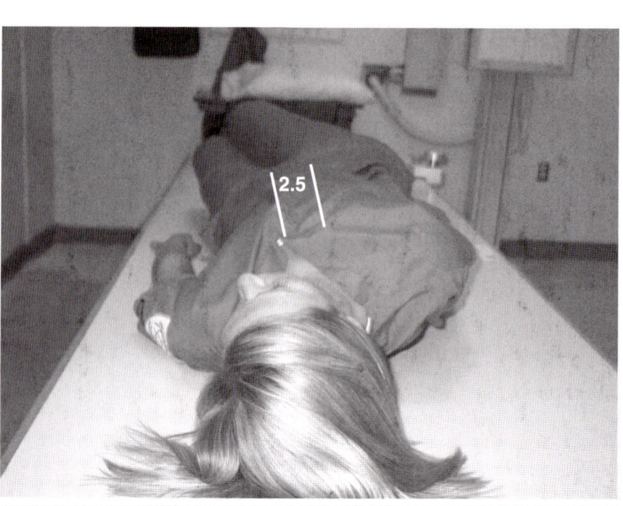

FIGURE 5-9

Using the *1-inch for every 10°* rule for an average patient, a 25° oblique for an IVP requires recentering the x-ray beam 2½ inches upside from the patient's midline.

Courtesy of Quinn B. Carroll

CASE STUDY

Case Study #2: Laws Projection for TMJ

A tightly collimated field is used to obtain a Law's view of the right TMJ. The patient's face is rotated downward toward the tabletop 15°, and the x-ray tube is angled 15° caudally. From the easily visible upside TMJ (just anterior to the tragus of the ear), what centering point will compensate for both the CR angle and the head rotation in this projection?

ANSWER: *From the upside TMJ, center the crosshairs of the light field 1½ inches superior, and then also 1½ inches posterior to this upside TMJ (Figure 5-10). This will place it just at the upper back "corner" of the ear. This centering will project the downside TMJ right in the middle of a tightly collimated field (Figure 5-11).*

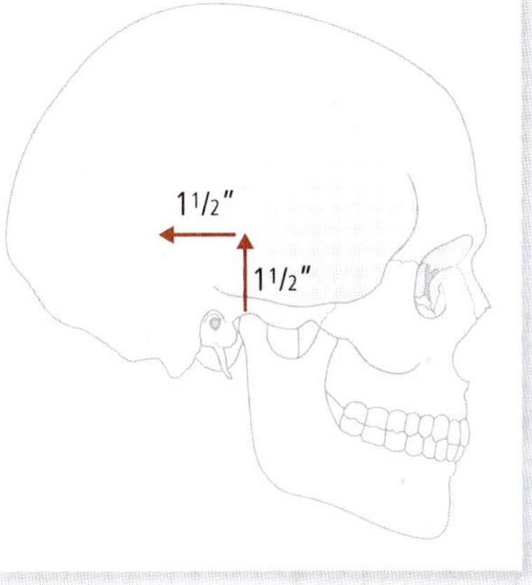

FIGURE 5-10

Using the *1-inch for every 10°* rule, the Laws projection for the TMJ (or mastoids), that employs a 15° caudal angle and 15° of head rotation, requires centering of the CR 1½ inches superior and 1½ inches posterior to the upside TMJ. See Figure 5-11.

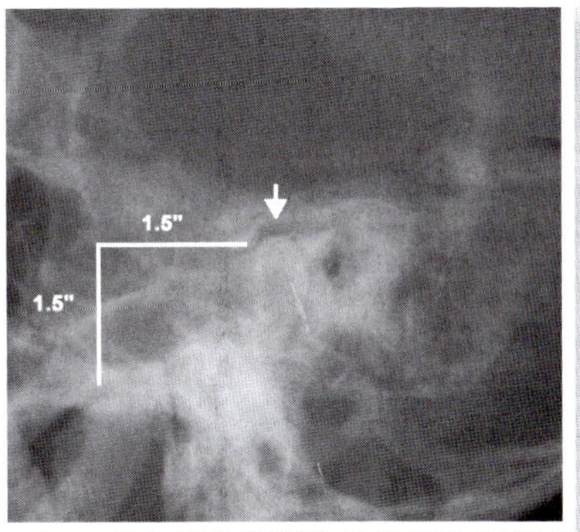

FIGURE 5-11

A radiograph of the TMJ using the *1-inch for every 10°* rule as diagramed in Figure 5-10 places the downside TMJ of interest right in the center of the collimated field (arrow). Note that the view of the magnified upside TMJ also follows the rule: It is projected 1½ inches anterior and 1½ inches inferior to the centered downside TMJ.

Carroll, Q. Evaluating Radiographs, 1993, Figure 199, Courtesy of Charles C Thomas, Publisher, Ltd., Springfield, Illinois.

ADJUSTING FOR PATIENT SIZE

A corollary rule is easily established to adjust the shift rule when dealing with very large patients: *From the average 22-centimeter torso thickness in AP, for every additional 5 centimeters of body thickness, add 1 inch to the centering shift rule.* Experimentation demonstrates a reliable

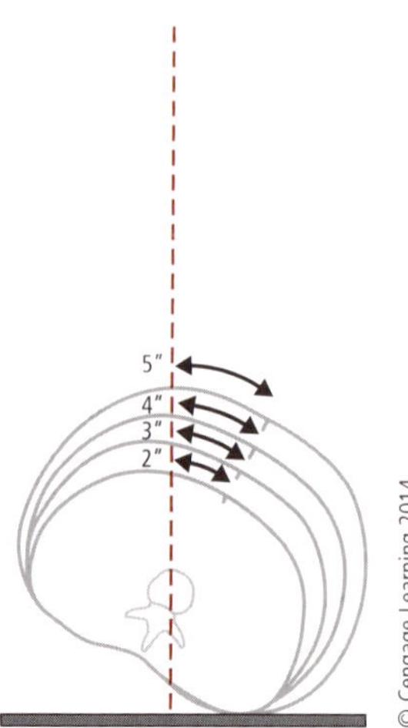

FIGURE 5-12

Experimentation establishes a reliable progression of adjustments to the shift rule for increasing patient thicknesses: For every added 5 centimeters of torso thickness, recenter 1 additional inch farther upside.

progression of adjustments to the rule for increasing thicknesses in the torso, shown in Figure 5-12. This can be accurately rounded for both British and metric units as follows:

British Rule

From the average 22-centimeter torso thickness in AP, for every additional 5 centimeters of body thickness, add 1 inch to the centering shift rule of thumb.

Metric Rule

From the average 22-centimeter torso thickness in AP, for every additional 4 centimeters of body thickness, add 2 centimeters to the centering shift rule of thumb.

BEST PRACTICE TIP

British Rule

From the average 22-centimeter torso thickness in AP, for every additional 5 centimeters of body thickness, add 1 inch to the centering shift rule of thumb.

Metric Rule

From the average 22-centimeter torso thickness in AP, for every additional 4 centimeters of body thickness, add 2 centimeters to the centering shift rule of thumb.

Practical Application Examples of Adjusting the Rule for Patient Size

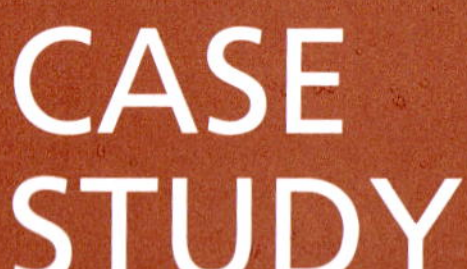

Case Study #3: AP Oblique for IVP on a Large Patient

Full abdominal survey views are being taken during an IVP series using 14-inch × 17-inch (35-cm × 43-cm) cassettes. The supine patient is rotated 30° into a right posterior oblique (right AP oblique) position. Using the shift rule of thumb for an average patient, the lengthwise crosshair in the light field would normally fall about 3 inches upside from the midline of the patient's stomach. This large patient, however, measures 32 centimeters in AP. This is 10 centimeters thicker than average. Which way, and by how much, should you recenter the CR to compensate for this patient's size?

ANSWER: *As illustrated in Figure 5-13, you should add about 2 inches to the upside shift (1 inch for every 5 cm). This places the*

CASE STUDY

adjusted central ray 5 inches upside from the midline (xiphoid process). This should project the central ray to exit close to the spine posteriorly. ■

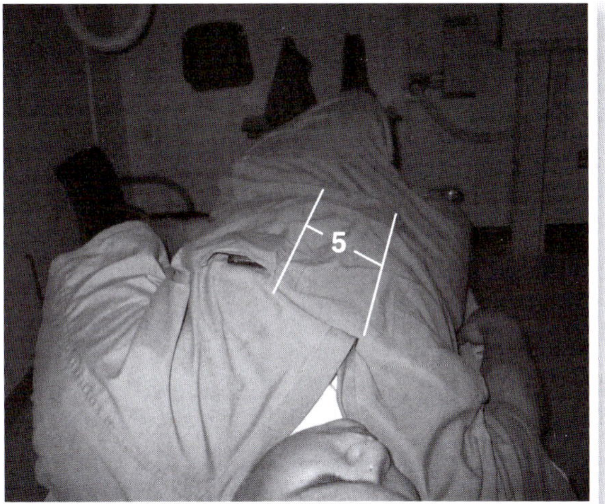

FIGURE 5-13
Application of the shift adjustment rule illustrated in Figure 5-12. This large patient is 32 centimeters thick in the torso, 10 centimeters thicker than average. Add 2 inches (1 inch for every 5 cm) to the normal 3" upside centering for a 30° oblique. This results in a total upside shift of 5 inches from the midline to the CR for this patient.

Courtesy of Quinn B. Carroll

NOTE FOR OBESE PATIENTS: Beware of using soft-tissue landmarks, such as the navel, to localize the abdominal surface midline, particularly on hypersthenic patients. When an obese patient is rolled up into an oblique position, the soft tissue of the belly will fall sideways, shifting toward the downside. The navel will not be a reliable landmark. As discussed in Chapter 1, bony landmarks are always more reliable. In this case, the xiphoid process is recommended.

Why Not Just Use Downside Exit Points?

In some positions, the radiographer can see downside landmarks, and there is clearly no need for the rules for shift in this chapter. A good example is the Rhese position for the orbital or optical foramen: When this position is done correctly with the acanthiomeatal line perpendicular to the tabletop, and the chin and nose is in contact with the table, the forehead will be raised off of the table about ½ inch. One can squat at the head of the table and sight down from above the patient's head, and clearly see the downside eyebrow. The x-ray beam is simply centered to *exit* the midpoint of the downside eyebrow.

In most positions, however, such downside centering landmarks cannot be clearly seen, so their locations can only be estimated by palpation without actually seeing them, or by trying to visualize them from the observed upside anatomy. In all of these cases, the rules presented in this chapter will prove to be helpful.

Practical Application Example for Flexion/Extension

CASE STUDY

Case Study #4: AP Apical Lordotic Chest

Intentionally using a lordotic position to specifically demonstrate the apices of both lungs, the radiographer positions the patient upright at the chest board, but in AP position and leaning back into the board at about 20°. Normally on a routine AP chest, the radiographer would center the 14-inch × 17-inch field at a midsternum point halfway between the sternal notch and the xiphoid tip. Based on the degree at which the patient is leaning back, which way and by how much should you recenter the CR from this point?

ANSWER: *From this point, for the 20° lordotic position the centering point will lie 2 inches lower.* ■

VALUE OF SECTIONAL ANATOMY TRAINING FOR ROUTINE CENTERING

If a radiographer were able to perfectly visualize the internal organs of the body in relation to each other, and the way that different anatomy shifts when the body is rotated or otherwise moved, centering landmarks and rules of thumb for adjusting them would all be unnecessary. Since none of us can be perfect in this respect, especially taking into consideration all of the different types of body habitus, then surface landmarks and adaptive rules of thumb become essential to minimizing repeated exposures.

Even with these helpful aids to positioning, one just cannot avoid the necessity to develop at least a moderate ability to visualize these anatomical relationships from a cross sectional frame of reference. A great example is found in radiography of the urinary system, when comparing oblique positions for the kidneys to oblique positions for the urinary bladder, as discussed in the next section.

When centering for an oblique projection for the kidneys, which lie posteriorly within the abdomen, the rule of shift for recentering the central ray toward the upside must be followed, as was shown in Figure 5-9. However, this rule of thumb will *not* apply for the oblique projection of the bladder. This is because the bladder lies *anteriorly* within the pelvis, just behind the pubic bone, and so it shifts *with* the anterior surface toward the patient's right when rotating the torso to the right, as shown in Figure 5-14. Note that the central ray must still be shifted toward the upside, only not as far. For a 45° obliquity of the body, the rule would normally place the central ray 4½ inches upside. But, as shown in Figure 5-14, since the bladder lies anterior, the correct side-to-side centering point is shifted to the upside by only about 2 inches from the surface midline.

The "1-inch for every 10°" rule of thumb applies only to "deep" anatomy, that is, anatomy in the midline or toward the downside of the body. For organs close to the upside surface, shift the centering upside less than usual, depending on how deep the organ of interest lies, when the body is rotated.

Always assess side-to-side centering by going to the head-end of the x-ray table and sighting down the body from above. With an ability to visualize the anatomy in cross section from this viewpoint, accuracy in positioning is achieved.

Figure 5-14 shows the cross sectional relationships of the urinary anatomy from the head-end of the table or "from the head down." Figure 5-15 and Figure 5-16 show the gastrointestinal organs in cross section from this viewpoint. These diagrams are unique in that they show the *entire* organs and related systems, all of which must be included on projections taken for UGI and LGI series. (An actual cross-sectional image only includes portions of this anatomy within the "slice" taken.) A great exercise is to try to resketch these diagrams by memory. If you can do so, you have developed the ability to visualize the anatomy and greatly enhance your positioning skills. These diagrams are also used in Chapter 10.

BEST PRACTICE TIP

The "1-inch for every 10°" rule of thumb applies only to "deep" anatomy, that is, anatomy in the midline or toward the downside of the body. For organs close to the upside surface, shift the centering upside less than usual, depending on how deep the organ of interest lies, when the body is rotated.

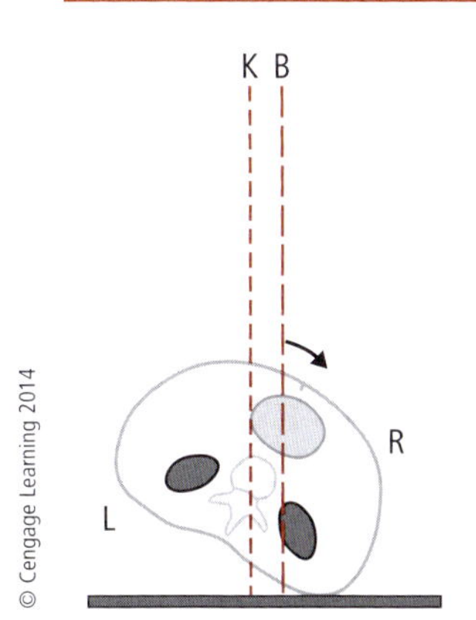

FIGURE 5-14

The bladder does not follow the shift rule because it lies so anterior in the body. Upside shift for the bladder is only about 2 inches B. The shift rule is useful, however, for all midtorso and posterior anatomy, such as the kidneys K.

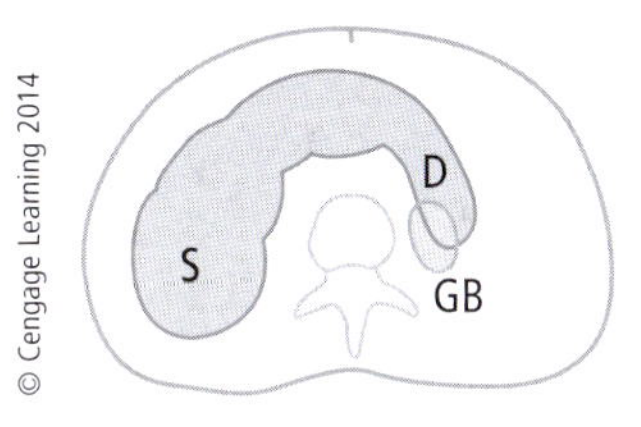

FIGURE 5-15

Cross-sectional diagram of UGI anatomy and gallbladder. The ability to visualize this diagram, while sighting down from the head of the table, greatly aids side-to-side centering.

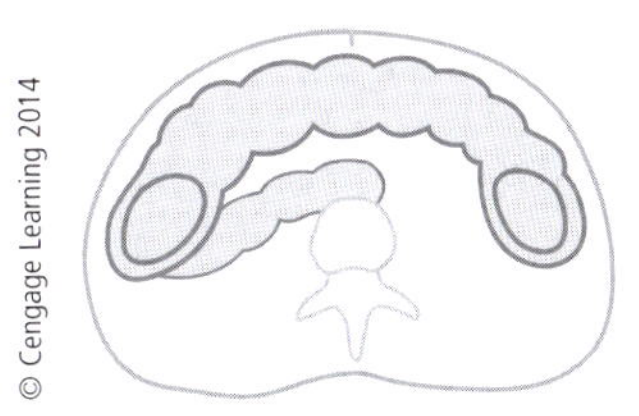

FIGURE 5-16

Cross-sectional diagram of LGI anatomy. The ability to visualize this diagram, while sighting down from the head of the table, greatly aids side-to-side centering.

SUMMARY

1. Always identify two points to define a positioning line.
2. To properly evaluate a position, the radiographer's viewpoint must be square and centered to the patient. The radiographer must see all planes and lines *end-on* and from a *straight* viewpoint.
3. The radiographer must view positioning lines and planes at the same *vertical level* that the patient or anatomy is on.
4. At least two different viewpoints, perpendicular to each other, are required in order to properly evaluate all positioning planes necessary for a position.
5. In torso and head positioning, for every 10° of average body part obliquity, tilt, flexion, or extension, the radiographer must adjust CR centering by 1 inch. (For every 5°, shift the centering by ½ inch.) Shift the centering towards the *upside*.
6. For large patients, for every additional 5 centimeters of body thickness beyond average, add 1 inch to the centering shift rule of thumb.
7. Shift the CR upside less for organs that lie more anterior.
8. Learning to visualize organs from a cross-sectional viewpoint is most helpful in centering.

CRITICAL THINKING CHALLENGE 5.1

BUILDING UP AN AP ODONTOID VIEW

A student is performing a "coned" AP projection for the odontoid. The first attempt came out with the occipital bone superimposing the odontoid process, and the student asks a radiographer for help in determining the correct adjustment in positioning or CR angle for the repeated exposure. The radiographer states, "Just build the patient's head up on a sponge and angle the CR 5° cephalic. It always works for me."

What are the flaws in this approach, if any? Is an additional repeated exposure likely? Is there a way to make the proper correction that is simpler, quicker, and easier on the patient?

REVERSED LATERAL "SPOT" VIEW OF L5–S1

CRITICAL THINKING CHALLENGE 5.2

A radiographer is performing a "spot" lateral projection of the L5–S1 joint space with the patient lying on his left side. The first attempt, taken with a vertical CR, came out with the joint space closed, and a repeated view using a 5° caudal angle only came out worse. A colleague offers the following advice: "Stand the patient up at the chest board, still use the 5° caudal angle, and just turn the patient around and do a right lateral instead of a left lateral projection."

Will this approach improve the view of L5–S1? Is there another way of achieving the same type of correction without as much trouble for the patient? Point out any flaws in this approach that might result in further repeated exposures.

DETERMINING THE ANGLE FOR A LATERAL "SPOT" VIEW OF L5–S1

CRITICAL THINKING CHALLENGE 5.3

A student is performing a "spot" lateral projection of the L5–S1 joint space. The first attempt came out with the joint space closed, and a radiographer is trying to help a student determine the correct CR angle for the repeated exposure. The radiographer prints a hard copy of the AP view of the lumbar spine for this particular patient, and carefully draws two lines, one across the two iliac crests, and one across the top of the L5 vertebral body. He then measures the angle formed between these two lines to determine the degree of "tilt" of L5 relative to the pelvis. He instructs the student to angle caudally by this amount for the "spot" lateral projection.

Is this an appropriate method to determine the CR angle for the "spot" lateral projection of L5–S1? If not, what are the flaws in this approach?

(Answers to Critical Thinking Challenges are found in the Appendix.)

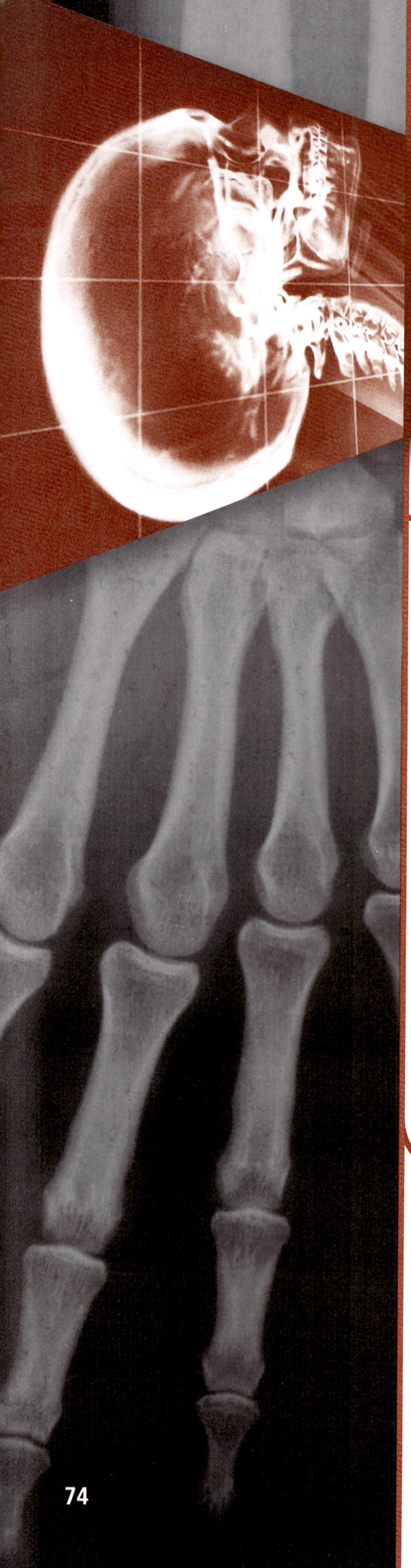

CHAPTER 6

Adapting Positions to Digital Equipment

OUTLINE

OBJECTIVES

Upon completion of this chapter, you should be able to:

1. Give examples of procedures that might be performed without a grid on modern digital radiography (DR) units.
2. Describe the general kinds of mobile (portable) unit DR detectors and how to handle them safely during mobile procedures.

Continues

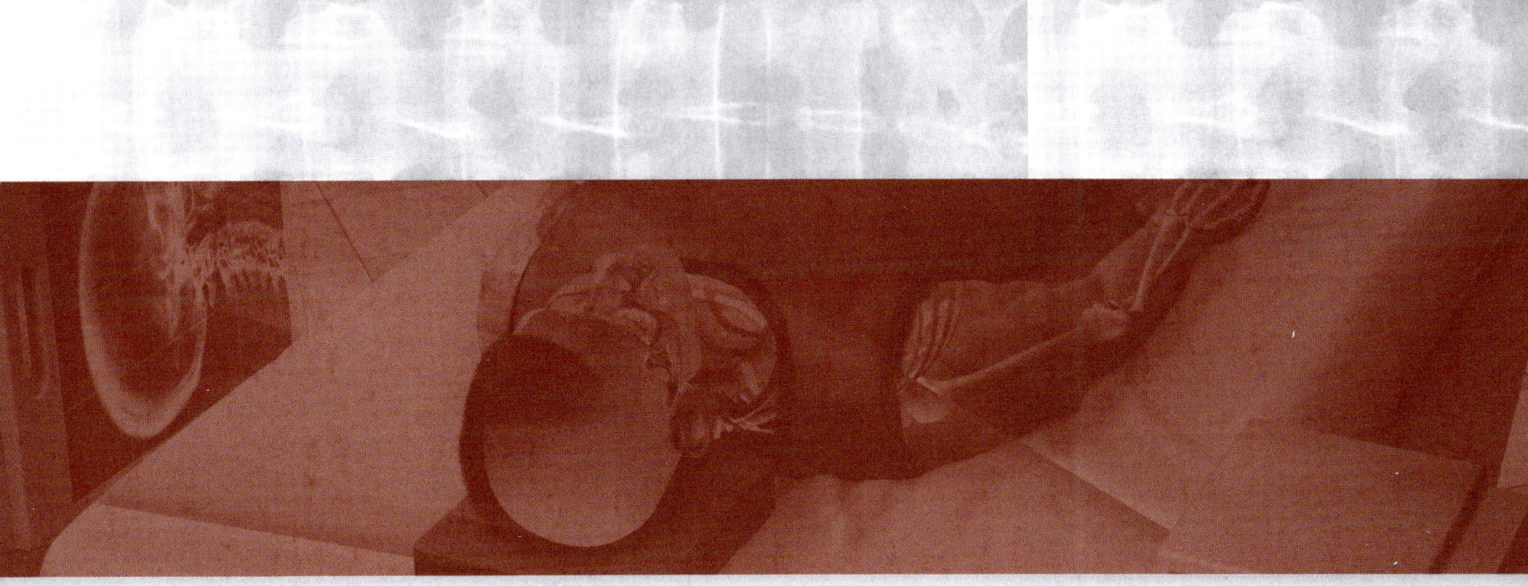

OBJECTIVES *continued*

3. Describe how a horizontally placed upright DR detector can be used to obtain AP and oblique projections of the skull, facial bones, and cervical spine with minimal movement for a trauma patient.
4. Explain the value of specific types of filters for digital imaging in axiolateral projections of the hip and cervicothoracic spine.
5. Describe modified projections of the axiolateral hip, wheelchair "sunrise" knee, and transaxillary shoulder for a built-in DR detector.
6. Describe a modified projection for the AP chest on a gurney using the upright Bucky detector.

INTRODUCTION

Computed radiography (CR) units allow all of the flexibility and portability of the older film/screen systems, because the CR cassette can be carried anywhere in the room and can be placed tabletop or in the gridded Bucky tray. Newer digital radiography (DR) systems use a cordless DR detector that can also be removed from its clamps in the table Bucky so that it can be used tabletop (Figure 6-1). These cordless detectors use radio waves to transmit their data to the display system. Manufacturers have significantly reduced the weight and thickness of these detectors with newer units, but they are still often more cumbersome and awkward to use than CR cassettes. You must take great care handling DR detectors because they are extremely expensive, and you must not drop them.

Many DR detectors are still thicker than CR cassettes (Figure 6-1***B***). This presents additional positioning problems such as the degree to which a backboard must be moved to slide the detector under it during a trauma series, which we will discuss later in this chapter.

Manufacturers are designing DR units so that different grids equipped with handles can be easily switched in and out of the "Bucky" unit or detector panel, as shown in Figure 6-2. A very important point

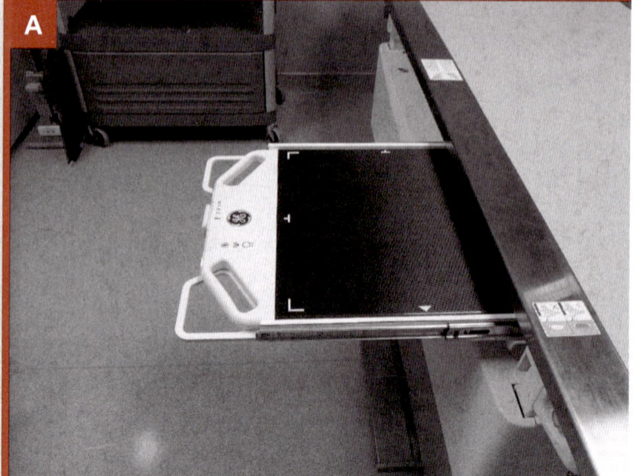

Courtesy of Quinn B. Carroll

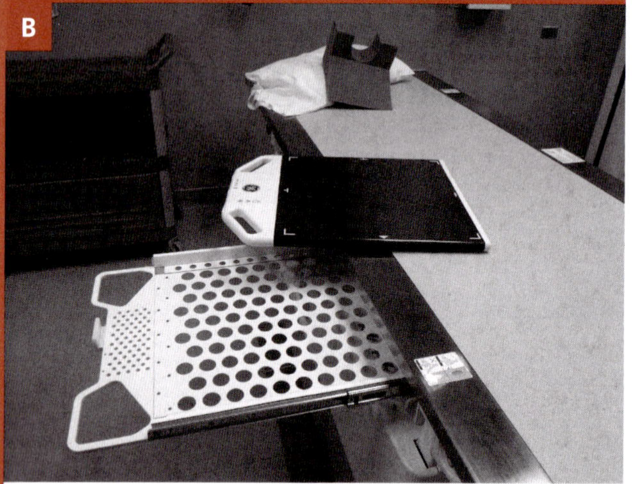

Courtesy of Quinn B. Carroll

FIGURE 6-1

This GE unit features a lightweight cordless DR detector in the Bucky tray **A**, that can be removed for tabletop work, **B**. Image data is sent to the display unit by radio waves.

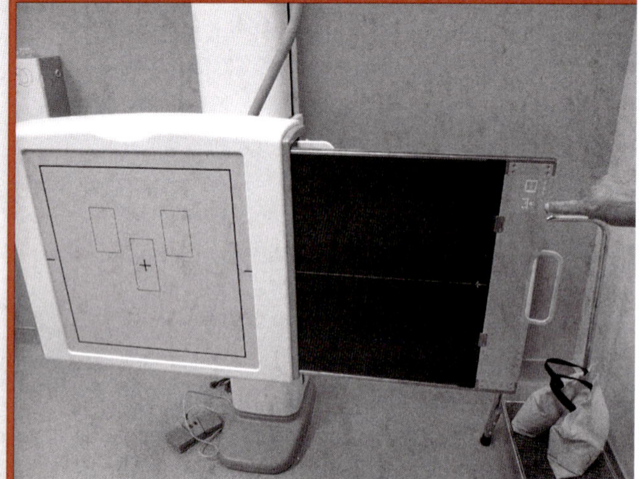

Courtesy of Quinn B. Carroll

FIGURE 6-2

Grids designed for different distances are equipped with handles for easy removal from the Bucky.

to remember in trauma and other adaptive situations is that by *removing the grid* in the DR detector entirely, you can achieve several angled positions. Modern DR and CR systems are generally very capable of correcting for the effects of moderate amounts of scatter radiation during the exposure and for the use of high kVp levels.

As described more fully in the next chapter, there is a number of body parts that are conventionally imaged with a grid, but in fact can be done *nongrid* with only minimal production of scatter radiation, especially on average or smaller-than-average patients. These include all skull, facial bone, and sinus work; the cervical spine; the shoulders; and the knees. Chests can also generally be done nongrid, as well as the thoracic spine (with the exception of the swimmers projection). By removing the grid from the DR detector, many projections using beam angles in any direction, including double angles can be achieved. When removing the grid, the general rule is to reduce the technique to about one-third of the usual grid technique for any particular anatomy.

PORTABLE DR DETECTORS

There are several different styles of portable DR detectors on the market. Some of them have the power/information cord attached, while the newer versions are cord-free. The substantial weight of all of these detectors makes them more cumbersome and hazardous to use during mobile radiographic procedures than conventional film cassettes were. For example, the corded Canon detector in Figure 6-3 weighs 10.5 pounds and the accompanying grid weighs an additional 5.4 pounds, for a total of nearly 16 pounds (7.3 kg). The GE detector in Figure 6-3 weighs 14.5 pounds and the grid weighs 3.6 pounds for a total of just over 18 pounds. The Canon detector has the conventional rectangular dimensions of 35 centimeters × 41 centimeters (14 inches × 17 inches), whereas the GE detector is 41 centimeters (16.1 inches) square.

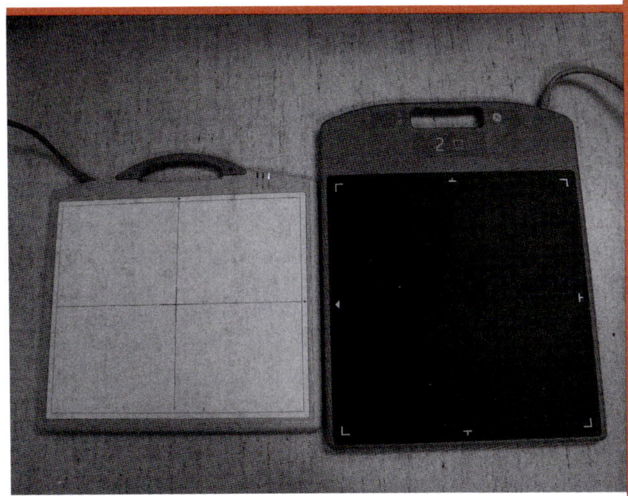

FIGURE 6-3
Corded DR detectors, left: GE; right: Canon.

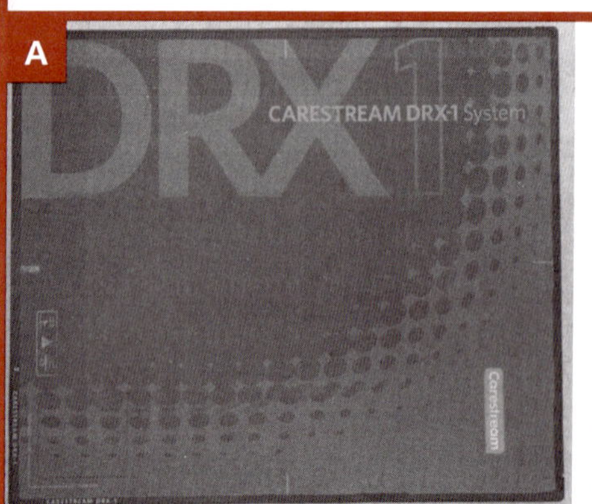

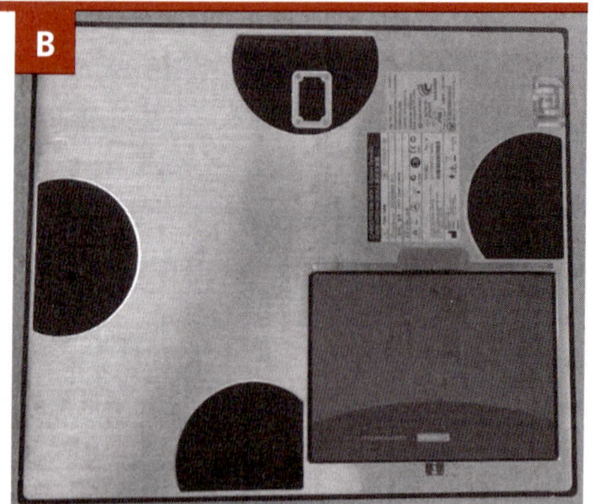

© Dennis Bowman

© Dennis Bowman

FIGURE 6-4
Cordless DR detectors:
A. CareStream, **B**. Canon.

Cordless detectors are available with an ultrathin battery enclosed for power (Figure 6-4). These send their data to the mobile unit by radio. (Many mobile DR units are now also equipped to send their images by radio into the PACS system, allowing quick access for physicians to "portable" radiographs right after they are taken.) All of these cordless detectors weigh around 8 pounds without their grids, and about 13 pounds with the grid. Most of the grids for these systems can also be used with CR cassettes. Not only are these much lighter than the corded versions, in addition to eliminating the added weight of the cord itself, but the awkwardness and safety issues associated with the cord (such as tripping over it or catching it on equipment and furniture) are removed.

Because of the weight of corded detectors, some radiographers resist using them to avoid injury to their shoulders when performing upright AP chests, where poor body mechanics such as reaching far out with the weight are often unavoidable. The safest way to place the detector behind the patient is to *make sure the handle is on the top* and let the detector slide straight down (Figure 6-5A). This allows the radiographer to take advantage of the weight of the detector. It is much more difficult to try to slide the detector from the side, because, with gravity removed from the equation, it takes pure muscle power to push the detector across (Figure 6-5***B***).

ADVANTAGES OF A HORIZONTALLY PLACED UPRIGHT DR DETECTOR

Most of the new "upright Bucky" detectors developed for DR units allow for the entire detector panel to be rotated down into a *horizontal* position, effectively creating a smaller "table" that can be positioned at nearly unlimited levels, well above or well below the vertical range of the standard x-ray table (Figure 6-6). This allows the radiographer to achieve a number of innovative positions. With the upright detector horizontal and raised to level higher than the x-ray table, patients in

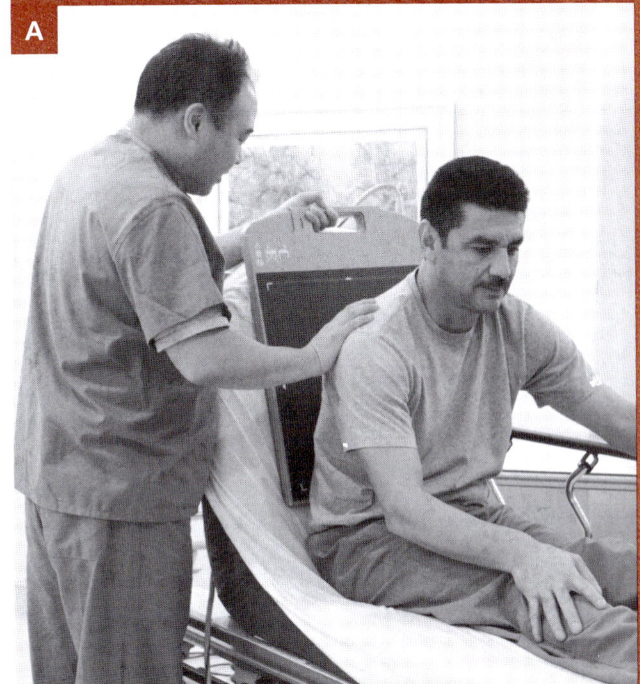
A

© Dennis Bowman

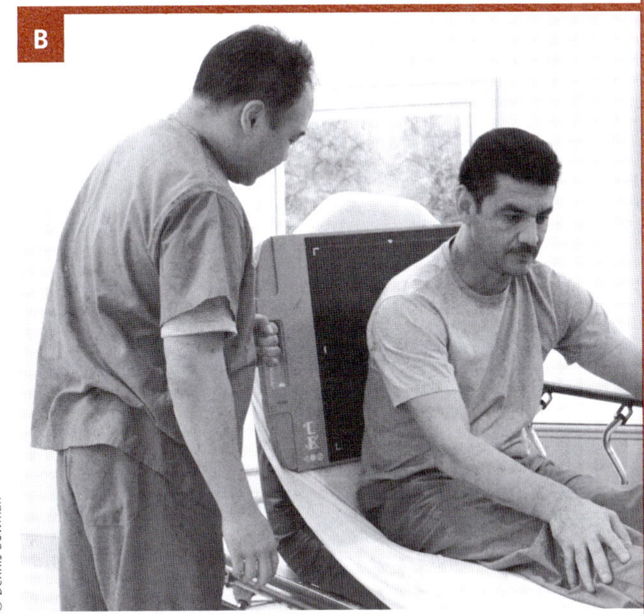
B

© Dennis Bowman

FIGURE 6-5
For mobile procedures, it is both safer and easier to place heavy DR detectors behind the patient by sliding them down from above, with the handle up **A**, rather than sliding them in from the side **B**.

wheelchairs can easily place their arm onto the detector for hand, wrist, forearm, or elbow series without needing to get out of the wheelchair. With the horizontal detector lowered as shown in Figure 6-6, a patient in a wheelchair can have her ankle imaged without getting out of the wheelchair.

Trauma AP and oblique projections for the skull, facial bones, and cervical spine can also be achieved *with minimal patient movement* as described in the following section.

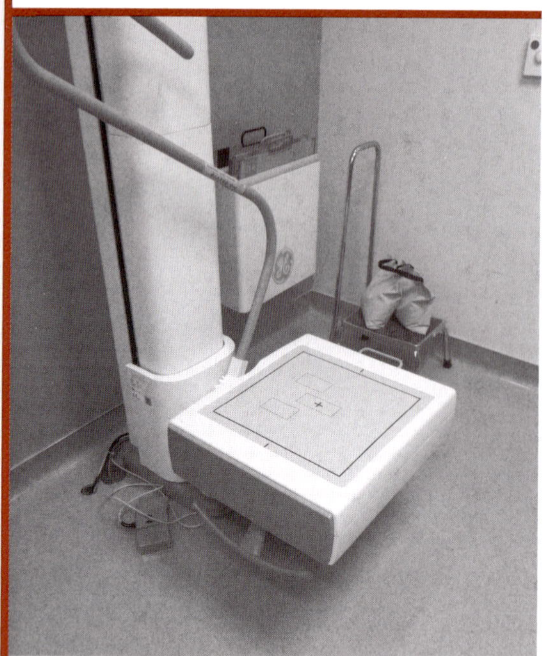

Courtesy of Quinn B. Carroll

FIGURE 6-6

Most upright DR detectors can be rotated down into a horizontal position, and vertically moved through a wide range of levels. This allows for a number of innovative positions to be achieved. Here, the detector is low enough to position an ankle with the patient still in a wheelchair.

TRAUMA PROJECTIONS FOR SKULL, FACIAL BONES, AND CERVICAL SPINE

Note that when a trauma patient is brought in on a stretcher (gurney) and supported by a backboard, *a horizontally positioned upright DR detector can be raised to precisely match the height of the gurney, such that the trauma backboard can be slid off the head of the gurney directly onto the DR detector with no significant movement of the patient* (Figure 6-7).

With CR (or the older film/screen) cassettes, in order to slide a cassette up under the supine trauma patient for AP projections of the skull and C-spine, some slight movement of the backboard (and thus the patient's neck) was not uncommon, even though the gurney pad could be compressed as the cassette was slid in. DR detectors can be an inch or more in thickness, and are often thicker than CR cassettes or film/screen cassettes, (Figures 6-1***B*** and 6-4). This makes it nearly impossible to slide the DR detector up under a backboard without lifting the backboard up and moving the patient's neck.

With the upright DR "Bucky" placed into horizontal position, the DR detector can sustain a limited amount of weight, certainly enough to support the patient's head and neck. With the detector at the correct level, the backboard can be slid right up off of the gurney *without any vertical movement*. As will be demonstrated, this allows several positions to be achieved *without any lifting of the backboard at all*. This is ideal and is strongly recommended over the older practice of sliding cassettes or detectors up under the backboard.

Figure 6-7 shows a patient on a backboard carefully slid from the stretcher into position over the horizontal DR detector for an AP projection of the skull or facial bones. The positions for AP projections of

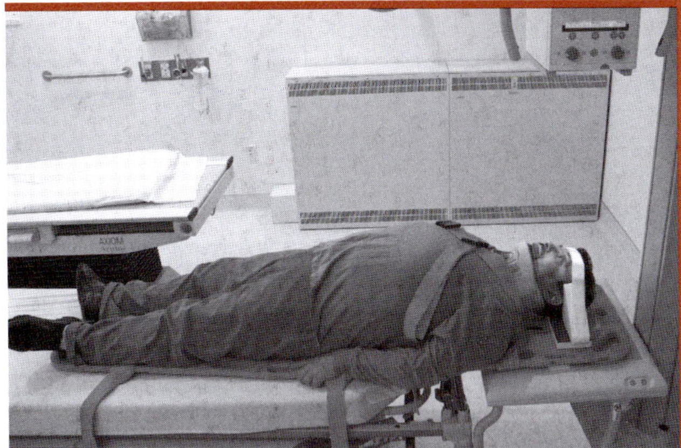

FIGURE 6-7

Trauma patient positioned for an AP projection of the skull with minimal movement of the patient, by sliding the head-end of the backboard over a horizontally placed upright DR detector carefully positioned at the same level as the backboard.

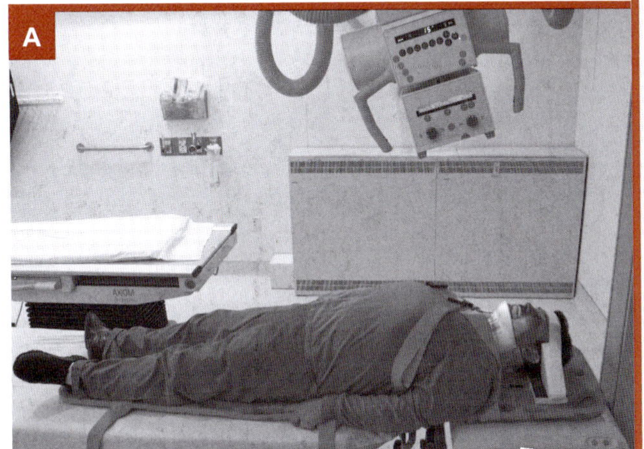

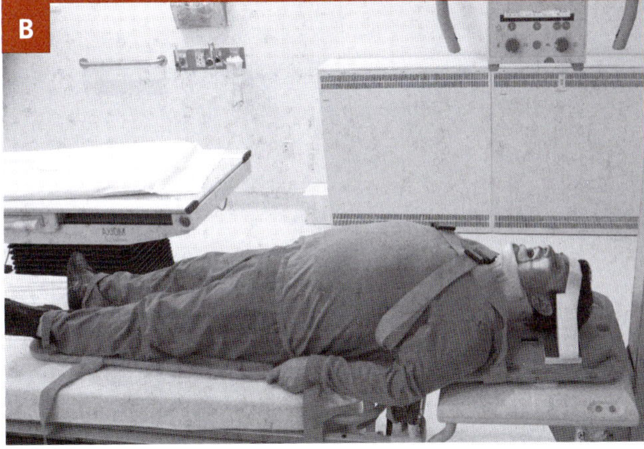

FIGURE 6-8

Trauma patient positioned for **A** an AP projection of the cervical spine, and **B** an odontoid projection, both with minimal movement of the patient, by sliding the head-end of the backboard over a horizontally placed upright DR detector.

the cervical spine and open-mouth odontoid are shown in Figure 6-8, using the same approach.

An oblique projection of the cervical spine is shown in Figure 6-9, using the horizontally placed upright DR detector. In this particular case, the grid has been removed to allow for a 45° transverse angle to be placed on the x-ray beam. *Note that if there is room, the gurney (stretcher) could be brought in sideways (parallel) to the upright Bucky, along the wall, with the backboard then extended over the horizontally placed*

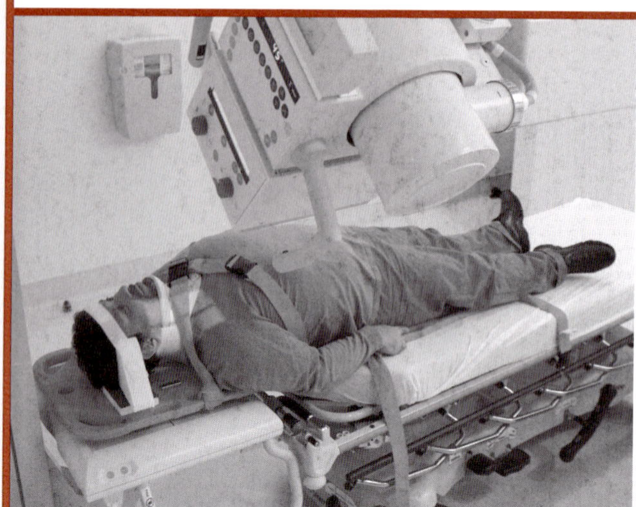

© Dennis Bowman

FIGURE 6-9
Trauma patient positioned for a modified oblique projection of the cervical spine with minimal movement of the patient, by sliding the head-end of the backboard over a horizontally placed upright DR detector. For this projection, the grid must be removed and a transverse angle placed on the x-ray tube.

detector from the side, such that the grid could be left in place and the beam angled 45°along the grid strips. These approaches allow the trauma oblique C-spine projection to be obtained without moving the patient.

All of the AP positions shown in this section (and perhaps other projections as well) can also be obtained with the gurney brought up from the side of the upright Bucky, along the wall—just adapt any tube angles and the position of the gurney accordingly to the orientation of the grid lines to prevent grid cut-off, or remove the grid.

Before using this configuration to support the patient's head on any particular x-ray unit, make a simple test to ensure that the horizontally placed detector can support an equivalent weight—for example, two or three sandbags can be placed on the detector. Never leave a patient unattended with the backboard still slid over the detector and the detector bearing the weight of the patient's head.

ADAPTING LOWER EXTREMITY LONG BONE SERIES FOR FIXED DR EQUIPMENT

With the image receptor built into the table for fixed DR units, for very tall patients it will not be possible to fit the entire leg or femur within the 17-inch length of receptor plate available. It will often be necessary to take two views, upper and lower, for each position in this series. Include about 2 inches past the nearest joint space in each view.

For mobile DR units, you can still arrange the IR plate diagonally, as used to be done with conventional film cassettes, in order to fit larger legs within a single view.

VALUE OF SPECIFIC COMPENSATING FILTERS

Even in the digital environment, there are still a few procedures that are especially difficult to produce with proper contrast and a good balance of brightness (density) across the area of the image. Two of these are the swimmers projection of the cervicothoracic spine and some axiolateral inferosuperior hips (cross-table lateral or Danelius-Miller projection), especially when the contrary thigh cannot be fully abducted out of the way. Due mostly to the large volume of scatter-generating soft tissue through the path of the central ray, the anatomy of interest in these images often present low contrast, even with good collimation. For this reason, special compensating filters are strongly recommended.

The swimmers/lateral hip Ferlic filter (Figure 6-10), works extremely well for both of these projections. This filter compensates for the thickest and thinnest parts of the anatomy so that balanced exposure is achieved across the image. The swimmers/lateral hip filter is an invaluable piece of equipment that every radiology department should have. As demonstrated in the swimmers and hip images in Figures 6-11 and 6-12, the

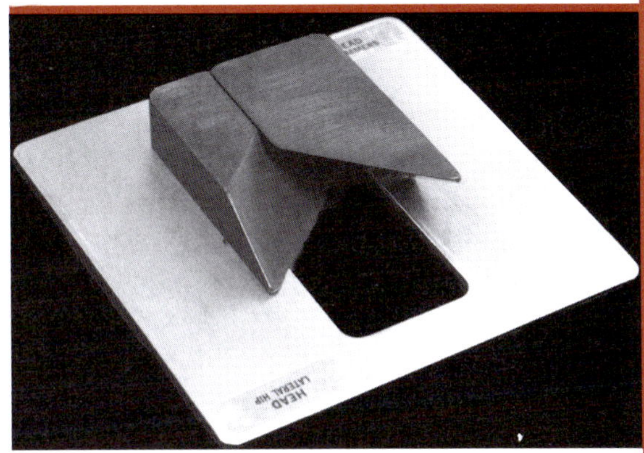

FIGURE 6-10
The Ferlic filter.

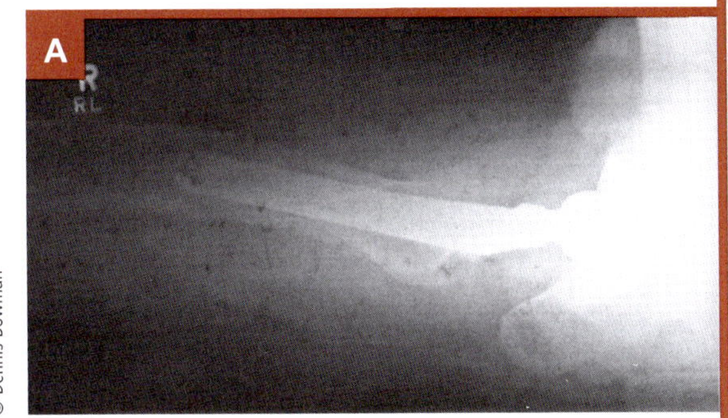

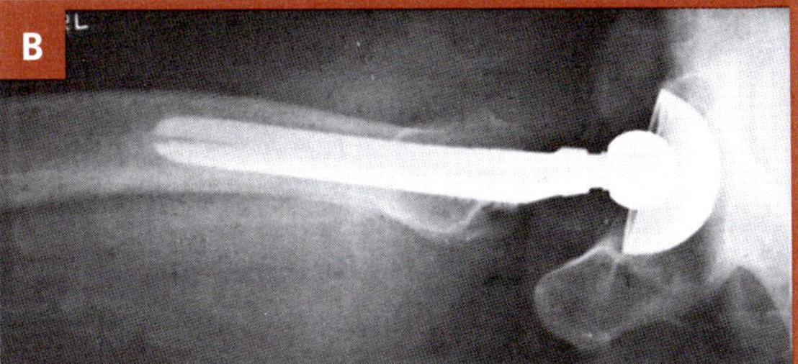

FIGURE 6-11
Cross-table lateral views of the hip in which the contrary thigh was not well abducted out of the way: **A** without using the Ferlic filter and **B** with the Ferlic filter added.

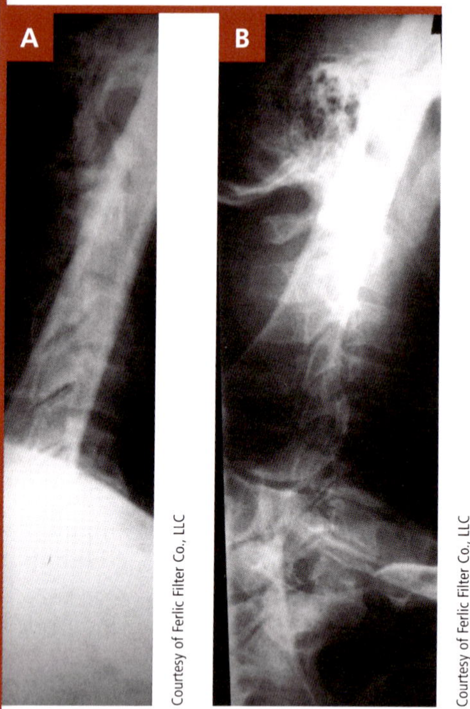

FIGURE 6-12
Swimmers views of the cervicothoracic spine: **A** without using the Ferlic filter and **B** with the Ferlic filter added.

degree of improvement is impressive. (See also Figure 6-14.) This demonstrates how significant the use of a filter can be on some projections using digital imaging.

ACHIEVING SPECIFIC PROJECTIONS WITH FIXED DR UNITS

Axiolateral (Cross-Table Lateral) Hip with Fixed Upright Detector/Tube Linking Armature

DR units that have the x-ray tube and an upright detector fixed in alignment by a linking armature are becoming increasingly common. Such units are shown in Figure 6-13, with a simple table on wheels in between. There is no Bucky tray in the table itself—the only detector is in the upright "Bucky." The x-ray tube can only be moved a limited distance, 6 to 10 inches (15 to 25 cm) in or out from its detente SID. Because of this configuration, it is impossible to get the necessary 45° cephalic angle needed for the axiolateral (cross-table) projection of the hip without creating an excessive OID with attendant magnification. In Figure 6-13, the table is rotated 15°, and another 15° is obtained by rotating the patient into a diagonal position across the table, for a total equivalent angle of 30°. But in this configuration, even with the patient on the edge of the table, the center of the affected hip is already 14 inches from the detector, a substantial OID. If the SID is increased to 60 inches, the table can then be angled another 15° to obtain the

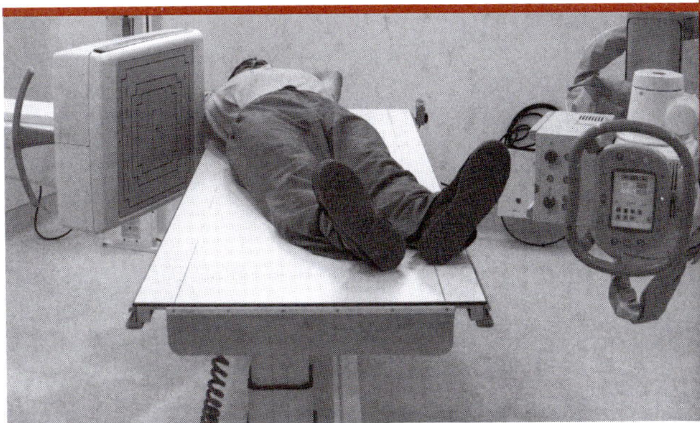

FIGURE 6-13

On this fixed-armature upright unit, with the table rotated on its wheels 15° and the patient rotated another 15°, the OID created for a cross-table hip projection is already at 14 inches.

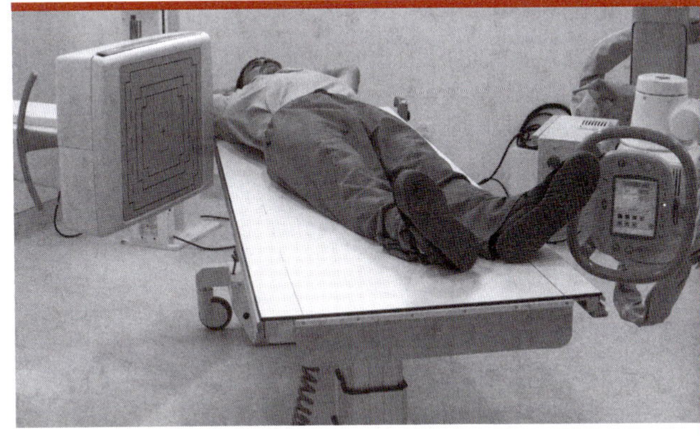

FIGURE 6-14

To obtain a 45° angle for the cross-table hip projection on the fixed-armature upright unit, the OID created is now an unacceptable 20 inches.

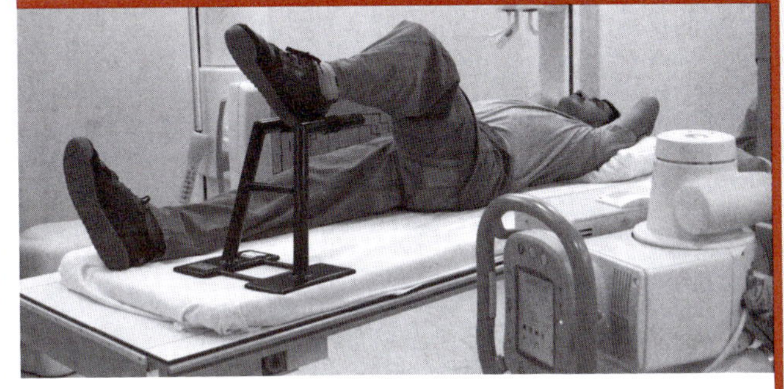

FIGURE 6-15

To obtain a 45° angle for the cross-table hip projection on the fixed-armature upright unit, the x-ray tube must be extended to a SID beyond the reach of the patient's foot. Therefore, an anchor-leg stabilizer is recommended to support the unaffected leg, with use of the Ferlic filter.

correct total of 45°, but the OID for the affected hip is now a completely unacceptable 20 inches (Figure 6-14).

Because a full 45° is not possible, the femoral neck will be foreshortened. The tube is now so far away that it is impossible to place the uninjured foot on the tube. Because of this, the other leg cannot be properly flexed out of the way even if an anchor-leg stabilizer is used (Figure 6-15). This means that the best that can be done is to rotate the table enough that the two femoral heads are not superimposed. The best advice may be to simply avoid using this type of unit for trauma hip series.

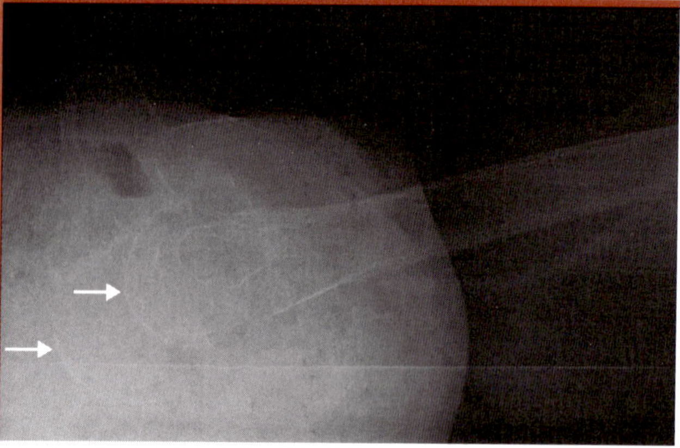

Courtesy of Quinn B. Carroll

FIGURE 6-16

A cross-table hip view taken with the configuration in Figure 6-13 shows insufficient desuperimposition of the femoral heads (arrows), and poor balance of brightness (density) because a Ferlic filter was not used.

When these units are used, there will always be considerable density overlap from the unaffected side, and as discussed in the previous section, a Ferlic filter is indispensable in keeping the distal femur from being overexposed. Figure 6-16 presents an image where the table was not angled enough and the two femoral heads overlap (arrows). It is also apparent that the distal femur is overexposed because a Ferlic filter was not used.

15/15/15 Wheelchair "Sunrise" Knee with Built-in Detector

In a department that only has a built-in DR detector, it may be impossible to perform the "sunrise" axial projection of the knee and patella. If the patient is able to climb up on the table, lie on her stomach, and bend her knees at least 45°, the Hughston method can be used to obtain a good axial patella view. The following adaptation of the "sunrise" projection is for a patient who cannot get out of the wheelchair.

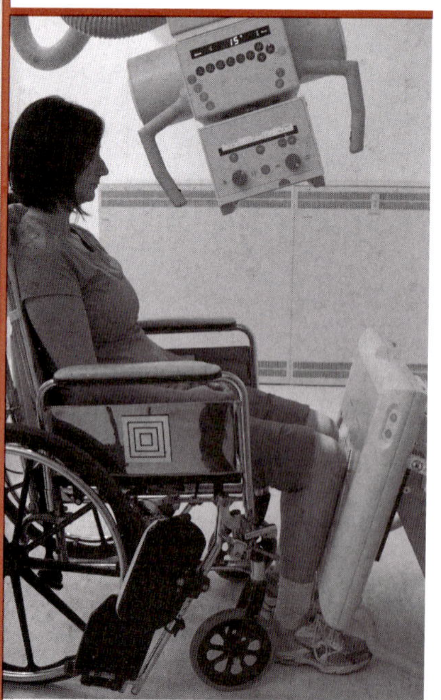

© Dennis Bowman

FIGURE 6-17

The wheelchair "sunrise" projection for bilateral axial patellas, with the IR tilted 15° away from the x-ray tube, the lower legs 15° back to match, and the beam angled 15° distally.

As shown in Figure 6-17, the patient can be wheeled directly up to the IR that has been tilted 15° *away* from the patient. This projection can be done with CR or DR, as long as the system has a *grid that can be removed and the IR can be angled*. The projection employs three different 15° angles: First, angle the top of the IR 15° away from the patient. Then angle the x-ray tube 15° *distally* (toward the patient's knees). Finally, adjust the patient's lower legs parallel with the IR (which means the feet are pulled back so the lower legs are 15° from vertical). Either

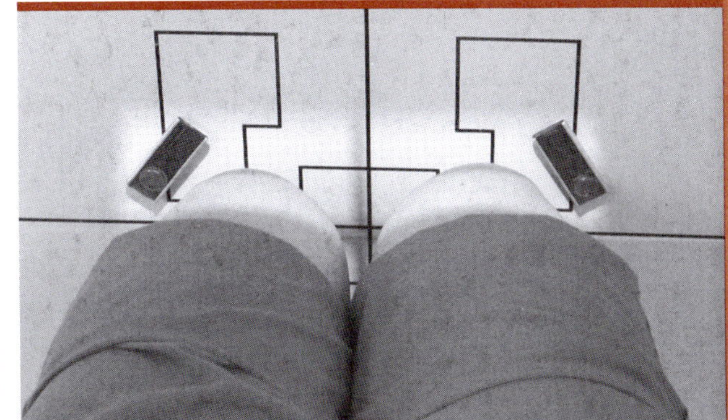
© Dennis Bowman

FIGURE 6-18

Centering for the wheelchair "sunrise" projection, over the bases of the patellas.

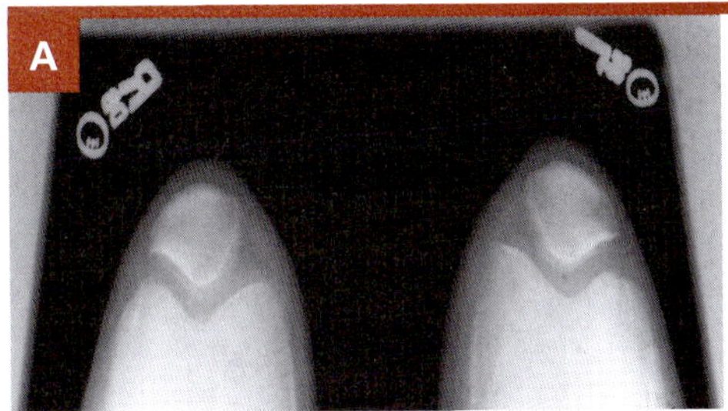
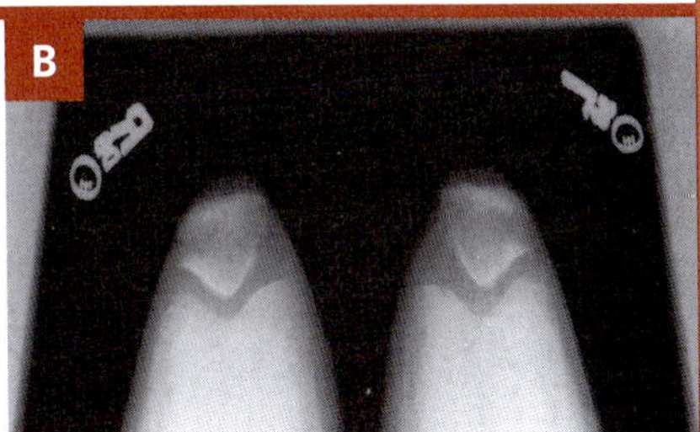

FIGURE 6-19

Two examples of the wheelchair "sunrise" view for bilateral axial patellas.

Courtesy of Community Hospital of the Monterey Peninsula, Diagnostic and Interventional Radiology.

the unilateral patella or a bilateral patella projection as shown in Figure 6-18 can be taken. The CR is centered to the level of the bases of the patellas (Figure 6-18).

Figure 6-19 demonstrates the resulting images of the two different patients: The tibial plateau is demonstrated in profile and the femoropatellar joint space is open. The intercondylar sulcus (trochlear groove) is seen slightly superimposed in Figure 6-19*A* and perfectly in profile in Figure 6-19***B***. There is some elongation distortion of the patella on these images.

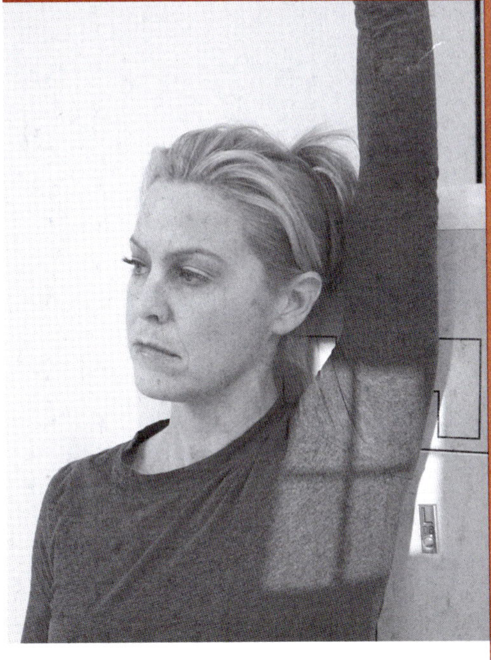
© Dennis Bowman

FIGURE 6-20

For the AP inferosuperior transaxillary shoulder (Walker method), it is best to raise the arm straight up.

AP Inferosuperior Transaxillary Axial Shoulder—Walker Method

In a department that does not have movable or portable detectors, the normal inferosuperior axial (axillary) shoulder may be impossible to perform. This new projection will produce similar results: Start with the patient standing, sitting, or supine. Lift the arm as vertical (straight above the head) as possible (Figure 6-20). It is alright to place the

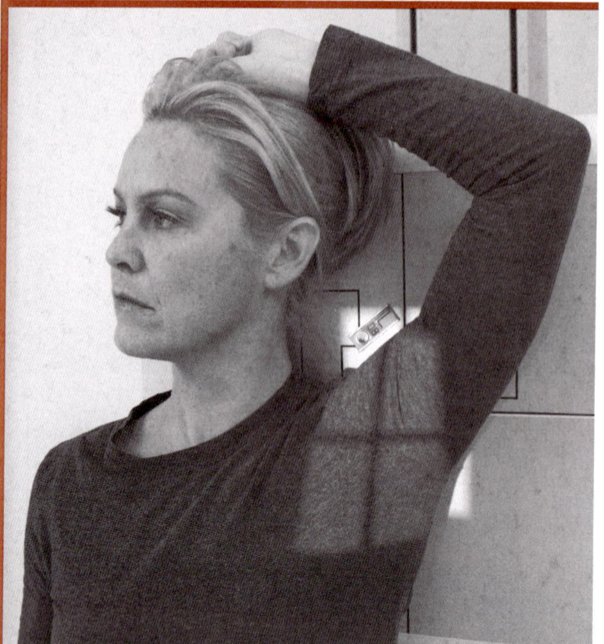

FIGURE 6-21

For the AP inferosuperior transaxillary shoulder (Walker method), the forearm can be rested on the head if needed.

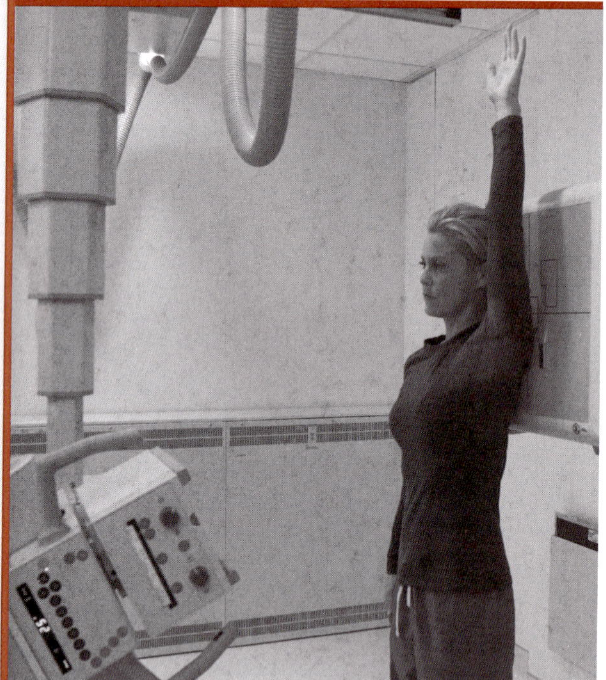

FIGURE 6-22

AP inferosuperior transaxillary shoulder (Walker method) uses an upward beam angle averaging 25°, centered to the humeral head.

patient's forearm on top of the patient's head as the goal is just to get the humerus vertical (Figure 6-21).

On small patients, 10 to 12 centimeters shoulder thickness, angle the x-ray tube 20° cephalad. For medium patients, 12 to 15 centimeters shoulder thickness, angle 25° cephalad, and for large patients, 15 to 17 shoulder thickness, angle 30° cephalad (Figure 6-22). The central ray is centered to the midaxilla and humeral head so that the glenohumeral joint is centered. As described in Chapter 2, be aware that with each 5° of cephalad angle, the CR should be centered a ½ inch lower from the starting point in the midaxilla.

Figure 6-23 demonstrates the proximal humerus in lateral position with a clear view of the glenohumeral joint space. The coracoid process is well visualized but superimposed over the clavicle. The glenoid cavity is seen almost in profile.

AP Chest on a Gurney using an Upright Bucky Detector with Extended Arm—Vanderzwaan Method

This AP chest projection can be taken with any system (CR or DR), but can only be used with a Bucky detector that has an extra-long arm that attaches the IR to the floor post as shown in Figure 6-24. Compared to using a portable IR plate, the built-in IR allows a better grid system

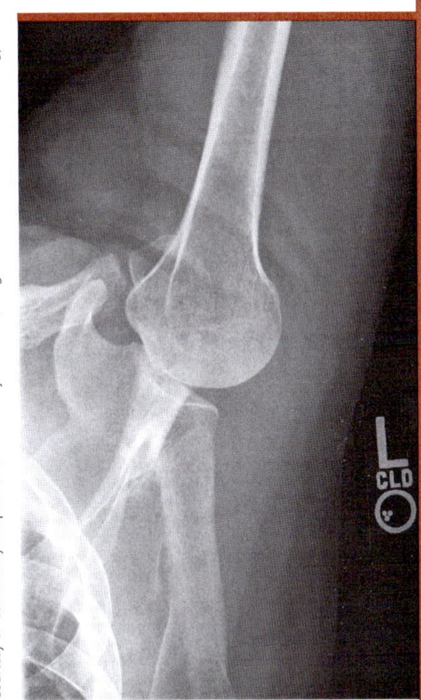

FIGURE 6-23
AP inferosuperior transaxillary shoulder view using the Walker method.

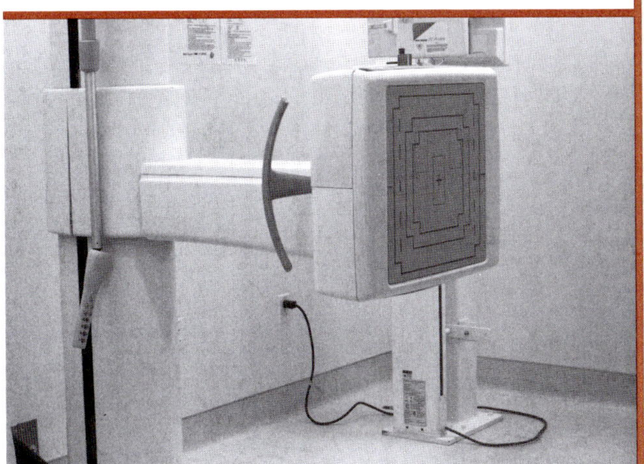

FIGURE 6-24
Many newer upright DR units have an extended arm, allowing the Vanderszwaan method to be used for an AP chest projection.

and the use of the AEC. This position adapts the AP chest projection for a fixed IR system with the extended arm.

Start with the gurney lined up with the IR and the x-ray tube. Pull the IR up so the bottom is about 2 feet above the gurney. Next, slide the patient to the top of the gurney, then sit the patient up as vertical as possible as shown in Figure 6-25. If the patient can hold himself up, have him grab both side rails of the gurney to keep his body upright, (Figure 6-26). If he is unable to do this, you will need an extra person to help keep the patient in this upright sitting position.

Now bring the head of gurney down so it is flat, and immediately drop the IR down so it is somewhat centered to the patient's back (Figure 6-27). Quickly back up the gurney so that the patient's back is

FIGURE 6-25

Vanderzwaan method for AP gurney chest: Start with the IR well above the gurney, then sit up the gurney.

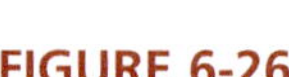

FIGURE 6-26

Vanderzwaan method, step 2: Have the patient grab the rails.

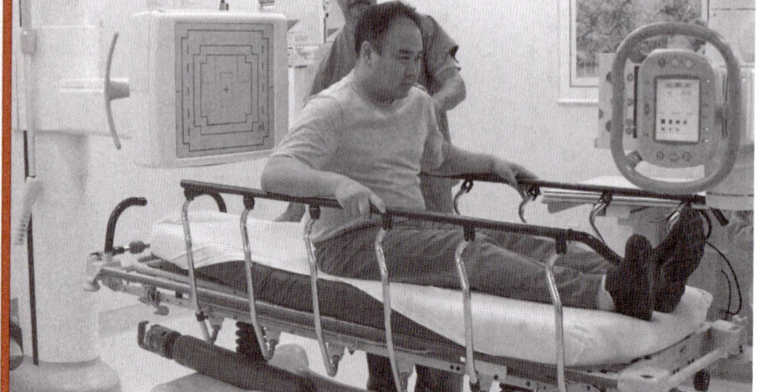

FIGURE 6-27

Vanderzwaan method, step 3: Lower the head of the gurney all the way down, then bring the IR down to its vertical centering point.

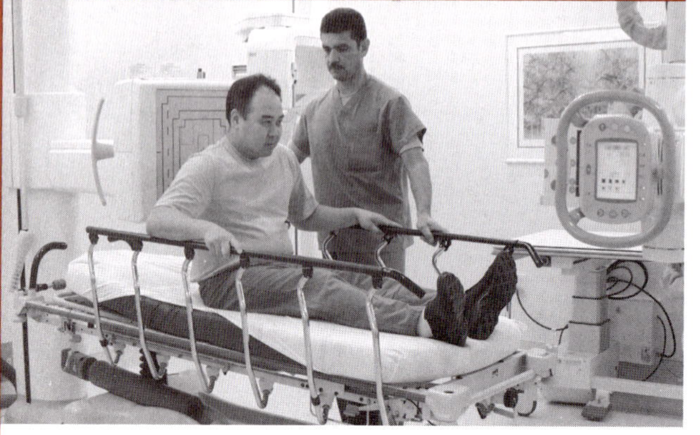

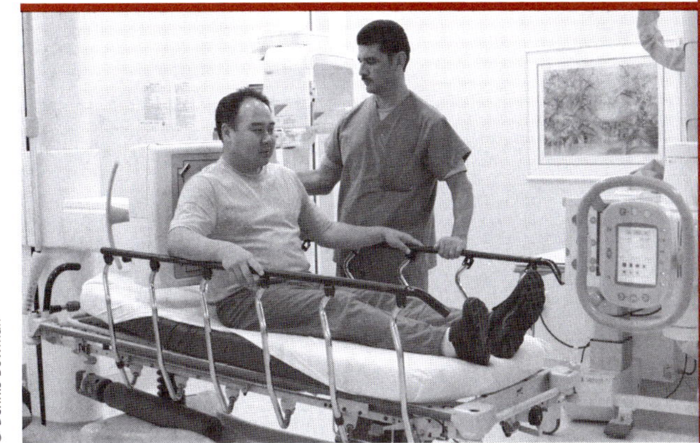
© Dennis Bowman

FIGURE 6-28
Vanderzwaan method, step 4: Back the gurney until the patient's back is in contact with the IR. Lock the gurney wheels.

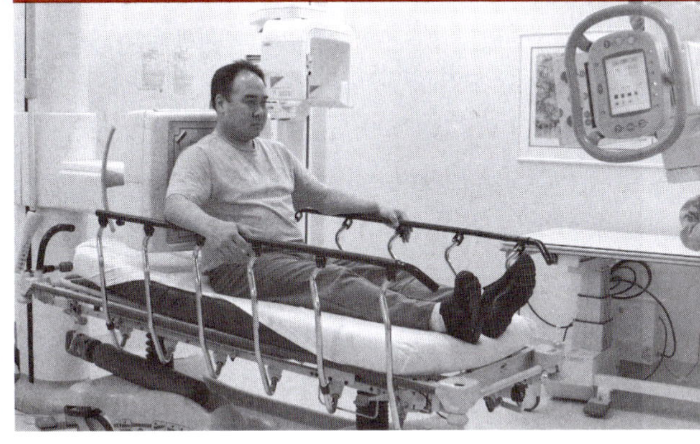
© Dennis Bowman

FIGURE 6-29
Vanderzwaan method, step 5: Center and collimate the x-ray beam for the exposure.

touching the IR (Figure 6-28). Do not forget to lock the gurney wheels. At this point, center the CR as for any AP chest (Figure 6-29). If the patient is leaning back, a caudal angle will be needed to match the degree of the coronal plane (see the section on mobile chest radiography in Chapter 7 to determine proper tube angle).

SUMMARY

1. A number of procedures conventionally done with a grid can be performed on modern DR units *nongrid,* which allows for various angled projections to be achieved. DR grids are easily removed.
2. DR mobile detectors can be very heavy and the radiographer must use good body mechanics in handling them, as well as extra caution for DR detectors with cords attached.
3. With the upright DR detector placed in a horizontal position, AP and oblique projections of the skull, facial bones, and cervical spine can be obtained with minimal movement for a trauma patient on a backboard. Distal upper extremity projections can also be obtained without getting a patient out of a wheelchair.

4. Both the axiolateral inferosuperior hip projection and the swimmers projection of the cervicothoracic spine are improved by using the Ferlic filter with digital x-ray units.
5. For fixed DR units, the leg or femur may not fit within the length of receptor plate available, and it will be necessary to take two views, one for each end joint, including 2 inches past the joint.
6. For some fixed DR units, the x-ray tube and detector are aligned and the table is movable. On such units, the best that can be done to obtain an axiolateral (cross-table lateral) projection of the hip is to angle the tube enough to desuperimpose the two hips and use the Ferlic filter to balance exposure through the various tissue thicknesses.
7. With a built-in DR detector, a sunrise projection of the knee can be obtained with the patient sitting in a wheelchair by using 15° angles on the x-ray tube, the upright detector, and the lower leg.
8. With a built-in detector, an inferosuperior transaxillary projection of the shoulder can be obtained by using the Walker method.
9. With a built-in detector, an AP chest projection can be obtained for a patient sitting on a gurney by backing the gurney up to the upright detector.

CRITICAL THINKING CHALLENGE 6.1

CROSS-TABLE LATERAL HIP PIN WITH A FIXED DR DETECTOR

A radiographer is performing a cross-table lateral hip with a possible dislocation, using a built-in DR detector system. The patient has a very long pin in the affected hip. The largest detector area available is already being used.

What two positioning tips will help ensure that the entire pin will be included within this view? ■

CRITICAL THINKING CHALLENGE 6.2

WALKER SHOULDER PROJECTION ON A LARGE PATIENT WITH A FIXED DR DETECTOR

A student is performing a Walker method projection for the shoulder as described in this chapter. The patient is very large, measuring 35-centimeters thick in AP projection.

Compared to an average patient, how much cephalic angle will be needed on the CR and how much lower than normal will the CR need to be centered? ■

USE OF A STEP SPONGE FOR AN OBLIQUE HAND

CRITICAL THINKING CHALLENGE 6.3

The "step" sponge has been designed by a manufacturer specifically to stabilize the oblique position of the hand. Figure 6-30 shows a cross section of the sponge design, with the placement of the thumb (T) and four fingers indicated on each step. (To answer this question, if such a sponge is available, actually use it as described and observe the results.)

Describe at least two disadvantages to using this sponge as indicated by the manufacturer. Also, how could the sponge still be used for stabilization and obliquity, but in such a way as to correct for these disadvantages?

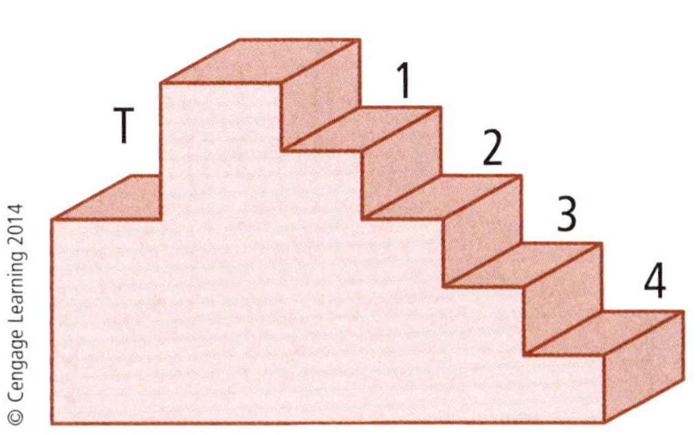

FIGURE 6-30
Use of a Step Sponge for an Oblique Hand.

OBLIQUE PROJECTION ON A PATIENT WHO MUST REMAIN ON THE SIDE

CRITICAL THINKING CHALLENGE 6.4

A patient comes in from the emergency department (ED) lying on his right side on a gurney. Due to injuries on both the anterior and the posterior surfaces of the body, the ED has requested that the patient be kept on his right side if possible. A lumbar spine series has been ordered with oblique views preferred. You have obtained lateral views by sliding detector plates under the patient, and you have obtained an AP projection using the upright Bucky with a horizontal beam.

Can either oblique projection of the lumbar spine be obtained while maintaining the patient in the right lateral recumbent position? If so, how?

(Answers to Critical Thinking Challenges are found in the Appendix.)

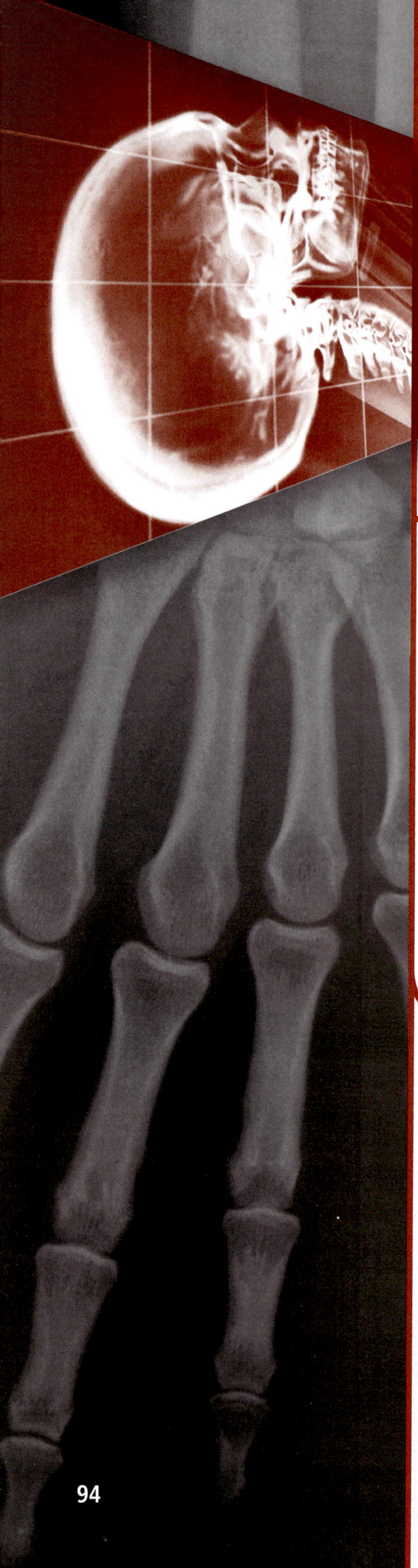

CHAPTER 7

Great Tips for Trauma and Mobile Radiography

OUTLINE

OBJECTIVES

Upon completion of this chapter, you should be able to:

1. Specify the priority of objectives in trauma positioning, because some factors must be compromised in order to ensure that the most important diagnostic objectives are achieved.
2. List those anatomical procedures normally done with a grid, that can be performed nongrid and tabletop in order to allow for transverse angles as needed for trauma positioning.
3. Describe how a gridded cassette or DR detector can be used so as to allow transverse angles as needed for trauma.

Continues

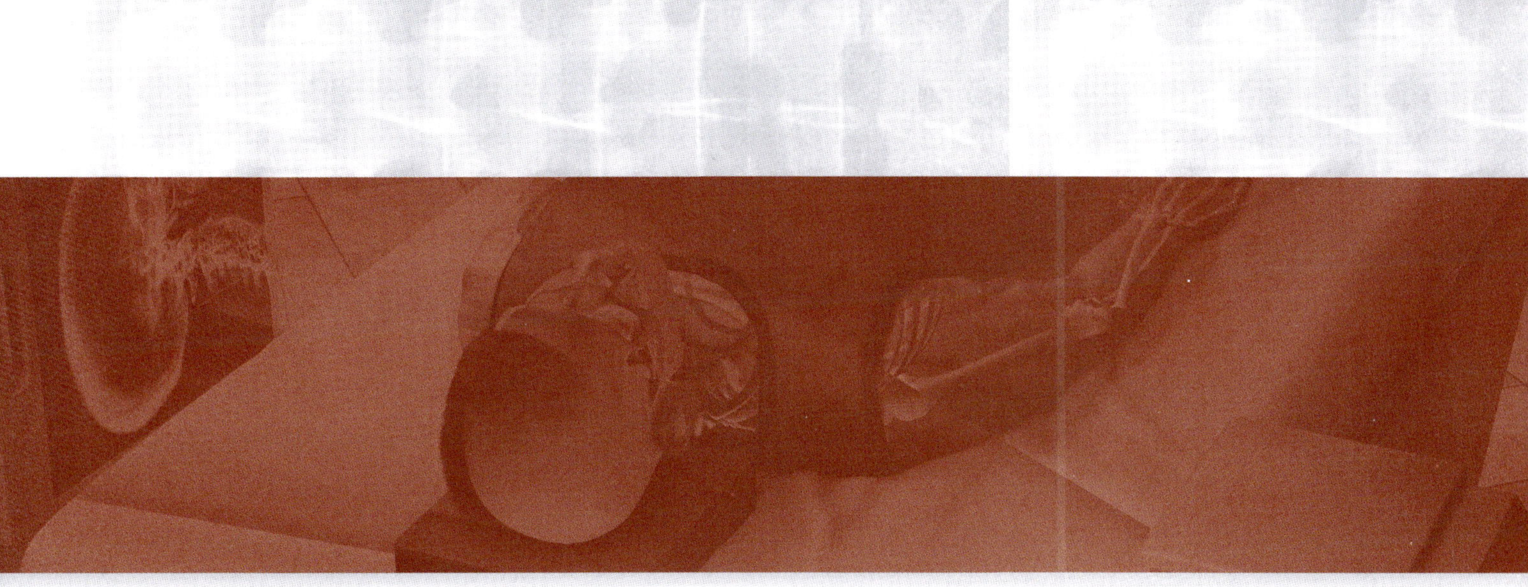

OBJECTIVES *continued*

4. Describe how the upright Bucky can be used to allow transverse angles on recumbent trauma patients.
5. Explain the adaptations in IR centering, CR centering, and SID that will minimize grid cut-off for horizontal-beam projections.
6. State the rule-of-thumb adjusting radiographic technique for 10-inch increments in changing the SID.

TRAUMA AND MOBILE RADIOGRAPHY

This chapter presents a number of generic concepts that are broadly applicable to various trauma situations, mobile radiography, and other circumstances in which radiographic positioning must be adapted to obtain the best possible images for diagnosis.

All trauma radiography involves *trade-offs* between desirable factors. By definition, trauma circumstances are less than ideal, and some aspect of the final image will therefore be sacrificed. We are forced to choose which factor will be sacrificed: a slight increase in unsharpness and magnification, a slight loss of contrast, some distortion of the anatomy, the closing off of a joint space, or the clipping of some anatomy. In the recommendations that follow, it is assumed that *inclusion of related anatomy* normally takes precedence, followed by accurate anatomical presentation (such as opening a joint of interest). Some unsharpness or loss of technical quality is often tolerated because a sufficient diagnosis for screening purposes can be made. By comparison, it is certainly not tolerable for related anatomical structures to be entirely *missing* from the view. Table 7-1 lists trauma radiography priorities.

TABLE 7-1

TRAUMA RADIOGRAPHY PRIORITIES

1. Inclusion of pertinent anatomy
2. Accurate anatomical presentation
3. Technical Quality

Advantages of a Horizontally Placed Upright DR Detector

Many new DR rooms include an upright unit that allows the detector panel to be rotated down into a horizontal position. This allows for a number of adaptive positions to be developed, many of which are very beneficial in trauma cases. In particular, head and neck series can be obtained *without sliding a detector or cassette under the backboard* for a patient on a gurney (stretcher). This is accomplished by sliding the entire backboard off the head end of the gurney onto the supporting detector panel in horizontal position. These positions for the head and neck were fully discussed and illustrated in Chapter 6.

Immobilization ("Brat") Boards

Most pediatric radiographers are familiar with the "brat board," a thin radiolucent board to which a small infant can be secured with straps or *mummified* using sheets, such that the body, legs, and arms are completely immobilized. With this arrangement, obliques and even laterals can be obtained by simply rotating the board.

ALTERNATIVES WHEN GRIDS PREVENT TRANSVERSE ANGLES

Many trauma positioning adaptations require the use of a transverse central ray angle *across* the bed, gurney, or table. The table Bucky tray cannot be used for this, because severe grid cut-off results from angling transverse to the strips of the table grid. The CR cassette or DR detector, whether used in conjunction with a stationary grid or not, must be placed "tabletop." There are two very workable options to consider, as discussed in the next paragraph.

First, many procedures that are normally done with a grid *can be done nongrid* with only minimal presence of scatter radiation. Bear in mind that, because the air in the lungs produces almost no scatter radiation regardless of the kVp used, a nongrid approach can be used not only for chest projections, but also for the ribs, sternum, and thoracic spine (except the swimmers-type projections of the cervicothoracic vertebrae, which include significant shoulder tissue). For the average patient's body, the skull, cervical spine (except the swimmers projection), shoulders, knees, and femurs produce only a small amount of scatter radiation, an acceptable level for trauma radiography even without a grid. For average or small patients, simply do these projections *nongrid*, using one-third of the grid technique (one-quarter for a 12:1 ratio grid). This makes the full range of central ray angles available to you, including transverse angles and double angles.

BEST PRACTICE TIP

For average and small patients, chests, ribs, AP and lateral T-spines, all C-spines, skulls, shoulders, knees, and femurs can all be radiographed in trauma situations without a grid by using one-third the usual technique.

For average and small patients, chests, ribs, AP and lateral T-spines, all C-spines, skulls, shoulders, knees, and femurs can all be radiographed in trauma situations without a grid by using one-third the usual technique.

On large patients, the upper thigh can present a problem, and on *very* large patients the knee and femur, shoulders, or neck may cause visible deterioration of the image. But, the only portion of the body for which grid use should be considered generally compelling is the abdomen and pelvis. (The author has even performed the mobile *abdomen* projection nongrid on very thin patients. It is the *thickness* and *type* of tissue, not the particular body part, that is at issue.) This was true *prior* to the advent of digital imaging; the ability of digital processing to restore image contrast lost to the remnant x-ray beam makes it even more applicable now.

Second, consider whether the image receptor can be placed tabletop such that the grid lines run *crosswise* under the patient rather than lengthwise, as shown in Figure 7-1. A transverse angle of the CR can then be applied, running parallel to the grid strips. For example, when performing a modified oblique projection of the lumbar spine, as shown in Figure 8-35 in the next chapter, a 45° transverse angle is used, allowing the patient to remain supine and unmoved. In this instance, a CR cassette or DR detector with a grid can be placed *on the tabletop* with the grid lines running crosswise to the table to allow for this angulation of the beam. The field can be collimated to the usual size side to side, using only the central portion of the image receptor.

Third, do not forget the possibilities created by placing a recumbent patient on a gurney (stretcher) against the *upright Bucky*. The grid lines in the upright Bucky run vertically. When a recumbent patient is placed against it, this translates to a *transverse* orientation of the grid lines relative to the patient, whether he is lying on his back or on his side. It

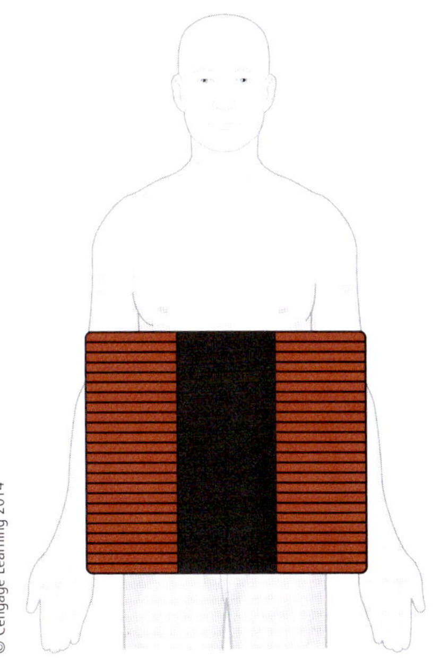

FIGURE 7-1

Placing the next larger size gridded IR plate "tabletop" but crosswise allows transverse angles to be used for adapted positions, with the angle running parallel to the grid strips. Shown here is the grid orientation and collimation for a modified (angled) oblique for the lumbar spine, using a 14- × 17-inch (35- × 42-cm) grid placed crosswise, but with a tightly collimated field (black area).

is common practice to perform decubitus ("cross-table") laterals and decubitus frontal (AP and PA) projections at the upright Bucky. But, various *trauma oblique projections* can also be obtained at the upright Bucky, especially if the patient can be rolled onto his side on the gurney. The central ray can then be angled up or down, transverse to the patient, without causing grid cut-off. Case Study #1 at the end of this chapter illustrates this concept.

HORIZONTAL BEAM PROJECTIONS

Whenever the patient is recumbent and a horizontal beam is used, problems can arise with clipping off the downside anatomy. On a cross-table lateral skull projection, part of the occipital bone at the back of the skull can be cut off at the bottom of the cassette or DR detector. On the cross-table lateral C-spine, the spinous process of C7 can be clipped. The cross-table lateral view of the chest may be missing the crucial posterior lung surfaces where fluid may be collecting.

There are two distinct causes for this cut-off: the edging on the CR cassette or DR detector panel, and the divergent geometry of the x-ray beam. A contributing factor is the increased object-to-image receptor distance (OID) inherently created by many lateral positions, which, in turn, may be exacerbated by any space left between the patient's body and the cassette to the patient's side. These will each be discussed.

Lowering the Image Receptor (IR)

Any type of CR cassette or DR detector must have supportive and protective edging. Unfortunately, when the image receptor (IR) is stood on end, this causes the imaging plate or active matrix array (AMA) inside to be lifted up off of the tabletop surface by an amount that may seem small but can be significant. As shown in Figure 7-2, *even if there were no beam divergence*, this results in clipping the bottommost ½-inch or more of the anatomy. This is not normally an issue for a cross-table lateral chest because sufficient "padding," in the form of muscles and fat, is present behind the ribs to also lift the anatomy of interest (the lungs) above this level and include them completely within the view. The same does not apply, however, to the posterior skull where only a small thickness of skin and tissue separates the occipital bone from the tabletop surface.

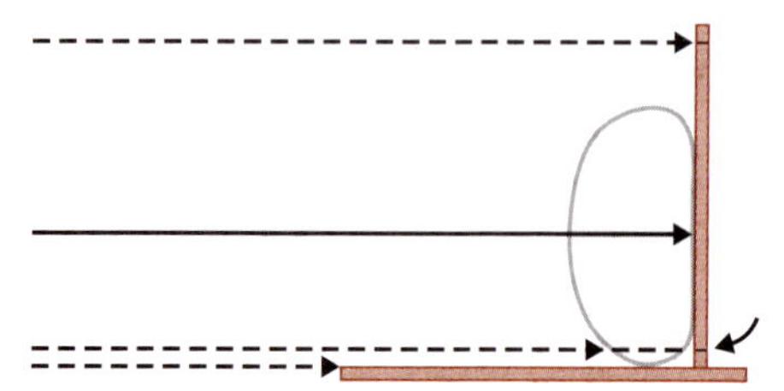

FIGURE 7-2

Even *without* beam divergence problems, downside anatomy can be clipped by the ½-inch metal edging on most cassettes and imaging plates (arrow).

The only solution is to either build up the patient with a pad or to lower the cassette or detector itself below the tabletop surface or backboard. There are several ways of accomplishing this. A popular "quick fix" is to drop the IR onto any supporting surface

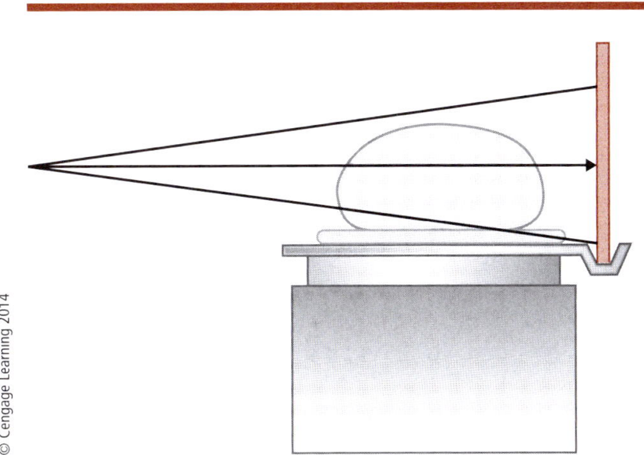

FIGURE 7-3

Even when a lower surface behind the table is used to hold the IR plate lower than the tabletop, a pad may be necessary to build the patient up so that normal beam divergence does not project the bottommost anatomy into the tabletop before it reaches the plate. (Observe the bottom diverging line, which just misses the tabletop with a pad in place.)

behind the back edge of the table (Figure 7-3). Note that if the patient is thin, if no pad is used to build the patient up, or if there is an OID gap left between the patient and the IR as in Figure 7-3, downward beam divergence may *still* result in clipping the down-most anatomy. Using tape to hold the IR vertically in place behind the table is risky, because the slightest movement of the patient against the IR may topple it to the floor. CR plates cost upwards of $1,000 each, and DR detectors cost much more. It is best to use a mechanical IR holder. If one is not available or cannot be used in a particular situation, have the patient or an assistant hold the IR in place. Whenever a pad can be placed under the patient, use a commercial cassette holder designed for the purpose, with the bottom panel of the holder placed under the pad and supported by the tabletop.

Many "floating" x-ray tables have a secure surface under the back portion of the table itself to rest the base of a cassette holder on. By floating the tabletop out laterally, the surface area supporting the cassette holder can be maximized for a steady, secure balance (Figure 7-4*A*). Often, especially with the table moved out as described, the holder can be pulled back an inch or so to allow the bottom edge of the IR to be lowered below the level of the table as shown in Figure 7-4*B*. This is ideal.

By reversing the projection across the table, the IR can be lowered and stabilized by placing it vertically in the Bucky tray (Figure 7-5). Bracing the IR against the edge of the table, the Bucky clamp can then be closed until it comes in contact with the back plate of the IR for some stability. Better still, use a commercial cassette holder placed *in the Bucky tray* for maximum stability.

Note that it is often advantageous to *leave a trauma patient on the gurney (stretcher)* rather than moving them to a table. With the typical layout of the gurney, a plastic backboard provides a firm surface to support the patient, while the pad beneath provides an opportunity to lower the IR as follows: The IR is clamped vertically into a proper cassette holder. The bottom plate of the holder itself can then be slid *under the stretcher pad*, where the weight of the patient ensures its

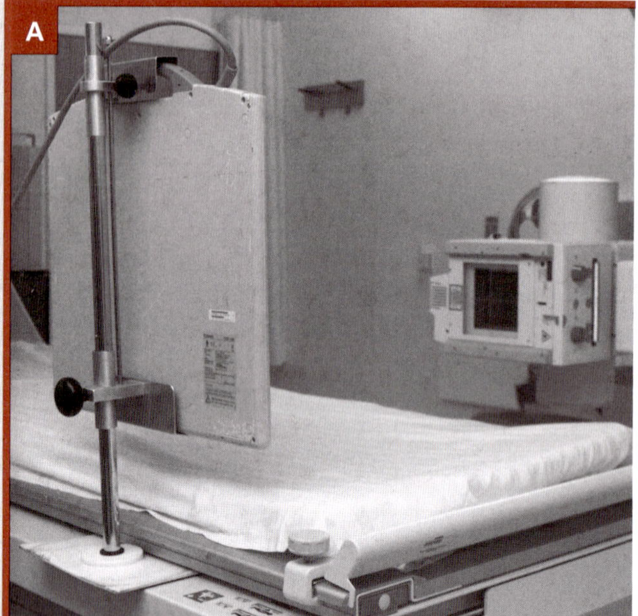

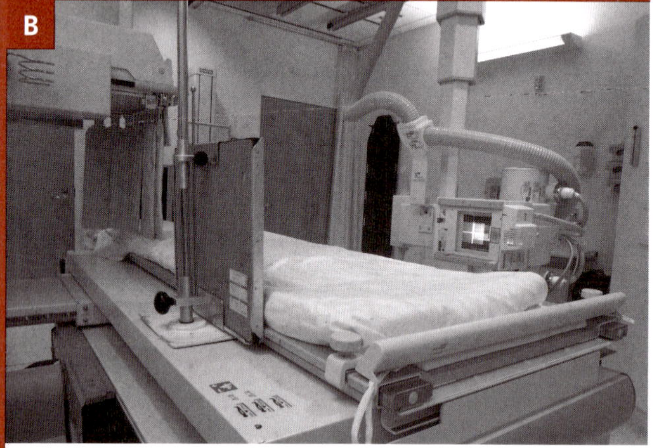

FIGURE 7-4

By floating some tabletops laterally, sufficient surface can be exposed to support a cassette holder, **A**. Bringing the clamps down, the cassette can be stablized behind the table and below the table level, **B**.

© Dennis Bowman

© Dennis Bowman

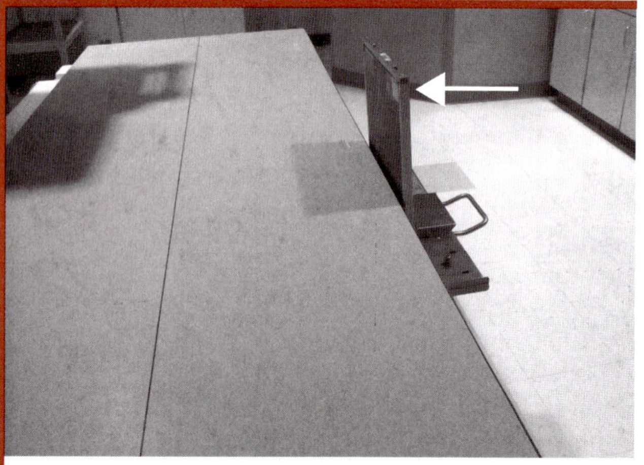

FIGURE 7-5

By reversing the projection across the table, the IR plate can be lowered and stabilized by placing it vertically in the Bucky tray and using the Bucky clamp and table edge as shown. (Better still, place a cassette holder in the Bucky tray.)

Courtesy of Quinn B. Carroll

stability (Figure 7-6). Many holders allow further vertical adjustment for the level of the CR cassette or DR detector.

Now, this may result in a troublesome space between the patient and the IR, increasing the OID. First, bear in mind that for many procedures such as the lateral cervical spine, a 6–8-inch OID already exists from the midline of the body to the shoulder where the cassette or IR plate would have been positioned. For the C-spine, an additional 2 inches, for example, would represent a relatively minor increase in distance of 25%–35%. This trade-off can be well worthwhile when it makes the difference between including or clipping off anatomy of interest. On a case-by-case basis, the radiographer must decide which issue is more important: slight magnification and blur, or the risk of clipping the bottom of C7.

Increasing Distance

Figure 7-7 shows how normal divergence of the horizontal x-ray beam causes downside anatomy to be projected into the tabletop surface before the image reaches the IR. *This is independent of the cassette edge problem*—It is the tabletop surface in this case that is "in the way." Any solution to this must somehow reduce beam divergence. And, there are only two ways that can be achieved: recentering and increasing distance.

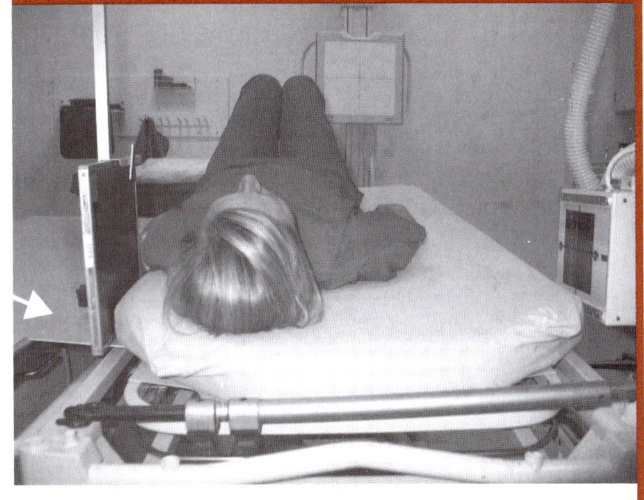

FIGURE 7-6
For the trauma patient on a gurney (stretcher), a cassette holder can be placed *under the gurney pad* to lower it, as shown on this cross-table C-spine (arrow). (If possible, slide the patient until the shoulder is in contact with the imaging plate.)

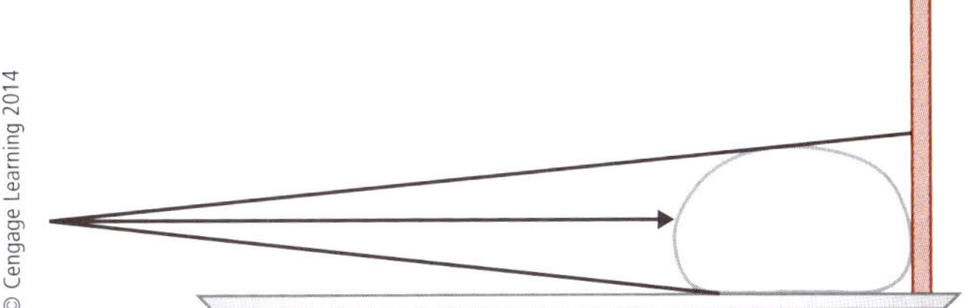

FIGURE 7-7
With normal cross-table projection geometry, unless a pad is used, the bottommost anatomy is projected into the tabletop by downward diverging beams before it reaches the IR plate, resulting in some cut-off.

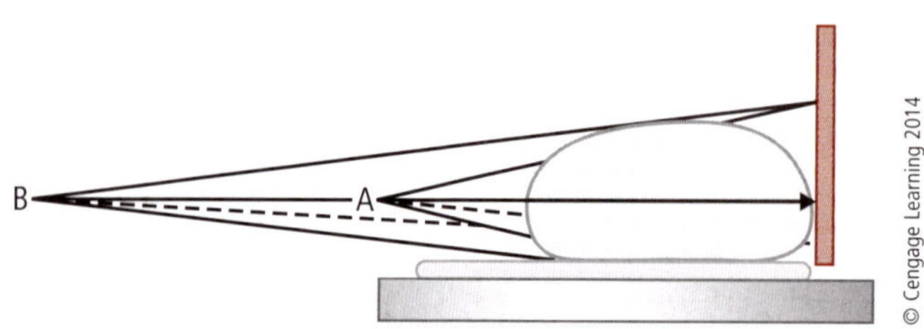

FIGURE 7-8

For cross-table projections, increasing the SID, as in B., is effective in reducing the amount of divergent cut-off (dotted lines).

Figure 7-8 illustrates how increasing distance (SID) causes the downside anatomy to fall within lesser divergent rays of the beam. For an object set at a specific distance from the central ray location, the farther the x-ray tube is moved back, the more parallel to the CR is the ray that passes through this anatomy.

Because increasing the SID also leads to improvements in sharpness and magnification, the only reason remaining for radiographers *not* to try this adaptation is the question of setting technique: There is often a lack of confidence in how to compensate the mAs for various distances, and we almost never have the time nor the inclination to do inverse square law mathematics in a clinical environment. So, the following rule, more fully discussed in the last chapter, is offered as a very helpful guideline:

> For every 10-inch change in SID, adjust mAs by at least one-third (35%).

Lower Vertical Centering

Finally, a helpful "trick of the trade" many radiographers have learned is to vertically *recenter the x-ray beam lower than normal* such that those rays passing just above the surface of the table are less divergent due to their proximity to the central ray, as shown in Figure 7-9. Downside anatomy close to the tabletop is then projected only slightly downward toward the IR plate, and more anatomy is included within the resulting view.

To do this, the field will have to be opened up vertically so that the upper portion of the anatomy is not clipped off (Figure 7-9). A *very* slight increase in distortion of the upper anatomy will occur due to the more divergent beams at the top. Also, the lowest portion of the actual beam is "wasted" because it misses the IR plate, and if done on a radiographic table, this portion of the beam may produce a slight increase in scatter radiation. As mentioned at the beginning of this

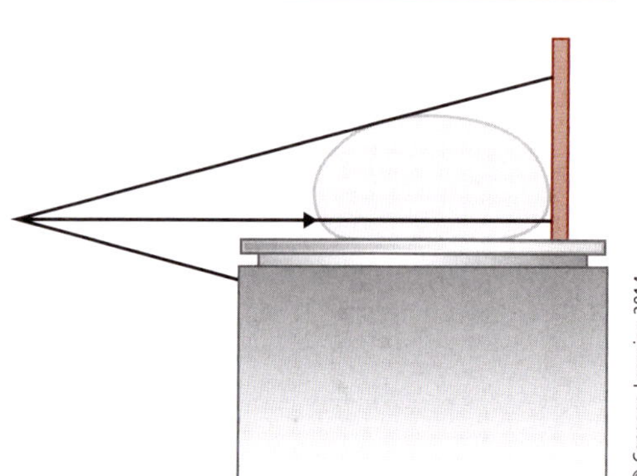

FIGURE 7-9

For cross-table projections, to further reduce downside cut-off from beam divergence, center the CR *vertically lower* than normal, shown here somewhat exaggerated, then open the field to compensate.

chapter, both of these are completely acceptable trade-offs for including related anatomy that might have otherwise been clipped.

On some CR systems, because this type of off-centering would prevent the inclusion of all four sides of the collimated field on the cassette, it may adversely affect histogram analysis and the resulting image. However, many of the newer CR systems are much more resilient against this effect.

The use of a grid *can* limit this recentering option, if the grid is placed with its lines running horizontal. For lower-ratio grids, the CR can be off-centered an inch or two without visible grid cut-off occurring. When a grid is used for the cross-table *lateral* skull, it should be positioned with the grid lines running vertically. This allows vertical off-centering as desired with no deleterious effects. More to the point, most of these trauma positions, including the skull, the C-spine, and the chest, can be done *nongrid* with only the slightest effects of scatter radiation. Complete latitude in positioning and centering is then allowed.

These three options—lowering the vertical position of the IR, increasing the distance, and vertically lowing the centering of the field—provide the radiographer with considerable armament in dealing with horizontal beam projections. It is not necessary to *radically* change any one of them if they are used in combination. For example, a relatively small adjustment to centering (1 or 2 inches lower), when combined with a small increase in distance (10 inches) can save a projection that might otherwise have been repeated.

For horizontal beam projections, the risk of clipping downside anatomy is minimized by combinations of increased SID, centering vertically lower, and lowering the image receptor (IR).

BEST PRACTICE TIP

For horizontal beam projections, the risk of clipping downside anatomy is minimized by combinations of increased SID, centering vertically lower, and lowering the image receptor (IR).

Correctly Taping an IR for Cross-Table Work

When performing cross-table (horizontal-beam) projections, especially when working alone, it may be necessary in some situations to tape the IR in place in order to secure it in a vertical position. There may be no other alternative if a mechanical IR (cassette) holder is not available. Whenever possible, some kind of stretchy tape such as rubber tape should be used instead of paper tape. The perfect width is 1 inch. Attach one end of the tape to the side of the x-ray table (not the table pad or sheet because they can move). Bring it over the patient and stick it to the top of the IR (making sure the IR is straight), and then down the other side, taping it to the opposite side of the table (Figure 7-10*A*). Stand back for a proper perspective to check if the IR is perfectly straight. If not, lift the tape off of it (the reason stretchy tape is preferred), straighten out the IR, and let the tape back down. Next, fold the tape side to side on top of itself over all the areas that are above the patient's body (Figure 7-10***B***). This way, the tape does not have any sticky side open and cannot accidentally "stick" to the patient, possibly moving or angling the IR.

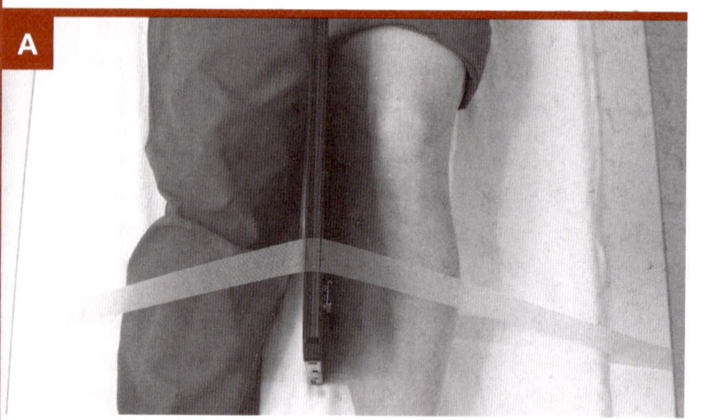

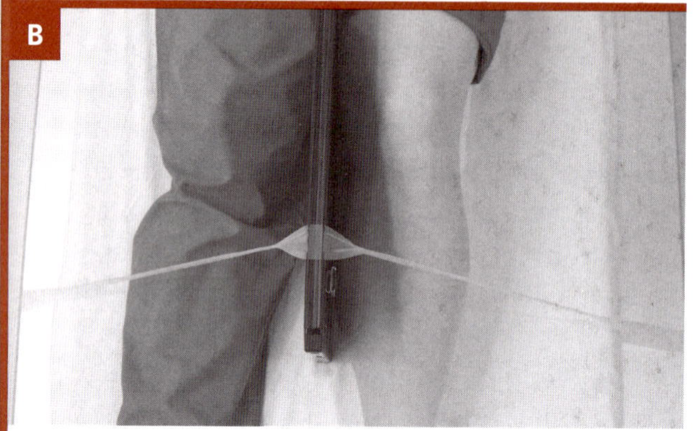

FIGURE 7-10
Stretchy tape can be attached to each side of the table to secure an IR in place for horizontal-beam projections **A**. Once the IR is adjusted to true vertical, fold the tape so that no sticky surface is exposed over the patient **B**.

COMPENSATING ANGLES FOR TRAUMA CASES

In general, if a patient can get into a true AP position, oblique and lateral projections can be taken without having the patient move. The cross-table lateral is fairly straightforward, but for different modified oblique projections the radiographer will need to develop the ability to visualize and determine which way to angle the tube. To do this, the radiographer must first imagine what the angle would look like if the patient was able to rotate the body part into the correct oblique position. For example, let us consider an internal oblique position of the ankle.

Figure 7-11*A* shows what the patient would look like if she were able to correctly oblique her ankle. The radiographer will need to visualize how the CR is entering and exiting the body part. Here, we see the CR entering more toward the lateral side, and exiting on the medial side. In effect, the CR is angled *lateromedially*. To maintain this relationship with the leg in AP position, Figure 7-11*B* demonstrates that the tube would need to be angled *lateromedially* to maintain the proper angle.

Double Angles

Examples of double angles include the oblique cervical spine (45° transverse, and 15° cephalic) or the Clements-Nakayama modification for the cross-table hip projection (25° cephalic, and 15° downward toward the floor). When a trauma patient is brought into a fixed

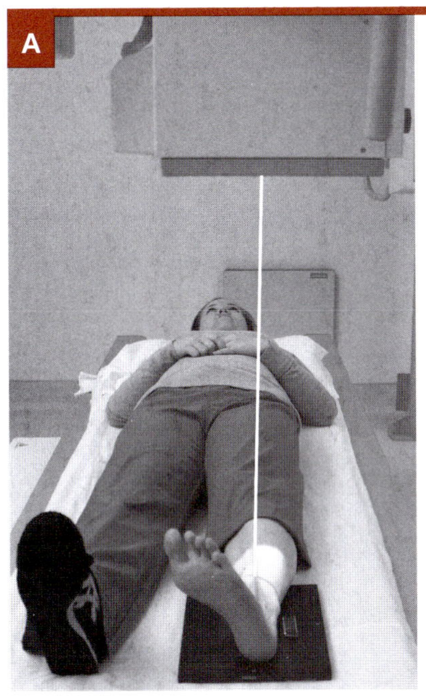

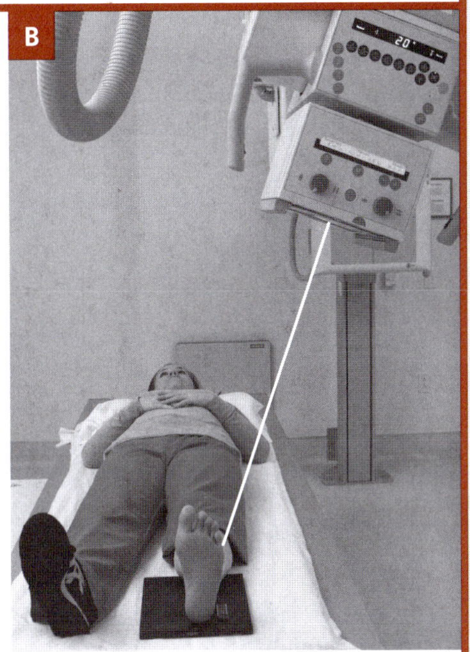

FIGURE 7-11

Example of compensating an angle for an oblique ankle position. Because the routine position results in the CR passing obliquely from the lateral to the medial side **A.**, the correct angle when the patient is left in AP position to achieve the equivalent view is a *lateromedial angle* **B**.

radiographic room, it can be very difficult and sometimes impossible to place a double angle on the ceiling-mounted x-ray tube for a supine patient who cannot be moved. For example, the swivel movement on most ceiling-mounted x-ray tubes only locks into 45° and 90° positions, so that when it is left swiveled at 30°, for example, it may drift in its rotational movement and it can be very difficult to get it to stay in place.

In some cases such as the oblique C-spine, the more crucial of the two angles can be employed, and radiologists may accept the resulting views without the refinement of the second angle. But, it is not necessary to settle for such compromised views. *To achieve double-angle positions in the fixed radiographic room, bring a mobile unit into the room.* Nearly all modern mobile units allow quick and easy angulation of the x-ray tube in all directions.

If the second, less critical angle needed happens to be a "lateral" angle, that is, it would normally be angled directly from the side of the patient, this type of angle can be obtained by *swiveling the gurney (stretcher) so that it is somewhat "diagonal" relative to the rest of the room*, or by *swiveling the patient on the x-ray table, such that the patient lies somewhat "diagonal" across the table.*

To achieve double-angle positions in the fixed radiographic room, bring a mobile x-ray unit into the room. Secondary "lateral" angles can be achieved by swiveling the patient on the table, or swiveling the gurney (stretcher).

BEST PRACTICE TIP

To achieve double-angle positions in the fixed radiographic room, bring a mobile x-ray unit into the room.

BEST PRACTICE TIP

Secondary "lateral" angles can be achieved by swiveling the patient on the table, or swiveling the gurney (stretcher).

Vertical Angles with an Upright Bucky

Although the need to use such an approach will be rare, it is worth noting and remembering that oblique projections for several anatomical series may be obtained when the patient is in a recumbent, lateral decubitus position (on his side) on a gurney and it is contraindicated or undesirable to move him from this position. This can be accomplished by moving the gurney up against an upright Bucky detector and employing *vertical* angles on the x-ray tube as the projection warrants.

CASE STUDY

Case Study #1: Oblique Projection on Patient Who Must Remain on Side

A patient comes in from the emergency department (ED) lying on his right side on a gurney. Due to injuries on both the anterior and the posterior surfaces of the body, the ED has requested that the patient be kept on his right side if possible. A lumbar spine series has been ordered with oblique views preferred. You have obtained lateral views by sliding detector plates under the patient, and you have obtained an AP projection using the upright Bucky with a horizontal beam.

Can either oblique projection of the lumbar spine be obtained while maintaining the patient in the right lateral recumbent position? If so, how?

ANSWER: *Yes. As illustrated in Figure 7-12, a lumbar spine projection equivalent to a right posterior oblique position is obtained by angling the x-ray beam downward 45° with the patient lying on his right side. A similar projection equivalent to a left posterior oblique position can be obtained by angling the beam upward. However, because the gurney may get in the way, the amount of angle may need to be compromised by reducing it somewhat.*

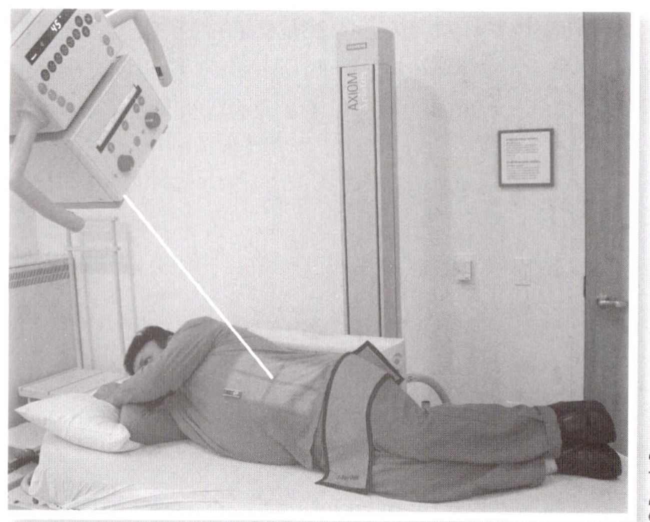

© Dennis Bowman

FIGURE 7-12
With the patient recumbent on his right side, the equivalent of an RPO lumbar spine is obtained by using the upright Bucky and angling the x-ray beam downward.

Figure 7-13 demonstrates a projection of the left ribs or chest equivalent to a right posterior oblique position. Other oblique projections, such as an SI joint, may also be obtained in this way.

CASE STUDY

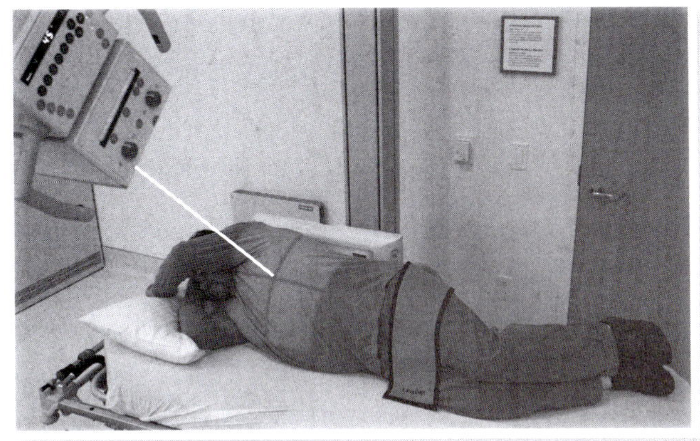

FIGURE 7-13
An RPO ribs or chest projection is obtained by using the upright Bucky and angling the x-ray tube vertically.

SUMMARY

1. Inclusion of the anatomy of interest within the view, and accurate presentation of that anatomy, always take precedence over small increases in fog, distortion, magnification, or unsharpness that may result from the positioning adjustments required to achieve these objectives.
2. For infants, when the patient is properly secured, immobilization boards facilitate oblique positions by simply moving the board.
3. All thoracic and skull anatomy, cervical spines (except the "swimmers" projection), shoulders, and femurs *can* be done nongrid. Therefore, transverse angles can be employed for trauma positioning in all these areas by using the imaging plate tabletop.
4. Transverse angles can be used in trauma radiography by placing a gridded cassette *crosswise* on the tabletop or gurney (stretcher).
5. Transverse angles can often be achieved on a recumbent patient by placing the gurney (stretcher) against the *upright Bucky.* If the patient can be rolled onto his side, oblique projections can be obtained by angling the tube vertically.
6. For horizontal-beam projections, combinations of lowering the plate, centering vertically lower, and increasing the SID all help to minimize grid cut-off.

7. For every 10-inch change in the SID, adjust the technique by at least one-third (35%).
8. To achieve double-angle positions in the fixed radiographic room, bring a mobile x-ray unit into the room.
9. Secondary "lateral" angles can be achieved by swiveling the patient on the table, or swiveling the gurney (stretcher).
10. Oblique projections can be obtained on patients lying on their side by using the upright Bucky detector and angling the x-ray beam *vertically*.

CRITICAL THINKING CHALLENGE 7.1

TRAUMA EXTERNAL OBLIQUE ELBOW

An elbow series is being done on a trauma patient who is unable to straighten the arm out. An AP projection using the "split the difference" method (see Chapter 8) has just been completed, and an external oblique view is required, but the patient has a shoulder injury and cannot roll the arm out into this position.

In which direction and by how many degrees will the x-ray tube be angled in order to obtain an equivalent projection to the external oblique position? ■

CRITICAL THINKING CHALLENGE 7.2

HEAD POSITION FOR A CALDWELL SKULL PROJECTION

On a Caldwell view taken for an orbit series, the petrous ridges are seen to be properly placed in the bottom one-third of the orbit. The radiologists asks for a modified version of this view where the petrous pyramid will be projected just below the bottom of the orbit so that the entire orbital rim can be visualized.

Knowing that the petrous bones are posterior to the middle of the cranium and the orbit is much close to the image receptor (IR) with the patient in PA projection, does the patient's head need to be extended more or flexed more to achieve this position? ■

SERIES MODIFICATION FOR TANGENTIAL FOREIGN BODY

CRITICAL THINKING CHALLENGE 7.3

A patient reports to the ED with a "pellet-gun wound to the belly." The ED physician believes the pellet is embedded only ½-inch or so beneath the skin, and requests an abdomen series with a "profile" view of the wound added. The wound is located on the anterior right corner of the patient's abdomen.

Give a precise and complete description of the "profile" view you would take. Also, would you use automatic exposure control (AEC)? Why or why not? If choosing manual technique, how the technique would compare to that used for the AP projection? ■

(Answers to Critical Thinking Challenges are found in the Appendix.)

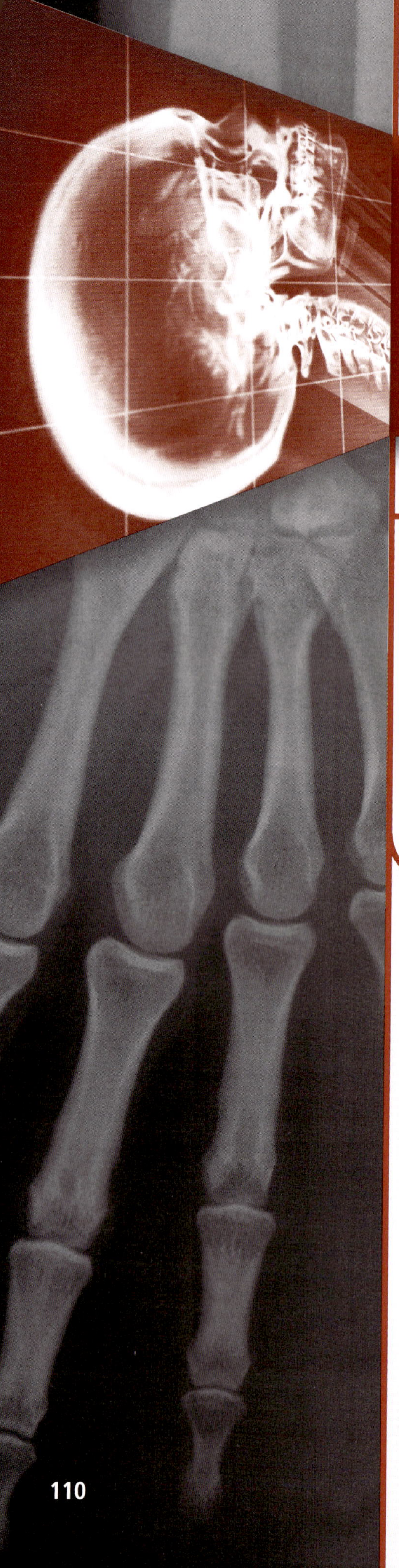

CHAPTER 8

Specific Trauma and Mobile Positions

OUTLINE

OBJECTIVES

Upon completion of this chapter, you should be able to:

1. State the three rules to minimize clipping of C7 for the screening cross-table cervical spine.
2. Describe several recommended adaptations for obtaining nonlordotic and well-centered AP projections of the chest for adults and infants.
3. Describe recommendations for facilitating and achieving higher quality radiographs on trauma and mobile projections of all anatomical portions of the body.
4. Describe recommendations for facilitating and achieving higher quality radiographs on newborn intensive care infants and general pediatrics.

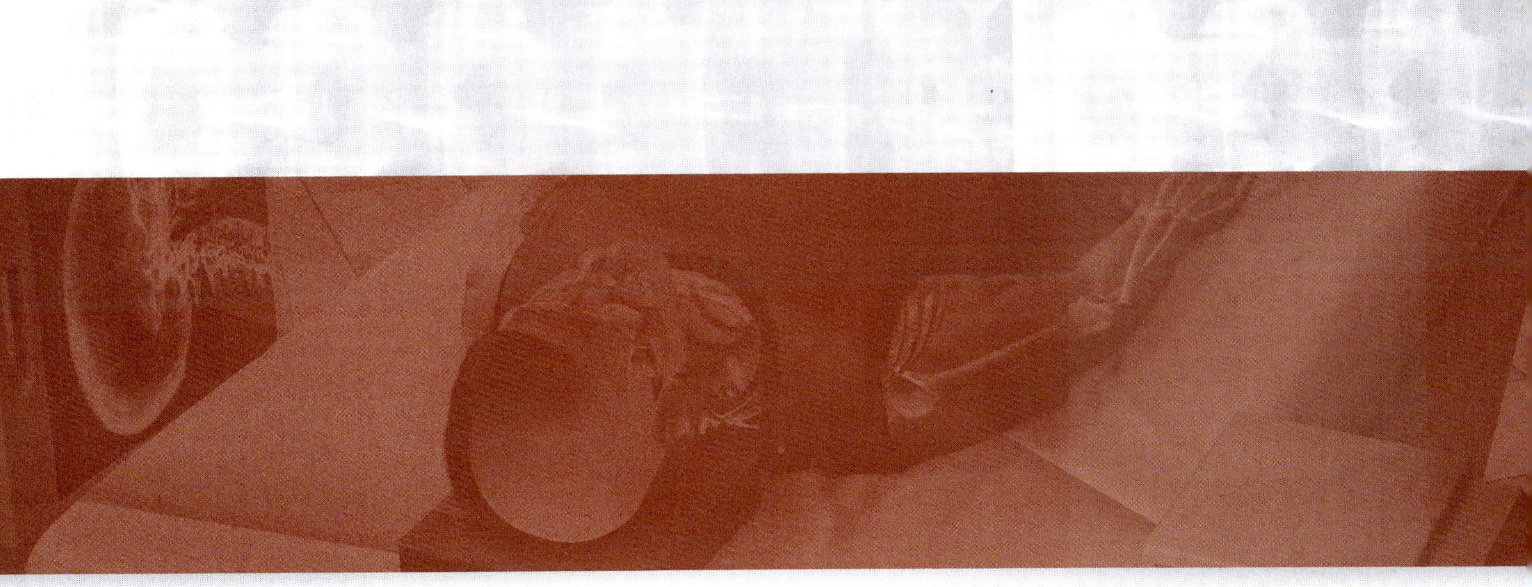

TRAUMA AND MOBILE RADIOGRAPHY

This chapter will present specific positioning recommendations for common trauma and mobile procedures, with several adaptations and aids that are not included in most positioning atlases. The adaptations are firmly grounded in the general principles presented in Chapter 1. These ideas are designed to improve efficiency, reduce repeat rates, and minimize inconvenience for both the radiographer and the patient.

Note that this chapter does not include skull positioning. All positions of the head, including the skull, sinuses, and all facial bones, are covered in the next chapter. Trauma skulls present some unique challenges, and so a special section in Chapter 9, *Adapting Skull Positions: Routine and Trauma,* is devoted to better understanding how to determine more specific and accurate corrections.

This chapter is not organized in anatomical sequence, but in an order based on the most frequently requested mobile procedures and the most problematic trauma situations. We therefore begin with the ubiquitous cross-table lateral cervical spine for trauma screening. Next, mobile and trauma chest projections are covered. Other routine procedures are each considered, and then the chapter ends with some helpful guidelines for newborn intensive care (NBICU) situations and general pediatrics.

THE SCREENING CROSS-TABLE LATERAL C-SPINE

The importance of a good cross-table lateral C-spine for trauma screening cannot be overstressed. As intimated in Chapter 7, it may be necessary to lower the level of the image receptor (IR) to get all of the downside anatomy within the view, in this case the entire spinous process of C7. **This projection can be done *nongrid* with an appropriate technique correction and this is recommended to allow centering flexibility,** except on the largest patients.

The main challenge for the cross-table lateral C-spine is how to ensure that C7 is not obscured on this projection by the superimposition of the shoulders. The following three tips minimize this probability:

1. Center lower than usual anatomically (superior-to-inferior on the *patient*), such that the central ray (CR) skims just above the shoulders. When the CR is normally centered at the level of the thyroid cartilage, those rays that pass through C7 diverge downward substantially, and project C7 down into the shoulder that is against the IR. As shown in Figure 8-1, centering lower results in C7 falling within a less divergent beam, so it is not projected downward as much. Less of the shoulder superimposes the vertebra. The field will need to be opened so that the upper cervical vertebrae are included within the view. *Do not center the IR itself more caudally*. The level of the IR should be centered to the thyroid cartilage as usual. The upper chest will receive some "wasted" radiation, but this is a viable trade-off in order to get C7

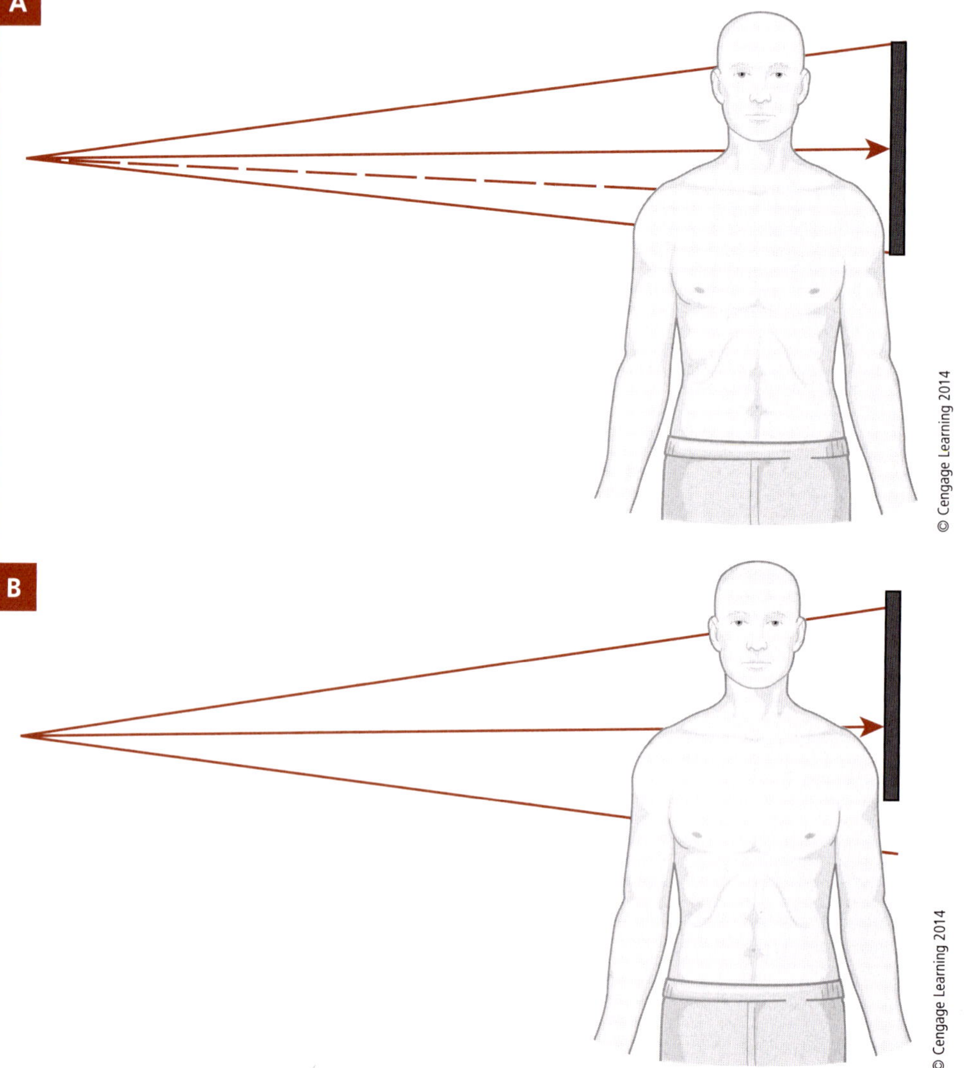

FIGURE 8-1

Routine centering for the cross-table lateral C-spine **A** projects C7 downward into the shoulder nearest the IR plate, from normal beam divergence (dotted line). To reduce this effect, center the CR *anatomically lower* such that the CR just skims over the shoulders **B**. Open the field to compensate (*do not* center the plate lower).

in view. This recentered projection is illustrated in Figure 8-2. (As previously mentioned, on *some* CR systems, because this type of off-centering prevents the inclusion of all four sides of the collimated field on the cassette, it may adversely affect histogram analysis.)

2. If there is room to do so, increase the source-to-image receptor distance (SID) to the maximum feasible distance. As shown in Figure 8-3 and as discussed in the last section, this further reduces the divergence of those rays that pass through C7 at a fixed location below the CR. (Increase mAs by at least 35% for every 10-inch increase in SID.)
3. Depression of both shoulders is required, but it is important to understand that it is the *downside* shoulder, the shoulder against the IR, that primarily obscures C7 because of the complications of beam divergence, as shown in Figure 8-3. Be sure to apply traction by grasping the forearms *above* the wrist, *not by grasping the hands.* This will avoid patient injury. Apply even traction first, then as your assistant begins to rotor the x-ray tube, *apply slight additional traction to the downside shoulder against the IR.*

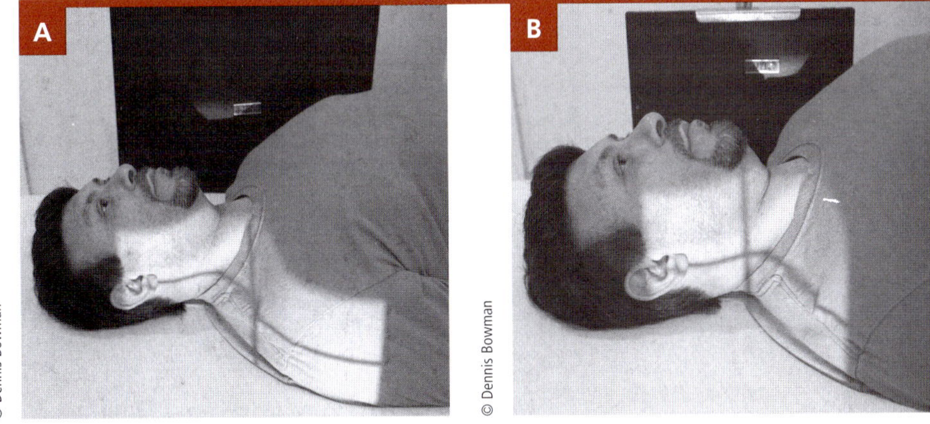

FIGURE 8-2

Cross-table lateral C-spine taken to minimize divergence of C7 into the shoulder by centering just above the shoulders **A**. Conventional centering and collimation are shown in **B** for comparison.

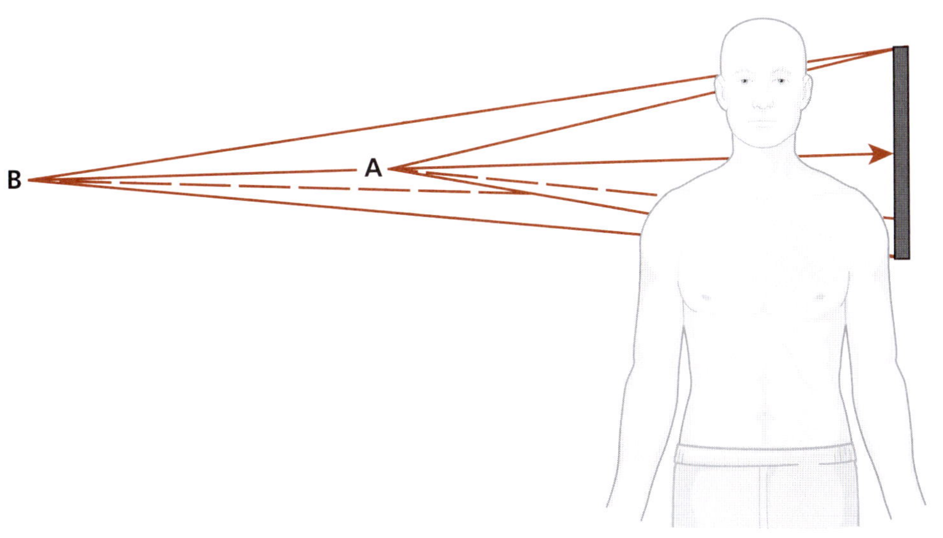

FIGURE 8-3

For the cross-table lateral C-spine, increasing the SID (B), is effective in reducing the amount of divergent cut-off (dotted lines).

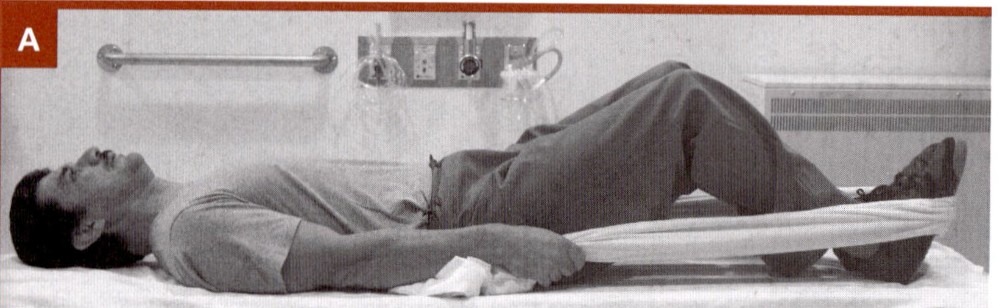
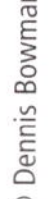

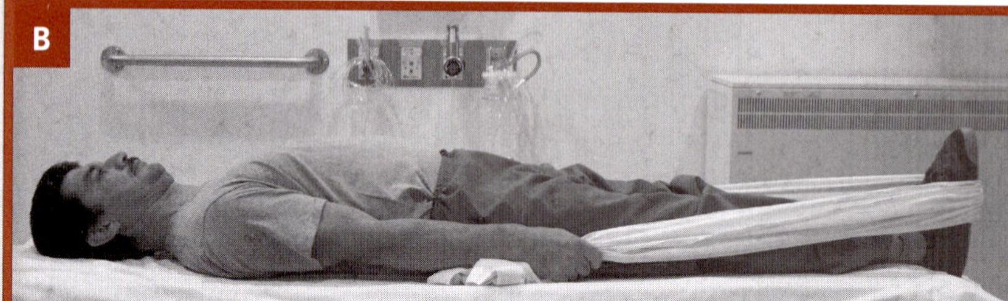

FIGURE 8-4
For the cross-table lateral C-spine, some trauma patients can pull their own shoulders down by bending both legs to position a rolled-up sheet against the bottom of the feet **A**, and then extending the legs while relaxing the shoulders **B**.

BEST PRACTICE TIP

For the cross-table lateral C-spine, to minimize the probability of clipping C7, center the CR lower anatomically (closer to the shoulders), increase the SID when possible, and apply slight additional traction to the "downside" shoulder (closest to the IR).

Using all three of these rules in combination will greatly improve your chances of obtaining a passable view of the cross-table C-spine on the first attempt.

For the cross-table lateral C-spine, to minimize the probability of clipping C7, center the CR lower anatomically (closer to the shoulders), increase the SID when possible, and apply slight additional traction to the "downside" shoulder (closest to the IR).

How the Patient Can Depress His Own Shoulders for the Cross-Table Lateral C-Spine

If the patient is willing and able, this method will allow the radiographer to exit the room during exposure, or perform the procedure when assistance is not available. Start by rolling up a sheet and having the patient hold it tightly in each hand. Have the patient bend his legs as much as possible and place the rolled up sheet against the bottom of his feet (Figure 8-4*A*). The patient then fully extends his arms and readjusts the sheet in his hands so that there is no slack. When you are ready to make the exposure, have the patient fully exhale, relax his shoulders, and then extend his legs all the way while keeping the sheet taut (Figure 8-4*B*). Observe to make sure that the patient does not move his neck off-center to the IR plate in this process. If done correctly, this can pull a patient's shoulders down 1–3 inches for an ideal projection like the one shown in Figure 8-5.

THE MOBILE AND TRAUMA CHEST

Projections of the AP and lateral chest seem so simple in concept that much is often taken for granted in obtaining these views in mobile and trauma situations. In reality, a number of complications arise from reversing the standard projection (AP rather than PA), from compromised

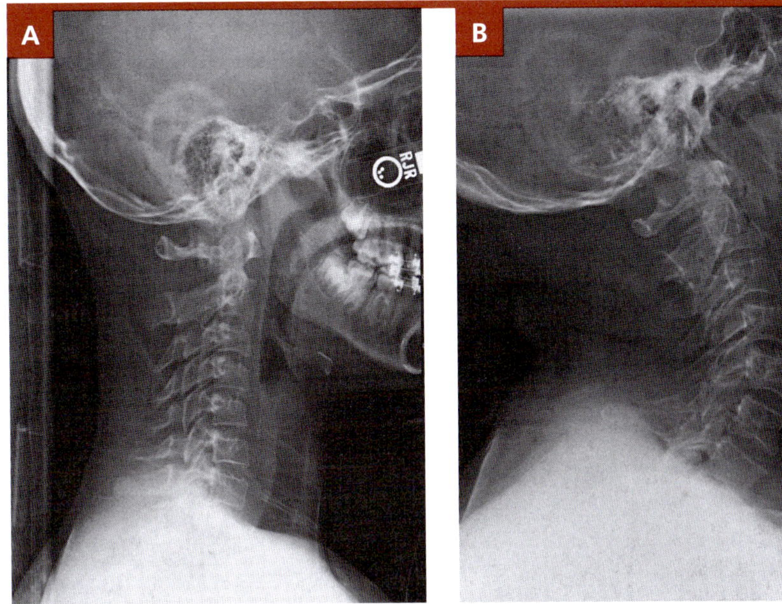

FIGURE 8-5

Two examples of cross-table lateral C-spine images on trauma patients with excellent desuperimposition of the shoulders to demonstrate C7.

Courtesy of Community Hospital of the Monterey Peninsula, Diagnostic and Interventional Radiology

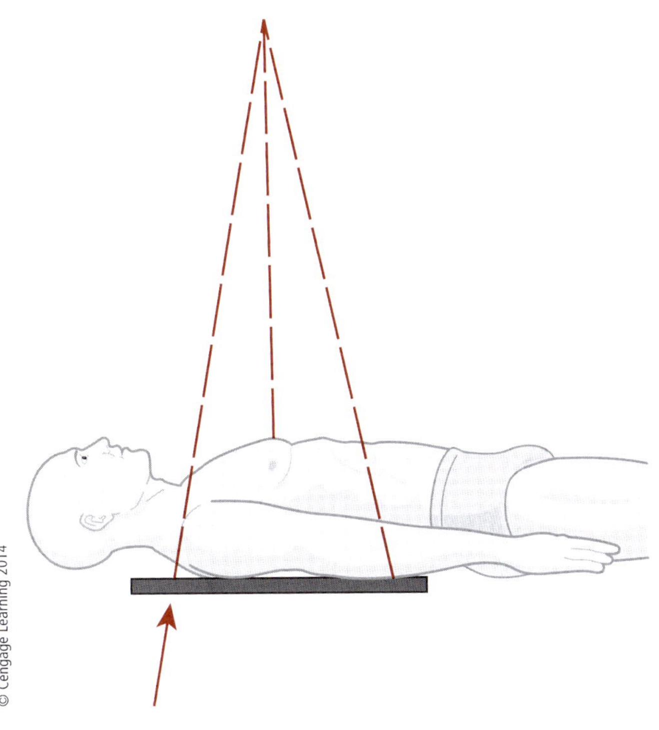

FIGURE 8-6

A supine AP chest projection at 40-inch (100-cm) SID shows substantial upward divergence for the upper half of the chest. This will cause unacceptable lordotic distortion unless a caudal angle is added to the central ray.

distances, and from the challenges of "working around" patient, equipment, and furniture.

There are several anatomical and geometric reasons for using a slight *caudal* angulation (relative to the IR) on all AP projections of the chest. Note that for a perpendicular x-ray beam with normal beam divergence, the apical portions of the lungs and upper bony thorax fall within beams that are effectively "angled" cephalic (Figure 8-6). This results in a *lordotic* distortion of the upper lungs, rib cage, and

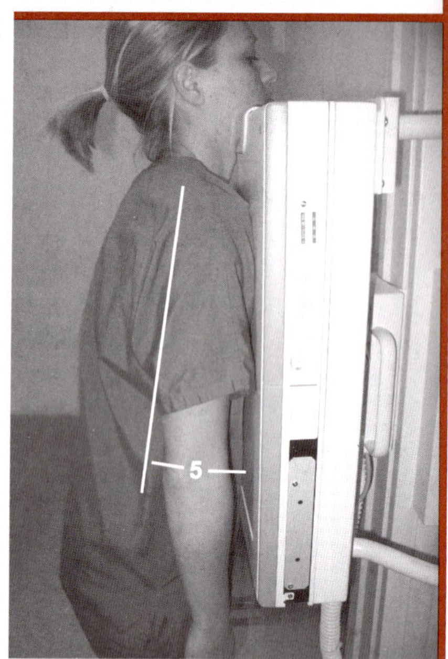

Courtesy of Quinn B. Carroll

FIGURE 8-7

On the routine PA chest, rolling the patient's shoulders forward against the IR plate causes the patient to effectively lean forward, placing the midcoronal plane at an approximate 5° angle. This is equivalent to a slight cephalic angle of the CR for the PA chest. It is also equivalent to a slight *caudal* angle of the CR for the AP chest as recommended in Figure 8-11.

clavicles. There is also a projected lordotic "straightening" of the normal curvature of the spine and ribs throughout. A caudal angle reduces these effects, and also better demonstrates the posterior bases and costophrenic angles of the lungs where small amounts of fluid will first accumulate.

If this principle holds true, one might question why a slight *cephalic* angle is not used on *PA* chests? Note that on the routine upright PA chest, ideally, the patient's shoulders are rolled forward until they touch the plate. Although the given purpose for this is to pull the scapulae laterally out of the lung fields as much as possible, you can see in Figure 8-7 that it also causes the patient to effectively lean forward slightly, placing the midcoronal plane at an approximate 5° angle. This is precisely equivalent to a 5° cephalic angulation of the beam relative to the IR.

Many positioning manuals recommend for the AP chest an angle *perpendicular to the sternum*, not perpendicular to the midcoronal plane. The lower sternum slants outward or forward relative to the spine and the midcoronal plane. Therefore, this approach accomplishes exactly the same thing as a caudal angle relative to the IR. All of these methods result in a projection "looking downward" somewhat over the dome of the diaphragm, so that small amounts of fluid accumulating in the posterior costophrenic angles of the lungs, which lie much lower than the anterior costophrenic angles, may be demonstrated. In addition, they prevent a lordotic projection that would present an abnormal straightening appearance to the ribs and spine.

Now, as described in Chapter 4, *the shorter the SID, the more extreme the x-ray beam divergence*. The effects of this on the 40-inch (100-cm) supine chest are illustrated in Figure 8-9 in the next section, but also apply to a sitting chest when done at any shortened distance. When performing mobile or trauma chests at 40-inch (100-cm) SID (as opposed to 72 inch or 180 cm), the effects of beam divergence are worsened. To compensate, at the shorter 40-inch (100-cm) SID, it is more critical to use the caudal angle, *and more caudal angle is needed*. At this distance, angle an *additional* 2°–3° *caudal to the sternum*.

Figure 8-8 illustrates *additional* geometrical factors that contribute to a subconscious tendency to produce an apical lordotic projection on the sitting AP chest. Namely, during the sitting position, the bottom of the IR often slides out a bit so that it is not flush against the back of the bed or wheelchair, such that it is slightly more angled than the back support, and the patient's derriere often does the same thing in relation to the IR plate—that is, the patient tends to slide out a bit so that his midcoronal plane is slanted more than the cassette or detector panel. Some added caudal angulation helps cancel out the effects of these tendencies.

Thus, we see that *both* the sitting chest and the supine chest present added geometrical problems that call for more caudal angle. For the sitting chest, there is a tendency for both the IR and the patient to slide out from the back support. For the supine chest, there is the added

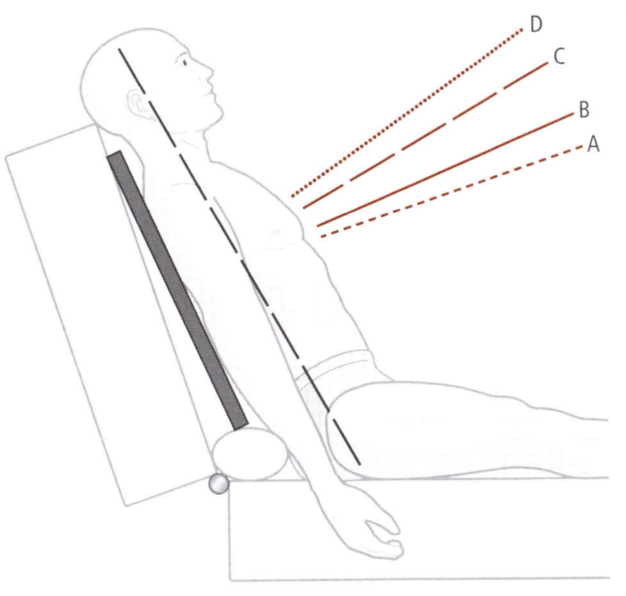

FIGURE 8-8

Common causes for lordotic views of the AP (D) chest include the subconscious tendency to angle the CR perpendicular to the back of the bed or gurney C or the plate B, neither of which is perpendicular to the patient's midcoronal plane as in A. Slight caudal angulation, perpendicular to the sternum, is always recommended on AP projections.

Image redrawn from Carroll, Q., Practical Radiographic Imaging, 8th Ed., 2007, Figure 32-2, Courtesy of Charles C Thomas, Publisher, Ltd., Springfield, Illinois

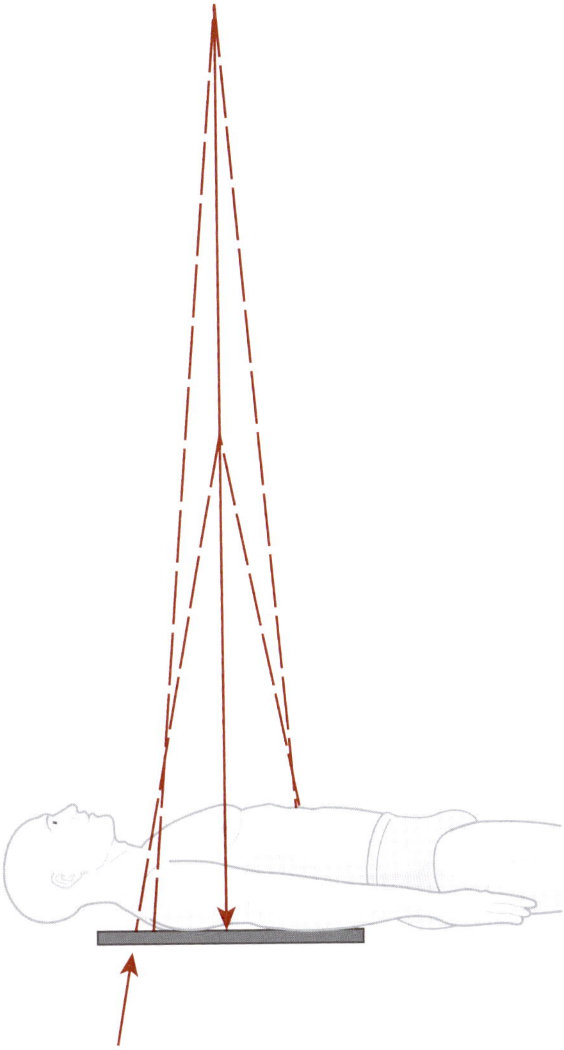

FIGURE 8-9

A reduced SID necessitated by supine AP chest projections results in upward projection of the shoulder shadows due to the increased beam divergence. Less of the IR plate or field light should be visible above the patient's shoulders than for a 72-inch PA chest.

BEST PRACTICE TIP

For the AP sitting projection of the chest taken at an SID of 72 inches (180 cm), always angle the CR perpendicular to the sternum.

If an SID of 40 inches (100 cm) cannot be avoided, angle downward an additional 3° to the sternum such that the CR appears slightly caudal to the patient's sternum.

beam divergence caused by a substantially reduced SID. When one adds all of these geometrical factors to the anatomical factors previously mentioned, the recommended total caudal angle falls at 5°–6° *caudal* relative to the IR for *any* 72-inch (180-cm) AP chest, and at 8°–9° *caudal* relative to the IR for *any* 40-inch (100-cm) AP chest—an angle that *includes* 3° caudal placement relative to the patient's sternum.

For the AP sitting projection of the chest taken at an SID of 72 inches (180 cm), always angle the CR perpendicular to the sternum. If an SID of 40 inches (100 cm) cannot be avoided, angle downward an additional 3° to the sternum such that the CR appears slightly caudal to the patient's sternum.

What about the issue of using a horizontal beam to demonstrate any fluid levels? Whenever it is feasible in mobile and trauma situations to sit the patient all the way up, this should be done so that a near-horizontal beam can be used to demonstrate fluid levels. Here, we define "near horizontal" as within 10° of horizontal. This allows some flexibility as trauma situations demand for the AP chest projection. With the IR plate perfectly vertical, a 5°–9° downward angle can still be used, and with the plate tilted 5° backward (a more common situation), the beam can still be angled 10° downward with reasonable results. Of course, by definition, most mobile and trauma patients will be too ill to sit up within 5° of vertical, and in these cases they must be radiographed supine or semierect using the geometry demonstrated in Figure 8-8 and Figure 8-10. Be sure to mark semierect and supine positions accurately so the radiologist knows what to expect in regard to the demonstration of any fluid levels.

The Supine Mobile Chest

When the AP chest projection must be taken with the patient *supine* on a gurney or bed, the SID is forcibly reduced to a range of 40–52 inches. This has implications for both *angulation* and *centering* of the x-ray beam. As described for sitting chest projections in the previous section, an *additional* 3° of caudal angle is needed to counter the effects of increased beam divergence.

BEST PRACTICE TIP

For the AP supine projection of the chest taken at 40 inches (100 cm), always angle the CR caudally 3° to the sternum, such that the CR appears slightly caudal to the patient's sternum.

This places the total CR angle at 8°–9° relative to the horizontal IR.

For the AP supine projection of the chest taken at 40 inches (100 cm), always angle the CR caudally 3° to the sternum, such that the CR appears slightly caudal to the patient's sternum. This places the total CR angle at 8°–9° relative to the horizontal IR.

Centering is also affected because, as shown in Figure 8-9, this reduced SID results in increased upward divergence of the shoulder shadows (due to normal magnification geometry of the entire chest). It then appears that there is less of the IR plate or field light extending above the shoulders, and inexperienced radiographers will tend to pull the CR cassette or DR detector plate up higher to compensate. This should not be done, as it only risks clipping off the bases of the lungs (which are also being projected further downward due to the same magnification geometry) at the lower edge of the IR.

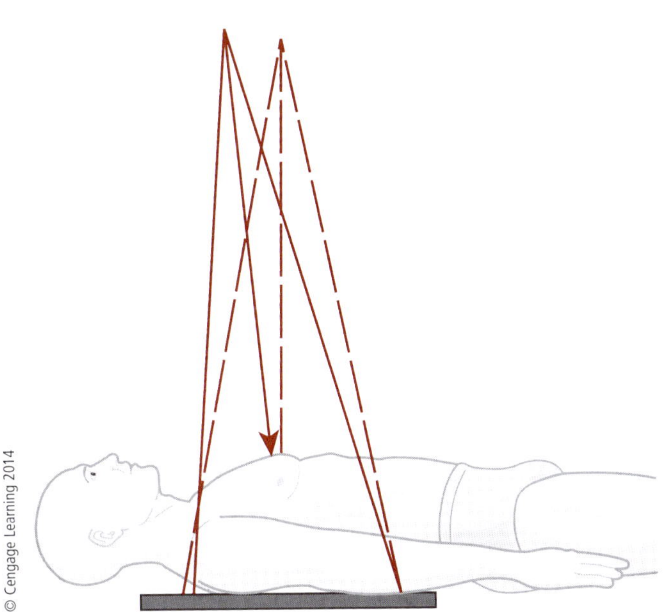

FIGURE 8-10
For supine AP chest projections, 5°–8° caudal angulation of the CR (solid line) minimizes the effect shown in Figure 8-12, and also ensures that a lordotic projection will not result.

At these shorter distances, *allow less of the IR plate and less field light above the shoulder shadows* than would normally be done at 72-inch SID. Note that while it is common to leave perhaps 1½ inches of the IR plate above the shoulders for a routine 72-inch PA chest in the department, for mobile AP chests the common practice is to leave only about ½ inch of the IR above the shoulders. Note too, that the use of a 5°–8° caudal angle on the x-ray beam reduces the upward divergence of the shoulder shadow, and so reduces the tendency to incorrectly pull the plate up too high. This is shown in Figure 8-10.

For the AP supine projection of the chest, allow less light field above the shoulder shadow than for a 72-inch (100-cm) sitting chest, only about ½ inch.

BEST PRACTICE TIP

For the AP supine projection of the chest, allow less light field above the shoulder shadow than for a 72-inch (100-cm) sitting chest, only about ½ inch.

Studies have demonstrated that most patients' lung fields are wider than they are long.[1] When there is any doubt, place the IR *crosswise*. Also, a fuller inspiration is usually achieved by exposing the image on the patient's *second* full breath. For very large chests or abdomens, if the image turns out poorly, try a 12-inch air gap technique (see Chapter 13). It really works!

Efficiency in Performing the Mobile Chest

There are many facets of the AP chest that bear discussion, such as placing the IR behind the patient correctly, measuring distance, collimation, and the side-to-side tube angle (which, when it is off, is the most distinct cause of grid cut-off). *A carefully planned order of operations will avoid repeating any move twice.* That order will always

[1] Bontrager, Kenneth. *Textbook of Radiographic Positioning and Related Anatomy*, 5th ed. (St. Louis, Missouri: Mosby, Inc., 2001).

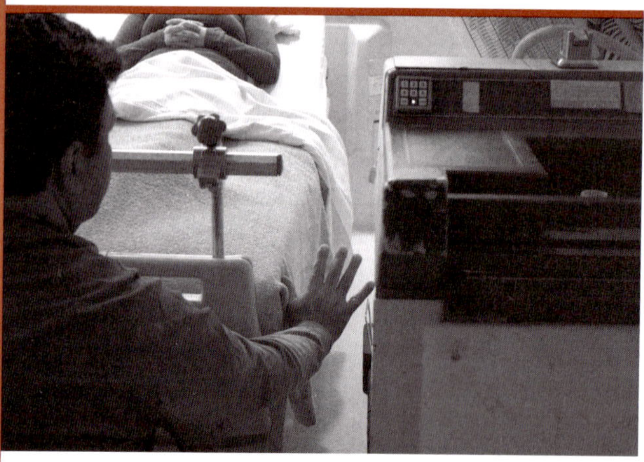

FIGURE 8-11
Mobile AP chest: Always start with the side of the mobile unit at least one hand-spread away from the side of the bed.

be the quickest and most efficient. The following sequence is strongly recommended:

1. When the mobile unit is brought into a patient's room, it is always best to keep the machine, bed, patient, and IR plate all at square (90°) angles to each other. By keeping the portable machine in alignment with the bed, you will be better able to see the side-to-side angle later on. If there is room, begin by parking the machine so that the side of the portable is at least 6–8 inches (about the distance of spread fingers) from the edge of the bed (Figure 8-11). This will allow the x-ray tube movement to cover the entire width of the bed so that if the patient is not centered on the bed, but is off to the right or left side, the tube position can be adjusted without moving the whole machine. For example, if the x-ray machine is too close to the bed, and the patient is off-center toward the x-ray machine, you may find that when the tube arm is swung out the tube will already be past the patient's midsagittal line (and the midline of any grid being used, causing grid cut-off). In this case, realignment of the general position of the mobile unit will be required, wasting time and effort.
2. Park the mobile unit so that the front edge of the tower is aligned with the bottom edge of the bed as shown in Figure 8-12. Most patients rest in bed with the head up approximately 25° (Figure 8-13). If the patient's bed is at this angle when you arrive and you follow this guideline, when the bed is later raised all the way up (to 60°), the IR will be close to 72 inches (180 cm) from the focal spot. The end of the bed moves in toward the tube as the bed is being raised. With the bed raised to 60°, the center of the x-ray tube will be about one foot (11 inches or 28 cm) from the foot panel of the bed. This forms a true 72-inch (180-cm) distance to the IR with the patient sitting at 70°.

   At this time, with the head of the bed still raised about 25°, swivel the vertical tube stand, bringing the x-ray tube around to the center area of the foot of the bed. Turn on the collimator light and center to the patient as a preliminary step. While the

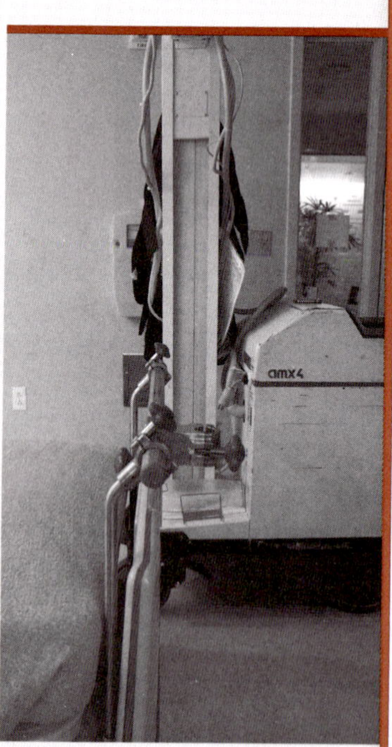

FIGURE 8-12
With the bed at a typical 25° angle as shown in Figure 8-13, placing the tower of the mobile unit at the foot of the bed will result in a 72-inch (180-cm) SID when the bed is fully raised.

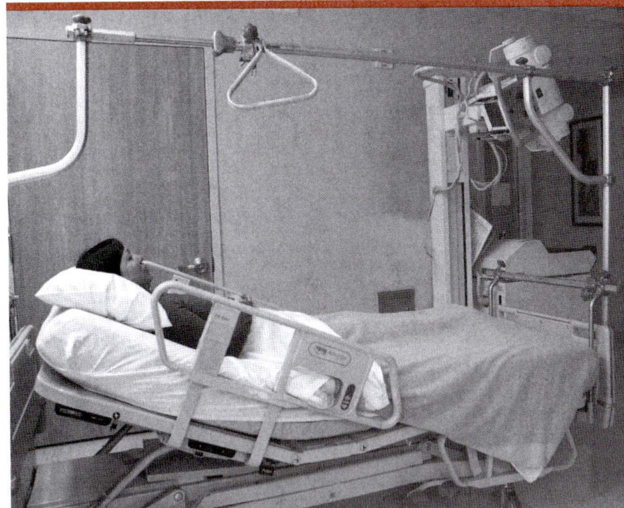

FIGURE 8-13

The patient's bed is most commonly positioned at a 25° angle.

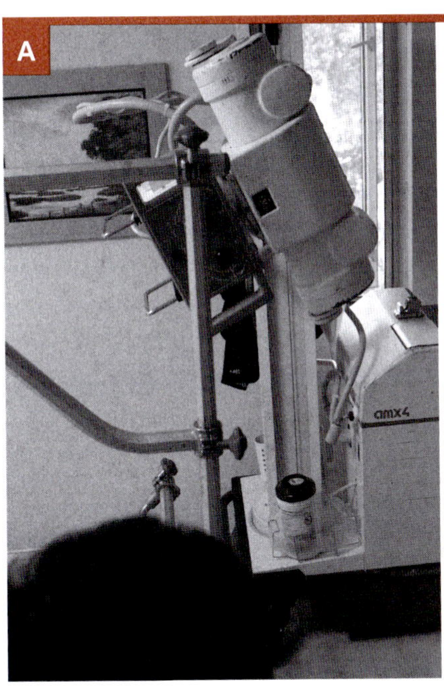

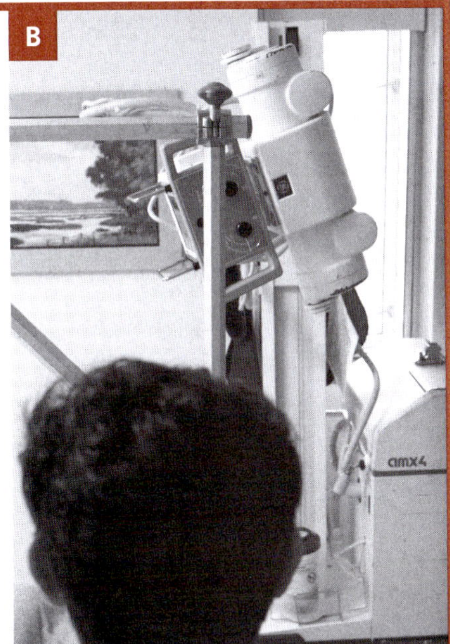

FIGURE 8-14

Standing directly to the side of the foot of the bed, the face of the collimator should appear in perfect profile **A**, rather than angled away or toward you **B**.

bed is still set at about 25°, align yourself exactly to the side of the foot of the bed as shown in Figure 8-14. From this vantage point, the face of the x-ray tube collimator should appear exactly parallel to the foot panel of the bed. For example, if you can see the surface of the window face of the collimator, the tube must be angled somewhat toward you (Figure 8-14*B*). The face of the collimator should be in lateral profile to your position.

3. Always assess the patient size and set the radiographic technique at the machine console prior to disturbing the patient. The technique used will vary between CR and DR systems, and will also depend on whether or not a grid is used.
4. After general tube alignment is checked and the technique set, the bed can be raised the rest of the way. Next, place the

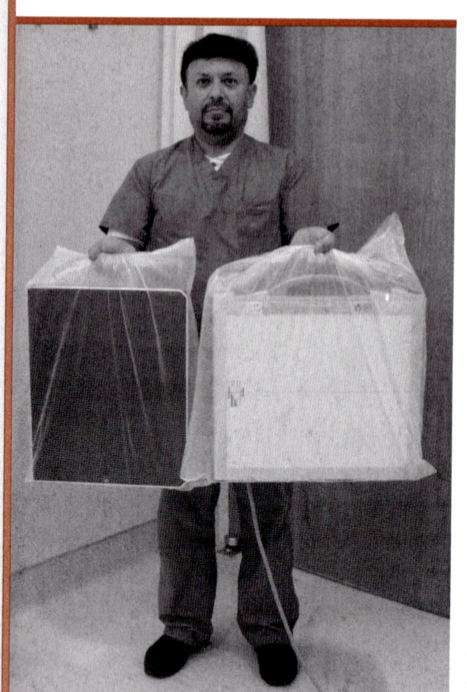
© Dennis Bowman

FIGURE 8-15

Ferlic SLIDER-ers™ *bags* can sustain the weight of modern DR detectors and greatly facilitate moving the detector behind or under the patient.

IR plate in a pillowcase or bag. (Ferlic SLIDER-ers™ bags are highly recommended. They are slippery, which facilitates moving the IR around behind the patient, and very durable. Figure 8-15 shows a $100,000, 16-pound DR detector and grid being supported by nothing but the SLIDER-ers™ bag.) All tethered DR detectors are too big to fit into a regular pillowcase, so some kind of plastic bag will need to be used.

5. To place the IR behind the patient, first assess how upright the patient can be tolerably raised. Most patients can sit up at 70°. (Most beds can be raised to 60°, and an additional 10° is obtained by placing a pillow behind the IR.) Lean the patient forward and place the covered IR behind the patient. (Remember that with heavy DR detectors, it may be easier to slide the detector *down* from behind and above the patient rather than in from the side.) Make sure the IR plate is centered side to side and top to bottom. Since the lowermost position of the patient's diaphragms is unknown, do not waste room at the top of the IR. It is recommended that ¾–1 inch of the IR plate be allowed above the top of the shoulders (Figure 8-16).
6. Side-to-side centering of the IR must be checked at two levels. At the top, make sure that the edges of the patient's shoulders are equidistant from the sides of the IR plate. To check the bottom, have the patient move her arms to the side, and place your palms against the sides of her ribcage with your fingertips touching the IR (Figure 8-17). Slide your hands to palpate the edges of the IR plate—they should fall off each side of the IR

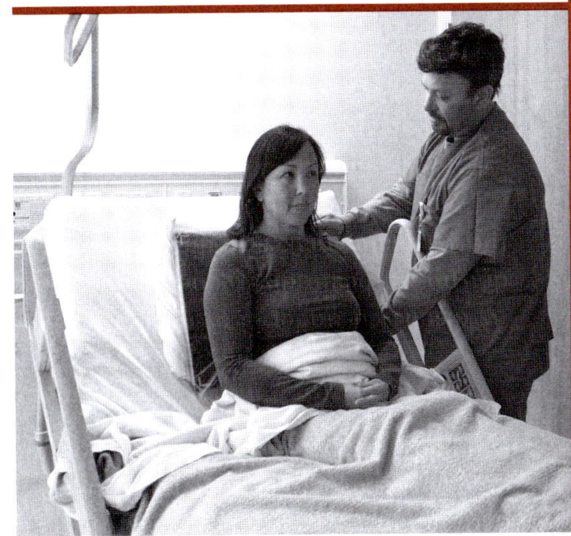
© Dennis Bowman

FIGURE 8-16
Allow ¾–1 inch of the detector above the patient's shoulders.

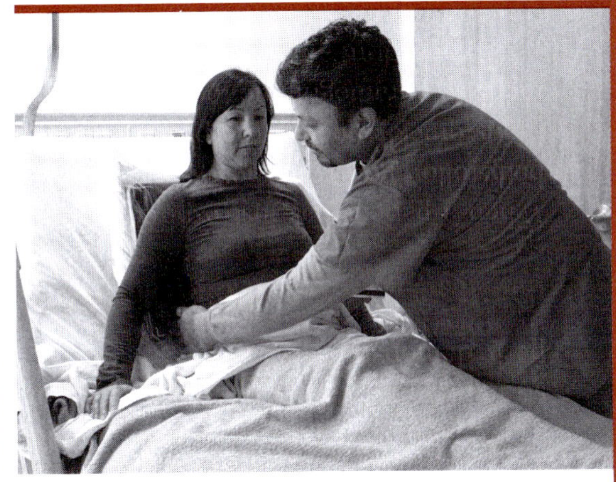
© Dennis Bowman

FIGURE 8-17
To check alignment of the bottom portion of the DR detector, place your palms against each side of the patient's ribcage, and then slide your hands outward equally to see if they "fall off" the detector at the same time.

at the same time. Adjust the IR plate as needed to place these edges equidistant from the patient's sides.

7. Adjust the height of the x-ray tube, and the angle perpendicular or slightly caudal to the patient's sternum as described in the previous section. Check the SID using the tape measure usually attached to the collimator (Figure 8-18), and correct the distance as needed by moving the *entire machine* forward or back, then recenter the tube vertically as needed, double-checking side-to-side alignment. As long as the patient is raised 50° or more, a 72-inch SID can be achieved. This is always the goal because the heart will be demonstrated with negligible magnification (about 3%, which is statistically insignificant and allows the radiologist to take measurements directly off of a proportional (14- × 17-inch or 35- × 43-cm) monitor screen.

In some areas, radiographers have gotten into the habit of bringing a mobile machine alongside the middle portion of the patient's bed, raising the bed only 45°, and then raising the

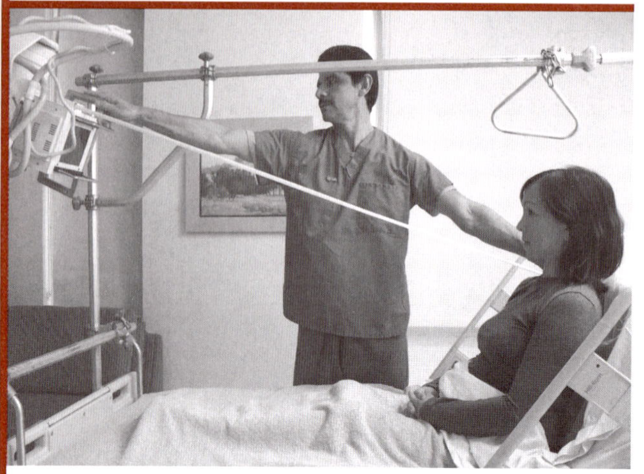
© Dennis Bowman

FIGURE 8-18
A final check of the SID can be made using the tape measure on the collimator. To adjust the SID at this time, the *entire mobile unit* must be moved forward or backward, then the tube must be adjusted vertically.

x-ray tube as high as it will go and angling 45° to match the bed angle. This is very poor practice for several reasons and should be discouraged. The important point for this discussion is that the resulting SID is about 55 inches (140 cm) and introduces an unacceptable degree of magnification of the heart for accurate diagnosis. A proper SID of 72 inches (180 cm) can never be achieved unless the mobile unit is backed up to the foot of the bed just as described in #2 above. By ensuring that the SID is a true 72 inches (180 cm), the following step #8 is greatly facilitated.

8. Next, it is *critical* to check the side-to-side angle in connection with side-to-side centering. It is common for the tube to be facing slightly toward the right or the left such that it is not perfectly perpendicular with the patient and the IR.

If you completely followed the procedure in step #2, the mobile unit was parked so that the front edge of the tower was aligned with the foot of the bed before fully raising the bed, and the alignment of the x-ray tube was checked at that time, so that now all that will be needed is to fine-center the light field to the patient. As you move the collimator to center the field, take care not to swivel the tube in any way, just push or pull it transversely—otherwise the alignment will be thrown off. This whole procedure is recommended.

However, in the event that you use any other SID (other than 72-inch or 180-cm), there is a *universal* method for checking proper alignment of the x-ray tube, in which you sight right down the central ray from behind the x-ray tube, using the center of the foot of the bed as a guide. The best vantage point from which to see this angle is to stand at least 5 feet (1½ m) directly back behind the tube so that you are exactly perpendicular to and centered to the tube face, sighting right down the CR as shown in Figure 8-19A. In this figure, you can see that the tube face is angled toward the right side of the patient. The further back at a distance you position yourself, the easier it will be to see if the tube face is parallel with the IR.

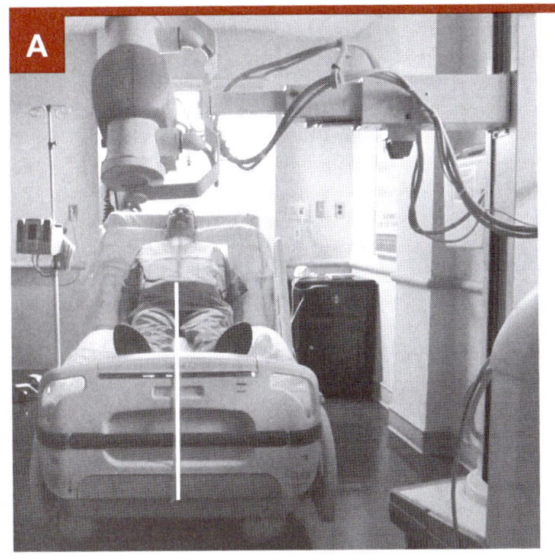

Courtesy of Quinn B. Carroll

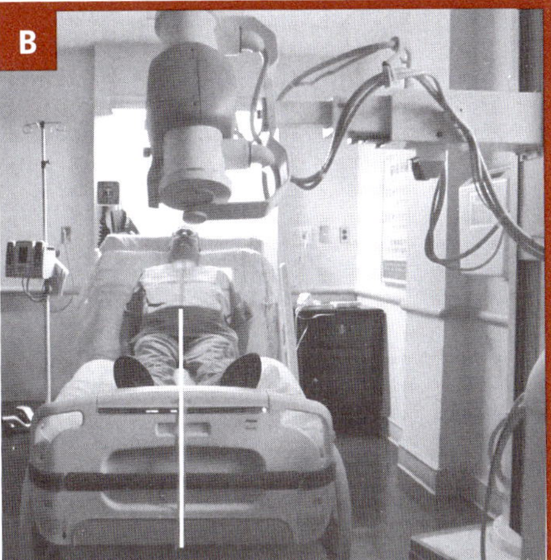

Courtesy of Quinn B. Carroll

FIGURE 8-19

To make a final check that the beam is not angled side-to-side, back up from the foot of the bed and visualize a line through its center. If the x-ray tube is not in this line **A**, *even though the field may be centered on the patient it indicates that the beam is angled and will result in a rotated view.* The tube must be recentered to this line **B**, and *then* re-angled side-to-side to bring the center of the field back to the center of the patient.

The patient is nearly always centered in the bed. When this is the case, just *be sure that the x-ray tube itself is centered to the center of the foot of the bed* before *adjusting the side-to-side angle,* as shown in Figure 8-19. It is a common mistake when working up close to the patient, to simply observe the centering of the light field on the patient's chest and *assume* that if the crosshairs of the field are centered, the central ray is perpendicular. In fact, when the crosshairs are not exactly centered on the patient, some radiographers will *angle* the x-ray tube to correct this, rather than recentering it, thus creating a slightly rotated view of the chest. This is avoided by keeping the tube centered to the foot of the bed while adjusting the side-to-side angle, because patients are nearly always centered in their bed.

Finally, adjust the vertical (head-to-foot) angle, then center the light field vertically. Once centered, the field may be collimated. The light field should appear symmetrical to the patient, as shown in Figure 8-20.

Many facilities now use a grid for AP chests on medium and large patients, so accuracy in angulation and centering becomes much more important. The conventional grid has the grid lines running lengthwise, which places them horizontally on crosswise placement (Figure 8-21*A*). This means that if the vertical (head-to-foot) angle is not perpendicular with the grid, grid cut-off will result. This is why a "short axis" or "decubitus" grid was developed, in which the grid lines run crosswise, as shown in Figure 8-21*B*. When the grid itself is placed crosswise behind the patient, there is freedom of movement

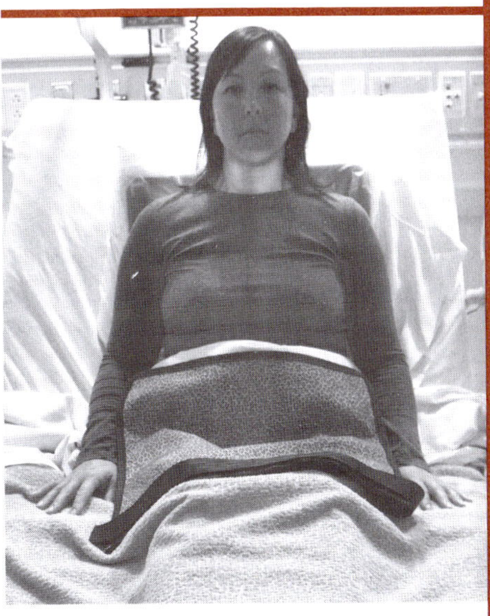

© Dennis Bowman

FIGURE 8-20

Final check with the field symmetrical on the patient.

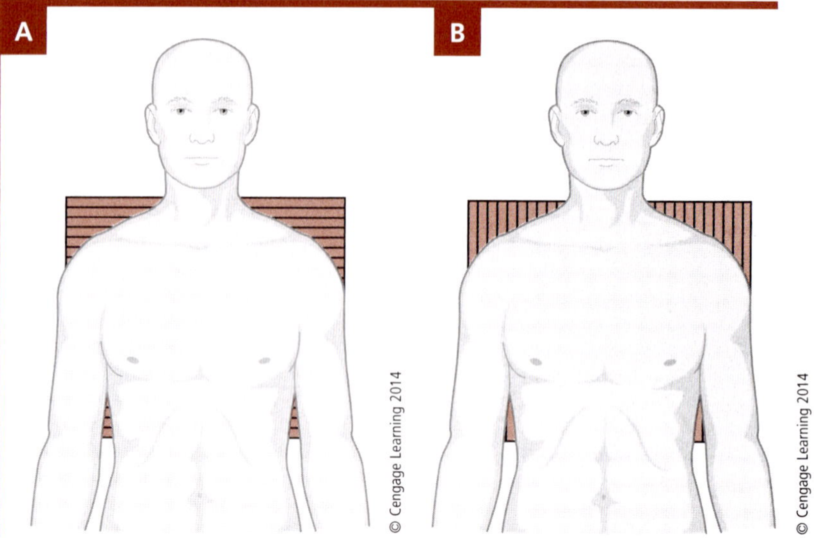

FIGURE 8-21

A conventional grid placed crosswise to the patient for an AP projection of the chest **A**, allows no flexibility for vertical angulation of the x-ray beam. The *short-axis* or *decubitus* grid **B**, is recommended to allow this freedom of movement.

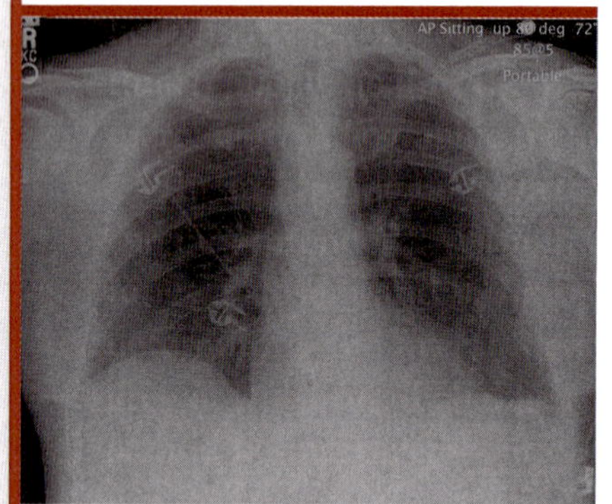

FIGURE 8-22

Properly positioned AP mobile chest radiograph, showing no lordotic distortion, and no rotation from improper side-to-side angulation of the beam.

Courtesy of Community Hospital of the Monterey Peninsula, Diagnostic and Interventional Radiology

in the vertical dimension, both for angling and for centering. Since downward (caudad) tube angulation runs *with* the grid lines, there will not be any risk of grid cut-off.

Figure 8-22 demonstrates a well-positioned and properly exposed AP chest image taken with a mobile unit, following all of these steps. Note that with the correct, slightly caudal angle on the central ray, no lordotic straightening of the ribs or spine is apparent, and all anatomy is properly demonstrated.

Postmortem Chest Technique

When a patient has just expired, within moments fluids throughout the body follow gravity to the lowest point. With the patient lying supine, chest fluids quickly pool in the posterior lungs across the entire lung field. An increase in radiographic technique is required to penetrate these fluids.

In addition, a postmortem chest is by definition an *expiration* chest (no pun intended). Without a full breath, the normal insufflation of the lungs is absent and *this* must be added to the accumulation of fluid in determining the overall density of the chest to be penetrated. The degree of this overall change is frequently underestimated. The mAs used should be increased by 35%–50% *on the first attempt*.

Lateral Chest with Patient Supine or Semisitting

As discussed under "Lowering the Image Receptor" in the Chapter 7, downward beam divergence, added to the imposition of the edging of the IR plate, makes it difficult not to clip the lowest portion of the downside anatomy on any horizontal beam projection. On the mobile lateral projection, the backs of the lungs may be clipped. On a gurney with pad and backboard, if possible, with the image receptor at the side of the pad, press the IR down below the level of the backboard. On a bed, have an assistant press the IR down into the mattress. If this is not feasible, center somewhat posterior on the patient and open the field vertically (ceiling to floor) to compensate.

Portable Abdomen

Positioning for the portable abdomen is completely different from the portable chest position. Since the bed is flat and the patient completely recumbent, a number of things can already be completed on the portable machine before the patient is even moved. It is best to park the machine at the foot of the bed so that assistants will have room to help roll the patient. Assess the patient and set the radiographic technique at the console. With the machine parked at the foot, swing the tube out so that the distance can be measured as shown in Figure 8-23*A*, and the tube checked to be parallel with the floor in both dimensions, Figure 8-23*B*.

Before rolling the patient up, the IR should already be lined up to the proper place where it will go underneath the patient (Figure 8-24). If the patient is rolled all the way up and the IR slid as far as it will go against the patient's back, at least ¾ of the patient's body will cover the IR when the patient comes back down. The IR or the patient will then need to be slid only a marginal amount to complete centering. If a Ferlic SLIDER-ers™ bag has been used, it is very easy to slide the IR.

Now the tube can be centered to the IR. If the patient is wide and the sides of the IR are not visible, place both hands under the patient and mark both the top and bottom of the IR (Figure 8-25). Estimate the midway point between your two hands and move one hand up to

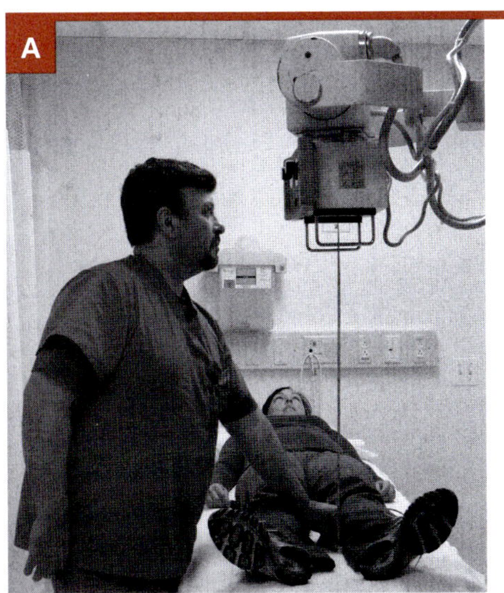

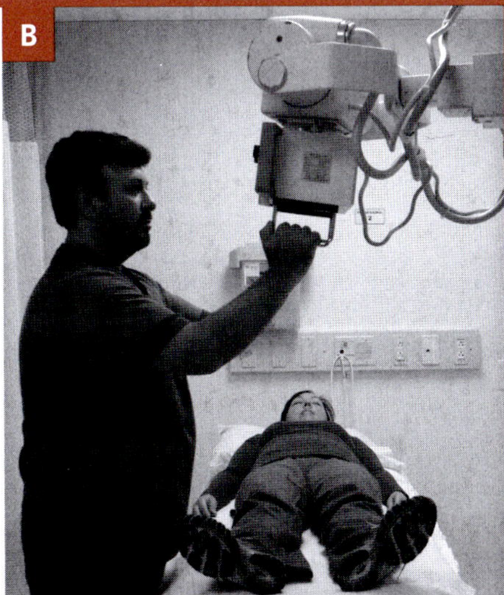

FIGURE 8-23
Mobile abdomen projection: Begin by measuring the distance **A**, then check that the face of the collimator is horizontal in both directions **B**.

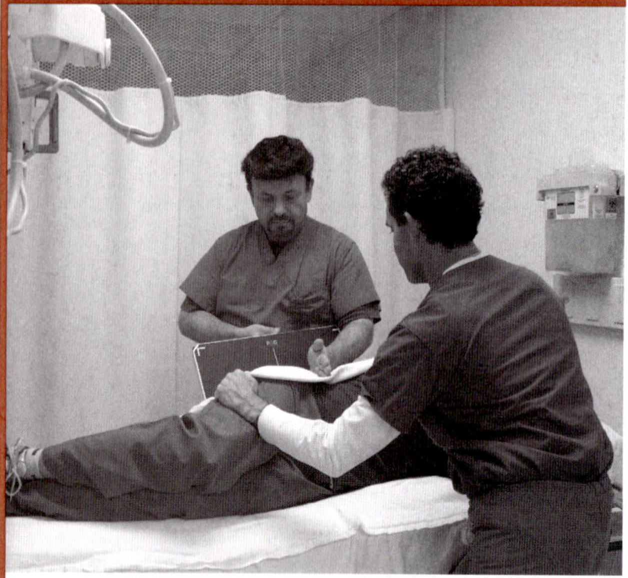

FIGURE 8-24
Mobile abdomen projection: Line the IR up with the iliac crest as it is slid as far as it will go under the rolled-up patient.

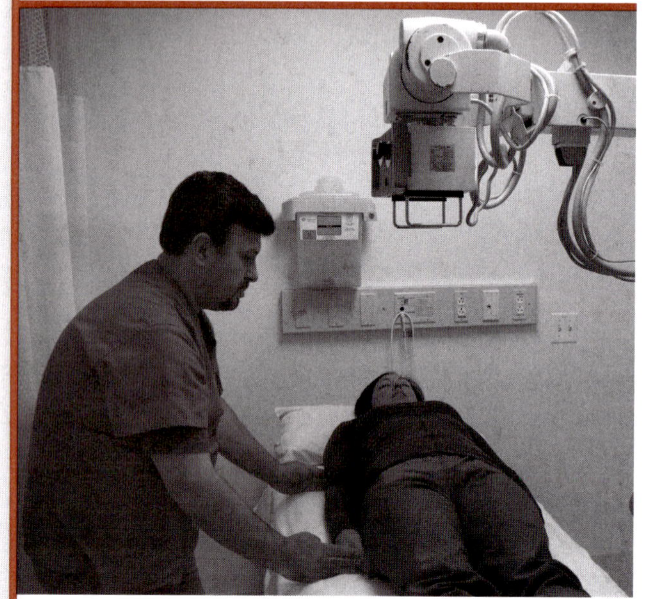

FIGURE 8-25
If the step in Figure 8-24 is followed, lengthwise centering of the x-ray tube can be determined by feeling for the top and bottom of the IR and finding the midpoint.

mark the middle. Using the other hand, move the tube until the CR is centered to your hand. Side-to-side centering and collimation can now be done.

TRAUMA POSITIONING TIPS FOR SPINE ANATOMY

Cervical Spine

All views of the cervical spine (except the swimmers or other views through the upper shoulder area) can generally be obtained nongrid, and this greatly facilitates cervical positioning for the trauma patient.

Trauma patients are typically lying on a gurney (stretcher) with a rigid backboard supported by the thick gurney pad. Often the IR plate can be carefully slid underneath the backboard without moving the patient or the backboard, by manually compressing the pad as the IR plate is slid in. Using this technique, it is significant to note that we are not limited to a single cross-table lateral projection, but that at least *three* cervical views can be obtained for initial screening of the trauma patient: the cross-table lateral, the AP, and the odontoid (see the following section). Indeed, even oblique C-spine views can be obtained with acceptable quality for trauma positions.

The cross-table lateral was discussed at the beginning of this chapter. A routine AP projection can be obtained but will not usually demonstrate C3 without raising the patient's chin.

The routine open-mouth "odontoid" projection for C1 and C2 may be attempted if the patient can open his mouth, but will very likely require some movement of the head to get a satisfactory view. The routine Fuchs method–for the odontoid – may be attempted if the patient can raise his chin until the orbitomeatal line (OML) is 35°–40° extended: Center a vertical CR just under the chin. When the patient cannot be moved, the following methods are recommended:

Modified AP: To demonstrate C3 through C7 *without moving the head*, increase the cephalic angle to 20°–25°. This desuperimposes the chin from C3. Slight distortion is acceptable because this view is still very valuable in the initial screening for displacement or fractures. (Note that for a normal, nontrauma AP projection of the cervical spine, a line from the mandibular mentum to the base of the skull is parallel to the CR. The added angulation here simply maintains this relationship.)

Modified Fuchs for Trauma Odontoid: Without moving the head, angle the CR 35°–40° cephalic (to the OML) and center just under the chin, collimating for a single vertebra (Figure 8-26). This projects the odontoid process nicely into the foramen magnum (Figure 8-27), and is sufficient to demonstrate alignment and gross fractures. (Small hairline fractures may be missed due to the upward-angled view, and the zygapophyseal joint between C1 and C2 is *not* demonstrated on this view, so more adequate projections *must* be taken after the patient is stabilized.)

Trauma Oblique: Angle 45° transversely and make the exposure *nongrid* (Figure 8-28). Most modern mobile units allow double angulation of the x-ray tube, so that a 15° cephalic angle can be added to the 45° transverse angle. If the machine does not allow

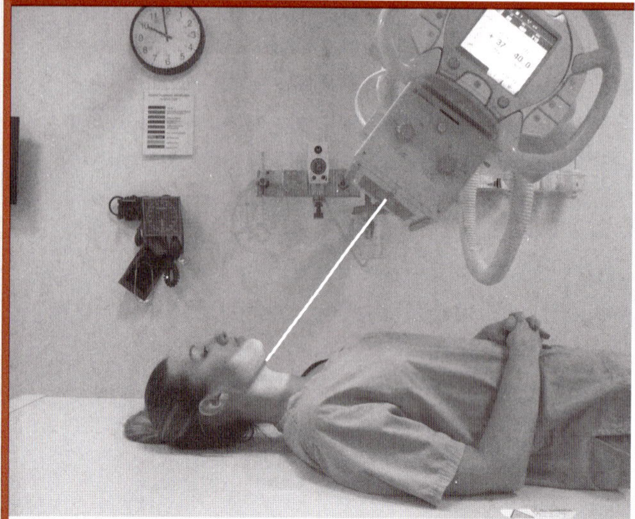

Courtesy of Quinn B. Carroll

FIGURE 8-26

Modified Fuchs position for the odontoid on a trauma patient, using 35°–40° cephalic angle centered just under the chin.

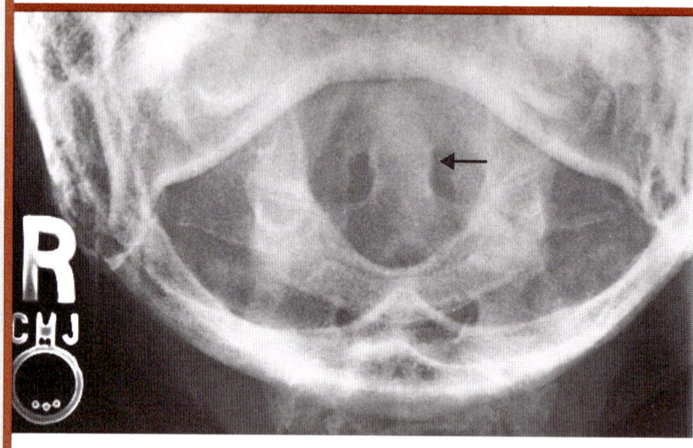

FIGURE 8-27

Modified Fuchs view of the odontoid (arrow).

Courtesy of Community Hospital of the Monterey Peninsula, Diagnostic and Interventional Radiology

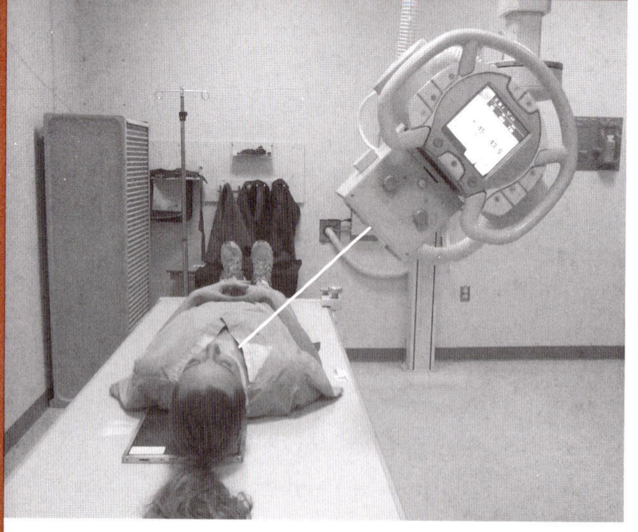

Courtesy of Quinn B. Carroll

FIGURE 8-28

Trauma oblique projection for the cervical spine, using transverse angulation.

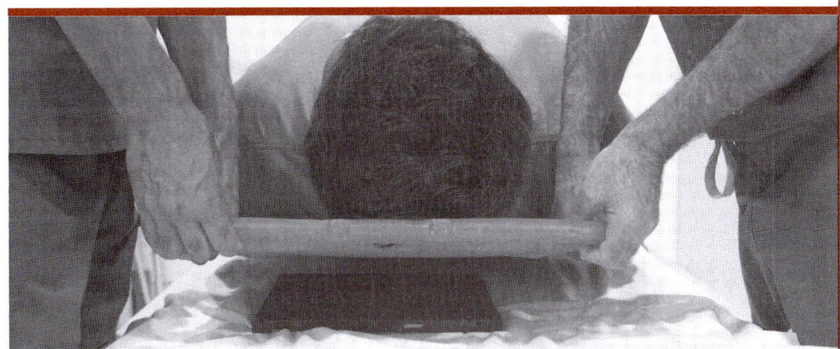

FIGURE 8-29

Placement of the IR under a backboard for the trauma oblique projection of the cervical spine: On the tube side, if the edge of the IR is placed directly below the side of the patient's neck, the opposite side of the IR will protrude by the proper amount to accommodate the angle of the beam (also shown in Figure 8-28).

double angulation, forego the usual 15° cephalic angle, which most radiologists will accept for a trauma position. (If using a grid, be sure to place it with the grid lines running *crosswise* to accommodate the angle.)

To maintain alignment with the CR, the IR plate must be accurately off-center, relative to the patient, in the direction the tube angle is facing. As shown in Figures 8-28 and 8-29, if the tube is angled from the right side, place the right edge of the IR so that it is even with the right edge of the patient's neck, with the rest of the IR plate protruding to the left side. Figure 8-29 shows this IR placement underneath the trauma backboard.

By leaving the x-ray tube at its normal *détente* height, magnification of the spine is reduced, which lowers the probability of clipping any anatomy of interest. However, because this is likely to result in an SID as much as 55 inches, *technique must be increased to compensate*. In a fixed x-ray room, swing the x-ray tube stand out 90° and angle the tube 45° laterally (Figure 8-30).

Center to the midcervical spine with the top edge of the collimated light field at the top of the ear (Figure 8-31).

With transverse angulation of the x-ray tube, lateral distortion will certainly be present in the image, as shown in Figure 8-32, but the view is sufficient for gross trauma screening.

Cross-Table Supine Reverse Swimmers: When the trauma patient lies supine, it is often more difficult to get the two shoulders raised and depressed enough, respectively, to fully

FIGURE 8-30

By leaving the x-ray tube at its normal *détente* height in spite of the angulation of the beam, magnification of the C-spine is minimized, which helps to include all vertebrae in the view. Technique must be increased by 35%.

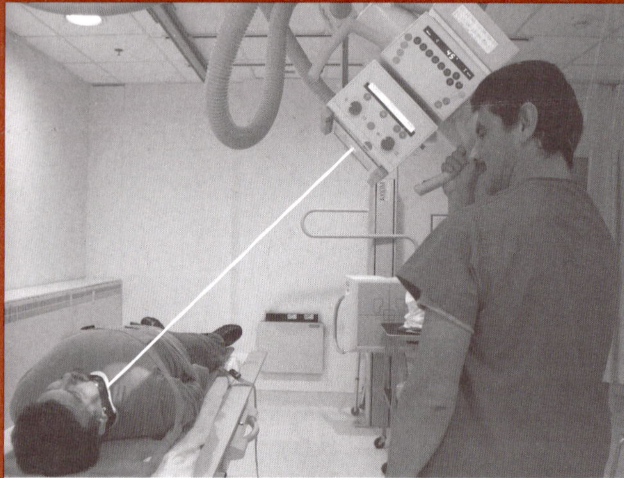

© Dennis Bowman

FIGURE 8-31

Trauma oblique C-spine: An 8 × 12-inch field can be centered with the top edge of the field at the top of the ear.

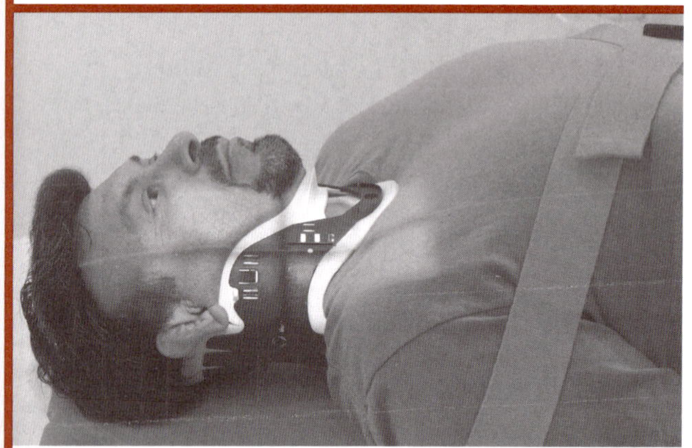

© Dennis Bowman

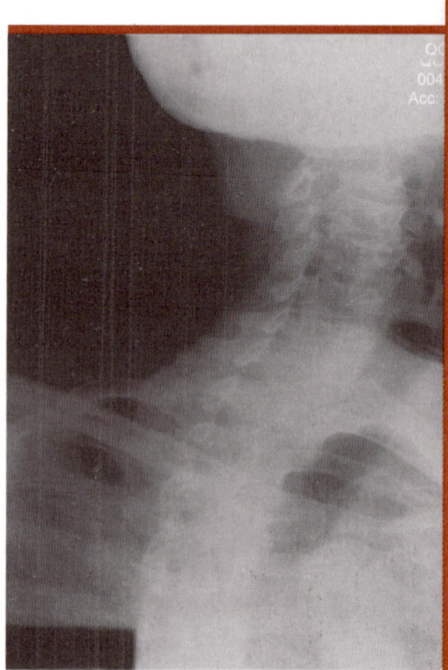

Courtesy of Quinn B. Carroll

FIGURE 8-32

Trauma oblique view of the cervical spine.

demonstrate the cervicothoracic vertebrae. For the standard swimmers projection, a 5° angle can be added to the central ray to help desuperimpose the shoulders from the spine. With the arm against the cassette or DR detector plate raised, use careful manual traction on the contrary arm to depress that shoulder, and angle 5° caudal as shown in Figure 8-33. Center the angled beam to the base of the neck.

There are occasions in which a swimmers projection is needed, but due to injury or pain the patient is unable to move the arm that would normally be raised above the head. This position can easily be reversed by placing careful traction on the arm that lies against the IR to depress that shoulder, and raising the opposite arm. Use a 5° *cephalic* angle, centered through the axilla, as demonstrated in Figure 8-34. Center the angled beam to the base of the neck.

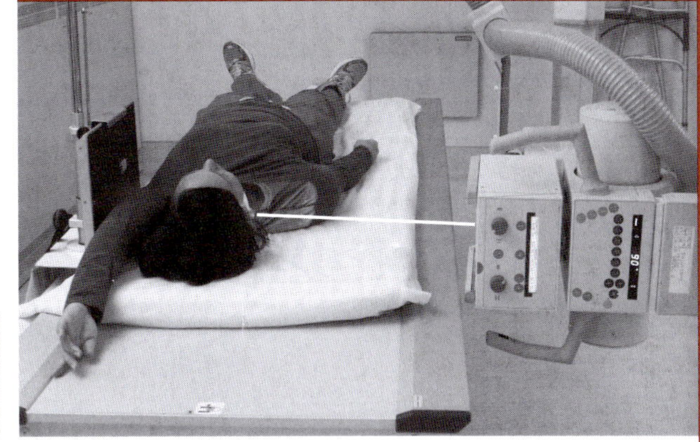

FIGURE 8-33
A cross-table swimmers projection, adding a 5° caudal angle to help desuperimpose the two shoulders.

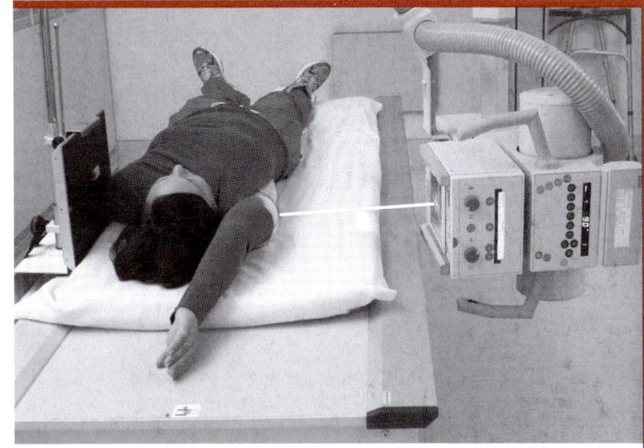

FIGURE 8-34
The alternate position, a reverse cross-table swimmers projection, using a 5° cephalic angle with the "upside" arm raised and the arm against the IR depressed.

Thoracic Spine

See Chapter 13 for significant technique tips for both the AP and lateral thoracic spine projections. Grids are not necessary on most patients for thoracic views.

For trauma screening, the AP chest view can be utilized. For a thin patient, a cross-table lateral projection of the T-spine can be difficult to obtain with the patient supine. The posteriormost spinous processes will likely be clipped, unless all of the recommendations for cross-table projections at the beginning of this chapter are taken into account.

Lumbar Spine

The cross-table lateral projection of the L-spine is not difficult to perform, but usually requires a grid, so vertical centering can become problematic. It is possible to obtain frontal and oblique views nongrid on thinner patients.

Trauma Oblique: Without moving the supine patient, angle 45° lateromedially, entering 4–5 inches lateral to the midsagittal plane (Figure 8-35). For thin patients, the exposure can be made *nongrid*. For large patients, place a gridded cassette

FIGURE 8-35

Trauma oblique projection of the lumbar spine, using a 45° transverse angle. Any grid used must be placed tabletop in a crosswise alignment for the grid strips.

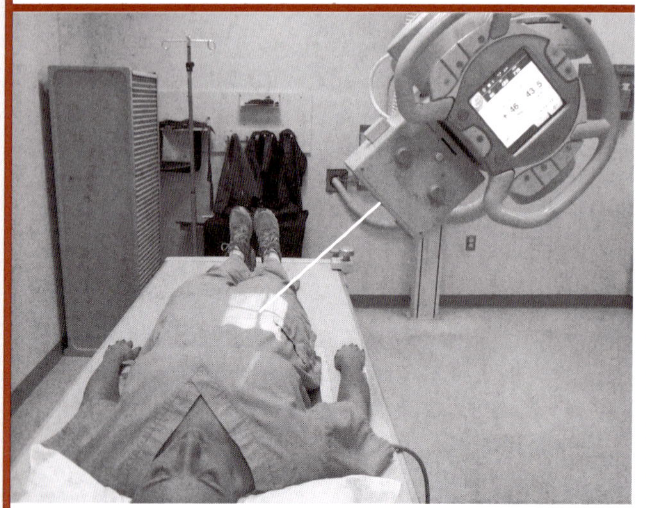

Courtesy of Quinn B. Carroll

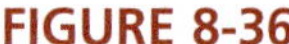

FIGURE 8-36

Projection for lumbar vertebral arches, using a 45° caudal angle.

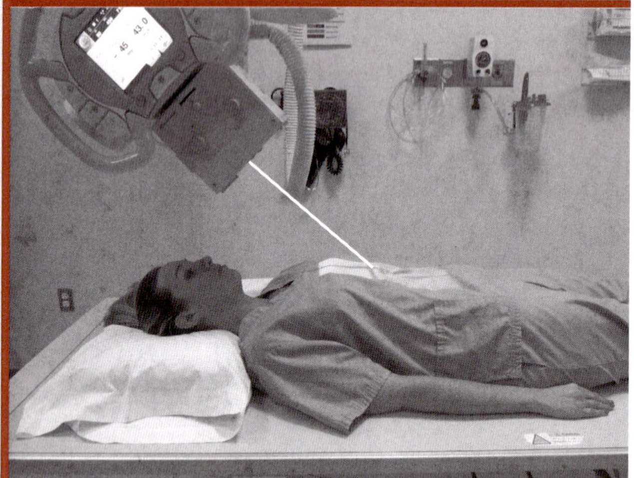

Courtesy of Quinn B. Carroll

crosswise on the tabletop and collimate side to side. (With CR, using the next larger plate size allows the plate to be placed crosswise while maintaining the lengthwise field length.)

Trauma Vertebral Arches of L-Spine: The laminae of the lumbar vertebral arches can be demonstrated with the patient supine by angling the CR 45° caudal, and centering 2 inches superior to the xiphoid process (Figure 8-36). Figure 8-37 is the cropped upper portion of a pelvic inlet view that demonstrates the effect of the 45° angle.

Trauma Oblique SI Joints: With the patient supine, angle 25°–30° lateromedially, entering just medial to the ASIS. For thin patients, do it *nongrid*; for large patients, place a gridded cassette *crosswise* on the tabletop and collimated side to side.

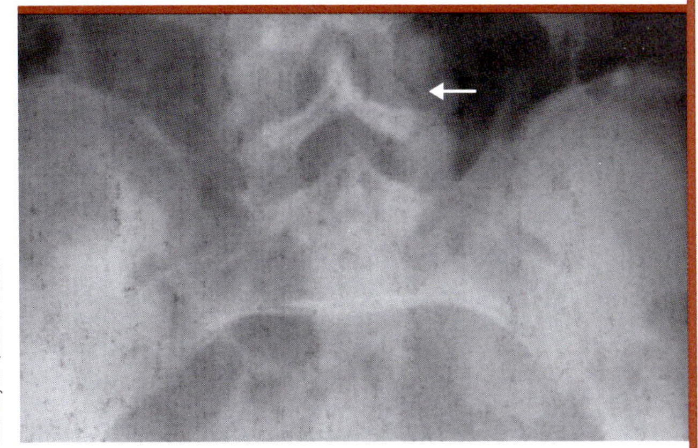

FIGURE 8-37
Pelvic inlet view demonstrating the lumbar vertebral laminae (arrow) by using a 45° caudal angle.

TRAUMA POSITIONING TIPS FOR TORSO ANATOMY AND GIRDLES

The trauma chest is discussed in an earlier section of this chapter. Trauma positions of the abdomen, including decubitus projections, do not require any changes in centering, angles, and so on from routine positions, nor do the routine shoulder series or single-view pelvis. These will not be discussed.

Trauma Unilateral Oblique Ribs: With the patient supine, angle 45° mediolaterally, *nongrid* (Figure 8-38). (The correct angle is mediolateral regardless of whether the projection is for posterior or anterior ribs, to avoid superimposition of the spine over the ribs. For a full discussion of routine rib positions, see Chapter 10.)

Trauma Oblique Sternum: With patient supine, use a right-to-left transverse angle of 20° through the sternum, *nongrid* (Figure 8-39).

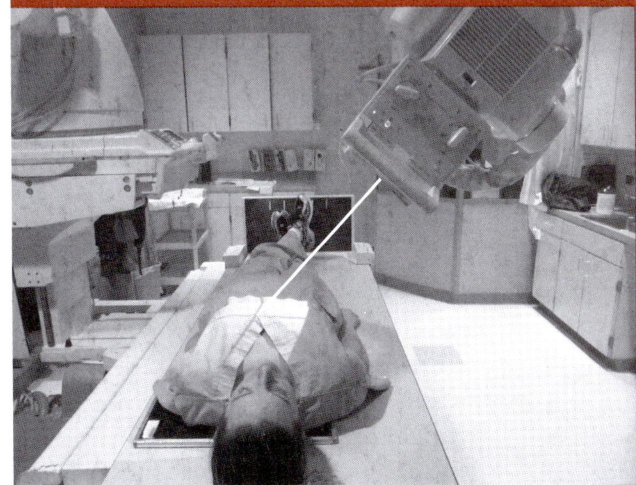

FIGURE 8-38
Trauma oblique projection of the ribs, using a transverse 45° angle.

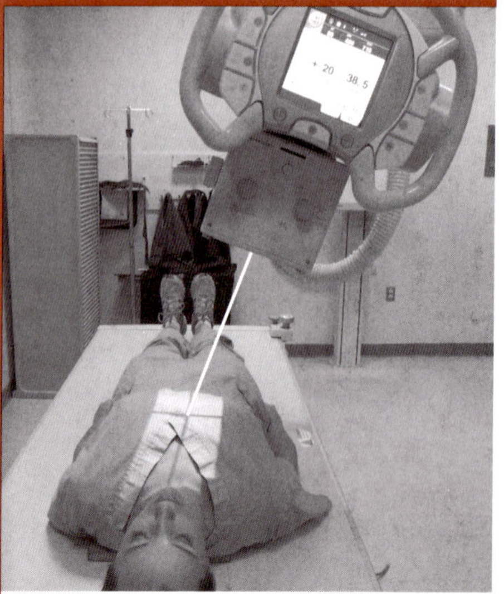

Courtesy of Quinn B. Carroll

FIGURE 8-39

Trauma oblique projection of the sternum, using a right-to-left transverse angle of 20°.

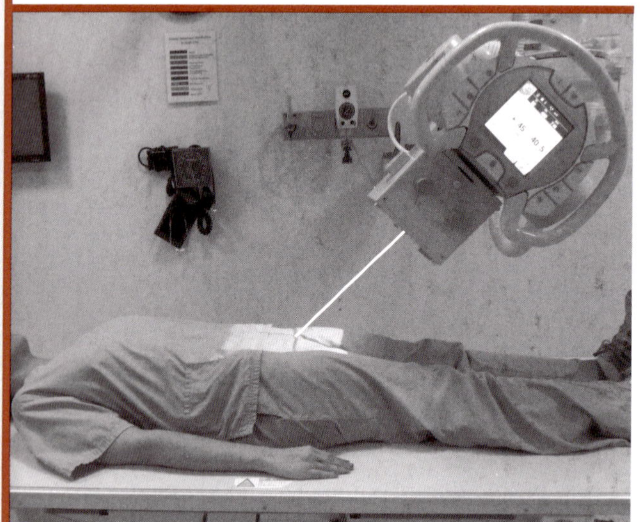

Courtesy of Quinn B. Carroll

FIGURE 8-40

Pelvic outlet projection, using a 45° cephalic angle.

Trauma Pelvis

Pelvic Outlet View: With the patient supine, angle the CR 45° (to 60°) *cephalic*, and centered to the symphysis pubis (3 inches inferior to the palpated ASIS), as shown in Figures 8-40 and 8-41. (This projection shows the femoral necks well.)

Pelvic Inlet View: With the patient supine, angle the CR 45° *caudal*, and center to the midsagittal plane at a level of the ASIS (Figures 8-42 and 8-43).

Modified Judet for Iliac Crests: When the patient's pelvis can be obliqued, bilateral views using the Judet position, shown in Figure 8-44, demonstrate fractures of each acetabulum and iliac wing from two viewpoints.

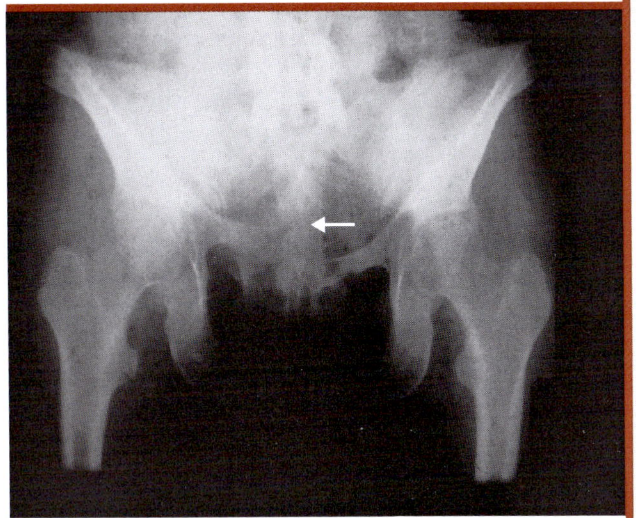

Courtesy of Quinn B. Carroll

FIGURE 8-41

Pelvic outlet view. Note face-on view of displacement of right pubic bone from fracture (arrow).

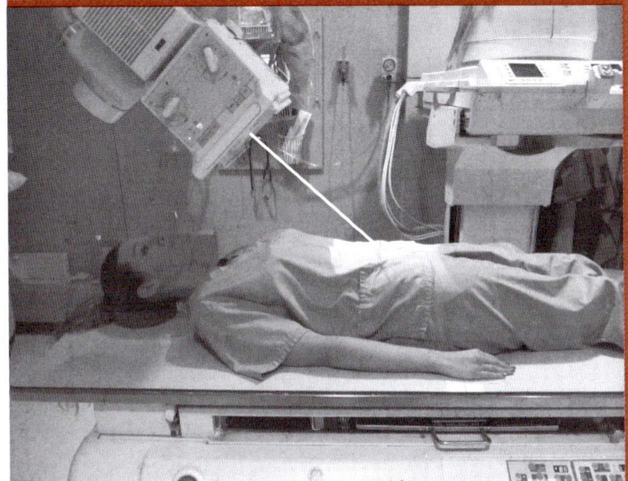

Courtesy of Quinn B. Carroll

FIGURE 8-42

Pelvic inlet projection, using a 45° caudal angle.

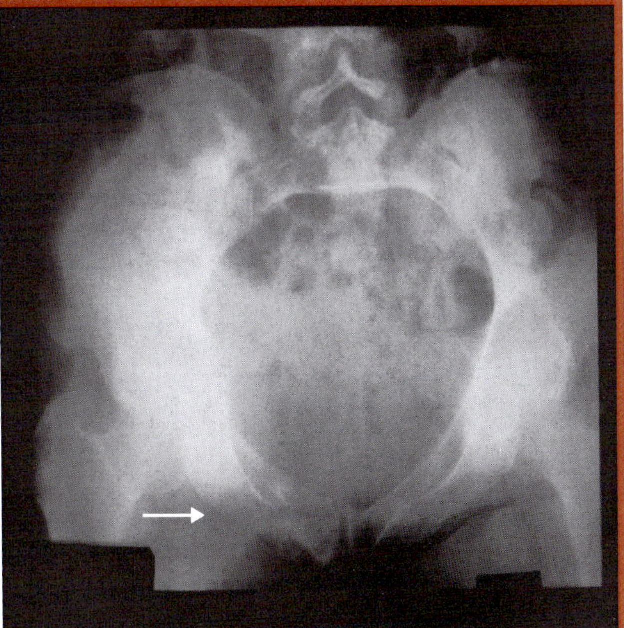

Courtesy of Quinn B. Carroll

FIGURE 8-43

Pelvic inlet view, showing end-on view of pubis with fractured right pubic bone (arrow).

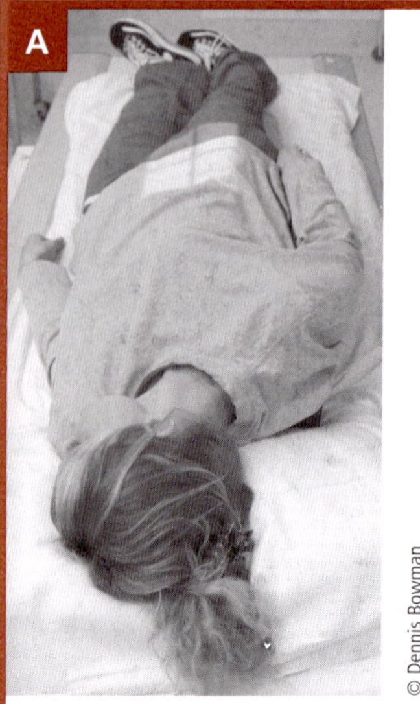

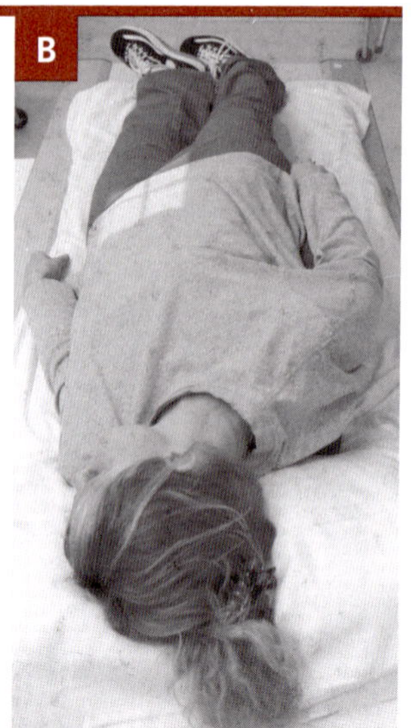

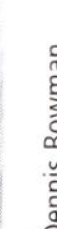

FIGURE 8-44

Judet position for iliac crests and acetabulum, using 45° of rotation, collimated and centered for **A**, the upside hip, and **B**, the downside hip.

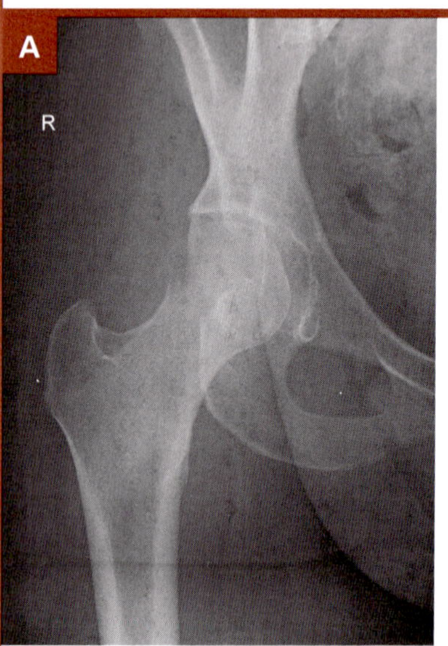

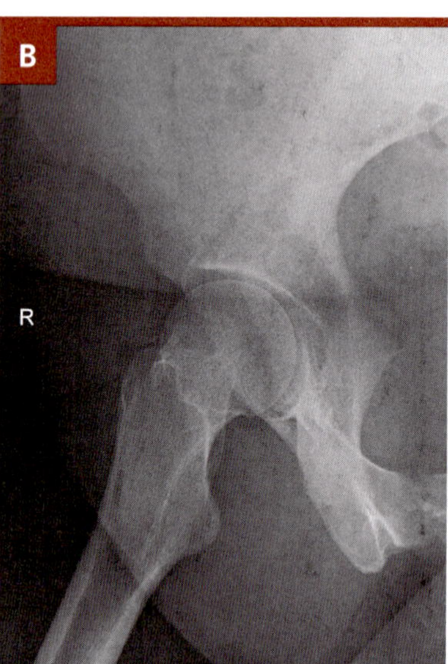

FIGURE 8-45

Collimated Judet views of the upside hip **A**, and downside hip **B**.

Courtesy of Community Hospital of the Monterey Peninsula, Diagnostic and Interventional Radiology

When the patient cannot be moved, a 45° transverse angle of the CR, as in Figure 8-35 but with the field opened, can be used if the gridded cassette is placed crosswise on the tabletop. One projection is taken with the CR angle directed mediolaterally, the other lateromedially. Sample views are provided in Figure 8-45.

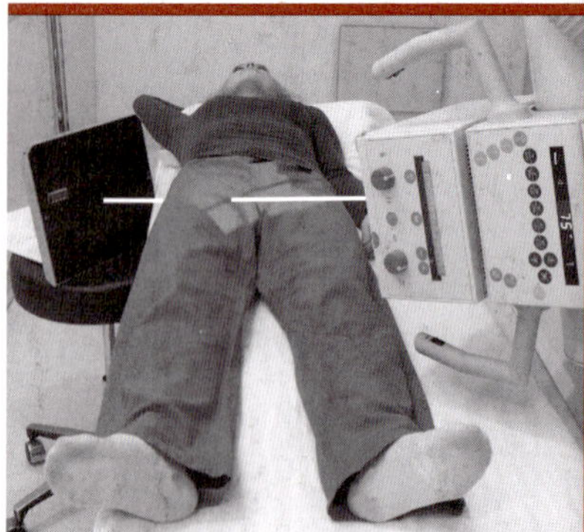

FIGURE 8-46

Standard Clements-Nakayama position for the trauma lateral hip, using 25° transverse and 15° downward angles.

Severe Trauma Lateral Hip: Patient Cannot Move Opposite Leg

Clements-Nakayama Method: Rest the CR cassette or IR plate against sponges at an approximate 25° angle from the midsagittal plane, and tilted back 15° (Figure 8-46), or have an associate hold the cassette in this position.

A horizontal x-ray beam is angled 25° cephalic from a cross-table lateral position, then angled 15° downward toward the floor, perpendicular to the cassette, and centered to the femoral neck.

Modified Clements-Nakayama Method: This is identical to the preceding position, only the CR is angled 25°–30° downward toward the floor (instead of 15°) to completely clear the contrary thigh (Figure 8-47). Keep the cassette or IR plate perpendicular to CR, and allow the affected side foot to remain in external rotation. A comparison of the two views is shown in Figure 8-49, along with an example (**C**) of how the view appears when a trauma patient typically has the leg externally rotated and the 25° modified method is used. Improved visibility of the affected femur is apparent with the 25° CR angle.

Note that this projection can be taken with the IR or CR cassette braced against the tabletop as in Figure 8-47, but this places the anatomy in the lower half of the IR (which can adversely affect digital image processing on some CR units). In order to center the anatomy to the IR, the cassette can be placed on a stool below the table level and braced against a cassette holder (Figure 8-48), and secured with a sandbag if needed. For this projection, the patient must be slid sideways to the edge of the table to avoid projecting the table itself onto the IR, which can also adversely affect digital processing. The views in Figure 8-49 were taken using this method.

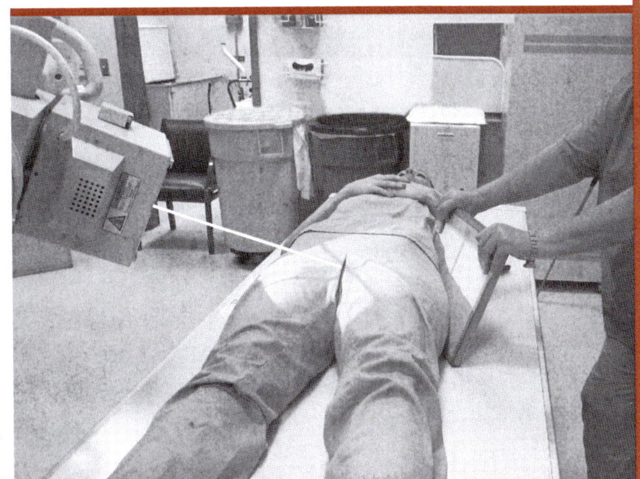

FIGURE 8-47
Modified Clements-Nakayama position for the trauma lateral hip, using 25° transverse and 25° downward angles.

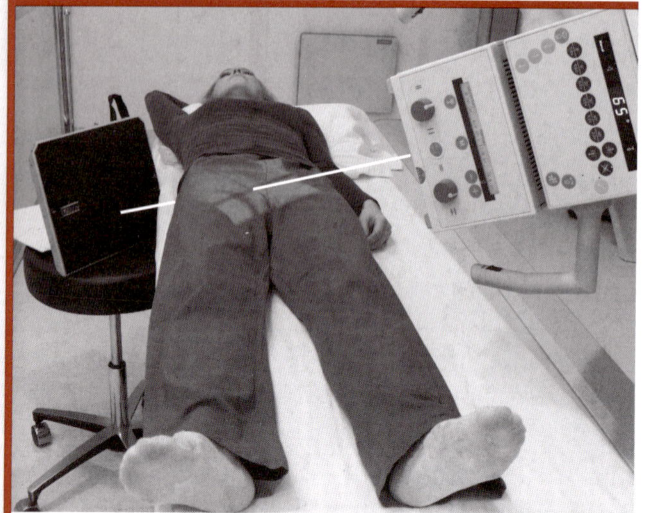

FIGURE 8-48

By securing the IR with sandbags on a stool below the level of the tabletop, the modified Clements-Nakayama projection can be taken with the field centered on the IR.

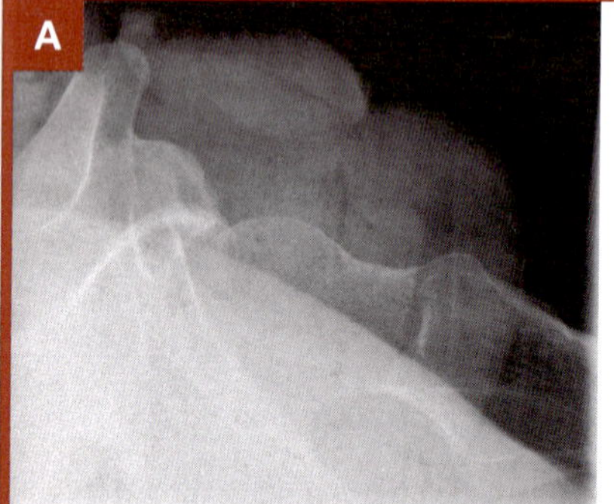

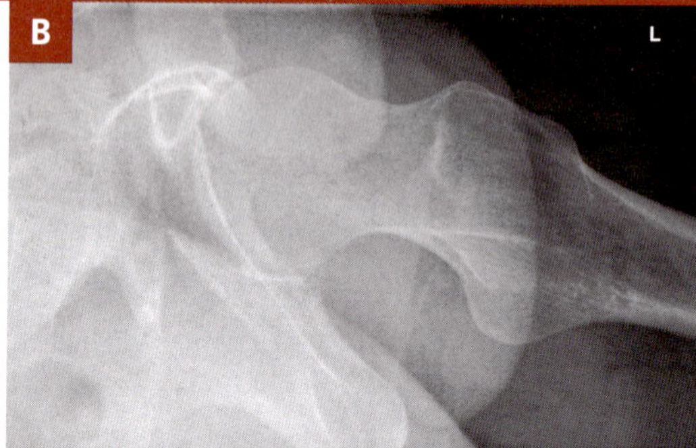

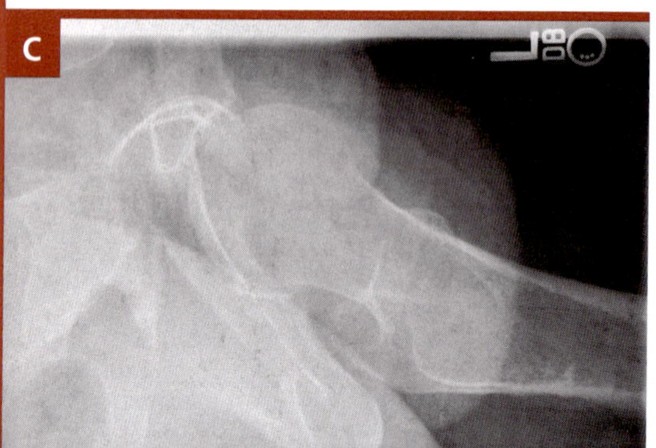

FIGURE 8-49

Comparison of Clements-Nakayama views, using **A** a 15° downward angle, and **B** a modified 25° downward angle. Note the improved visibility with the 25° angle. In view **C**, the 25° downward angle was used and the patient's leg was externally rotated.

Courtesy of Community Hospital of the Monterey Peninsula, Diagnostic and Interventional Radiology

Ferlic Filter: For cross-table lateral hip cases where the unaffected leg cannot be rolled out, the Ferlic filter is essential. Figure 8-50 demonstrates a cross-table lateral hip projection that had the unaffected leg superimposing the affected hip, but a Ferlic filter was used. Figure 8-51 demonstrates the Ferlic filter along with a newer hinged model, which opens to allow for light field centering.

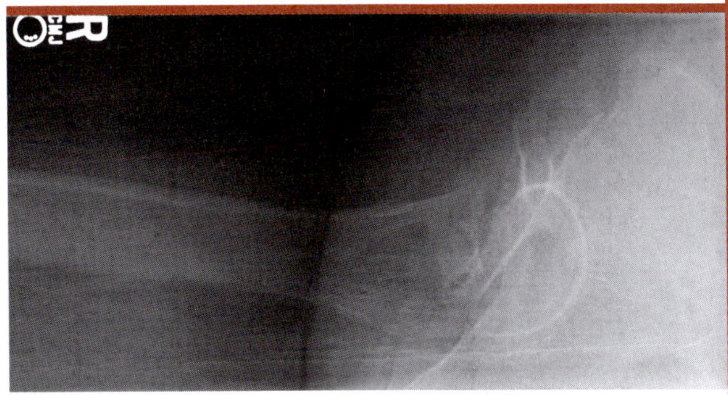

FIGURE 8-50

When the patient's contrary thigh cannot be moved out of the way for the cross-table lateral hip projection, use of the Ferlic filter can help even out the exposure.

Courtesy of Community Hospital of the Monterey Peninsula, Diagnostic and Interventional Radiology

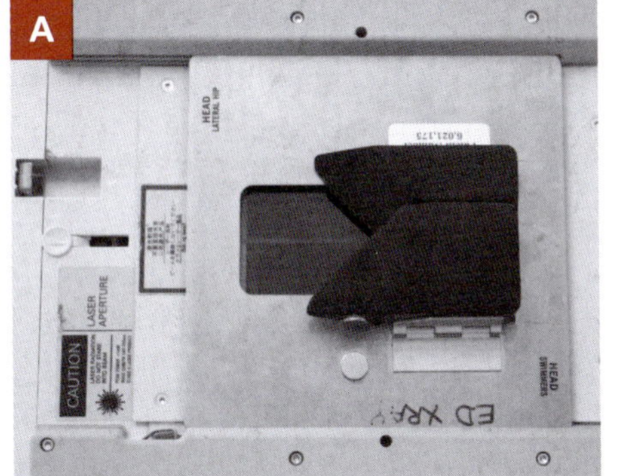

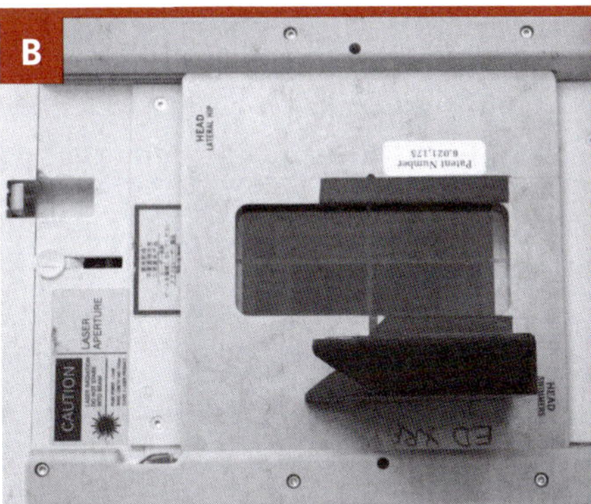

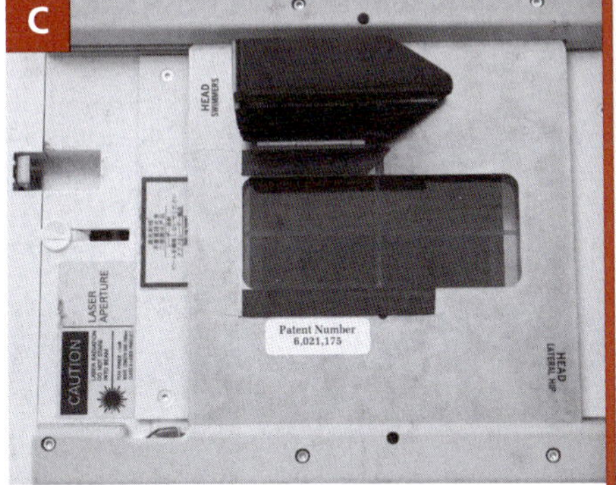

FIGURE 8-51

A. The conventional Ferlic filter.
B. The newer hinged filter with the hinge opened to allow the light field to shine through for centering.
C. The hinged filter closed after centering is completed.

Trauma Lateral Hip: Patient Can Move Opposite Leg

Many necessary components must come together to obtain a proper cross-table lateral projection of the hip. Most often, the IR plate will be gridded, since the hip in this projection is quite thick, even on smaller patients. The IR plate should be placed at a 45° angle to the patient (to match the angle of the surgical neck of the proximal femur). Because this can be difficult to ascertain, it may help to angle the tube 45°, using the angulation gauge for accuracy, then the IR can simply be placed parallel with the tube face (perpendicular to the CR).

Because of the extreme angle of the tube, the hip anatomy will be projected much more superior anatomically than is often expected, so the IR should be placed more superior than usual. A common practice is to place the top of the IR at the top of the iliac crest, but the top of the IR needs to be placed just under the lowest lateral (10th) rib to ensure that the acetabulum and surrounding bone structures are included. It is also helpful to have the patient grasp the end of the IR and pull it into the soft tissue of the waist as far as he can comfortably tolerate.

There are several methods in which to get the unaffected leg up and out of the way. The Anchor Leg Stabilizer™ (Figure 8-52) is a superb tool to use because it is both safe and sturdy. Without such an aid, the next best thing to do is to rest the patient's foot on top of the x-ray tube collimator (Figure 8-53). Always put a folded towel or pillowcase on top of the collimator box first, because it can get very hot from the lightbulb inside. Place the patient's foot on top of the collimator as the last step, just before making the exposure, because it can cause some patient discomfort. Most patients with a hip fracture can tolerate this position.

After the unaffected foot is placed on the collimator, have the patient roll out his knee so as to abduct the leg, as shown in Figure 8-53. This is very important because this is the part of the positioning that actually gets the soft tissue of the unaffected thigh and gluteal area

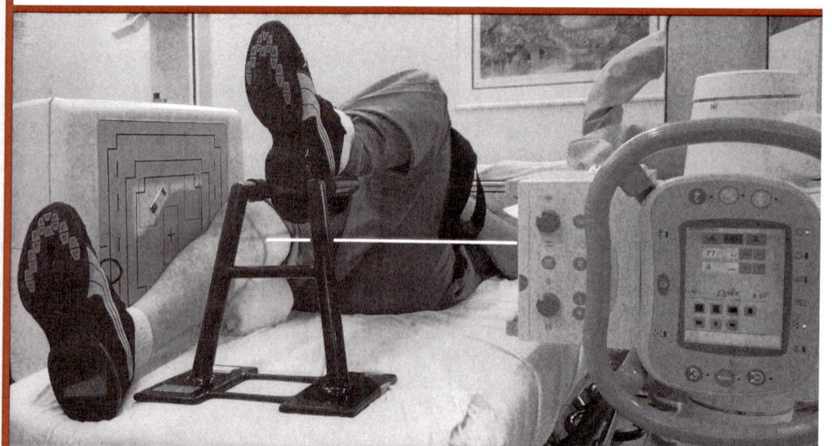

FIGURE 8-52
The anchor-leg stabilizer used to support the unaffected leg for a cross-table projection. Note that although the device provides support, the unaffected leg is not abducted well, so the Ferlic filter should also be used for this projection.

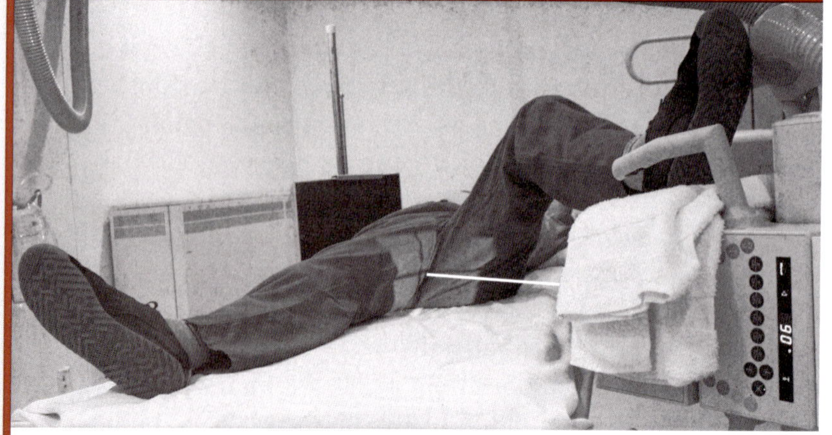

FIGURE 8-53
Cross-table lateral hip projection with the unaffected leg properly abducted to the side, and the foot resting on the x-ray tube collimator with towels for insulation.

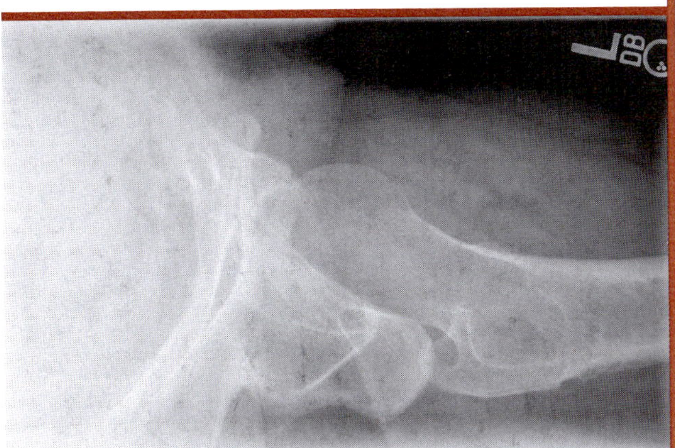

FIGURE 8-54

Cross-table lateral hip view showing good desuperimposition of tissues of the unaffected thigh due to proper abduction.

Courtesy of Community Hospital of the Monterey Peninsula, Diagnostic and Interventional Radiology

completely out of the way so that there is no superimposition, as illustrated in the radiograph in Figure 8-54. In cases where the unaffected leg cannot be rolled out, use the Ferlic filter as described in the preceding section.

TRAUMA POSITIONING TIPS FOR THE EXTREMITIES

Most views of distal and intermediate extremities are easily obtained without moving a trauma patient by using horizontal beam projections (HBPs) or cross-table projections for lateral views and various transverse tube angles for obliques. In radiographing patients "as they lie," the key skill involved is the ability to visualize the perpendicularity of the CR relative to the part and imaging plate. This ability is essential and has universal application for all trauma extremity radiography. An example of good beam perpendicularity using a trauma lateral forearm projection is given in Figure 8-55. We will avoid repeating this concept for each individual anatomical part. Our focus will be on those body parts and positions that present particular challenges for the radiographer.

Humerus

Upright "Sling" AP: When the patient is standing, all that is required is to rotate the entire body until the intercondylar line of the humerus parallels the plate (Figure 8-56).

Supine AP, Elbow Bent: When the patient is supine with the forearm resting on the belly, build up or hold up the wrist until a feasible transverse angle can be employed to get the CR perpendicular to the intercondylar line (Figure 8-57). (The IR can be left flat on the table for this position.)

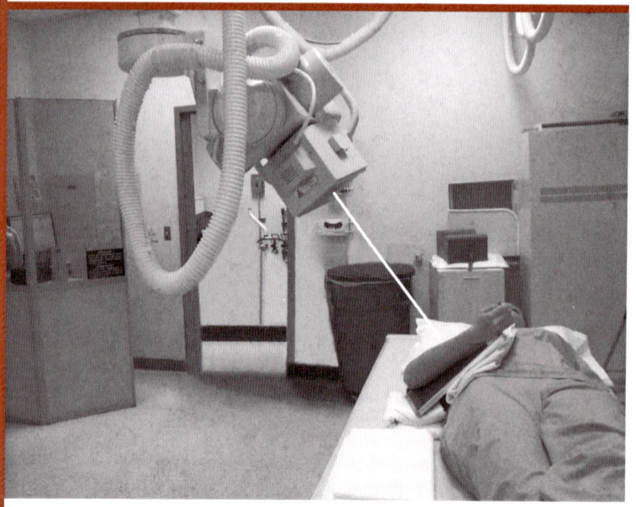

Courtesy of Quinn B. Carroll

FIGURE 8-55

Trauma lateral forearm demonstrating correct perpendicularity of the CR to the part and cassette plate. The ability to properly visualize this perpendicularity is essential and has universal application for all trauma extremity radiography.

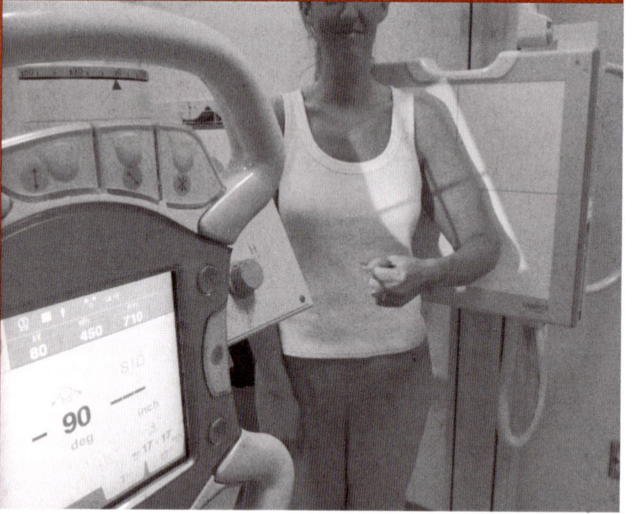

Courtesy of Quinn B. Carroll

FIGURE 8-56

For the standing AP "sling" humerus, simply rotate the patient's whole body as needed.

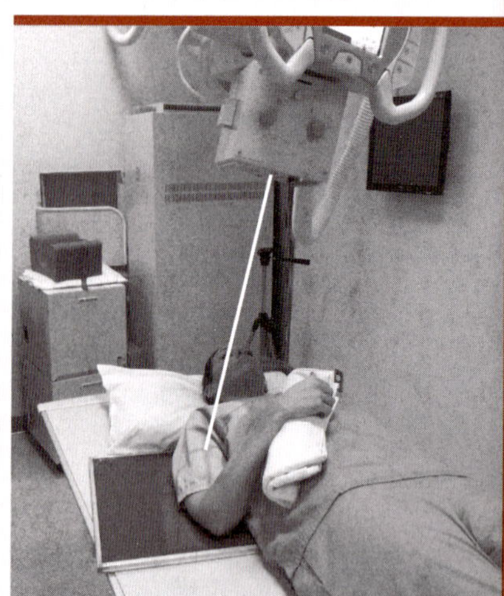

Courtesy of Quinn B. Carroll

FIGURE 8-57

For the supine AP "sling" humerus, bring the wrist up off the belly with supports until a feasible transverse CR angle can be used.

Lateral Projections

Lateral projections of the humerus present considerable challenges even for nontrauma patients. For the "internal rotation" method, some positioning atlases suggest merely pronating the hand. As can be seen in Figure 8-58A, this does not come close to placing the elbow and humerus into a true lateral position. Rather, for most patients, the hand must be internally rotated *well past pronation of the hand until the palpated epicondyles prove that* the intercondylar line of the humerus is perpendicular, as shown in Figure 8-58B. If the patient can freely move, a much easier approach is a mediolateral projection with the elbow bent 90° and the arm "to the square," as shown in Figure 8-59A. (*Note that* **any** *time the elbow is bent 90° and the shoulder, elbow, and wrist are all in contact with the table, the humerus is* guaranteed *to be in true lateral position, as shown in Figure 8-59***B**. *This concept will be used in the following discussion on trauma positions.*) Neither of these two positions, internal rotation nor the "arm to the square"

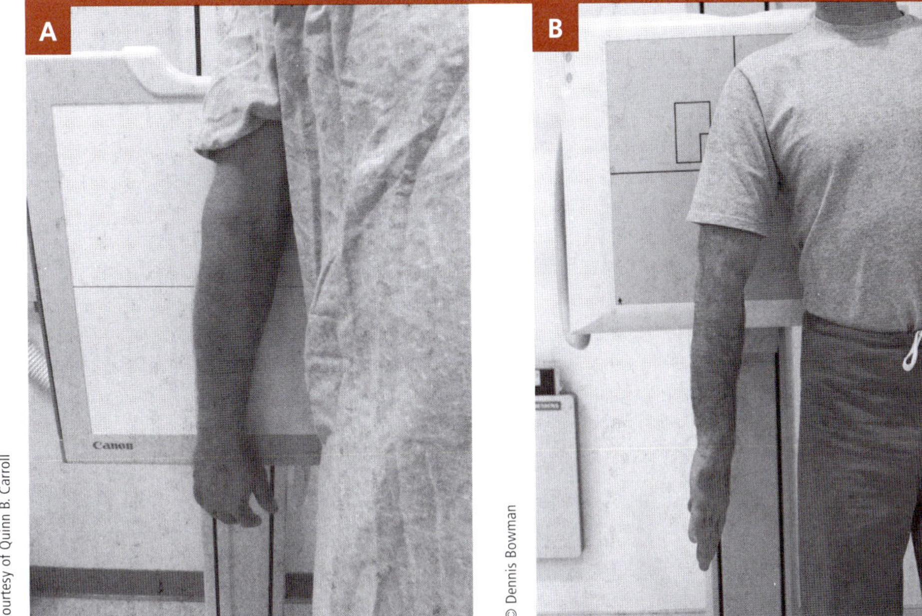

Courtesy of Quinn B. Carroll

© Dennis Bowman

FIGURE 8-58

Mere pronation of the hand, as recommended in many positioning atlases, does not place the elbow or humerus in true lateral position. In **A**, the wrist is completely pronated, yet the elbow remains far from lateral. Usually, the wrist must be internally rotated as far as possible **B** to obtain a true lateral humerus. (This method should not be used for serious trauma patients.)

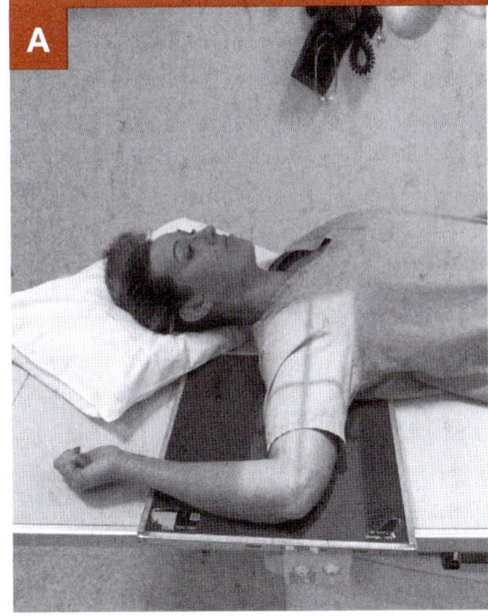

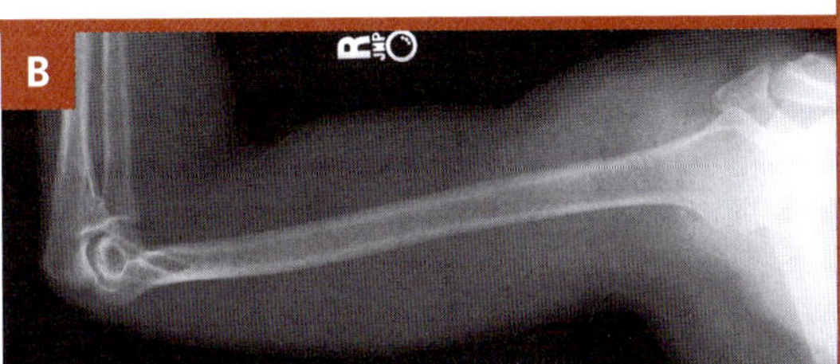

Courtesy of Quinn B. Carroll

FIGURE 8-59

The "arm to the square" approach shown in **A** produces a mediolateral projection that virtually guarantees a true lateral humerus **B**, because the shoulder, elbow, and wrist are all in contact with the table. This method should *not* be used for serious trauma patients.

Part B is Courtesy of Community Hospital of the Monterey Peninsula, Diagnostic and Interventional Radiology

position, is suitable for trauma patients. They are both fully discussed in Chapter 10 on routine positioning.

Each of the following positions for a trauma lateral humerus has advantages and disadvantages. They are given in order of preference considering ease of positioning, accuracy in obtaining a true lateral, and their ability to produce an unimpeded view:

First Choice: Upright "sling" position: The patient stands in a shallow anterior oblique position against the chest board or upright table (Figure 8-60). The elbow is flexed 90°, with the wrist, elbow, and shoulder all in contact against board. The collimator may be swivelled to slant the light field parallel to the humerus, allowing proper collimation. (Mark the view as a *mediolateral*

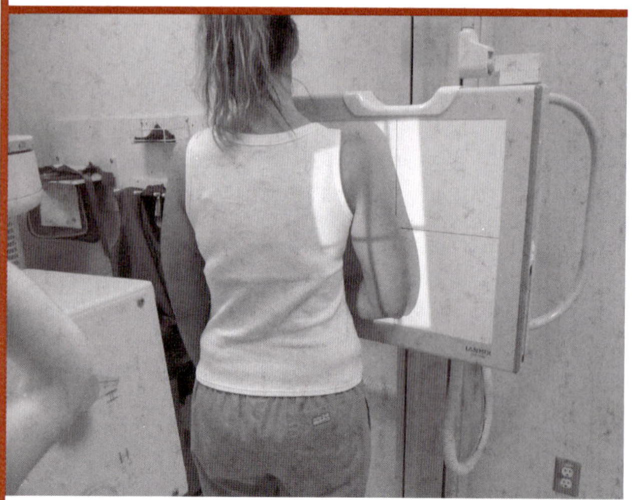
Courtesy of Quinn B. Carroll

FIGURE 8-60

The "sling" lateral position of the humerus, first choice for trauma patients if they can be done upright.

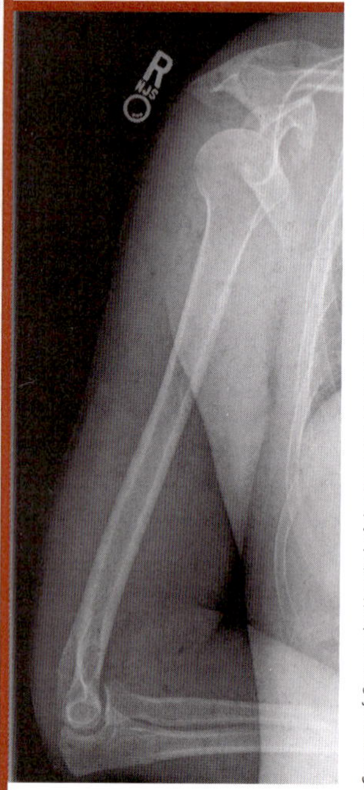

Courtesy of Community Hospital of the Monterey Peninsula, Diagnostic and Interventional Radiology

FIGURE 8-61

The "sling" lateral view of the humerus.

projection.) When the elbow is bent and the wrist, elbow, and shoulder are against the board, the resulting view is a true lateral with the humeral condyles perfectly superimposed (Figure 8-61).

Second Choice: Trauma supine lateral: The IR is slid under the patient's shoulder flat on the table in order to include the entire humerus. The CR is angled lateromedially to parallel the intercondylar line. This step must be carefully executed (Figure 8-62). A slightly distorted but true lateral view of the entire humerus results (Figure 8-63).

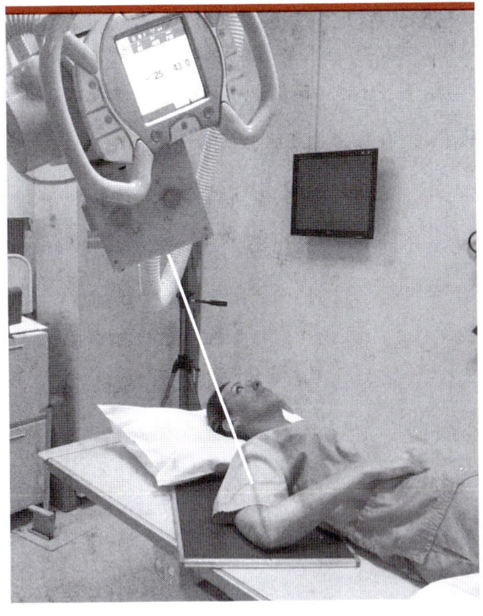

Courtesy of Quinn B. Carroll

FIGURE 8-62
Trauma supine lateral projection for the humerus, second choice for trauma patients, recommended when the patient cannot sit or stand.

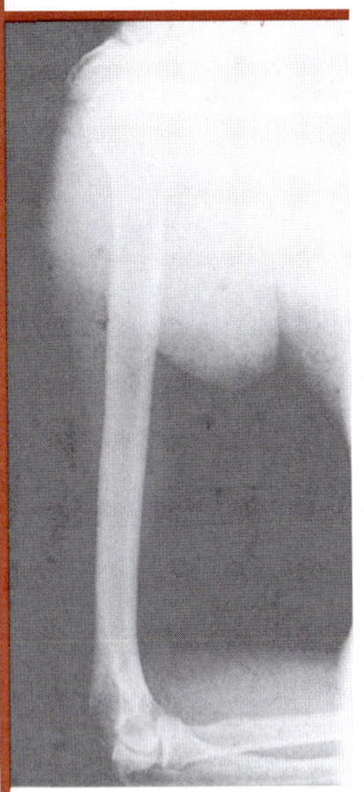

FIGURE 8-63
Trauma supine lateral view of the humerus.
Courtesy of Quinn B. Carroll

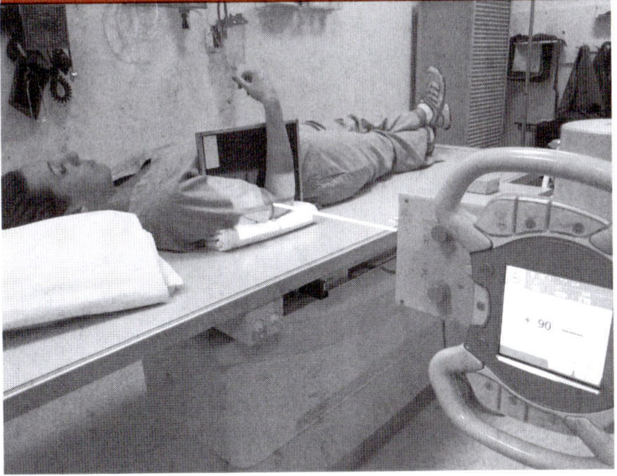

Courtesy of Quinn B. Carroll

FIGURE 8-64
Clipped trauma lateral projection for the humerus. Though popular, this approach should be a *last resort*, and if done should be combined with an additional transthoracic projection in order to also demonstrate the upper humerus.

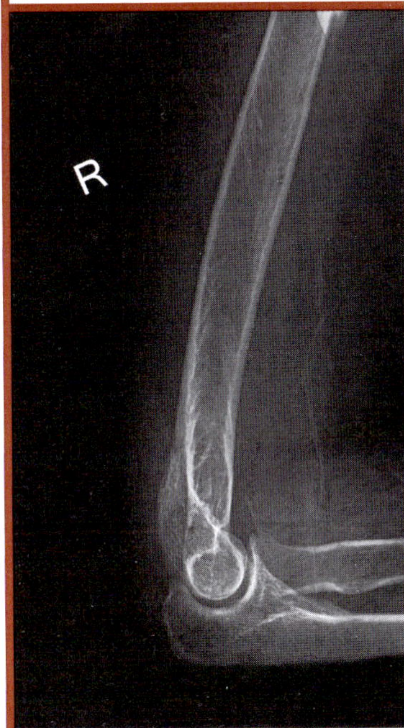

FIGURE 8-65
Clipped trauma lateral view of the humerus.
Courtesy of Community Hospital of the Monterey Peninsula, Diagnostic and Interventional Radiology

Third Choice: Clipped trauma lateral *combined* with transthoracic lateral or scapular Y: It is a popular first choice approach among some radiographers to simply slide the IR or cassette up into axilla as the supine patient lies (Figure 8-64), and make an exposure that is missing the upper humerus. Although it usually gives a true lateral view, this method should be a last resort because the entire humerus is not demonstrated (Figure 8-65). When it *is* done, an additional transthoracic lateral, cross-table transthoracic lateral, or scapular Y projection should also be performed to demonstrate the proximal humerus.

Transthoracic Lateral: Because it superimposes the proximal humerus with the thoracic organs and obscures the distal humerus with abdominal tissues under the diaphragm, the transthoracic humerus projection should also be considered a "last resort" approach. Positioning atlases often recommend leaving the hand in a "neutral" position as shown in Figure 8-66A. This may be unavoidable with a trauma patient, because the possibility of a humeral fracture precludes any forced rotation of the upper arm.

However, note in Figure 8-67A that it results in an *oblique* position of the humerus where the greater tuberosity is seen in semiprofile anteriorly. *If the patient himself can manage to fully supinate his hand, without*

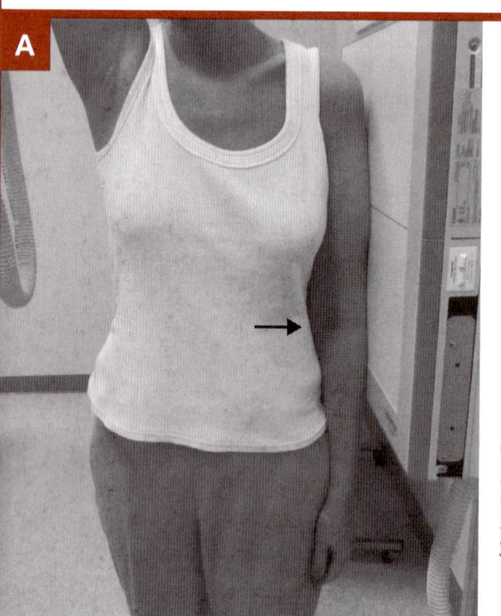

Courtesy of Quinn B. Carroll

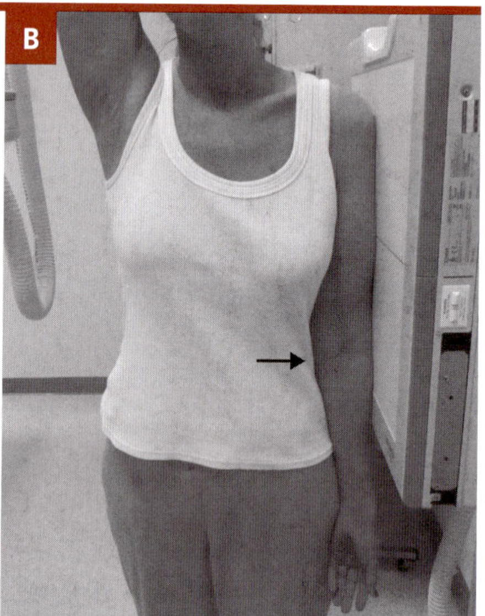

Courtesy of Quinn B. Carroll

FIGURE 8-66

For the transthoracic lateral projection of the humerus, when the hand is left in "neutral" position, it can be seen in **A** that the elbow is not positioned truly lateral. The patient can be asked to attempt rotating the hand into full supination as in **B**, *without* forcing it. If this is too uncomfortable, proceed with the hand in a neutral position. See Figure 8-67.

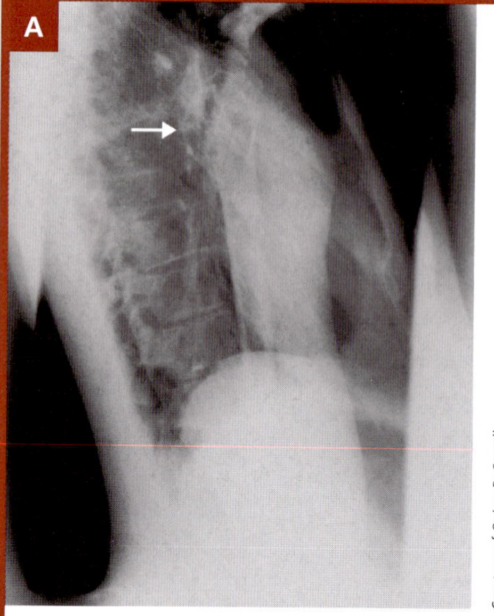

Courtesy of Quinn B. Carroll

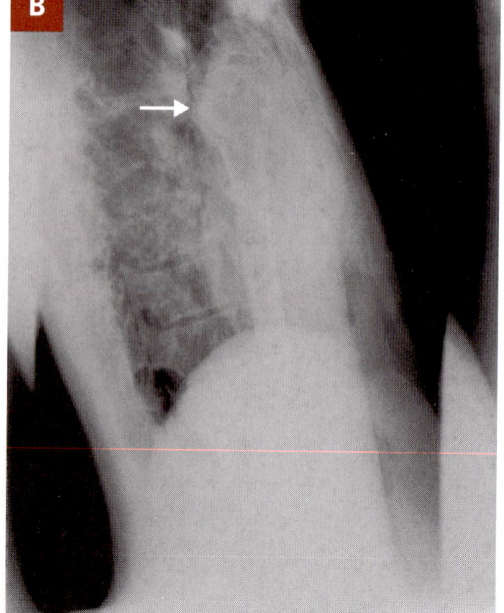

Courtesy of Quinn B. Carroll

FIGURE 8-67

A transthoracic view taken without supinating the hand results in an oblique position of the humerus itself **A**, with the greater trochanter in semiprofile anteriorly (arrow). Radiograph **B** was taken with the hand fully supinated and shows the head of the humerus in true lateral position with the lesser tuberosity extending posteriorly (arrow).

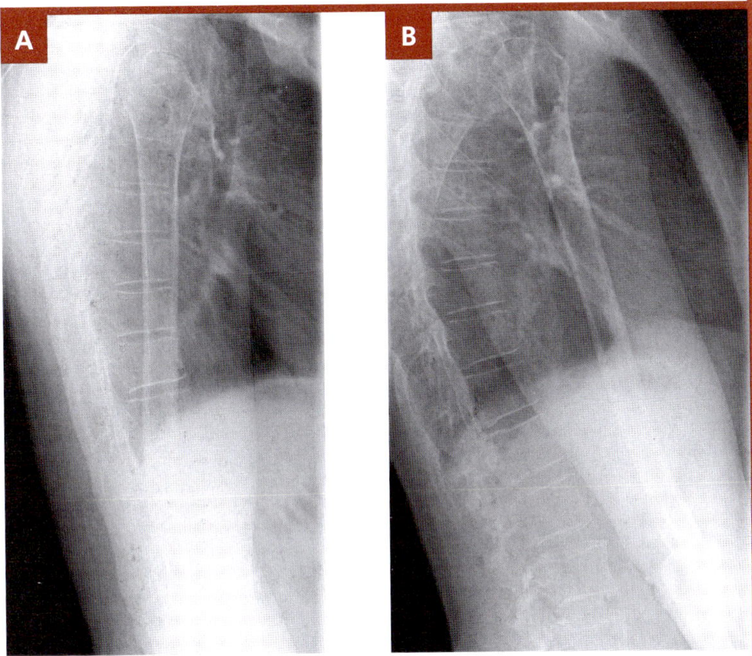

FIGURE 8-68
Transthoracic projections often superimpose the spine over the affected humerus **A**. By rotating the body 7°–10° with the upside shoulder pulled back, the humerus can be projected free of the spine **B**.
Courtesy of Community Hospital of the Monterey Peninsula, Diagnostic and Interventional Radiology

forcing it, as shown in Figure 8-66***B***, a true lateral view of the head and neck of the humerus can be obtained. Figure 8-67***B*** demonstrates the resulting radiograph with the head of the humerus in true lateral view, symmetrical in appearance and with the lesser tuberosity extended posteriorly (arrow).

The radiographer might demonstrate the desired position, and have the patient attempt to imitate it without force. If it is too uncomfortable using normal muscle control, proceed with the hand in a "neutral" position.

Note that if the patient can stand and can flex the elbow with the arm across her belly, the first choice "sling" method should be used. The transthoracic projection would only be necessary for an upright patient when she cannot flex the elbow.

If the patient is upright and in a true lateral position, and the affected arm is hanging straight down, the humerus can often be superimposed over the spine as shown in the radiograph in Figure 8-68*A*. Rotate the patient 7°–10° toward a posterior oblique position (upside shoulder pulled back). This positions the humerus anteriorly to the spine within the lung field for an unimpeded view, demonstrated in Figure 8-68***B***. Nothing of this nature can be done for the patient who must remain recumbent.

Trauma Series for Forearm, Elbow, and Wrist

Combined Views: A severely traumatized patient is most likely to be in supine position during a radiographic exam, with the wrist roughly pronated. Figure 8-69 illustrates a series of three projections designed to collectively demonstrate

FIGURE 8-69

A forearm, elbow, or wrist series with minimal movement of the trauma patient, using a DR plate: The horizontal projection in **A** produces a lateral view of the wrist and distal forearm, and that in **B** yields a *PA* view of the elbow. The combined view in **C** demonstrates the elbow in lateral position while the wrist is in PA position.

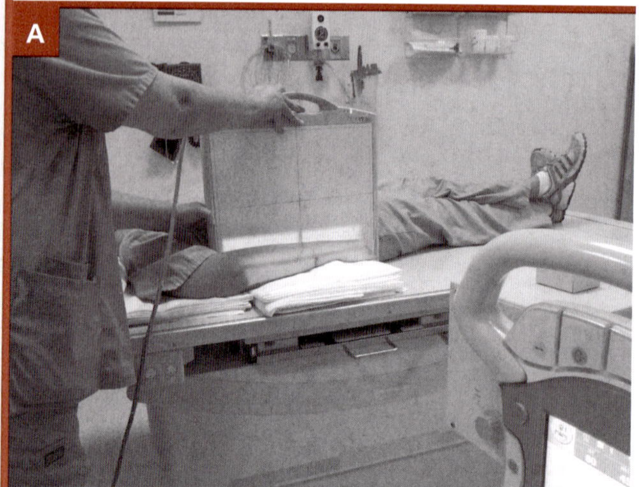

Courtesy of Quinn B. Carroll

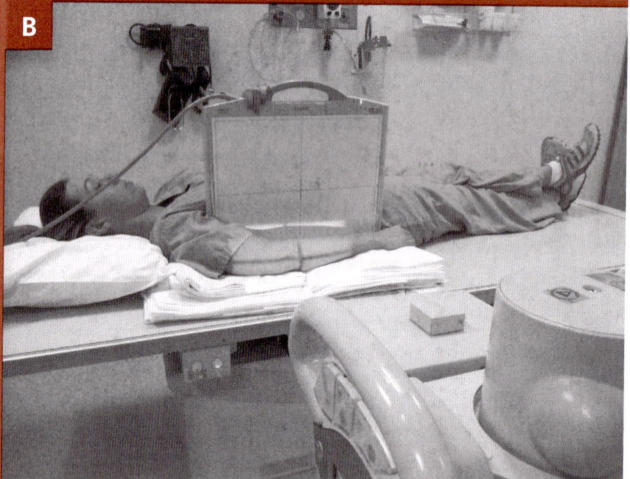

Courtesy of Quinn B. Carroll

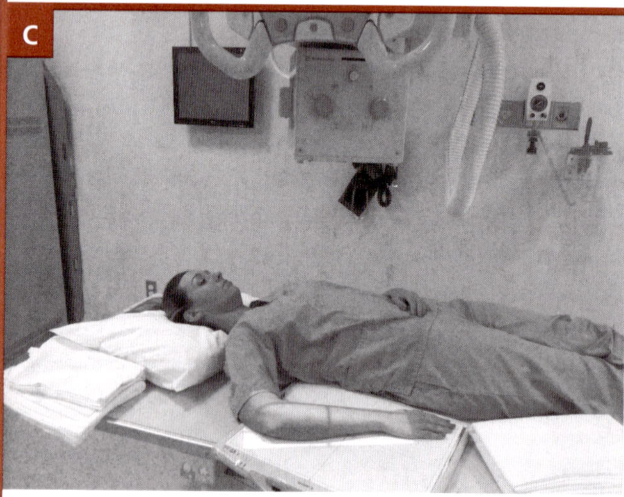

Courtesy of Quinn B. Carroll

frontal and lateral views of both the elbow-end and the wrist-end of the forearm, with minimal movement of the patient. To obtain the lateral wrist (**A**) and a *PA* (rather than AP) projection of the elbow (***B***), horizontal beam projections are used (in this case with a DR detector). Some building up of the arm off of the tabletop or backboard with sheets is necessary, and full pronation of the wrist. With slight abduction of the elbow away from the body as in (**C**), a projection from above can be used to obtain a combined view of the lateral elbow and PA wrist.

Elbow

Semiflexed AP: When the elbow cannot be straightened out, several books recommend alternately placing the forearm, and then the humerus, flat on the IR plate (Figures 8-70 and 8-71).

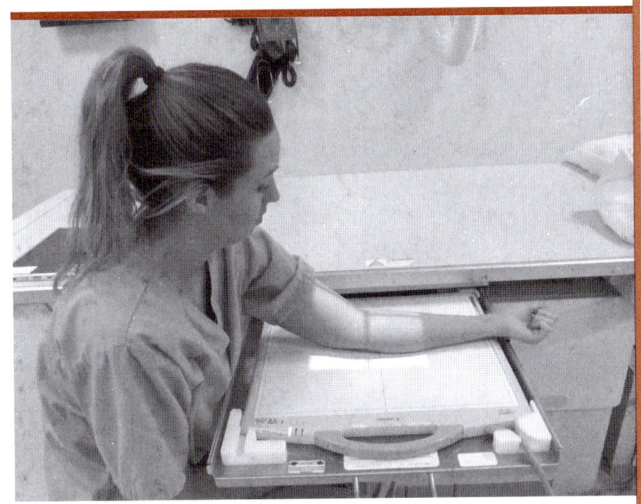

Courtesy of Quinn B. Carroll

FIGURE 8-70

Bent AP elbow with forearm parallel to IR, not recommended.

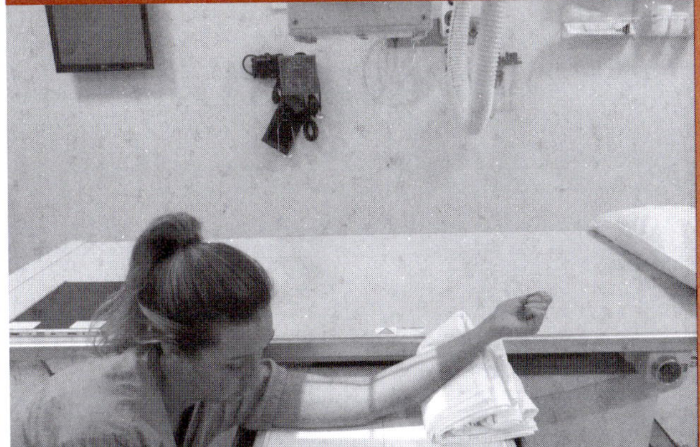

Courtesy of Quinn B. Carroll

FIGURE 8-71

Bent AP elbow for distal humerus, with humerus parallel to the IR, is *not* recommended.

However, if there is significant flexion, the second view results in superimposition of the upper forearm tissue over the elbow joint, capitellum, and trochlea of the humerus (Figure 8-72*B*). To better see these areas, as shown in Figure 8-72*C*, "split the difference" by resting the elbow on the CR cassette or DR plate with symmetrical angles formed between the limbs and the cassette (Figure 8-73). This position also works very well for internal and external oblique projections of the elbow.

Trauma Radial Head: It is of considerable diagnostic value to desuperimpose the head and neck of the radius

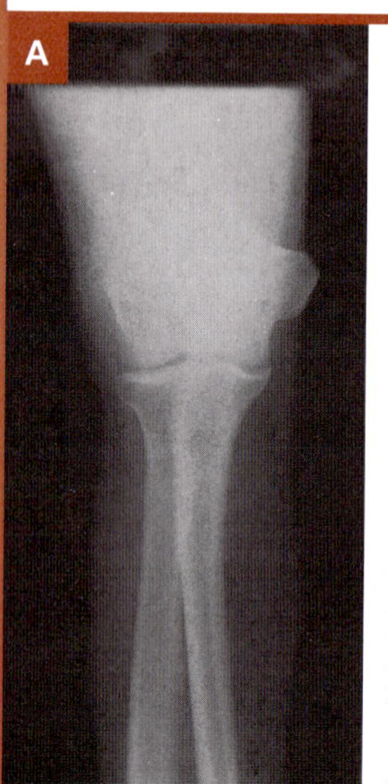

Courtesy of Quinn B. Carroll

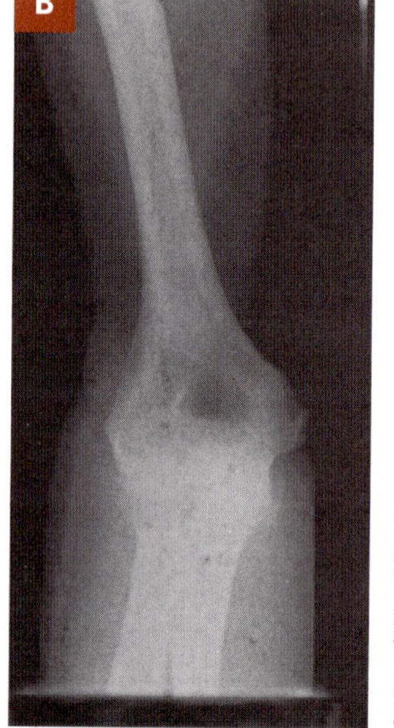

Courtesy of Quinn B. Carroll

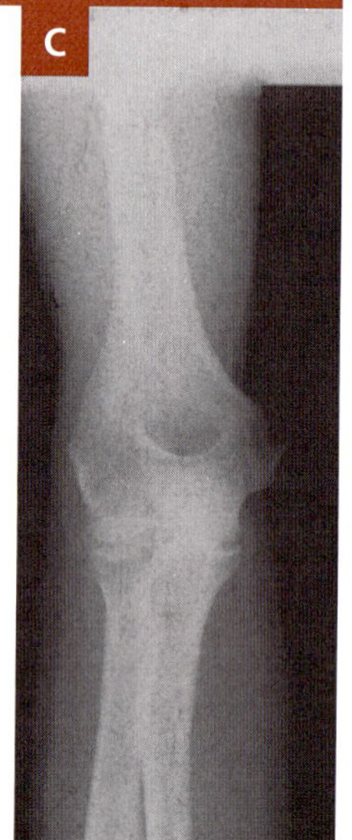

Courtesy of Quinn B. Carroll

FIGURE 8-72
Views of bent AP elbow, demonstrating **A** forearm parallel, **B** humerus parallel (*not* recommended), and **C** "splitting the difference," recommended for the distal humerus.

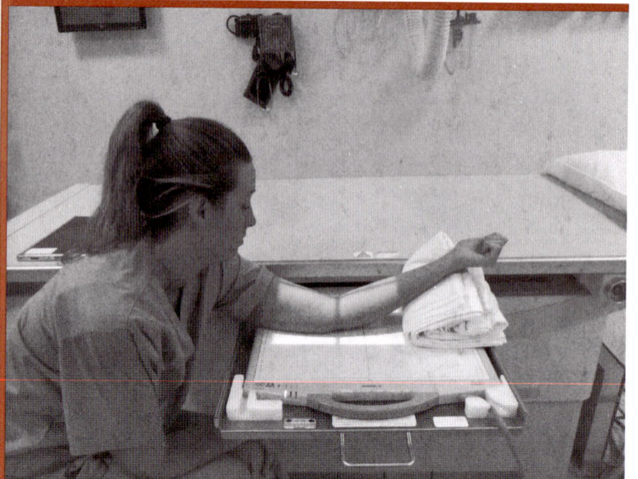

Courtesy of Quinn B. Carroll

FIGURE 8-73
Bent AP elbow for distal humerus, "splitting the difference," (recommended).

from the proximal ulna. Only two positions achieve this unobstructed view of the proximal radius: the external oblique elbow and the Coyle method. Rotating the elbow 45° externally is difficult even for a healthy patient. If the trauma patient can flex his elbow into a routine lateral position, the Coyle method is easy to do as follows: With the elbow flexed 90°, simply angle the CR 45° *proximally* toward the body, adjusting tabletop-tube distance to maintain a 40-inch SID (Figure 8-74). This replaces the external oblique, producing an unobstructed if somewhat distorted view of the proximal radius (Figure 8-75). (By reversing the angle *distally*, the coronoid process can be demonstrated, replacing the internal oblique position.)

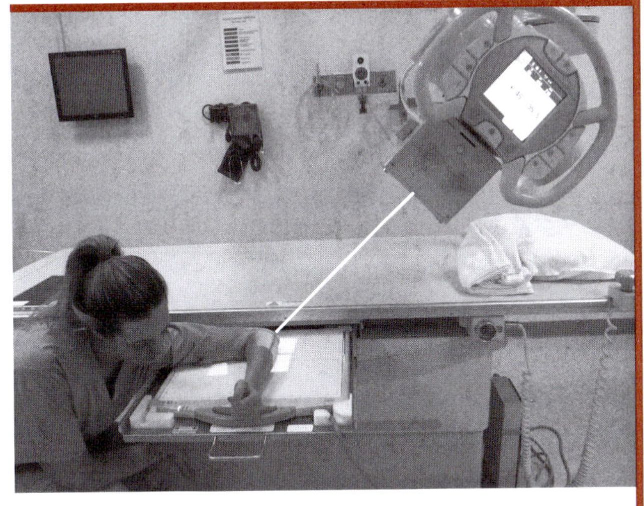

Courtesy of Quinn B. Carroll

FIGURE 8-74

The Coyle method for an unobstructed view of the proximal radius: Angle 45° proximally to a routinely positioned lateral elbow.

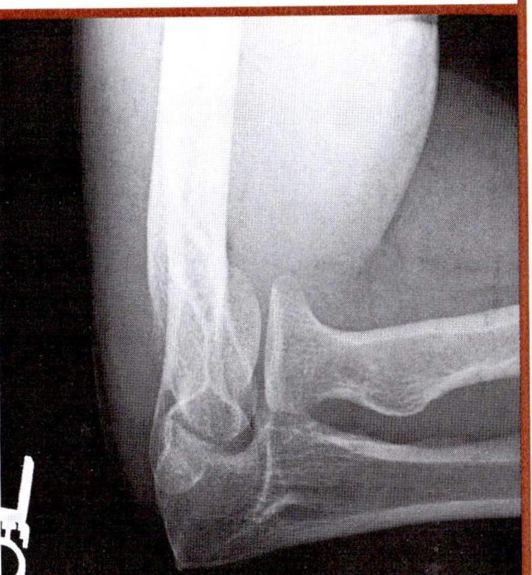

Courtesy of Quinn B. Carroll

FIGURE 8-75

View of the proximal radius using the Coyle method. Note the desuperimposition of the radial head.

Note that the Coyle method can also be used on a patient who lies supine by positioning the arm as shown in Figure 8-69C.

Fingers/Hand

Semiflexed AP: When the fingers cannot be straightened out, the hand must be radiographed in AP rather than PA position to take advantage of beam divergence. (See Chapter 4.) Several views may be needed in AP, to place each phalanx perpendicular to the CR in turn. Distal angulation can be increased in increments (Figure 8-76), or the wrist may be pulled up incrementally placing each set of phalanges parallel to the cassette plate in turn. Figure 8-76 shows a *bilateral* projection. Note that this position may also be used for a *unilateral* projection of a single hand.

Knee

Trauma patients on a gurney will often have, as they lie, the affected leg externally rotated as much as 40°–45° (Figure 8-77). Without moving them, an AP projection can be obtained by angling 45° medially, an "external oblique" view obtained with a vertical beam, and a lateral by angling 45° laterally as in Figure 8-77. In any case, use the intercondylar line in the knee as a guide.

Trauma Obliques: With the leg straight, both internal and external obliques may be obtained by angling the x-ray beam 45° medially, then laterally, with the cassette flat or, preferably, angled perpendicular to the CR. Figure 8-78 is an example using a

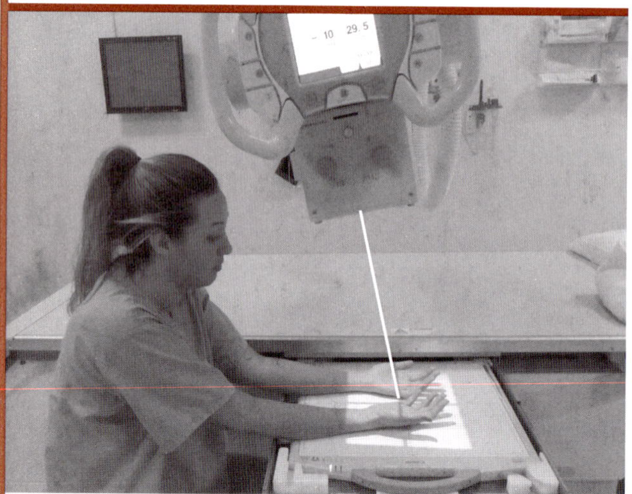

FIGURE 8-76

With hands semiflexed, increments of caudal angulation (15°, 25°, 35°) can be used to demonstrate each set of phalanges.

Courtesy of Quinn B. Carroll

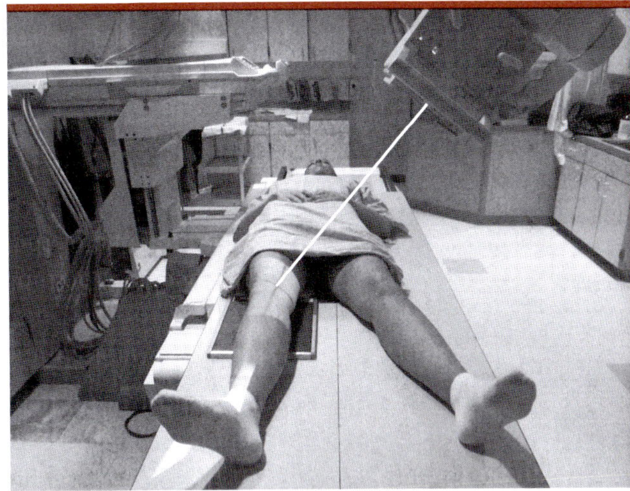

Courtesy of Quinn B. Carroll

FIGURE 8-77

Trauma lateral projection of the knee "as the patient lies" with 40°–45° of external rotation in the leg. (In this position, reverse the CR angle for an AP projection, and use a vertical angle for an oblique.)

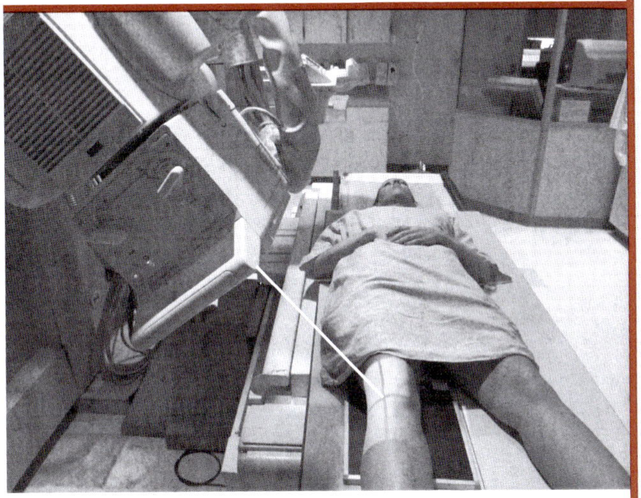

Courtesy of Quinn B. Carroll

FIGURE 8-78

Trauma "internal oblique" projection of the knee using a 45° medial angulation with the leg straight.

medial angle to produce the "internal oblique" view. Oblique views of the patella can be obtained identically with adjustments in collimation and cassette placement.

Note that these oblique views can also be achieved in cross-table fashion with the cassette vertical, by alternating mediolateral and lateromedial projections.

Trauma Lateral: The most common way to obtain a trauma lateral projection of the knee on a supine patient is to do it cross-table using a lateromedial projection. Remember that this is opposite to the routine mediolateral projection, so that the recommended 5° *cephalic* angle will now be *caudal*. Without the angle, although the view obtained may be passable, the larger medial condyle of the femur will obscure the knee joint proper.

In Figure 8-79, the tube swivel lock of a fixed unit is difficult to set at a 5° angle. To fully open the knee joint space, the patient lies slightly diagonal slanting the leg 5° away from the beam. This is equivalent to caudal angulation, which in a routine mediolateral projection would be equal to a 5° *cephalic* angle. This improves the view and is a good example of refined adaptive positioning skills.

Another great tip for refining this view is to remember that for the routine lateral projection of the knee, up to 45° of knee flexion is recommended. A great way to bend the knee correctly is to use a small towel. Fold it in half twice (quarters) and then roll it up. It will now be approximately the width of the knee, which is perfect for placement as a support under the back of the knee. The IR plate can now be placed directly against the knee on the lateral side without the towel bowing upward and superimposing the posterior knee (Figure 8-80). This also raises the knee to better center it to the IR.

If a good bracing device is available, such as the Ferlic anchor-leg stabilizer shown in Figure 8-81, and the patient can freely move the

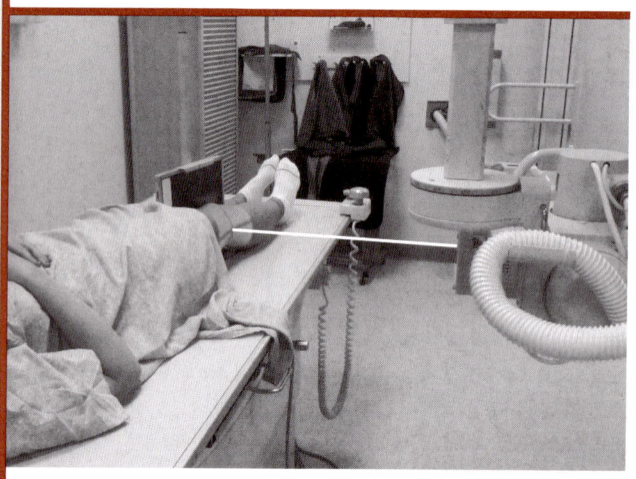

Courtesy of Quinn B. Carroll

FIGURE 8-79

Cross-table lateral position of the knee using lateromedial projection in a fixed unit room. Note that the patient is slanted 5° away from the beam. This is equivalent to 5° caudal CR angle, or a 5° *cephalic* angle for a routine mediolateral projection.

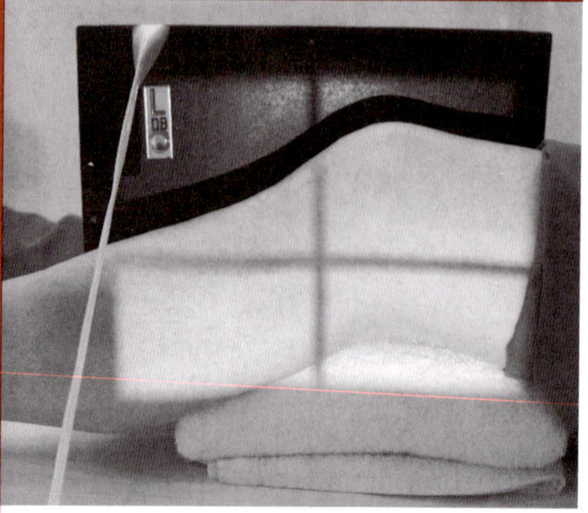

© Dennis Bowman

FIGURE 8-80

Cross-table lateral position of the knee with the added benefit of flexion and supported by a folded towel.

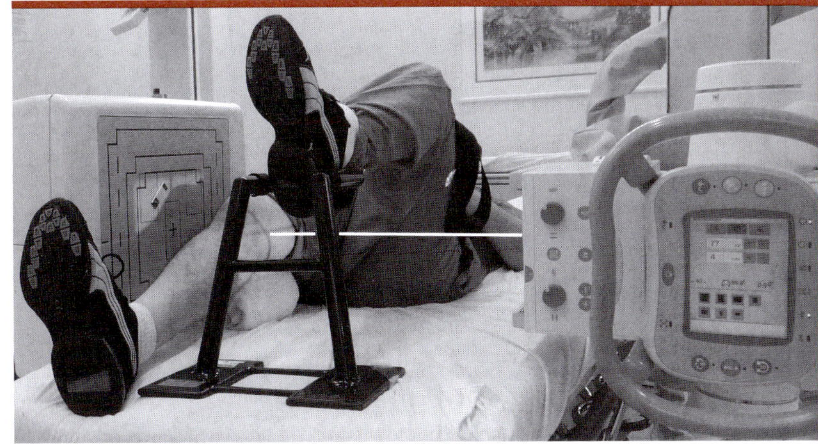

FIGURE 8-81

Mediolateral projection of the knee using the anchor-leg stabilizer to support the unaffected leg out of the way.

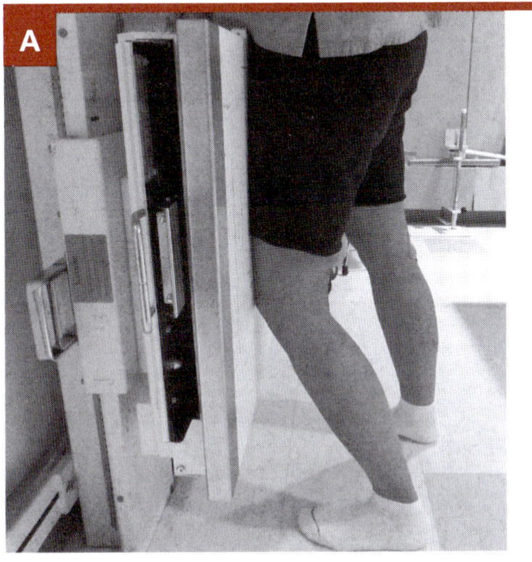

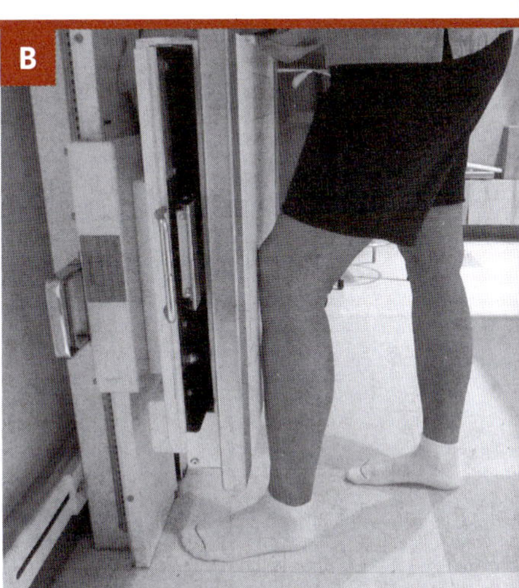

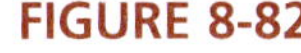

FIGURE 8-82

Two projections recommended for the semiflexed knee **A** with the femur parallel to the IR, and **B** with the lower leg parallel to the IR.

unaffected leg to place the foot on the stabilizer, a *mediolateral* cross-table projection can be obtained for the knee.

Semiflexed PA: When the patient cannot fully straighten out the leg, two views may be taken, one in PA projection with the femur parallel to the plate, and one in PA projection with the tibia parallel to the plate (Figure 8-82).

Ankle

Here, also, most views can be obtained with little or no movement of the patient by employing correct CR angles relative to the intermalleolar line, which lies approximately 15°–20° externally, and by using the cross-table approach for the lateral, shown for a foot in Figure 8-83.

Trauma Oblique: With the foot vertical, angle the CR 45° *lateromedially*.

Trauma Oblique Mortise: With the foot vertical, angle the CR 15°–20° *lateromedially* (Figure 8-83A), to demonstrate the talofibular joint space. If the foot is rotated out

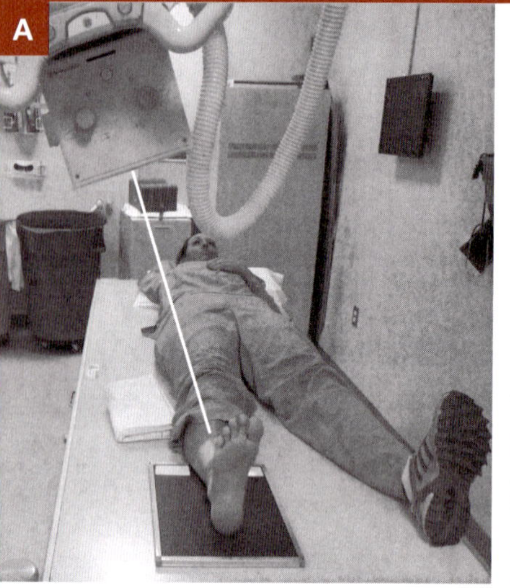

Courtesy of Quinn B. Carroll

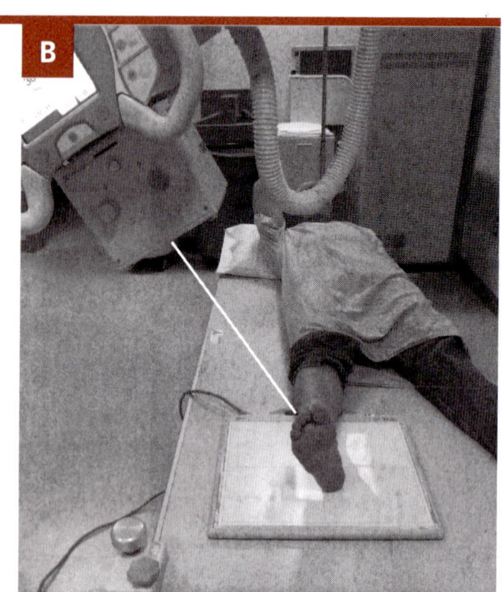

Courtesy of Quinn B. Carroll

FIGURE 8-83

Without twisting the foot internally from the AP ankle position **A**, an oblique ankle mortise projection can be obtained using a 15° lateromedial angle. In **B**, a 30° angle is used to compensate for 15° of external rotation "as the patient lies."

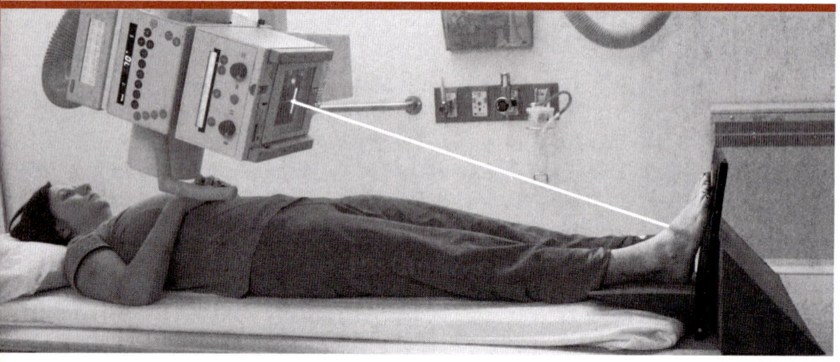

© Dennis Bowman

FIGURE 8-84

Trauma AP foot projection with the foot and cassette plate tilted 5° from vertical and the CR angled 20° downward from horizontal.

laterally only slightly, this amount can be added to the CR angle to compensate (Figure 8-83***B***).

Foot

Trauma AP: The trauma patient in supine position who cannot move the leg will require a vertically placed CR cassette or DR plate supported by sandbags or a holder. Do not forget the 15° caudal angle required relative to the plantar surface of the foot. In Figure 8-84, the foot is extended 5° and so the IR plate is tilted accordingly. The needed CR angle is now 20° downward from the horizontal.

Trauma Oblique: With the foot vertical, place the cassette or IR plate vertically against the plantar surface. Angle a horizontal beam 30° *lateromedially.*

Trauma Lateral: With the patient supine, use a cross-table projection for the lateral foot. Do not forget to build up the heel off the tabletop to avoid cut-off at the bottom edge of the cassette (Figure 8-85).

Courtesy of Quinn B. Carroll

FIGURE 8-85

Cross-table projection for a lateral foot, with the heel built up to avoid cut-off at the bottom edge of the cassette.

Calcaneus

The plantodorsal projection may be obtained as the patient lies, but a cephalic angle increased to 45° will likely be needed to compensate for normal dropping or flexion of the foot. The lateral can be done cross-table, but will need to be built up on sponges to avoid clipping the inferiormost portion of the heel.

Figure 8-86 demonstrates the utility of "oblique" views of the calcaneus, not found in most positioning atlases. Note that the bone is visible all the way up to the subtalar joint. These can be useful as optional views. They are easy to obtain if the leg can be rotated 45° internally and externally (Figure 8-87), while using a 40° cephalic angle centered to the level of the bases of the metatarsals.

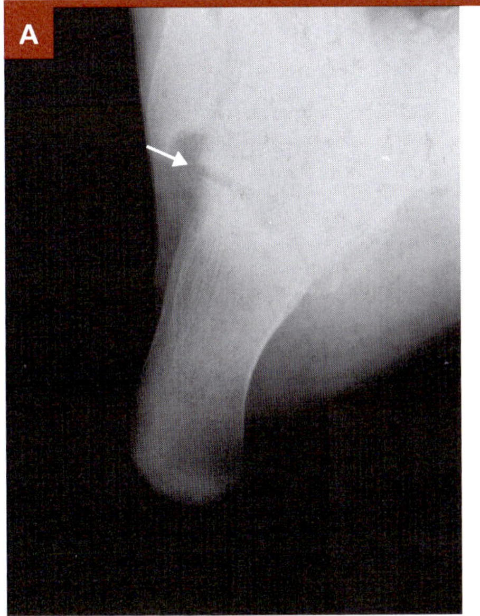

Courtesy of Quinn B. Carroll

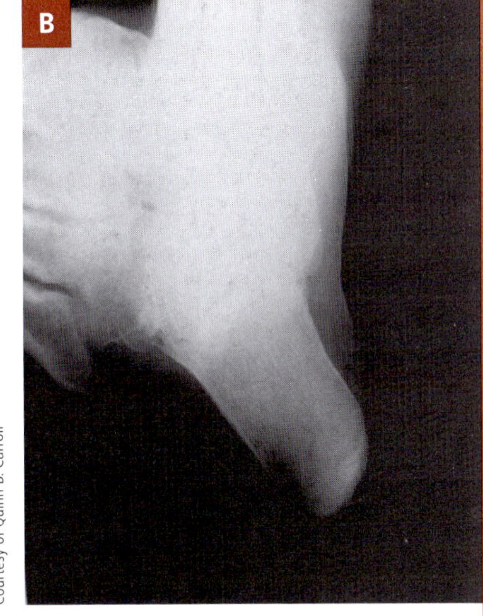

Courtesy of Quinn B. Carroll

FIGURE 8-86

Optional "oblique" views of the calcaneus demonstrate the upper portion of the bone well.

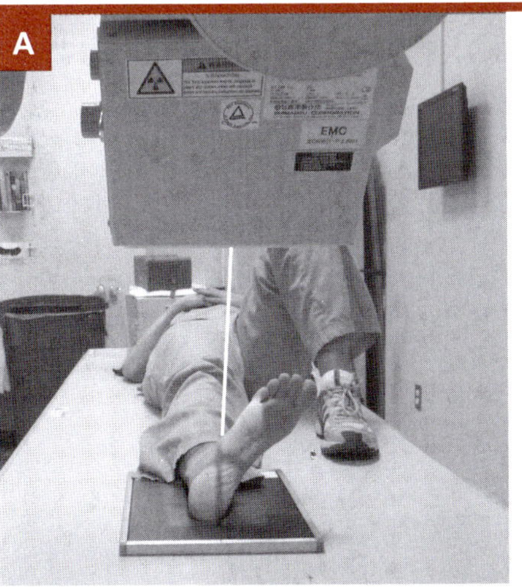

Courtesy of Quinn B. Carroll

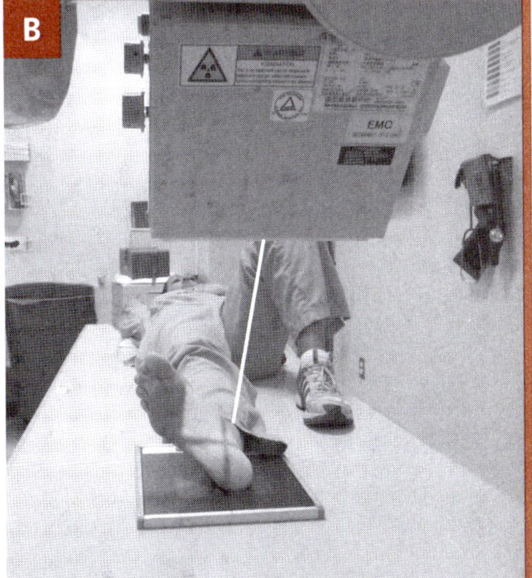

Courtesy of Quinn B. Carroll

FIGURE 8-87

Optional "oblique" projections of the calcaneus, using a 40° cephalic angle and 45° of **A** internal and **B** external rotation of the leg. See the radiographs in Figure 8-86.

TIPS FOR PEDIATRICS

The Newborn Intensive Care Chest and Abdomen

All of the challenges inherent in the radiography of small infants are redoubled in the newborn intensive care unit working with premature babies. Because the head of a newborn infant is much larger in proportion to its body than that of an adult, when a baby lies on its back the head is forced into flexion and the chin pushed down. Thus, a very common problem in obtaining a supine AP chest projection on a newborn is to get the baby's chin over the lung fields as shown in Figure 8-88.

Some radiographers allow the baby's head to fall off the top edge of the cassette or IR plate in order to bring the chin up a little. This frequently results in clipping the apices of the lungs from the view, and since only about ½ inch is gained in allowing the head to drop further back, the chin can still easily get over the lungs.

A 10°–12° wedge-shaped sponge can be very useful. As diagrammed in Figure 8-89, the sponge is placed on top of the imaging plate under the baby's back with the thickest end at the shoulders. This allows the child's head to fall off of the thick end of the sponge, *but the head is supported by the cassette or IR*, preventing hyperextension. This usually provides just the right amount of head extension to get the chin completely off of the chest.

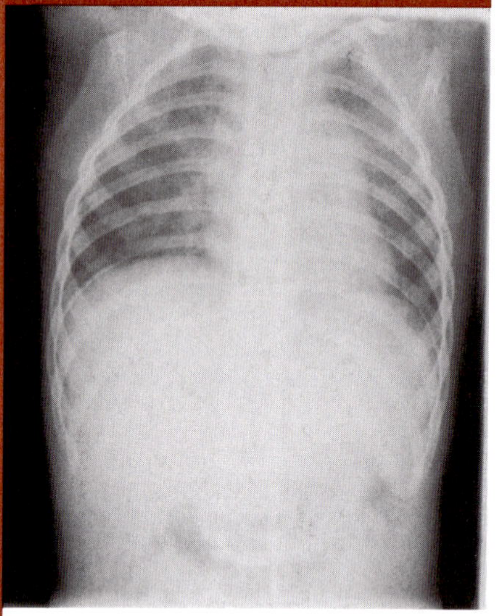

Courtesy of Quinn B. Carroll

FIGURE 8-88

Supine chest radiograph of a small child with his chin over the apices of the lungs, due to forced flexion of his proportionately large head when lying supine.

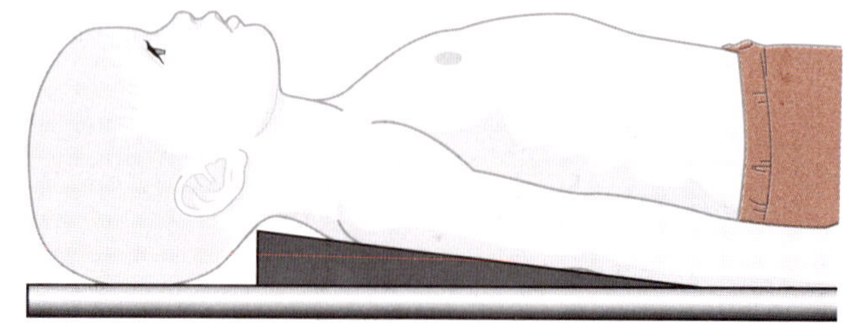

FIGURE 8-89

Recommended correction for the problem in Figure 8-88: Allow the infant's head to fall off the thick end of a wedge-shaped sponge, **but with the head supported by the cassette or IR plate.** This raises the chin, supports the head, and prevents a lordotic view because it is equivalent to a slight caudal angulation of the CR.

Note, also, that building up the shoulders in a supine position is equivalent to a caudal angle of the CR. This is just what is recommended early in this chapter for all AP projections of the chest to prevent a lordotic projection. If the sponge is a bit too much, a slight *cephalic* angle of the beam can be used to reduce the effect to that level desired. For example, with a 10° sponge, a 5° cephalic angle will cancel ½ of its effect. This leaves a net result equivalent to a 5° *caudal* angle, while still taking advantage of the original purpose of the sponge, namely, elevating the chin out of the way.

Regarding cleanliness, the wedge sponge can be wrapped in cellophane, which can be changed from patient to patient. This also prevents body fluids or iodine from soaking into the wedge sponge. Also, CR cassettes or other image receptors can often be wrapped in cellophane, taking care not to leave large wrinkles on the front.

Radiographers experienced in the NBICU know that the radiographic technique used for the AP chest also demonstrates the AP abdomen very well. Furthermore, since the newborn's torso is almost *round* in cross section, rather than oval like an adult, the chest measures nearly the same in lateral as in AP. Therefore, the same technique used for the AP chest in the newborn intensive care unit can frequently be used for the lateral chest.

Finally, the method used to hold and immobilize the newborn infant bears mention. With very small babies such as "premies," one can often pin both arms raised alongside the head with one adult hand, leaving the other hand free to hold the pelvis or upper thighs in place (Figure 8-90). This is essential because it is natural for the baby to writhe about trying to get free when it feels pinned down. Without firm immobilization, the baby will twist its hips and abdomen, causing a rotated view of the chest or abdomen. Holding the knees down will not suffice to prevent this twisting. One must hold down the pelvis for an AP chest, or the upper thighs for an AP abdomen as shown in Figure 8-90. A firm and proper grip will get it right the first time and

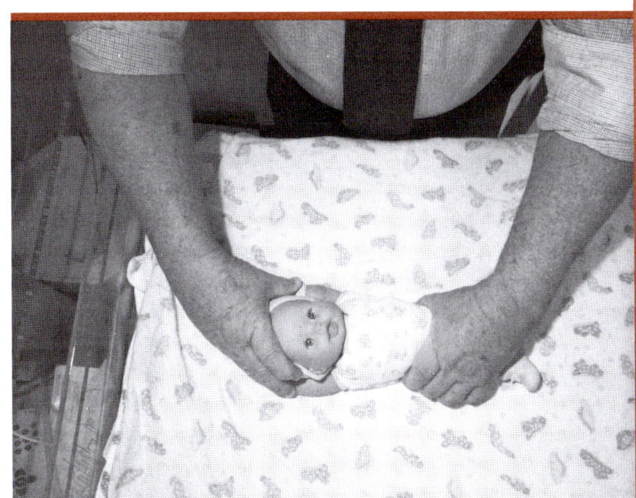
Courtesy of Quinn B. Carroll

FIGURE 8-90

Proper holding for a very small infant for the AP supine chest projection. The arms are raised and pinned against the sides of the head with one hand, and the pelvis is secured in true AP with the other hand.

prevent the trauma of a repeated exposure to the patient. These grips, and the importance of applying them firmly the first time, should be taught to assisting nurses.

On smaller infants, the assisting nurse or radiographer can hold both arms against the baby's head with one hand and the pelvis in a nonrotated AP position with the other hand, as noted earlier. On larger infants, the assisting nurse or radiographer may need both hands to firmly hold the baby's arms alongside its head (Figure 8-91), in order to keep the head close to true AP position. This is important because substantial rotation of the head can bring the shoulders into a twisted position, rotating the upper chest and apical portions of the lungs. In this case, the radiographer who is taking the exposure with one hand can use her free hand to pin the baby's pelvis in straight AP position.

Don't forget the utility of immobilization boards. Whenever the infant can be properly secured to an immobilization board without interfering with IV or other lines, oblique and even lateral projections are greatly facilitated by simply moving the board into position.

General Pediatrics

For chest radiography, a newborn infant up to about 3 months old should be done supine with great care to guard against the infant rolling over and off of the table or other safety issues. Perhaps the safest approach is to "papoose" the baby with a sheet or secure the baby to a "brat board," made of a radiolucent plastic material. But, one must be mindful of artifacts that are likely to show up, especially at the low kVp techniques used for such small infants. Too many wrappings of a sheet, or "brat boards" that are not radiolucent, may result in artifacts that hinder particularly the visibility of fine trabecular lung markings. A parent can be involved in holding the infant down if complete and clear instructions are given, or another radiographer should assist if available.

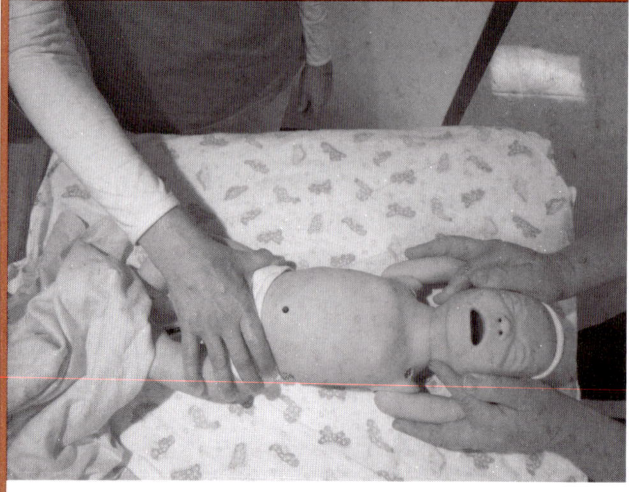

Courtesy of Quinn B. Carroll

FIGURE 8-91

For a large infant, an assisting nurse or radiographer can use both hands to pin the arms alongside the head and keep the head straight. The radiographer making the exposure can use his free hand to secure the pelvis.

From 3 months to about 2 years old, a commercial restraining device such as the Pigg-O-Stat™ should be used with great care. The clamps on these devices must be closed firmly against the child, preventing twisting of the torso, but not so tight as to restrain their breathing. It is good policy to use enough firm restraints to "get it right the first time" so that the child is not subjected to the trauma of retakes. *These devices should not be used for infants who cannot yet hold their own head up*. Those babies should be radiographed supine. These devices should also not be used on children old enough to follow simple breathing instructions while being held in place manually.

For children old enough to follow the instruction to hold their breath, they should be seated straddled on a cassette holder that can be placed at the end of the radiographic table while an adult (with a lead apron on) helps hold the child in position. For the PA projection, the child is instructed to "bear-hug" the CR cassette or IR plate, which pulls the scapulae to the side and leans the torso forward as desired, Figure 8-92*A*. A nonrotated lateral can then be procured by having the child sit facing the assistant who holds the child's arms well up out of the lung fields (not just forward, but *up* and out, as shown in Figure 8-92***B***), and who calls for the exposure when ready. In all cases, good collimation should be used. The eyes should never be included within the field for a chest radiograph. Proper shielding of the gonads is also strongly recommended.

Specifics for "working around the patient" to position are already given throughout this book and can be applied for pediatrics as well as for trauma.

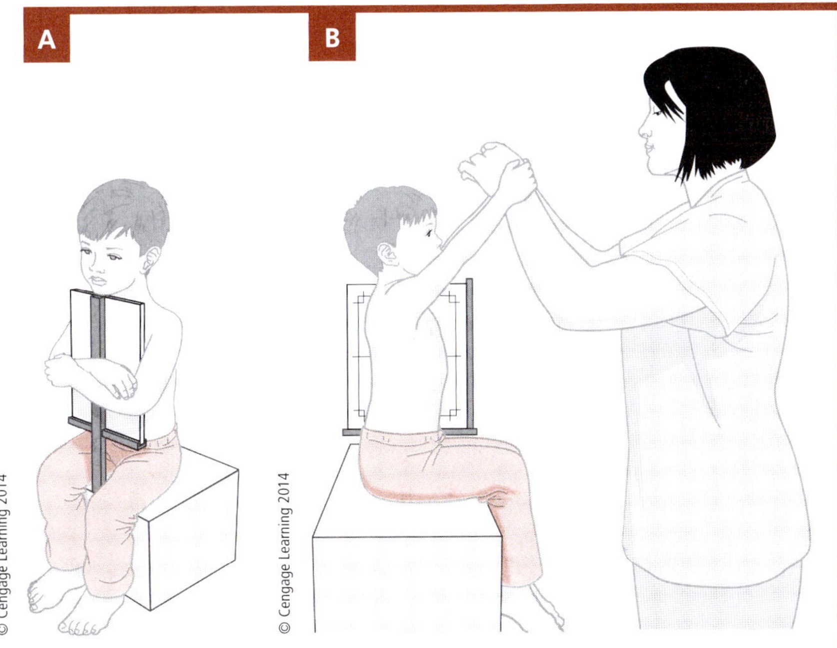

FIGURE 8-92

For small children who can follow directions, the PA chest is best obtained by using a cassette-holding device that allows the child to "bear hug" the detector or cassette **A**. The same device can then be used for the lateral projection, pulling both arms of the child up and forward out of the lung fields, while watching the centering over the IR **B**.

As described for NBICU infants earlier, the torso of a newborn is essentially round in shape, so that the same technique can be used for the lateral chest or abdomen projection as for the AP or PA. By the time a child is 6 months old, the torso is about 4 centimeters wider than it is thick, and technique must be approximately doubled when changing from the AP to the lateral projection. Many radiographers simply go up 9 to 11 kVp, (which is equivalent in the range of 60–70 kVp), while leaving the same mAs. By the time a child is about 6 years old, the technique must be increased by about three times when changing from the AP or PA to the lateral, just as with an adult patient.

SUMMARY

1. For the screening cross-table cervical spine, to minimize clipping of C7, center lower, increase the SID, and depress the *downside* shoulder (against the IR) a little more.
2. For all AP projections of the chest, including supine projections, always angle the CR slightly caudal in relation to the IR and the midcoronal plane, such that the CR is perpendicular to the patient's sternum.
3. For AP projections of the chest, allow less field light above the shoulder shadows.
4. Use of a wedge sponge, wrapped in cellophane for cleanliness, is highly recommended for AP chest projections on infants and in the NBICU, to get the chin out of the way and prevent a lordotic exposure.
5. Recommendations for each specific procedure are presented throughout this chapter.

CRITICAL THINKING CHALLENGE 8.1

ALLEGED EFFECT OF SID ON CR ANGLE

A student is setting up an oblique C-spine using a 72-inch (180-cm) SID. The assisting radiographer mentions that with a 40-inch SID, a 15° cephalic CR angle is needed due to the high divergence of the x-ray beam, but with the increased SID that angle is no longer warranted.

Is the radiographer correct? Why or why not?

CRITICAL THINKING CHALLENGE 8.2

MAGNIFICATION ON THE OPEN-MOUTH VIEW OF C1/C2

A clinical instructor explains to a student why the open-mouth projection of C1 and C2 should *not* be done at 72-inch SID. She states that by keeping the SID at 40 inches, or even by reducing it to 30 inches, the open mouth is magnified so that the distance between the upper and lower teeth is increased and more of C1 and C2 are demonstrated. A radiographer later tells the student that "It really doesn't make any difference, because at shorter distances C1 and C2 *themselves* are magnified along with the open mouth, so they 'fill it up' just the same."

What is the flaw in this reasoning by the radiographer? Or is it accurate to say that the magnification of C1/C2 and of the open mouth effectively cancels each other out at different SIDs? ■

CRITICAL THINKING CHALLENGE 8.3

STANDING THORACIC SPINE LATERAL

A student is performing a standing thoracic spine lateral projection on a wide, broad-shouldered patient with a radiographer observing. Because of where the control panel and table are located in this room, it is very difficult to get to and see the left side of the Bucky. The student decides to perform a right lateral projection instead of the (usual) left lateral so that it is easy to see the light field at the back of the spine. The radiographer tells the student that the lateral needs to be a left, just like it is done when the patient is lying on the table.

Is the radiographer correct? Why or why not? ■

(Answers to Critical Thinking Challenges are found in the Appendix.)

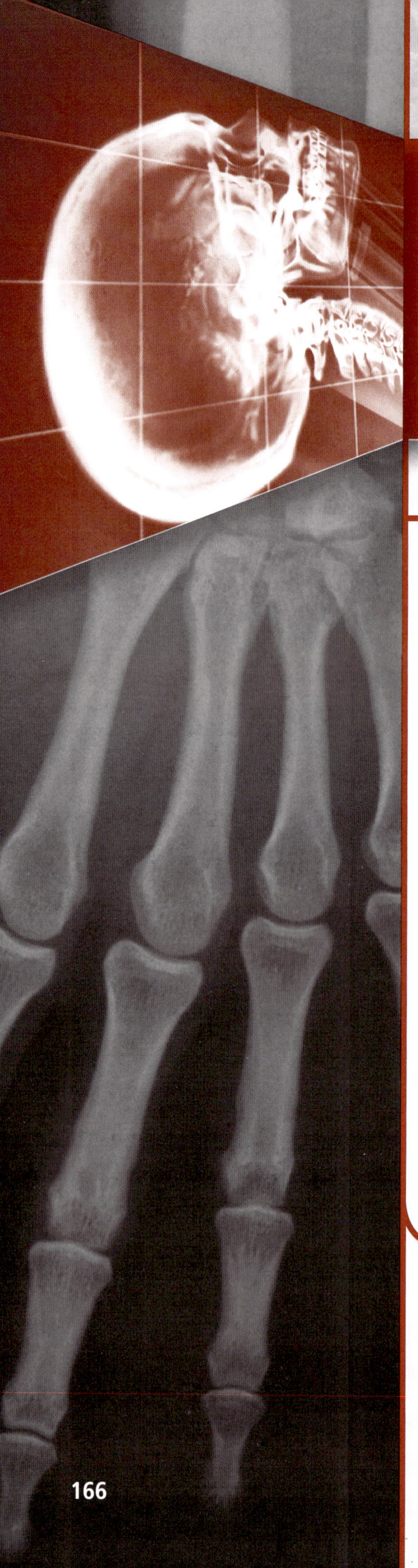

CHAPTER 9

Adapting Skull Positions: Routine and Trauma

OUTLINE

OBJECTIVES

Upon completion of this chapter, you should be able to:

1. Describe when an alternative general approach to positioning should be used rather than compensating by angulation, and give two examples of changing the general approach.

Continues

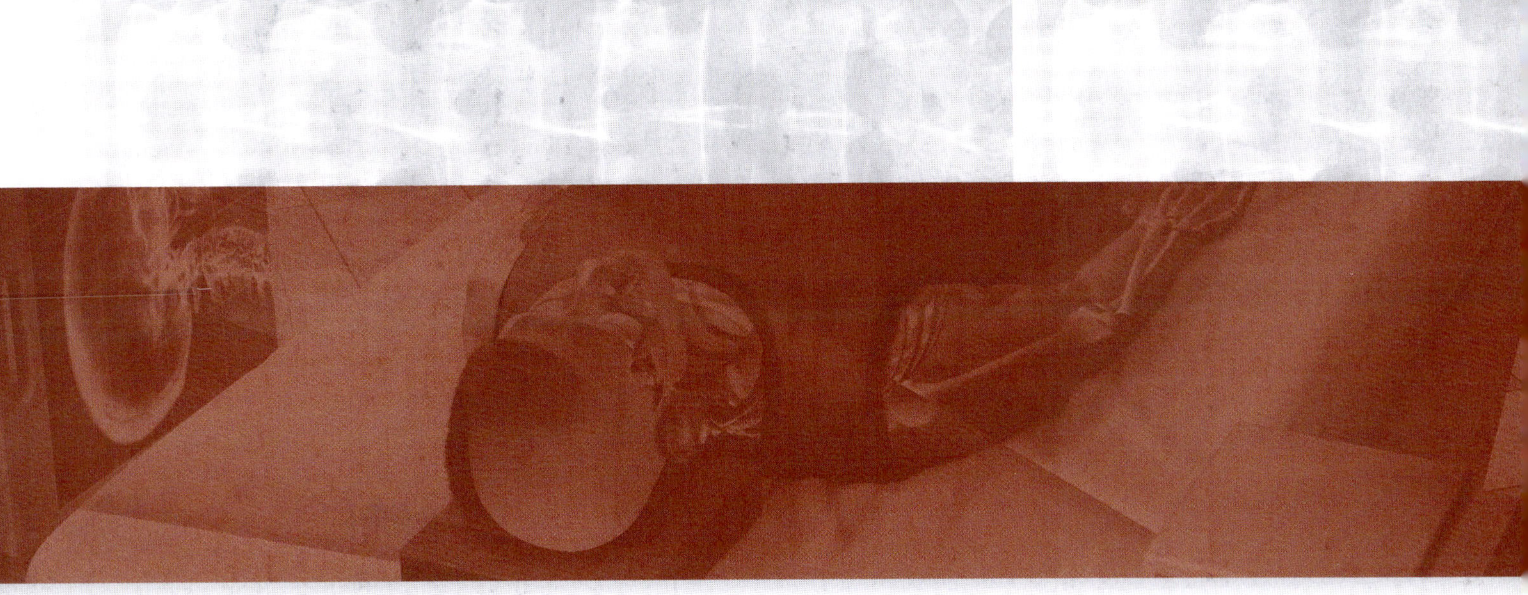

OBJECTIVES *continued*

2. Memorize the average degrees of arc for six skull landmark lines, and using these figures, state the compensating angles needed for various degrees of head flexion and extension for AP, PA, Caldwell and reverse Caldwell, Waters and reverse Waters, and Townes and reverse Townes positions for the skull. Apply these concepts to trauma situations.
3. Explain how to eliminate head tilt from a lateral head position, both for situations where the chin is lower than the forehead and those where the chin is higher than the forehead. Apply this to trauma situations.
4. Describe how head tilt for lateral skull positions may be compensated for with angulation of the CR. Apply this to trauma situations.
5. Describe how tube angulation may be used to compensate for skull rotation. Apply this to trauma situations.
6. Describe two ways to facilitate the submentovertex (SMV) position for the skull.
7. Explain two adaptive methods for obtaining a bilateral projection of the zygomatic arches.
8. List ways to simplify the Rhese, reverse Rhese, and oblique lateral mandible positions.
9. List the priorities for cross-table lateral (horizontal beam) projection of the trauma skull.
10. Describe four alternative ways to obtain a cross-table lateral (horizontal beam) projection of the trauma mandible.
11. Describe the periorbital and trauma oblique projections for the mandible and facial bones.
12. State the rule for adjusting the CR angle for frontal projections of the skull on infants and toddlers.
13. List the steps to turning an upright patient's head into true lateral while maintaining all planes parallel to the image receptor.

REVERSING POSITIONS, CHANGING VENUES

The essence of trauma and mobile radiography is to "work around the patient" by using angulation and positioning of the x-ray tube, moving the equipment rather than the patient. By observing the rotation, flexion/extension, and tilt of the body part, angulation must be added to the direction of the CR until it lines up properly with the designated landmarks and anatomical lines. The required angulation may be transverse, caudal, or cephalic; or for extremities, "distal" or "proximal." For the extremities in general, we are *unlimited* in the inventive use of beam angles. If one can properly visualize anatomical lines such as the intercondylar line (between the *palpated* condyles) of the humerus, one can perform accurate trauma projections.

However, for head procedures and some torso procedures, there is a practical limit to how much the tube can be angled before distortion of the projected anatomy reaches unacceptable levels. This limit falls at about 45°. If the compensating adjustments to any existing tube angle results in a total angle greater than 45°, the radiographer should consider whether there are any alternative positions—reverse positions, upright methods using the chest board, and so on—that the patient can tolerate, that would require less beam angle.

For trauma skull and torso projections, if a compensated angle would exceed 45°, consider alternative general positioning approaches (reverse, upright, and so on).

BEST PRACTICE TIP

For trauma skull and torso projections, if a compensated angle would exceed 45°, consider alternative general positioning approaches (reverse, upright, and so on).

The following case study provides a classic example for applying this principle:

CASE STUDY

Case Study #1: Modified Townes

A Townes projection has been ordered on an ambulatory patient. Placing her supine on the table, you find that she cannot flex her chin down, even using sponges, and the orbitomeatal line (OML) remains extended about 20°. The 20° of caudal angulation to compensate, added to the original 30° required by the position, would result in extreme distortion of the skull. This would be from a total caudal angle of 50°. What whole different approach to this position will accommodate a reasonable tube angle such that distortion is minimized, and achieve the correct projection of all of the anatomical structures relative to each other?

ANSWER: *Reversing the position on the table alone does not* solve *the problem. However, if the patient can be* seated *upright facing the chest board, she can be* bent at the waist, *resting her forehead against the board. Doing so, you estimate the OML to now lie 5° flexed from the horizontal. By adding 20°–25° of upward (cephalic) angle on the CR, you can achieve a* reverse

Townes or Haas view upright. *This makeshift position is illustrated in Figure 9-1. Note that for this situation,* **both reversing the position and changing venues** *from the table to the chest board were required to finally achieve the desired result. This is the essence of trauma positioning skill.*

CASE STUDY

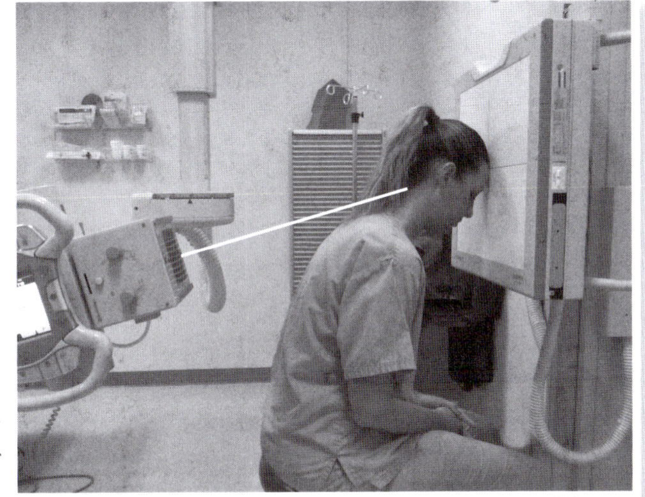

Courtesy of Quinn B. Carroll

FIGURE 9-1

To obtain the equivalent of a Townes projection on a patient who could not tuck down her chin beyond 20° of extension, it was necessary both to position her upright so she could bend at the waist, and also to reverse the position. (In this particular case, the resulting head position was flexed about 20°, added to 10° cephalic angulation of the CR.)

ESTIMATING DEGREES OF FLEXION/EXTENSION

A few universal rules can be adopted to help the radiographer accurately adjust beam angulation in trauma situations for *any* of the frontal projections of the skull, sinuses, and facial bones: These include the AP and PA, the Caldwell and reverse Caldwell, the Waters and reverse Waters, the Townes and reverse Townes, and all their variations for sinuses, sella turcica, TMJs, and so on. These are simple ideas that greatly enhance our ability to estimate not only in which direction, caudal or cephalic, to adjust the beam angle, but *by how many degrees*, with impressive precision.

The student may note that *most* of the landmark lines used for skull positioning violate *paradigms 2 and 3* in Chapter 1, that is, they are essentially based on soft-tissue landmarks rather than true bony landmarks and are also visually observed rather than physically palpated. In a practical sense, this is the best we can do for skull positioning, because it is not feasible to be "poking at" the patient's face to ascertain these landmark points. They are also easily observed, and those lines drawn close to the center of the face (the GML, OML, IOML, NML, and AML, to be discussed shortly), are quite reliable. However, the mentomeatal line (MML) varies a great deal and although it is still useful, the radiographer must be conscientious of the compensations that will be needed from patient to patient.

Practicing radiographers may take for granted that the critical landmark lines of the skull will always fall into place, without carefully observing them, when simplified positioning rules are followed. For example, it is often assumed that for the PA skull or sinus, placing the patient's forehead and nose against the tabletop will automatically bring the OML perpendicular to the plate. But for the patient with an unusually large nose, placing the forehead and nose against the board causes significant hyperflexion, as much as 8°–10° in some cases. The opposite is also true for patients with a small "button" nose, who will likely end up 5° extended. The landmark lines of the skull *must* be carefully observed. Most of the recommendations in this chapter depend entirely upon one's ability to correctly define these lines as a starting point.

The OML is often identified in a sloppy manner by "eyeballing" the general area of the midorbit. It must be observed correctly by taking mental note of the actual outer canthus (junction) of the eyelids. Then, in accordance with the guidelines fully discussed at the beginning of Chapter 5, an imaginary line can be extended to the external auditory meatus (EAM), defined by two distinct points and seen from a proper viewpoint with the positioner's eyes at the same level as the patient.

BEST PRACTICE TIP

For the PA projection of the skull, when the head is flexed or extended, simply angle the beam until the CR parallels the carefully observed OML.

For the routine PA skull or sinus position, when the patient's chin is extended or flexed, an accurate adjustment is easily made by simply observing the OML and angling the CR parallel to it.

For the PA projection of the skull, when the head is flexed or extended, simply angle the beam until the CR parallels the carefully observed OML.

For all the remaining views that involve angles relative to the OML, a simple system of estimation can be derived by memorizing the following three relationships:

1. The acanthiomeatal line (AML) lies, on average, about 27° from the OML.
2. The infraorbitomeatal line (IOML) lies, on average, about 7° from the OML.
3. The *nasomeatal line* (NML) lies, on average, about 17° from the OML.

Now examine Figure 9-2 in which the two conventional lines are illustrated with another midpoint line between them, extending through the bulb of the nose at 17°. This is easily visualized as an angle exactly midway between the AML and the IOML.

We shall identify this as the nasomeatal line (NML).

Naturally, the considerable variation in the size and shape of different noses can skew the placement of the NML. This is easily overcome, however, for patients with unusual noses by simply visualizing the NML as the *midpoint between the IOML and the AML.* In spite of the fact that this is a soft-tissue landmark by name, the landmarks near the center of the face upon which it is based are surprisingly consistent, and by using the method of splitting the difference between the AML and the IOML in order to visualize it, the NML is found to vary only by +/−2° between different patients. It is therefore an extremely practical landmark line. Memorize the angles listed for these three lines. You will find them *extremely* useful in the discussion that follows.

With these three lines in mind, most angles needed for frontal positions can be estimated within a degree or two of perfect accuracy. This includes adaptations for all routine and reversed positions for the Townes, the Caldwell, and the Waters methods as well as the AP and PA projections. Note the pattern for these lines—7°, 17°, and 27° for the IOML, NML, and AML respectively—that makes it easier to commit them to memory: They all end with 7 and go up by 10° each step.

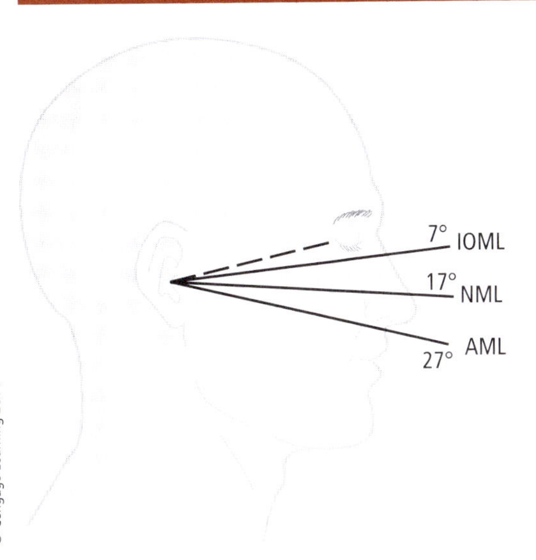

FIGURE 9-2
Angles for three landmark lines *essential* for adapting skull positions. From the orbitomeatal line (OML; dashes), IOML = 7°, the line NML = 17°, and the AML = 27°.

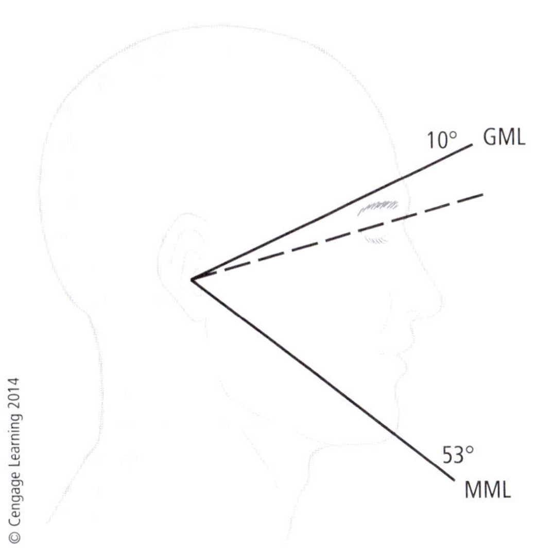

FIGURE 9-3
Angles for two additional landmark lines also useful in adapting skull positions. From the OML; dashes, the *average* glabellomeatal line (GML) = 10°, and the average mentomeatal line (MML) = 53°.

It is also useful to know the degrees of arc for two other landmark lines of the skull: the glabellomeatal line (GML) and the mentomeatal line (MML). These two lines are illustrated in Figure 9-3. Because the jaw and the forehead vary greatly in shape, these lines are somewhat less reliable than those in Figure 9-2, but are still very useful to know.

HOW TO TURN AN UPRIGHT PATIENT'S HEAD LATERAL

A patient is generally unable to maintain his body in the PA (or AP) position and, at the same time, rotate his head 90° into a true lateral position for a skull, facial bones, sinus, or mandible series. This means that the patient's body will have to rotate into an oblique position to some extent. When the patient is upright, attempting to turn the head all the way lateral without rotating the body at all will result in unacceptable head tilt. With substantial body rotation, as the planes of the skull are kept parallel to the IR, an OID "gap" is often unavoidable (Figure 9-4*B*). However, this gap must be minimized as much as possible, and to achieve this, the following approach is recommended.

To begin, with the patient still in PA (or AP) position, have him rotate his head as far as he can without straining (Figure 9-4*A*). Then, keeping the head, neck, and torso in position so that none of the body or head planes become tilted, rotate the entire body toward an oblique position as shown in Figure 9-4*B*, until the head is in true lateral position (Figure 9-4*C*).

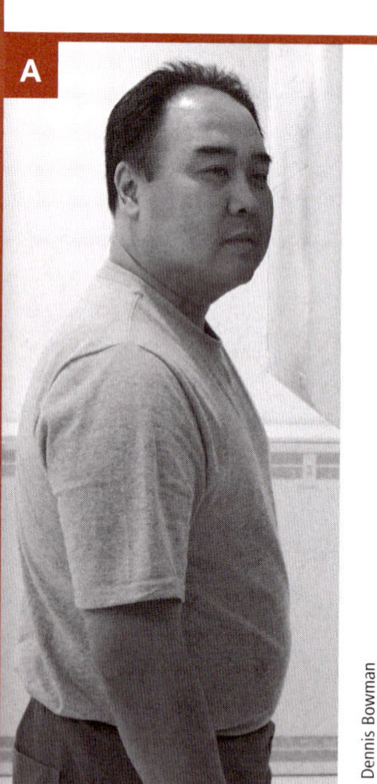

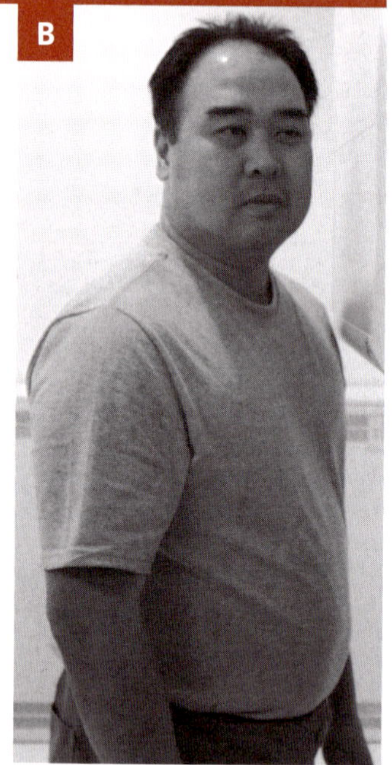

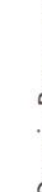

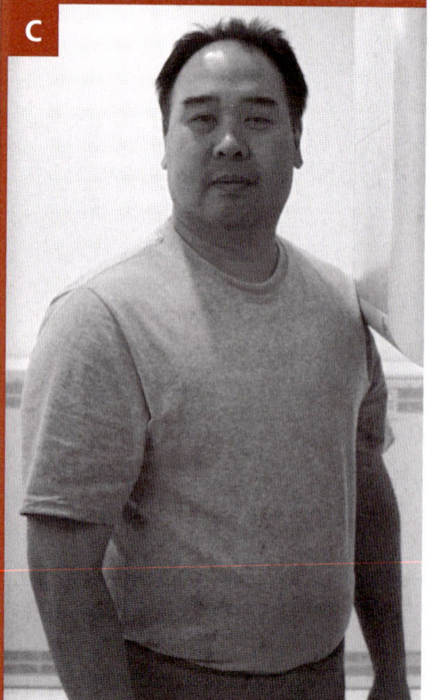

FIGURE 9-4

To turn a patient's head into lateral, with the patient in PA or AP position, begin by rotating the head as far as the patient can without straining **A**. Then, turn the entire body into oblique position **B**, until the head is in a true lateral position, even though some OID gap may result **C**.

Some magnification due to the OID gap will be unavoidable, but it is more important to keep the position parallel to the IR, and the patient will easily be able to hold this true lateral position.

For a recumbent patient, the same *principles* of keeping the planes of the head parallel to the IR should be followed, so the body will be lying in an oblique position that must be properly and well *supported* by placing the downside arm extended alongside the body and the upside arm flexed, as described in nearly all positioning atlases. The upside hand is placed on the table to support the raised upside shoulder. In this position, it is again common for an OID gap to be created, and in order to keep the planes of the head all parallel to the tabletop, a sponge or other radiolucent support is strongly recommended to support the patient's head.

ADAPTING ROUTINE SKULL POSITIONS

Head Rotation

See Chapter 5 for essential considerations in evaluating and correcting rotation. Any compensation of the x-ray beam direction for rotation requires a *transverse* angle. In fixed radiographic rooms, it is not usually an option to disengage the transverse lock that keeps the x-ray tube perpendicular to the grid in the Bucky tray. However, remember that although head radiography is generally done in the Bucky, *skull positions can be done with the CR cassette or DR detector plate tabletop* without producing substantial scatter radiation. If the standard angle lock is not already being used for a cephalic or caudal angle, the entire x-ray tube can be swiveled 90° and then angled transversely using the regular lock, provided the IR plate or cassette is tabletop and nongrid. Modern mobile units allow double angulation of the x-ray tube, in both directions simultaneously, so that with any position it is easy to adopt a small transverse angle when the patient's head is slightly rotated.

Remember the general rule that, when the patient cannot be placed in perfect alignment (parallel or perpendicular) with the IR plate, it is critical to align the CR *with the anatomy, so as to pass straight through it*, even though this may result in an angle relative to the IR plate. Relative tilting of the IR plate is always secondary in importance, while the relationship between the CR and the anatomy is always paramount.

Frontal Skull Projections with Hyperflexion or Hyperextension

PA Skull, Sinus, or Facial Bones

When the patient's head is flexed too much or extended too much, you may simply angle the CR cephalic or caudal until it is *parallel to the OML*. Although this is a simple matter conceptually, it is essential that you identify the OML accurately as discussed in the previous section.

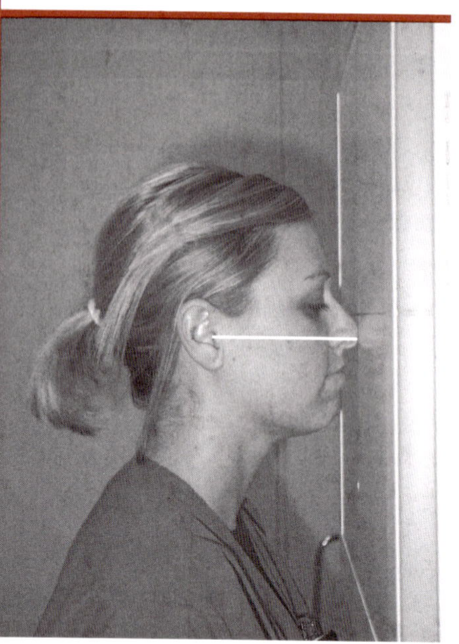

Courtesy of Quinn B. Carroll

FIGURE 9-5
Caldwell position for sinuses, to demonstrate fluid levels. The NML is roughly perpendicular to the plate, placing the forehead and chin equidistant from the plate. The NML is located midway between the IOML and the AML (see Figure 9-2).

Caldwell for Sinuses

When a Caldwell projection is done upright for a sinus series, 15° of *head extension* should be used rather than a caudal angle. By keeping the CR horizontal, the demonstration of any fluid levels in the sinuses is assured. This is strongly recommended.

An additional help in estimating 15° of head extension is that the *NML*, a line drawn from the EAM through the *tip of the nose*, will be roughly perpendicular to the tabletop. As shown in Figure 9-5, this places the *forehead and chin equidistant from the table*. Neither the chin nor the forehead touches the tabletop.

Caldwell (PA Axial) for Skull or Facial Bones

In PA projection, hyperflexion of the head requires additional *caudal* angle added to the normal 15°. Head extension requires a *cephalic* angle. Use the landmark lines in Figure 9-2 to determine the exact amount of angle needed to compensate in Case Study #2 and Case Study #3.

CASE STUDY

Case Study #2: Caldwell for Facial Bones

The patient's chin is slightly up, and it is uncomfortable for her to tuck her chin any further. You estimate that the *IOML* is perpendicular to the plate, as shown in Figure 9-6. What is the corrected tube angle for a proper Caldwell projection?

ANSWER: *See Figure 9-2. The head is extended about 7°. The extension is equivalent to the needed angle, so the amount will be subtracted from it. The tube should be angled 15° − 7° = 8° caudal.*

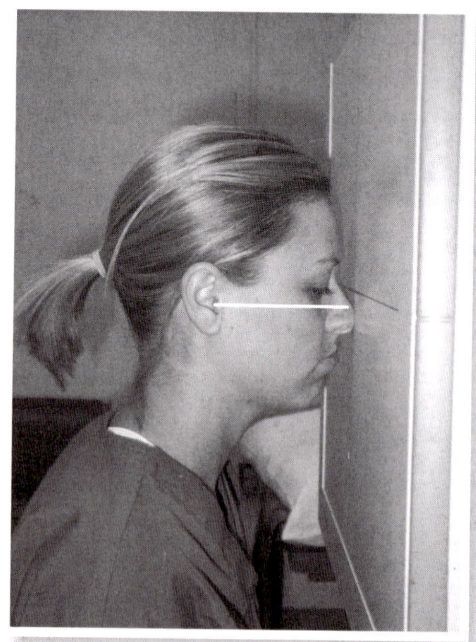

Courtesy of Quinn B. Carroll

FIGURE 9-6
How much is the head extended? For a Caldwell for facial bones, what degree and direction of CR angle is needed to compensate?

Case Study #3: Caldwell for Facial Bones

The patient has a large nose resulting in some hyperflexion when the forehead touches the tabletop. He is shaky, so you want to keep the forehead braced against the table rather than using head extension and only having his nose resting on the tabletop. You estimate that the horizontal is a line midway between the *OML* and the *GML*, as shown in Figure 9-7. What tube angle is needed for an adapted Caldwell projection?

ANSWER: *See Figure 9-3. The GML lies approximately 10° from the OML. Therefore, a line midway between the GML and the OML lies at about 5°. Flexion works against the needed angle, so the amount must be added to it. The tube should be angled 15° + 5° = 20° caudal.*

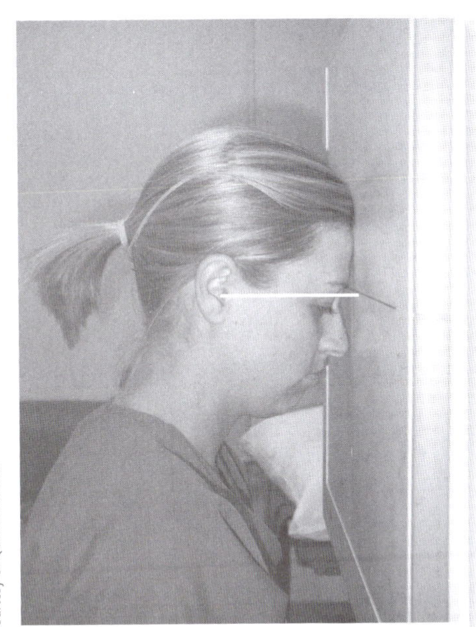

Courtesy of Quinn B. Carroll

CASE STUDY

FIGURE 9-7
How much is the head flexed? For a Caldwell for facial bones, what degree and direction of CR angle is needed to compensate?

Townes (AP Axial) for Skull

When a patient is lying supine, it is natural for the head to drop back into a somewhat extended position. Few patients can lie supine and, while resting their head back against the table, tuck their chin enough to place the OML perpendicular. (This is especially difficult for trauma patients.) Yet historically this is how the Townes position has been taught, with an accompanying 30° caudal angle.

A much more realistic approach is to allow for some extension of the head and simply compensate the angle of the CR. The degree of head extension must be *added* to the 30° relationship between the CR and the OML. (This is because in an AP projection, head extension *cancels out* caudal angulation.)

If the *IOML* (instead of the OML) is placed perpendicular, the extension of the head is about 7°, (see Figure 9-2). Therefore, a 37° caudal angle can be used with the *IOML* perpendicular (Figure 9-8). This achieves the same projection, but is much easier for both patient and

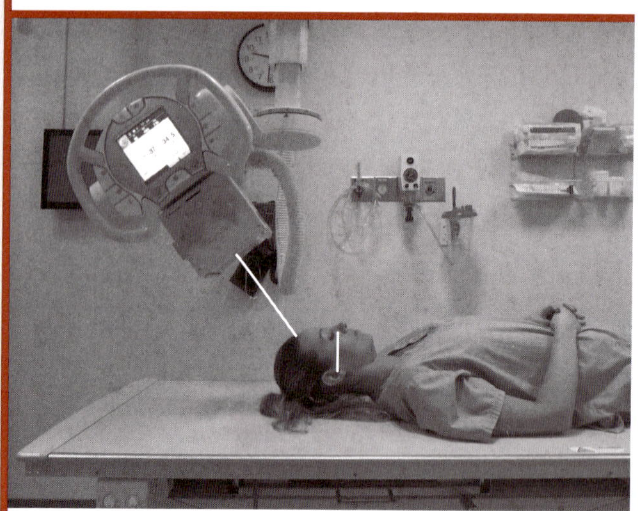

Courtesy of Quinn B. Carroll

FIGURE 9-8

Placing the IOML vertical and using a 37° caudal angle for the Townes projection is more realistic than trying to tuck the patient's chin down until the OML is vertical.

positioner. This method is strongly recommended as a routine approach to the Townes position.

Even when using this approach with the IOML perpendicular, you will still find a frequent need to build up the patient's head with sponges to some degree. This is especially true for patients with thick shoulders, or with kyphosis, because their head tends to drop back even more. Wedge-shaped sponges are recommended, because they can be simply slid in or out to adjust the thickness and degree of buildup.

Whenever the head cannot be ideally positioned with a landmark line perpendicular, small adjustments in the caudal angulation of the CR can be readily made by visualizing whatever line *is* perpendicular relative to the landmark angles in Figure 9-2, that is, by "splitting the difference" between these landmark lines. As an example, try the exercise in Case Study #4.

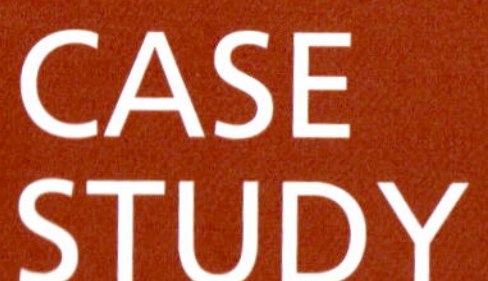

Case Study #4: Modified Townes

On an average patient, you estimate that the vertical is midway between the *IOML* and the *NML*, as shown in Figure 9-9. What CR angle should be used for a modified Townes projection?

ANSWER: *Splitting the difference between these two lines, the head is* extended *about 12° (halfway between 7° and 17°). In this case, the extension is* contrary *to the needed angle (extending the head cancels out the caudal angle). So, the amount will have to be added. The tube should be angled 30° + 12° = 42° caudal.*

CASE STUDY

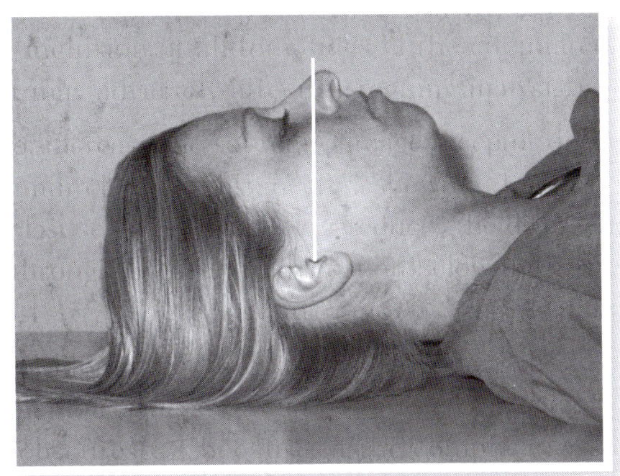

Courtesy of Quinn B. Carroll

FIGURE 9-9

How much is the head extended? For a Townes projection, what degree and direction of CR angle is needed to compensate?

The Special Case of the Waters (Parietoacanthial) Projection

The Waters position presents a special case that is somewhat more complicated than any of the other frontal skull projections. The complication arises from the fact that the angle of 37° typically presented in positioning atlases ***is NOT the angle of actual head extension.*** Rather, it is the angle *formed between the tabletop and the OML when the head is extended* 53° (Figure 9-10).

Remember that from the "starting point" in which the head is in true PA position, the OML is not at 0° but at 90° from the tabletop, placing it perpendicular. As the chin is then extended for a routine Waters

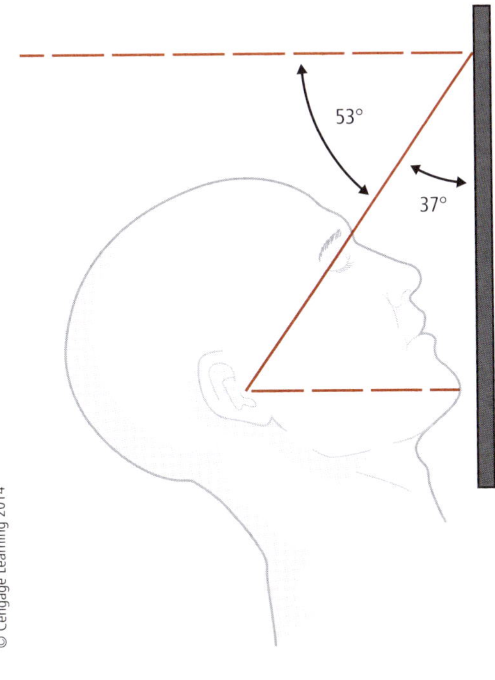

FIGURE 9-10

In the Waters position, extension of the head is 53° (not 37°), measured from the normal perpendicular position of the OML.

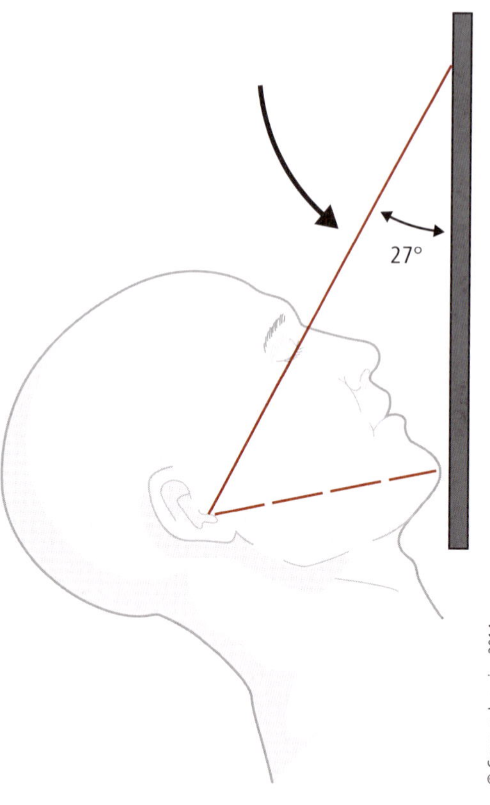

FIGURE 9-11

As head extension increases, the angle formed between the OML and the table is actually *decreasing*. Here, overextension reduces it from 37° to 27°.

projection, this angle is actually *decreasing* from 90° down to 37°. Ironically, overextension of the chin results in this angle being measured *less* than 37°, not more (Figure 9-11). This can be quite confusing for the positioner.

Recall that many positioning atlases recommend, as a starting point for the Waters position, extending the head until the *MML* is roughly perpendicular to the tabletop. Although this method is not very consistent due to great variations in the shape of the jaw, it is worth noting here that *on average*, the MML lies at a 53° angle from the radiographic baseline (OML) (see Figure 9-3). This represents the amount of head extension required.

Once it is understood that the actual degree of head extension for the routine Waters position is 53°, we can then apply the above landmark skull lines in adapting any Waters projection, as shown in Case Study #5 and Case Study #6.

CASE STUDY

Case Study #5: Waters for Facial Bones

On a patient who cannot fully raise her chin into position, you estimate that the *NML* is close to horizontal, as shown in Figure 9-12. What is the tube angle for an adapted Waters projection?

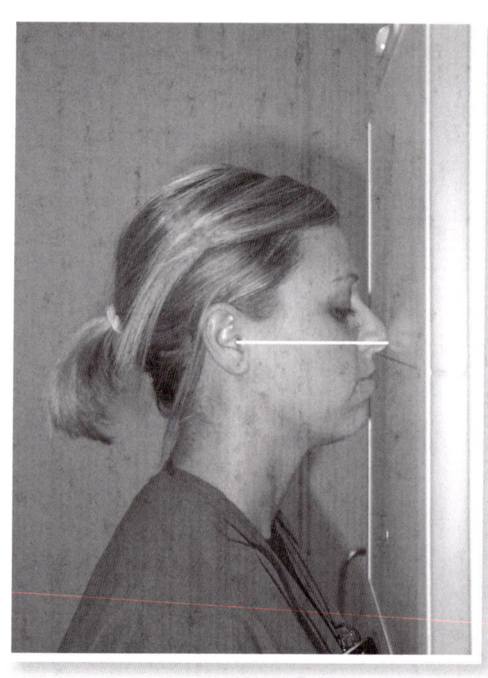

FIGURE 9-12

How much is the head extended? For a Waters projection, what degree and direction of CR angle is needed to compensate?

ANSWER: *See Figure 9-2. The head is* extended *about 17°. In a PA projection, head extension is equivalent to caudal angulation, so the amount of extension will be subtracted from the needed angle. The tube should be angled 53° − 17° = 36° caudal. (Note that this degree of angulation will not show air-fluid levels for a sinus series, and will also result in significant distortion. Yet, it can be and has been utilized in screening for fractures, foreign bodies, or other trauma to the facial bones and orbits.)*

CASE STUDY

Case Study #6: Waters for Facial Bones

An elderly, kyphotic patient cannot raise his chin at all. Placing him in a general PA position against the chest board, you estimate that the horizontal is a line midway between the *OML* and the *GML*, as shown in Figure 9-13. What tube angle is needed for an adapted Waters projection?

ANSWER: *See Figure 9-3. The GML lies approximately 10° from the OML. Therefore, a line midway between the GML and the OML lies at about 5°. The head is flexed 5°, which would be added to the normal 53° for a total of 58°.* ***However, note that this is well beyond the 45° limit discussed at the beginning of this chapter,*** *and will result in unacceptable distortion of the anatomy.* ***The position must be reversed,*** *so the patient can be leaned back at the waist.*

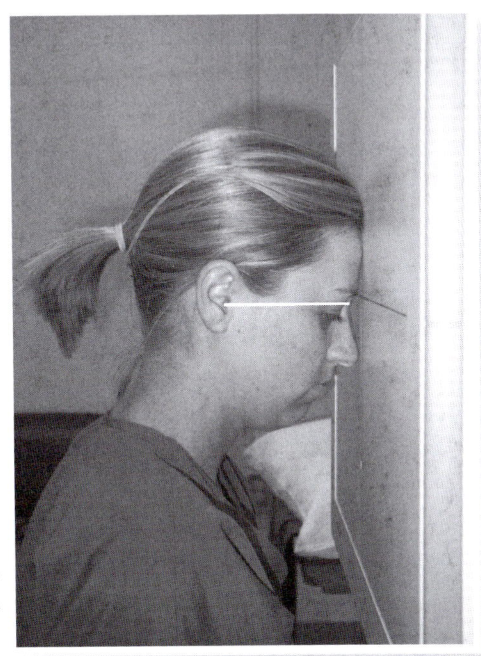

Courtesy of Quinn B. Carroll

FIGURE 9-13
How much is the head flexed? For a Waters projection, what degree and direction of CR angle is needed to compensate?

Different Positioning Line for the Waters Projection

The *MML* is frequently recommended as a landmark line for the Waters position, which, it is stated, should lie "approximately" perpendicular to the IR. Of all the landmark lines used in the skull, the MML is the most variable and unreliable, due to the tremendous variety in the shape of the mandible between different patients. Therefore, this line can be used as a "rough" starting point in positioning the Waters projection, but *never* should be used as a final criterion that the position is correct.

For this purpose, positioning atlases generally suggest use the OML, which must lie at a 37° angle from the IR plate surface or tabletop. But, to accurately assess this, an "angliner" or protractor is needed to actually measure the angle. (Furthermore, as was discussed in the preceding section, increasing head extension *reduces* the measured angle of this line, while flexion of the chin *increases* the measured angle, making the whole approach more complicated for the radiographer.)

A simplified, yet accurate, way to position a Waters view can be derived by establishing a new landmark line along the side of the face. A palpable landmark is the *bottom margin of the body of the zygoma, or cheekbone* (Figure 9-14*A*). This point lies just 2–2½ inches anterior to the EAM and *must be felt laterally on the cheek, not anteriorly*. A positioning line can be extended from the *top-of-the-ear attachment (TEA)* to this point on the lateral cheek (Figure 9-14*B*). We shall designate this as the *EZ* line (ear-to-zygoma line).

Recall that the TEA (top of ear attachment) is at the level of the petrous pyramids, which must lie below the maxillary sinuses in the final Waters view. As the patient extends the head, lifting the chin, the petrous ridge is moved downward while the maxillary sinuses are raised. Once the EZ line is perpendicular to the IR (horizontal for an upright position), the petrous bones should be projected directly under the maxillary sinuses and the patient is positioned correctly for a Waters projection (Figure 9-14*B*).

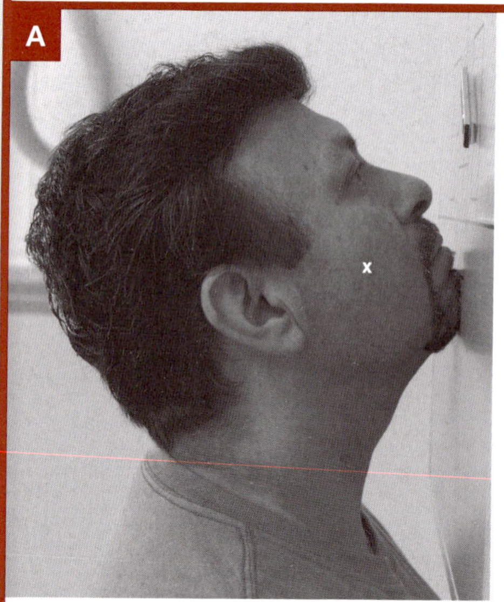

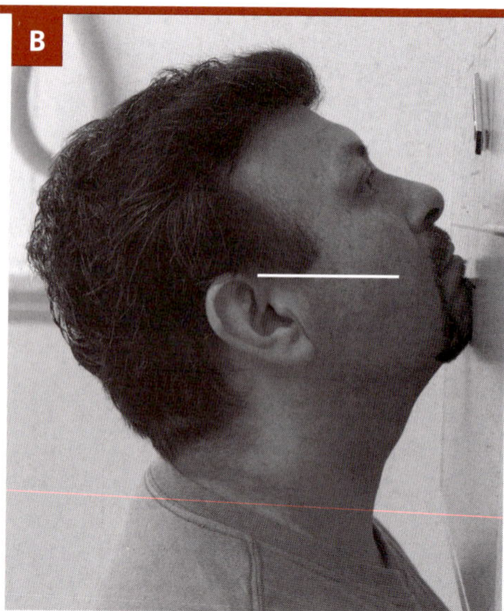

FIGURE 9-14

By palpating the bottom margin of the zygoma laterally **A** and observing the TEA and landmark line, the *ear-to-zygoma or EZ line,* is established. For a Waters projection, the *EZ line* should be perpendicular to the IR **B**.

Other Head Projections

Lateral Head Projections

Lateral head positions are particularly vulnerable to problems with both tilt and rotation, due to their connection with the position of the *shoulders*. The shoulders can vary widely in thickness and breadth, and they are placed in an oblique position of variable degrees, thus twisting the neck. Success in positioning any lateral projection of the head is very much dependent on fully appreciating this connection with the shoulders and the rest of the body.

As described in Chapter 5, tilt of the head must be assessed by squatting or bending down to the level of the patient, and observing the patient's facial landmarks from a frontal viewpoint. Rotation must also be observed by squatting or bending down to the level of the patient, but this time from the head of the table looking directly down on the top of the head.

Head tilt can be a particular problem. When the head is tilted with the *chin lower than the forehead*, many radiographers neglect the importance of the upside *elbow*, leaving it resting on the table (Figure 9-15A). This prevents the shoulders from being rotated up

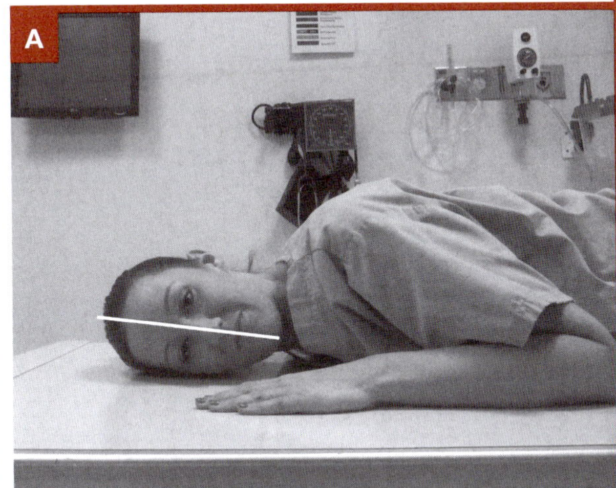
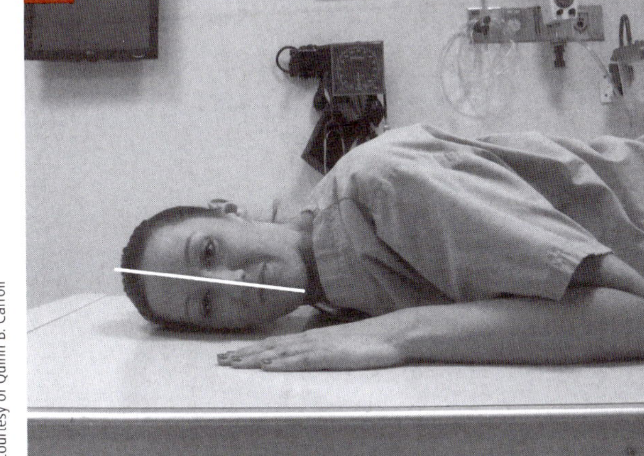

Courtesy of Quinn B. Carroll

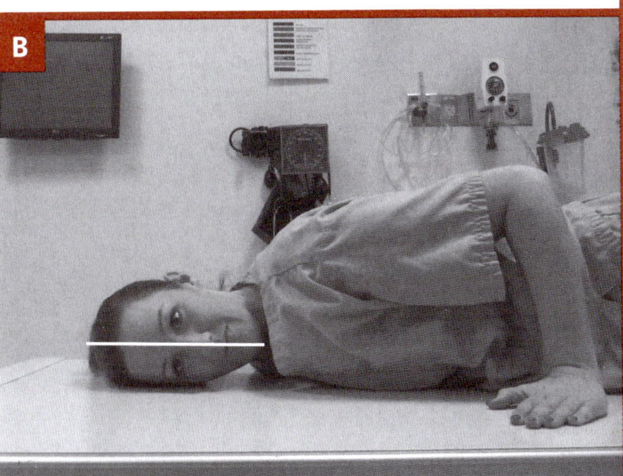

Courtesy of Quinn B. Carroll

FIGURE 9-15

Head tilt with the chin low often cannot be corrected as long as the elbow is left resting on the table **A**, because this prevents the *shoulders* from being rotated upward sufficiently. In **B**, *the arm and elbow are supported up off the table* allowing a steep obliquity of the shoulders, then the chin tucked, to eliminate tilt.

enough to, in turn, allow the chin to be properly elevated. Use the following key steps to eliminate this type of tilt:

Eliminating Tilt from Lateral Head Projections (Chin Low):

1. Get the patient's elbow off the table, supporting the arm up with the hand (Figure 9-15***B***).
2. Then, rotate the shoulders up into a steeper oblique as needed.
3. Finally, a small amount of remaining tilt can be eliminated by tucking the chin.

When the head is tilted with the *chin higher than the forehead*, frequently the case for patients with very large shoulders, a wedge-shaped sponge can be slid up under the parietal eminence until the midsagittal plane is built up parallel to the table (Figure 9-16). The *wedge* shape is specifically recommended, because the sponge can be slid in or out to adjust the degree of buildup. The magnification effects

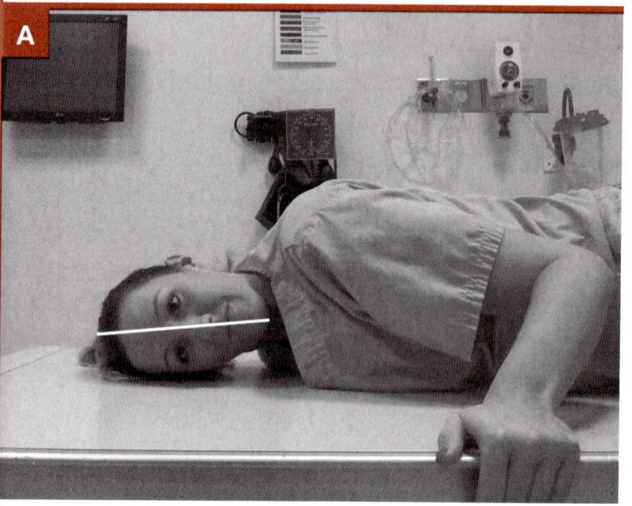

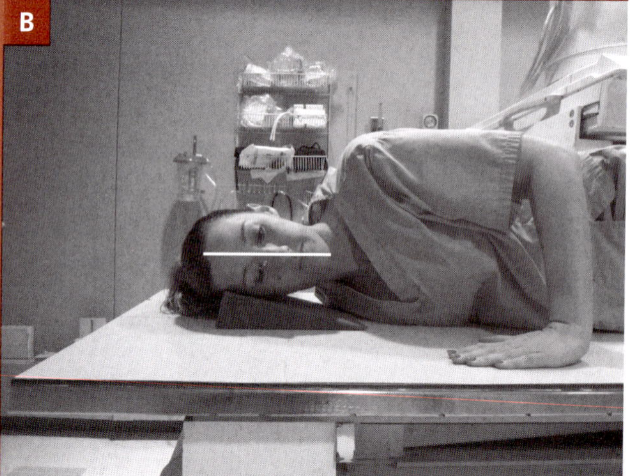

FIGURE 9-16

Head tilt with the chin high **A** can be corrected with a wedge-shaped sponge **B**. The *wedge* shape is specifically recommended, because it can be moved in or out to adjust the degree of buildup.

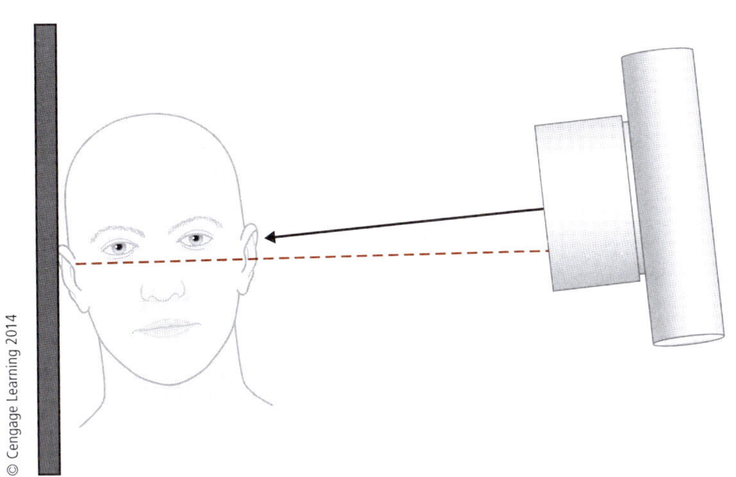

FIGURE 9-17
Head tilt with the chin high can also be corrected with slight caudal angulation as needed to place the CR parallel to the interpupillary line (between the eyes).

of the small OID gap created are insignificant and always secondary to proper alignment.

Alternatively, when the head is tilted with the chin high, simply angle the CR caudal until it lies parallel to the interpupillary line (Figure 9-17). (The interpupillary line is formed between the two pupils of the eyes.) As previously explained, the distortion effects of slight angulation against the cassette plate are negligible (even unmeasurable), and always secondary to alignment between the CR and the *part*. This correction is quick, easy, and handy when positioning sponges are unavailable.

Submentovertex (SMV)

Following are two approaches to the submentovertex (SMV) position that are easier to accomplish:

Supine SMV

This position is very useful for trauma patients or weak patients who can extend the head without injury. Use sandbags and sponges as needed, to hold the IR plate or cassette on the x-ray table at an angle tilted 20°–25° from vertical, as shown in (Figure 9-18). Rest the vertex of the patient's head against it, and gently extend the chin some 27°–32° such that the IOML parallels the plate. Angle the CR 20°–25° downward from the horizontal (65°–70° on the meter), such that it is perpendicular to the IR plate. (The shadow of the chin on the plate should be projected just above the broader shadow of the forehead.)

Sitting SMV

If a chest board or wall mount is unavailable, stand the x-ray table up for a vertical Bucky. Place a stool about 1 foot (30 cm) out in front of the table, perfectly centered. This allows the patient to gently arch his back without overstraining, until the vertex of the head is resting against the table (Figure 9-19). Cephalic angulation is then increased until the shadow of the chin is seen rising over the broader shadow of the forehead on the table.

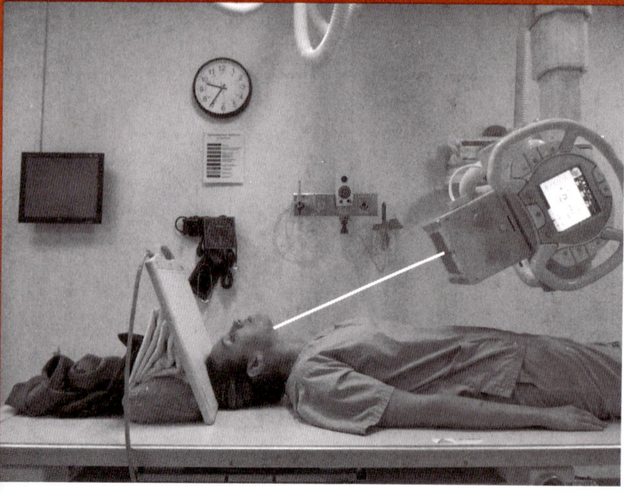

Courtesy of Quinn B. Carroll

FIGURE 9-18

SMV projection with the patient supine. The patient's chin is extended until the infraorbitomeatal line lies 20°–25° from vertical. The CR is angled downward 20°–25°, and the IR plate tilted to match.

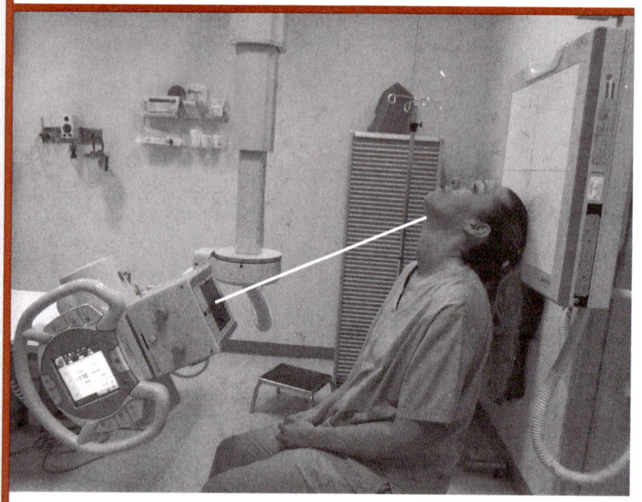

Courtesy of Quinn B. Carroll

FIGURE 9-19

SMV projection seating patient 1 foot away from the upright table or chest board, gently arching the back, and adding cephalic angulation as needed. In this case, the CR is *over angled* an additional 10° upward to demonstrate the zygomatic arches.

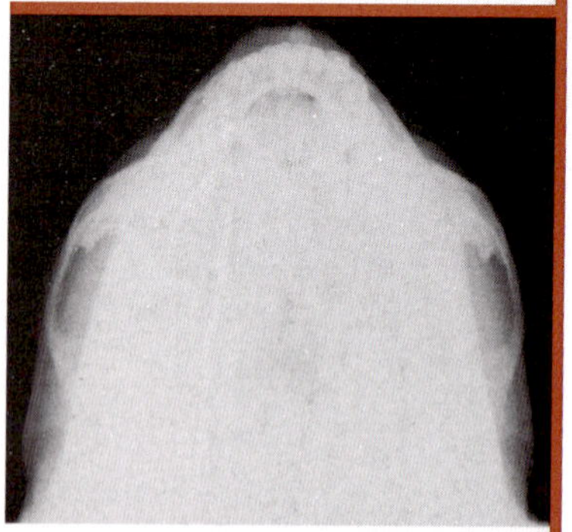

Zygomatic Arches

There are two adaptive methods in which easy bilateral views of the zygomatic arches can be obtained. Both are equivalent to the more difficult Mays method used for a single arch, but save time and effort. These methods are both based on the submentovertex projection of the skull described earlier.

Submentovertex with CR Overangled

In the submentovertex position, simply angle the CR cephalic 10°–15° *past* perpendicular to the *IOML* (Figure 9-19). On the cassette plate or tabletop, the chin shadow will be seen to rise 2–3 inches above the forehead shadow. With this approach, the projection of the arches only has to clear the *forehead* laterally, rather than the wider *parietal* portion of the head. Normal divergence of the x-ray beam provides a bilateral angle sufficient to do so (10°–12° along both sides of the face). By opening the field, both zygomatic arches are demonstrated in one exposure (Figure 9-20).

FIGURE 9-20

Bilateral SMV view of the zygomatic arches using an overangled SMV position.

Carroll, Q. Evaluating Radiographs, 1993, Figure 189, Courtesy of Charles C Thomas, Publisher, Ltd., Springfield, Illinois.

Submentovertex with SID Reduced to 30 Inches

In the submentovertex position, with the CR perpendicular to the IOML as shown in Figure 9-20, simply reduce the SID to 30 inches, and open the collimated field to restore the field size for a bilateral projection. As shown in Figure 9-21, the reduced distance results in 15° of beam divergence on both sides of the face. The resulting view is demonstrated in Figure 9-22. It is critical to ensure that there is no tilt in the head position, which will obscure the zygomatic arch on one side.

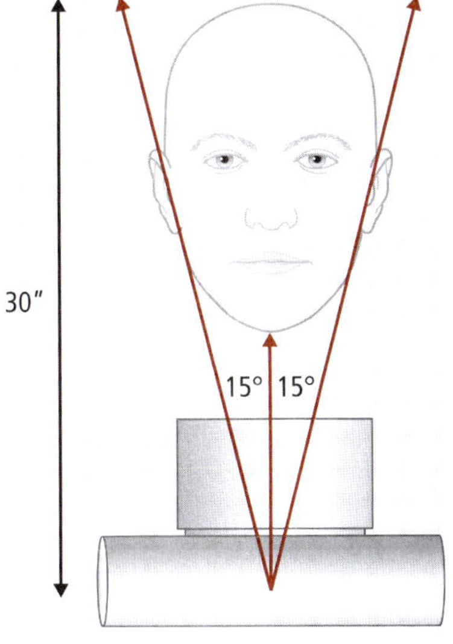

FIGURE 9-21

For the SMV projection, reducing the SID to 30 inches results in beam divergence equivalent to 15° on *both* sides of the face, making it possible to obtain a bilateral SMV view for the zygomatic arches.

Rhese Position for Oblique Facial Bones, Orbit, or Optic Foramen

Note that the *reverse* Rhese position, described in the following section, is recommended over the conventional Rhese method for ease of positioning, especially for screening of the orbit for foreign bodies and for the optic foramen. However, if a high-detail view of facial bones around the rim of the orbit is required, then the conventional PA Rhese should be used as described here.

With the body and the head in a PA oblique position, center the downside orbit over the midline of the table or IR plate. Head rotation of 53° can be closely estimated by starting with the head at 45°, then rotating it steeper by an estimated 8°. From the side of the table, adjust the AML perpendicular, resulting in a "3-point landing" with the chin, cheek, and nose against the table. *Note that in the proper Rheese position with the AML perpendicular,* ***the forehead does NOT touch the table****, but the downside eyebrow is raised ½-inch or so off the table.* Check again from the head of the table to see this. With the forehead raised, you can easily center the downside orbit by sliding the patient to the right or left until the midpoint of the downside eyebrow, which you can clearly see, is centered.

A *very* common mistake is to touch the forehead down to the table. Not only is this an incorrect position, it makes it impossible to see the downside eyebrow from the head of the table for centering purposes.

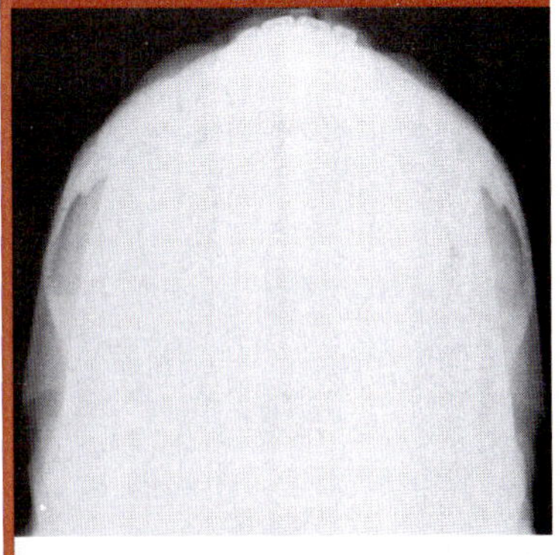

FIGURE 9-22

Bilateral SMV view of the zygomatic arches using a reduced 30-inch SID.

Carroll, Q. Evaluating Radiographs, 1993, Figure 188, Courtesy of Charles C Thomas, Publisher, Ltd., Springfield, Illinois.

Reverse Rhese Position for Oblique Facial Bones, Orbit, or Optic Foramen

This position is easier to obtain than the PA Rhese method, and is particularly useful for the optic foramen. The optic foramen, at the deep end of the orbital cone, lies almost midway through the head, so it is hardly magnified more in the AP projection than in the PA. Furthermore, with the AP approach the orbital rim is magnified, which only serves to move it farther away from the optic foramen. This is desirable, because it reduces the probability of superimposing the rim over the foramen from small errors in rotation of the head.

This position also serves well for screening of the orbit for foreign bodies (pre-MRI survey), and as a general facial screening view for

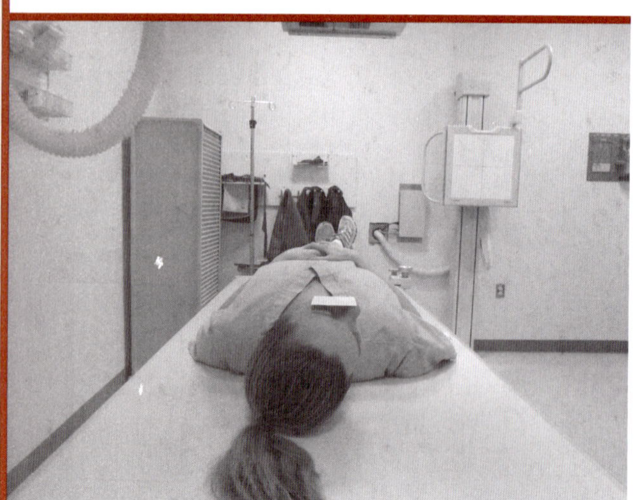
Courtesy of Quinn B. Carroll

FIGURE 9-23

Reverse Rhese position for trauma facial bones and orbit, using an index card to establish the "3-point landing". Simply adjust the head rotation and extension until the index card is horizontal in both planes.

trauma patients, although some magnification of the facial surface is present.

With the patient supine, further extend the head until the *AML* is vertical, then rotate the head 53° *away* from the side of interest. Head rotation of 53° can be closely estimated by starting with the head at 45°, then rotating it steeper by an estimated 8°. The "3-point landing" method can actually be used if you have access to an index card: Place the index card so that it touches the chin, the cheek, and the nose. Then simply adjust both rotation and extension of the head until the index card lies horizontal in both planes (Figure 9-23).

Slide the head to center the CR right through the middle of the easily observed upside orbit (have the patient close his eyes from the field light). Double-check rotation and extension, or the index card, before exposing.

This position can be further adapted for the supine trauma patient to minimize or eliminate movement of the head, as presented at the end of the following "Trauma" section.

Lateral (Oblique) Mandible

For this position, *head tilt is strongly recommended whenever it can be used instead of angling the CR.* (Many positioning atlases show a 25°–30° cephalic angle that can project the shoulder shadow into the mandible. The CR angle can also cause substantial distortion, and is more difficult to position.) Place the patient in a straight lateral body position *with the downside shoulder "in the way" against the chest board (or table)*. On the average patient, tilting the head from this position until it rests against the board will result in 25°–30° of head tilt exactly as desired. This allows a *horizontal* (or perpendicular) beam to be used (Figure 9-24). With no angle, simply center the CR just below and anterior to (by ½-inch each) the *upside* gonion (angle of the jaw).

For patients with very broad shoulders, with the body in true lateral position as described, the 30° of tilt may not bring the head to rest

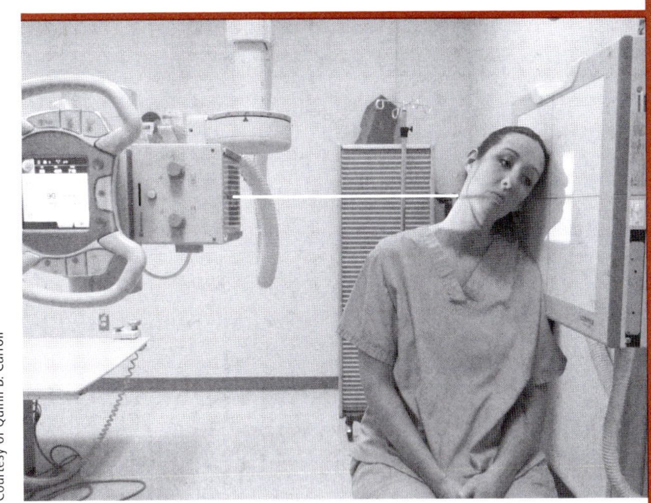

Courtesy of Quinn B. Carroll

FIGURE 9-24
Lateral (oblique) mandible position using 25°–30° of head tilt with a horizontal beam (no angle).

against the tabletop, leaving a gap. Simply oblique the *shoulder* position as needed to bring the head a bit closer to the table prior to tilting it.

When the head cannot be tilted a full 25°–30°, various combinations of tilt and CR angle can be employed. The head can be tilted 15° with the CR angled 15° cephalic. However, use as much tilt, and as little CR angle, as possible. Avoid using more than 15° of angulation, which can create problems with the upside shoulder being projected into the mandible.

Note that no *rotation* of the skull is recommended here as is common in positioning atlases. This is because more than 5°–8° of head rotation brings the downside gonion (the side of interest) back under the cervical spine, resulting in superimposition of the vertebrae over the ramus portion of the mandible. When specific interest is in the mentum, 45° of rotation places it parallel and closer to the plate. For interest in the body portion, 30° does the same. But, for interest in the ramus portion or for the general mandible, the 15° of rotation designated in many positioning atlases is *not* recommended. That is, placing the part more parallel is not worth getting the cervical spine superimposed over the posterior mandible.

TAMING THE TRAUMA SKULL

This section builds heavily upon the material presented in the first half of this chapter, and especially upon the landmark lines and their degrees of arc presented in Figures 9-2 and 9-3. Although most of the positions discussed are reversed and the CR angles are therefore in the opposite direction (cephalic instead of caudal and vice versa), the geometrical logic follows exactly the same process and uses the same landmarks. If you have difficulty following any of the case studies in this section, be sure to review the same position, unreversed, in the last section and then come back to it here. In addition to reversed positions, specific methods will also be presented here for other trauma situations such as the cross-table oblique mandible and the trauma orbit.

We assume that the typical trauma patient is found in a supine position and cannot be moved out of it because of their condition or attached equipment. Therefore, most frontal projections must be obtained in reverse, and lateral projections must be obtained cross-table (decubitus).

Head Rotation

As a patient lies supine on a stretcher or table, in a naturally relaxed position, the head is not often rotated. It should be checked, nonetheless, and correction should be made for slight rotation. If you are certain that the patient's head can be moved, it is best to carefully adjust the head itself. But, modern mobile x-ray units allow for double angulation of the x-ray tube, and the x-ray beam can be angled transversely until it lines up with the midsagittal plane of the head. Performing trauma skull radiography *nongrid* allows full leeway in angling the CR as needed. Remember that keeping the CR passing straight through the *anatomy* takes precedence over keeping the CR parallel to the cassette or IR plate.

For a more full discussion, see *Head Rotation* under "Adapting Routine Skull Positions" at the beginning of this chapter. See Chapter 5 for essential considerations in evaluating and correcting rotation in general.

Reversed Skull Positions with the Patient Supine

Before discussing specific adjustments, it is useful to better appreciate the *average* situation. As a trauma patient lies supine on a gurney (stretcher) or x-ray table without a pillow, the head naturally falls *back* to that surface such that the OML is *extended*. It is rarely a question *whether* the head will be extended, only how much! What can be derived from this is that *the compensating angle needed to produce an AP projection of the skull will nearly always be a caudal angle.*

In fact, leaving the tube vertical will typically result in a reverse *Caldwell* view, in which the petrous ridges fall roughly in the lower one-third of the orbits. This, in turn, is an indication of how much the head has been extended—an average of 12°–15°. For a proper AP projection, then, a caudal angle of 12°–15° will place the central ray approximately parallel to the OML and produce Figure 9-25.

BEST PRACTICE TIP

A caudal angle of 12°–15° will compensate for head extension on most patients for the supine, AP skull projection.

A caudal angle of 12°–15° will compensate for head extension on most patients for the supine, AP skull projection.

Patients with unusually large shoulders will require *more* caudal angulation because their head falls back more. Hypothetically, in all cases, a more accurate adjustment is easily made by simply observing the OML and angling the CR parallel to it. However, this line must be observed correctly by taking mental note of the actual outer canthus of the eyelids (rather than "eyeballing" the general area of the midorbit), as discussed in Chapter 5.

BEST PRACTICE TIP

For the AP (supine) projection of the skull, simply angle the beam caudal until the CR parallels the carefully observed OML.

For the AP (supine) projection of the skull, simply angle the beam caudal until the CR parallels the carefully observed OML.

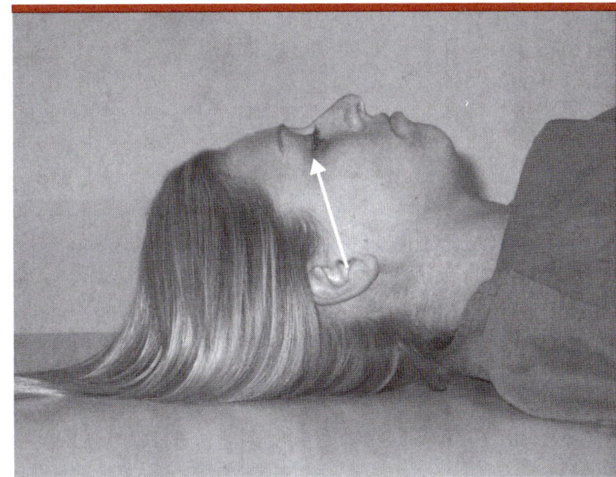

Courtesy of Quinn B. Carroll

FIGURE 9-25

Lying supine, the average patient's head will fall back into 12°–15° of extension. A 12°–15° caudal angle will be required for a proper AP projection of the skull. In all cases, angle the CR parallel to the carefully observed OML that passes through the outer canthus (junction) of the eyelids.

For all the remaining views that involve angles relative to the OML, a simple system of estimation can be derived by using the landmark lines taught at the beginning of this chapter. With these lines in mind, most angles needed for frontal positions can be estimated within a degree or two of perfect accuracy. By way of illustration, the following case studies are presented in order of increasing difficulty.

Reverse Caldwell Positions

All of the following examples will assume a trauma patient lying supine. Recall that since a routine Caldwell projection requires a caudal angle, the reverse Caldwell will require the equivalent of a *cephalic* angle. This, in turn, is equivalent to *extension of the head*, which raises the orbits and lowers the petrous pyramids relative to the orbits. For a *reversed* Caldwell, some combination of head extension and/or cephalic angulation will always be used.

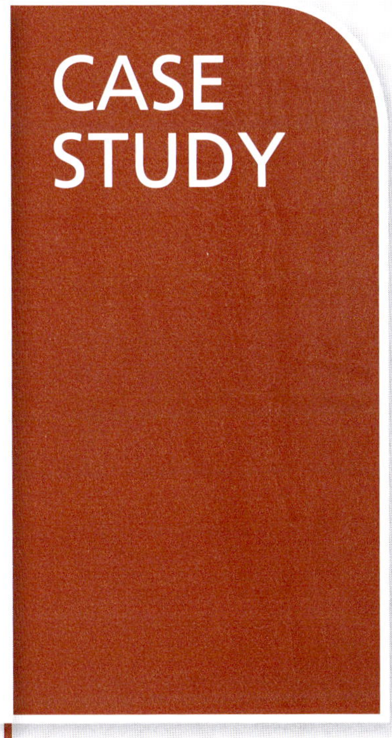

Case Study #7: Reverse Caldwell Projection #1

On an average patient lying supine, you estimate that the vertical is midway between the *IOML* and the *AML*. That is, the *NML* (See Figure 9-2) is vertical. This patient position is shown in Figure 9-26. What is the tube angle required for a reverse Caldwell projection?

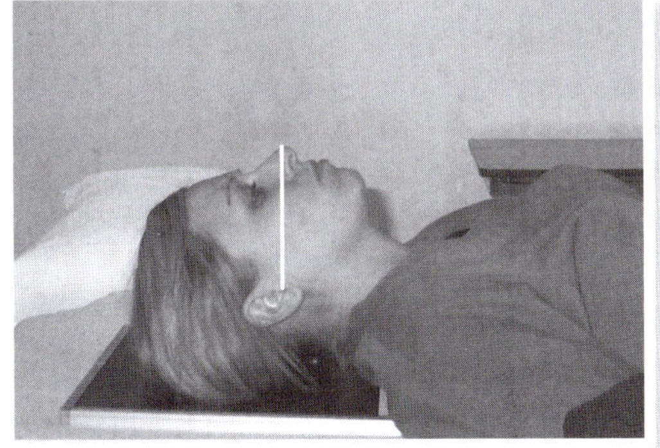

Courtesy of Quinn B. Carroll

FIGURE 9-26

How much is the head extended? For a reverse Caldwell projection, what degree and direction of CR angle is needed to compensate?

(continues)

CASE STUDY

ANSWER: *From Figure 9-2, the angle of this line (the NML) is 17°. The head is* extended *about 17°. With the patient supine, head extension is equivalent to the needed angle. Furthermore, this 17° is so close to 15° that for practical purposes,* ***no angulation of the CR is needed, because the head is already in position*****. Simply make the exposure with the CR vertical.**

(Technically, for those who wish to be precise, the amount of head extension will be subtracted from the tube angle: 15° – 17° = **minus** *2° cephalic, or in other words, 2°* caudal*. But, such a small adjustment is simply unnecessary.)* ■

Case Study #8: Reverse Caldwell Projection #2

On an average patient lying supine, you estimate that the vertical is one-third of the way from the *IOML* to the *NML*, as shown in Figure 9-27. What is the tube angle for a reverse Caldwell projection?

ANSWER: *The angle of this line would fall one-third of the way from 7° (for the IOML) to 17° (for the NML). The difference is 10°, one-third of which is 3°. Adding the 3° to the 7° IOML, the head is* extended *about 10°. Extension is equivalent to the needed cephalic angle, so the amount will be subtracted from it. The tube should be angled 15° – 10° = 5° cephalic.* ■

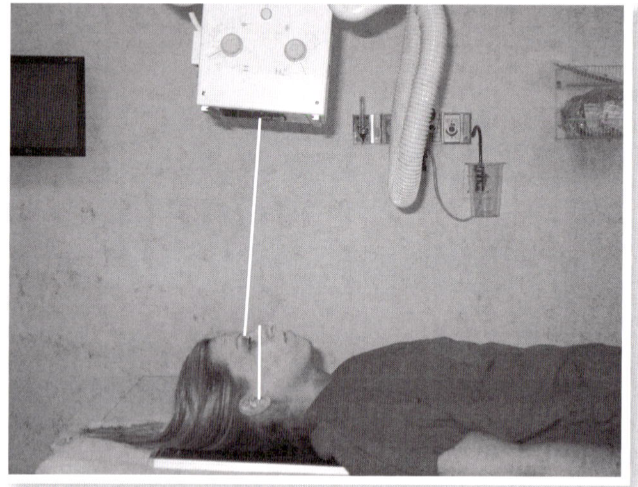

Courtesy of Quinn B. Carroll

FIGURE 9-27
How much is the head extended? For a reverse Caldwell projection, what degree and direction of CR angle is needed to compensate?

CASE STUDY

Case Study #9: Reverse Caldwell Projection #3

On a large-shouldered patient lying supine, the head falls way back. You estimate that the *AML* is vertical, as shown in Figure 9-28. What is the required tube angle for a reverse Caldwell projection?

ANSWER: *This patient is in a* hyperextended *position, with the head extended an estimated 27°. Unless a caudal tube angle is used to cancel out some of the over extension, the petrous ridges will be projected much too low, below the floor of the orbits. The head is overextended by 27° – 15° = 12° for the projection. This amount must be deducted by angling the CR 12° caudal (Figure 9-29).*

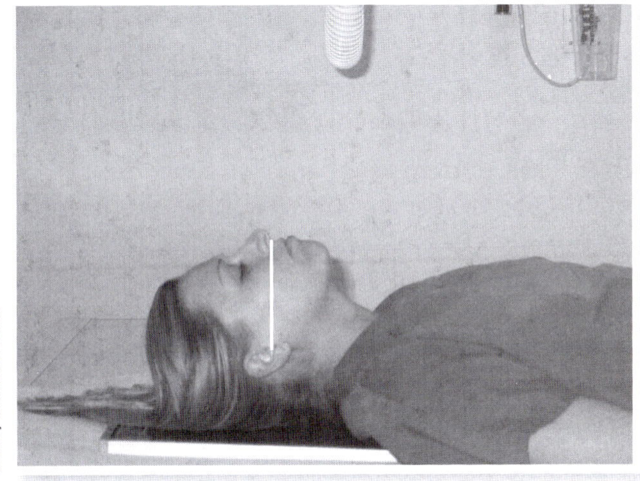

Courtesy of Quinn B. Carroll

FIGURE 9-28
How much is the head extended? For a reverse Caldwell projection, what degree and direction of CR angle is needed to compensate? What is the correct CR angle for a reverse *Waters* projection?

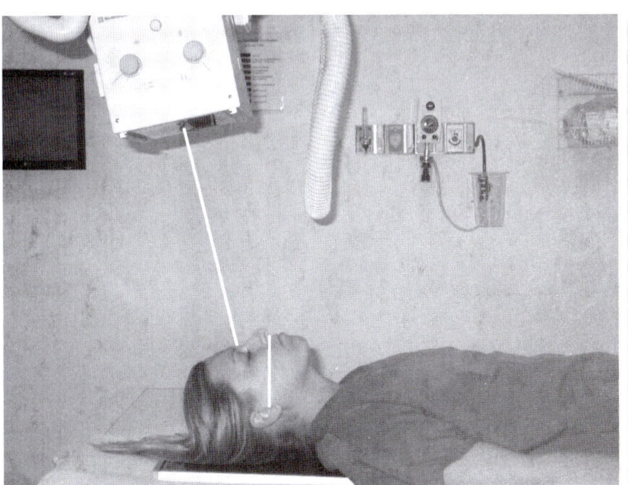

Courtesy of Quinn B. Carroll

FIGURE 9-29
With the acanthiomeatal line vertical, the correct CR angle for a reverse Caldwell projection is 12° *caudal.*

Reverse Waters Positions

The routine Waters projection also involves extension of the head (equivalent to angling caudally from behind the head). Therefore, a reverse Waters will also invert this angle to *cephalic*. ***Nearly all reverse Waters projections require cephalic angles.*** The combination of tube angle and head extension must add up to a total of 53°. Case Study #10 and Case Study #11 provide valuable practice in application.

AP Upright Waters with Poor Head Extension

Often a patient is unable to extend his head back enough to perform a proper Waters position. If the position is close enough that only a few degrees of adjustment are needed, the x-ray tube may be *slightly* angled caudally to compensate. As demonstrated in Chapter 5, keeping the CR close to horizontal is crucial for diagnosing air/fluid levels, but a range of + or −5° from a perfectly horizontal beam will suffice. If dropping the angle of the CR into a slight caudal angle will achieve the correct relationship between the CR and the anatomy, this may be allowed. However, if more than 5° of angulation would be required, it is better to opt for the following *reversed* position in order to be sure that air/fluid levels are properly demonstrated.

Instead of angling the x-ray tube, perform the exam in a reversed, AP position. Place a chair *with the back* 3–6 inches away from the IR. Have the patient sit and extend his chin as high as possible, then have the patient lean back in the chair, sliding the pelvis forward as needed, until the *EZ line* discussed above is horizontal and the OML is correctly positioned 37° from the tabletop or IR plate (Figure 9-30). Make sure to just annotate the image as an AP rather than a PA position, and if additional notes are provided for in the image or patient file, explain why the reversed projection was taken.

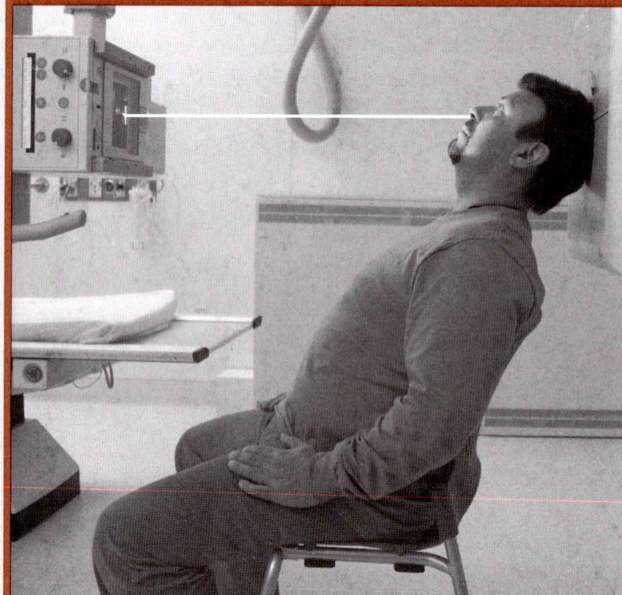

FIGURE 9-30

For an upright Waters projection, when the head cannot be extended to within 5° of the proper position, and demonstration of fluid levels is important (as for a sinus series), it may be better to reverse the position using a chair with a back to support the patient while leaning back. The *EZ line* should be horizontal.

CASE STUDY

Case Study #10: Reverse Waters Projection #1

With a large-shouldered patient, you estimate that the *AML* is close to vertical, as shown in Figure 9-28. What is the tube angle for a reverse Waters projection?

ANSWER: *See Figure 9-2. The head is extended about 27°. For a reverse position with the patient supine, head extension is equivalent to cephalic angulation. The amount of extension will be subtracted from the needed angle. The tube should be angled 53° − 27° = 26° cephalic (Figure 9-31).*

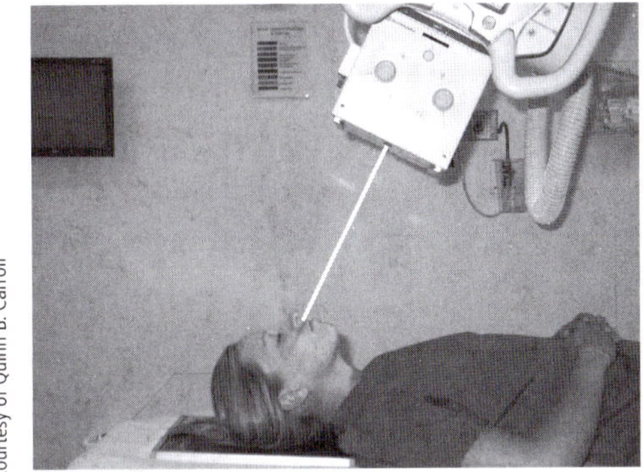
Courtesy of Quinn B. Carroll

FIGURE 9-31
With the acanthiomeatal line vertical, the correct CR angle for a reverse Waters projection is 26° cephalic.

Case Study #11: Reverse Waters Projection #2

On an average patient, you estimate that the vertical is midway between the *IOML* and the *AML*. What is the tube angle for a reverse Waters projection?

ANSWER: *Splitting the difference between the IOML and the AML, this is the* NML *that is perpendicular (see Figure 9-2). It lies at 17°. The head is extended about 17°. Extension is equivalent to the needed type of angle, so the amount of extension will be subtracted from the needed angle. The tube should be angled 53° − 17° = 36° cephalic (Figure 9-32).*

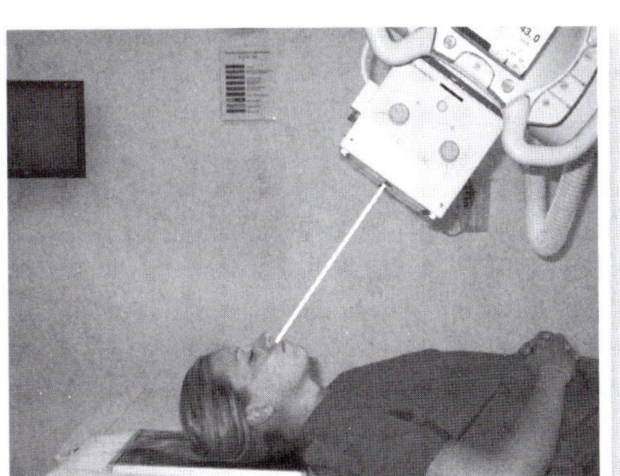
Courtesy of Quinn B. Carroll

FIGURE 9-32
With the nasomeatal line vertical, the correct CR angle for a reverse Waters projection is 36° *cephalic.*

With a little practice, and having memorized the degrees assigned to the IOML, the NML, and the AML, one can become skillful at reversing trauma skull projections of all types and in all situations. By estimating where the vertical or horizontal lies between any two lines, "midway from the IOML to the NML," or "one-third of the way," and so on, one can determine the actual head extension to within a couple of degrees of accuracy.

Cross-Table Lateral Projection

A persistent challenge with cross-table lateral projections of the skull is the tendency to clip the back of the occipital bone at the bottom due to normal beam divergence and to the edging of the IR plate or cassette. If you are *certain* the head can be gently moved, the head may be built up on a 1-inch sponge. This allows the vertically held cassette or IR plate to be placed in contact with the skull, avoiding an OID gap.

In many trauma situations, however, the head cannot be moved. Place the lower edge of the plate below the backboard or tabletop. As shown in Figure 9-33, this will result in an OID gap with some attendant magnification, but allows the entire cranium to be included in the view. This will be important if there is any probability of injury to the posterior occipital bone.

When an OID gap is unavoidable, magnification and blur can be reduced by using increased SID if possible. Increase the SID to about 50 inches and increase the mAs setting by one "step" (35%–50%), OR increase the SID to 72 inches and *triple* the mAs from a 40-inch technique. See "Horizontal Beam Projections" at the beginning of Chapter 7 for related essential information in minimizing the amount of occipital bone that will be clipped from the view.

When a lateral skull is ordered for trauma screening, proceed with it even if clipping some of the occipital bone from the view cannot be avoided. The view still provides critical trauma information to the

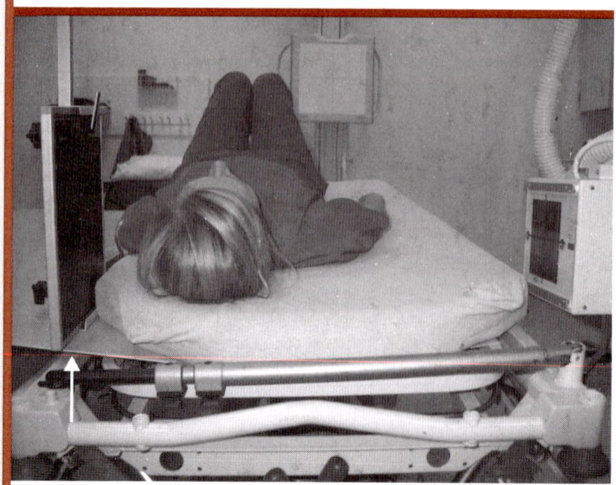

Courtesy of Quinn B. Carroll

FIGURE 9-33

For a cross-table lateral skull projection, placing the cassette plate (arrow) below the gurney pad ensures inclusion of the posterior occipital bone in the view, at the expense of some magnification.

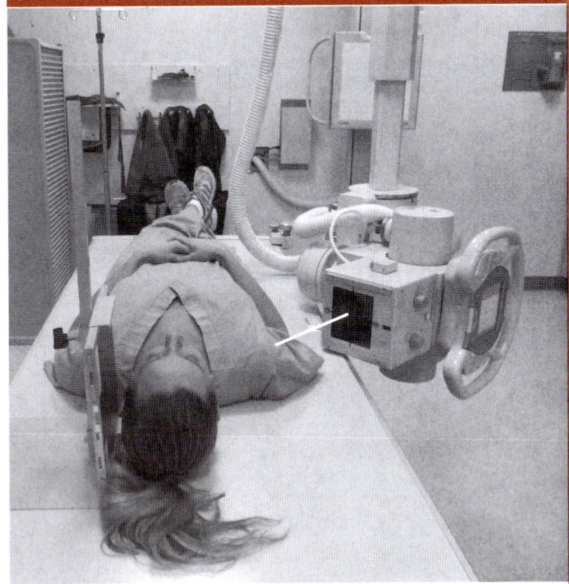

Courtesy of Quinn B. Carroll

FIGURE 9-34

For a cross-table lateral (oblique) mandible, using *only* a 25°–30° cephalic angle will project the "upside" shoulder into the mandible. The position must be adapted.

physician, such as basilar skull fractures bleeding into the sphenoid sinus. After trauma screening is completed, a lateral skull including the entire occipital bone may be obtained later on.

Cross-Table Mandible, Lateral (Oblique) Projection

For the cross-table trauma projection of the mandible, it is impossible to use a 25°–30° cephalic angle of the CR (Figure 9-34) because it projects the shoulder into the mandible (Figure 9-35). The position must be adapted.

There are at least three different approaches to obtaining a good lateral projection of the mandible with the patient lying supine. All three, however, require some movement of the head. (And, therefore, may require clearance from the ED physician when there is serious cervical spine trauma associated with the injury.) When the head absolutely cannot be moved, combinations or partial adaptations of these approaches must be used. This will be discussed after presenting the three general approaches.

Using Head Tilt

With a horizontal beam and the patient flat on their back, more than 15° of CR angle will project the "upside" shoulder into mandible. Never use more than about 15° of cephalic beam angulation. Rather, use a combination of head tilt (at least 15°) and up to 15° beam angle (Figure 9-36). The head is tilted toward the IR plate or cassette. The plate is not tilted nor angled, but kept parallel with the long axis of the body and table. Center the CR about ½-inch just below and anterior to the *upside* gonion (angle of the mandible).

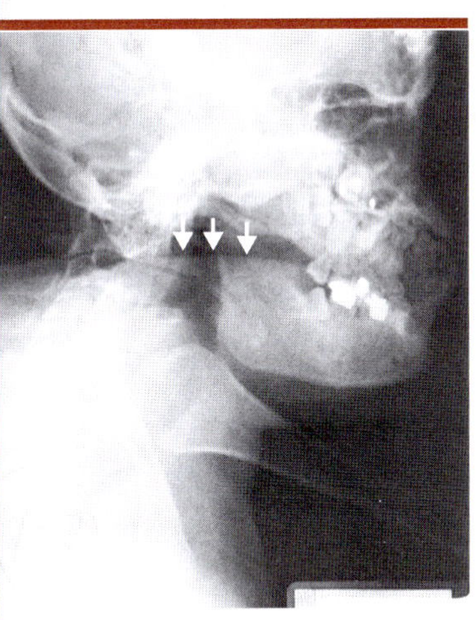

FIGURE 9-35

Cross-table lateral (oblique) mandible view using *only* a 25°–30° cephalic angle, showing the "upside" shoulder (arrows) projected into the mandible.

Carroll, Q. Evaluating Radiographs, 1993, Figure 197, Courtesy of Charles C Thomas, Publisher, Ltd., Springfield, Illinois.

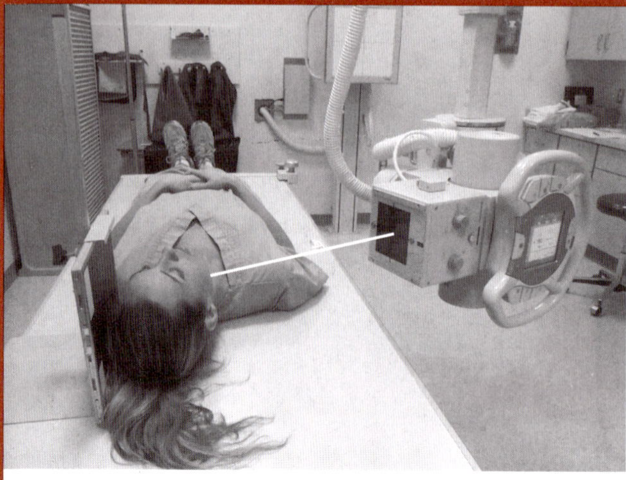

FIGURE 9-36
Cross-table lateral (oblique) mandible using a combination of head tilt (15°) and cephalic CR angulation (15°).

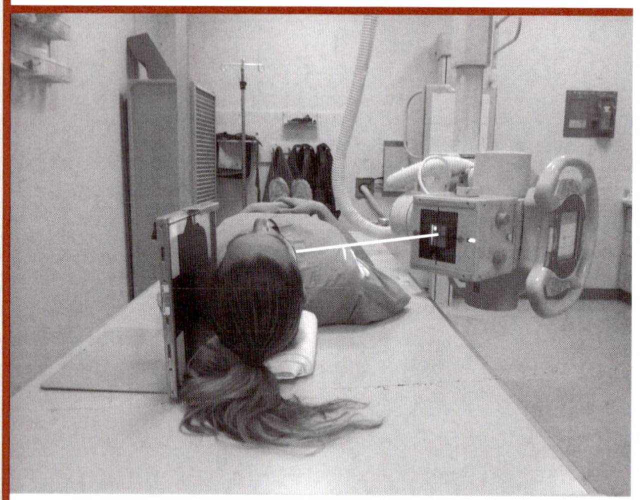

FIGURE 9-37
Cross-table lateral (oblique) mandible using elevation of the head on a sponge or towels, with a 25°–30° cephalic CR angle.

Using Head Elevation

If the patient's chest is not too thick, and the head can simply be built up using a 2-inch sponge, this can elevate the entire mandible above the obstructing shoulders and chest. Then a 25°–30° cephalic angle may be used to good effect with the horizontal beam directed ***above and over*** the chest as shown in Figure 9-37. The cassette or IR plate is not tilted nor angled. Center the CR about ½-inch just below and anterior to the *upside* gonion (angle of the mandible).

Using Head Rotation

Fairly minimal rotation of the head, only 15°–20°, can be used to effect, allowing a downward angulation of the beam over the patient's chest (Figure 9-38). The head is rotated toward the IR plate or cassette (it may already be rotated somewhat in that direction so that only a small increase in obliquity is required). In this case, tilt the

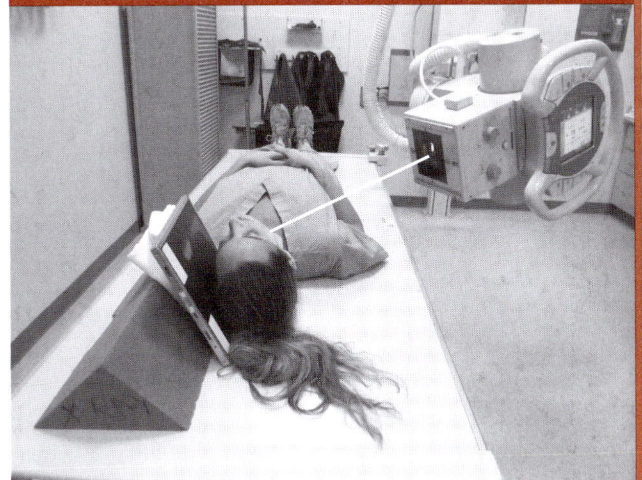
Courtesy of Quinn B. Carroll

FIGURE 9-38
Cross-table lateral (oblique) mandible using 15° rotation of the head and IR plate, with a double tube angle, 25°–30° cephalic and 15°–20° downward to match the head rotation.

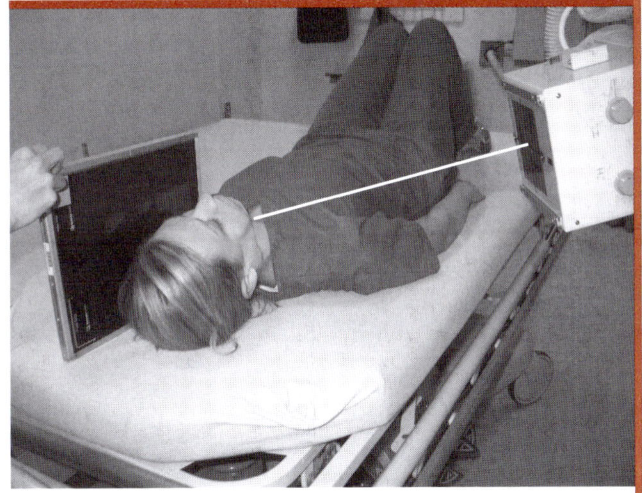
Courtesy of Quinn B. Carroll

FIGURE 9-39
Cross-table lateral (oblique) mandible without moving the trauma patient: A double angle is placed on the CR, 25°–30° cephalic and 15° downward, leaving the patient's head and the cassette plate straight.

cassette or IR plate back 15°–20° to match the head rotation and keep it parallel to the CR. A double angle is placed on the CR, downward to match the head rotation, and cephalic 25°–30°. Center the CR about ½-inch just below and anterior to the *upside* gonion (angle of the mandible).

Without Moving the Head

When the head cannot be moved, try to approximate the preceding method #3 as much as possible. Pull the x-ray tube up where the CR can clear the chest and shoulders, and angle the CR downward 15°–20° (Figure 9-39). Center the CR about ½-inch just below and anterior to the *upside* gonion (angle of the mandible). The cassette or IR plate is not tilted. This view will present some obvious distortion of the mandible, but will suffice in screening for fractures and trauma (Figure 9-40).

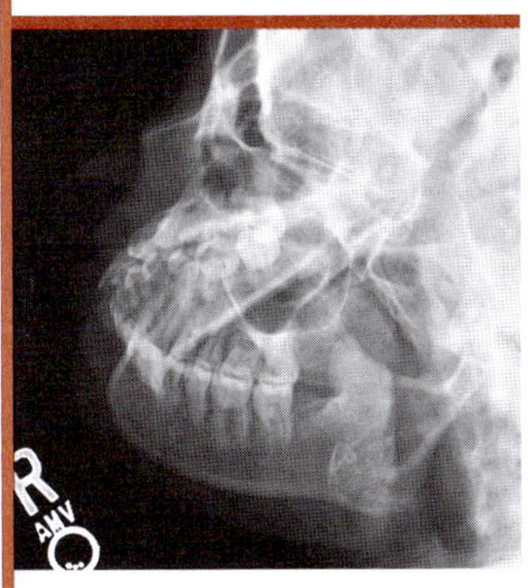

Courtesy of Quinn B. Carroll

FIGURE 9-40
Trauma cross-table lateral (oblique) mandible view.

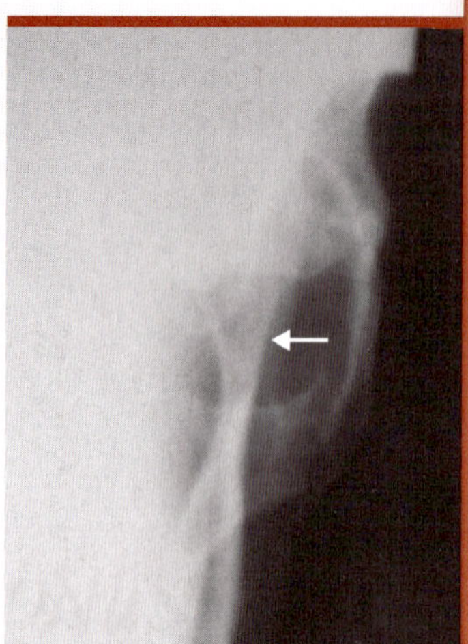

FIGURE 9-41

Periorbital view of mandibular condyle and orbital rims.

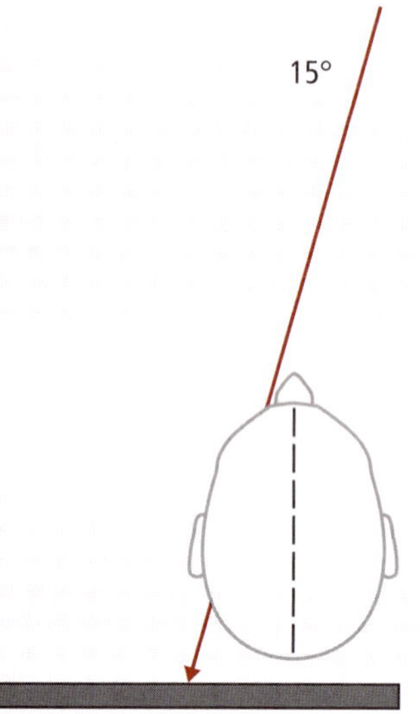

FIGURE 9-42

Diagram of peri-orbital projection for mandibular condyle and orbital rims.

Trauma AP Mandible

The AP projection of the mandible is identical to a reversed routine PA mandible, with the CR parallel to the OML and centered to the junction of the lips. Remember that the supine patient normally has the head extended, so that a caudal tube angle will be needed to parallel the OML.

Periorbital Mandibular Condyle/Facial Bones

An optional view can be obtained demonstrating the lateral and inferior rims of the orbit, the malar bone, and a nice frontal view of the mandibular condyle and head (Figure 9-41). A collimated beam is aligned parallel to the OML (remember to angle caudal as needed for a supine patient, or build the head up, to achieve this). The CR is then angled 15° *laterally* to the affected side and centered through that midorbit, shown in Figure 9-42.

Trauma Oblique Facial Bones or Reverse Orbit

This is effectively a modified, reverse Rhese position. With the patient supine, some extension of the patient's chin is assumed. If possible, extend the chin further until the *acanthiomeatal line* is vertical. If the chin is not extended enough, angle the beam *cephalic* until the CR is parallel to the *acanthiomeatal line*. If only one direction of angle can be used on the x-ray tube, such as for a fixed radiographic room, that lock must be reserved for the transverse angle required rather than used here to compensate for head extension. Mobile units usually allow double angulation, facilitating this projection.

With no rotation of the head (with the midsagittal plane vertical), use a **37° lateral (transverse) angle**. (This transverse angle is *not* 53° as listed in some references.) The CR is directed medially into the side of interest (for a right orbit, angle to the patient's left 37°), then center through the mid-right orbit (Figure 9-43).

In screening for facial fractures, this position not only gives a view of the orbit without the petrous ridge obstructing it, as well as the periorbital bones, but it also provides a beautiful tangential view of the *contralateral* zygoma (cheek) bone and lateral orbital rim, as demonstrated in Figure 9-44. For this reason, it is usually desirable to obtain *both* right and left oblique views for facial bone screening, and to open the collimated field to include both sides of the head in each view.

Note that in Figure 9-44 the full recommended extension of the head was not achieved, a typical situation for trauma patients. The petrous ridge (arrowhead) lies at about the level of the lower one-fourth of the orbit, indicating 17°–18° of chin extension, short of the 27° that would place the AML vertical. While the *optic foramen* (just right of the center of the orbit) is not opened as well as the full head extension would have achieved, the rim of the orbit and associated bones are well demonstrated all around its circumference. As an added bonus, on the *opposite* side of the face, the malar (cheek) bone is laid out in a

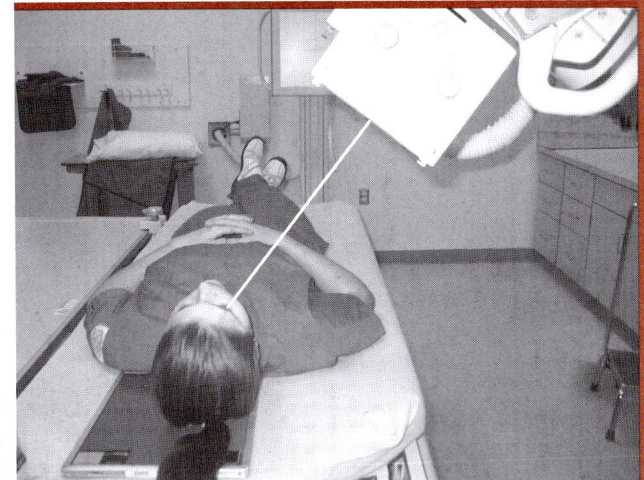

FIGURE 9-43
Trauma oblique facial bones/reverse orbit projection. With the chin extended, a 37° transverse CR angle is directed through the mid-orbit of the affected side.

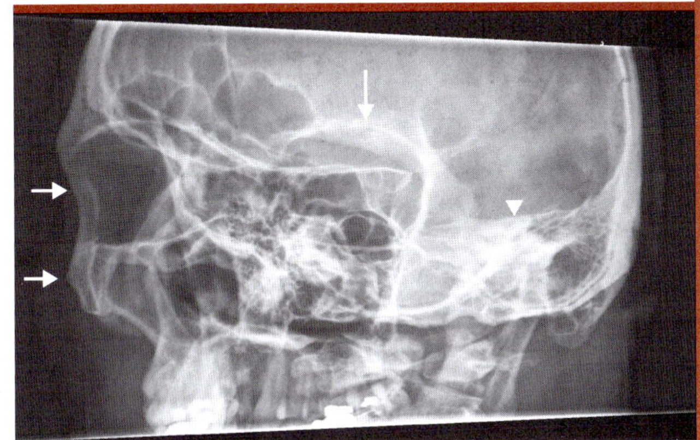

FIGURE 9-44
The trauma oblique facial bones view shows excellent visualization of the lateral orbital rim and malar bone of the far side (horizontal arrows) and the entire orbital rim of the centered side (vertical arrows), as well as the petrous pyramid of this side (arrowhead).

beautiful profile view, and the lateral rim and lateral wall of *this* orbit are very nicely demonstrated. The diagnostic value of bilateral views using this trauma oblique projection is readily apparent.

THE INFANT SKULL

Angled frontal projections of the skull include the Caldwell, the Waters, and the Townes projections and all their modifications. In all cases, the *purpose* of the CR angle is either to desuperimpose facial bones from portions of the cranium that need to be seen, or to desuperimpose the petrous portions of the skull from facial bones that need to be seen. For example, the Townes projection is primarily designed to demonstrate the occipital bone, but the facial bones are in the way, so we must effectively "look down over" the facial bones to see it, using a caudal angle. The Caldwell projection is primarily designed to demonstrate the frontal bone and its sinuses. In this case, the angle is designed to project the orbital plates, cribriform plate, and crista galli downward, so that the entire squamous portion of the frontal bone along with its sinuses can be clearly seen. The objective of a Waters projection is to extend the head to such a degree that the petrous portions of the temporal bones are brought down below the floor of the maxillary sinuses so they can be seen clearly.

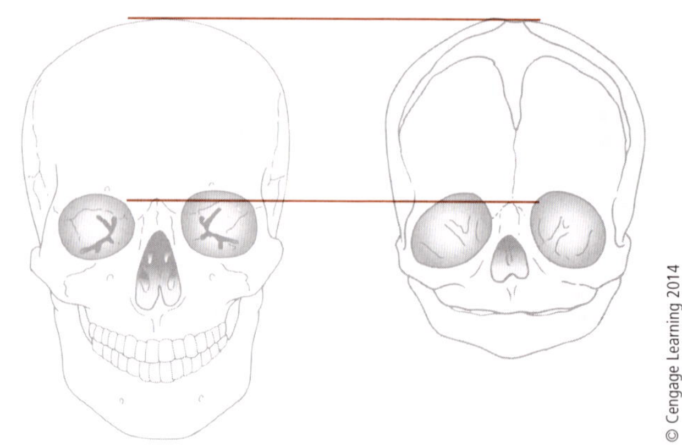

FIGURE 9-45

Adjusting for the size of the cranium, it can be seen that the entire facial mass for a small infant is proportionately much smaller. The facial bones are vertically "compressed." This means that the CR angles used for Townes, Waters, and Caldwell projections must be reduced.

BEST PRACTICE TIP

On average, for an infant, reduce the CR angle for all angled frontal skull positions by about one-third from that used for an adult.

Because angulation of the CR also results in some distortion of the anatomy of interest, only the minimum angle required to achieve the above objectives should be used. Figure 9-45 shows the relative proportions of the head of an infant compared to those of an adult skull, if the cranium were adjusted to equal size. Note that the entire facial mass of an infant is *compressed* vertically. Compared to an adult, a small child has a much smaller face (or a much larger cranium) proportionately. This has significant implications for positioning of all angled frontal projections in the head. Generally, it means that less angle is needed to desuperimpose facial features from the skull or vice versa on small children.

In Figure 9-46, we place some measurements on this relationship, using the angle formed between the AML and the OML. In **A**, we see the 27° angle previously discussed, formed between the OML and the AML on a typical adult. In ***B***, we see that for a 1-year-old toddler, this angle is reduced to about 22°. In **C**, for a newborn infant, the angle is only about 17°.

A valuable positioning rule can be derived from these measurements:

On average, for an infant, reduce the CR angle for all angled frontal skull positions by about one-third from that used for an adult.

A

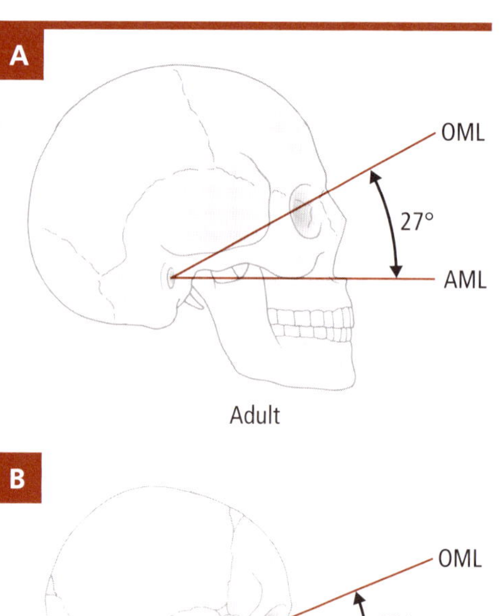

B

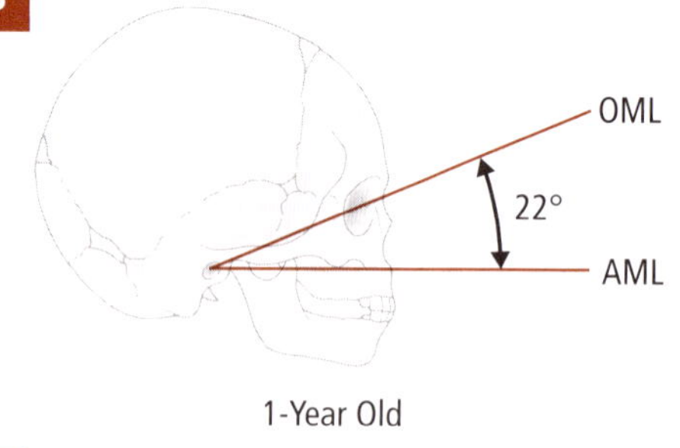

C

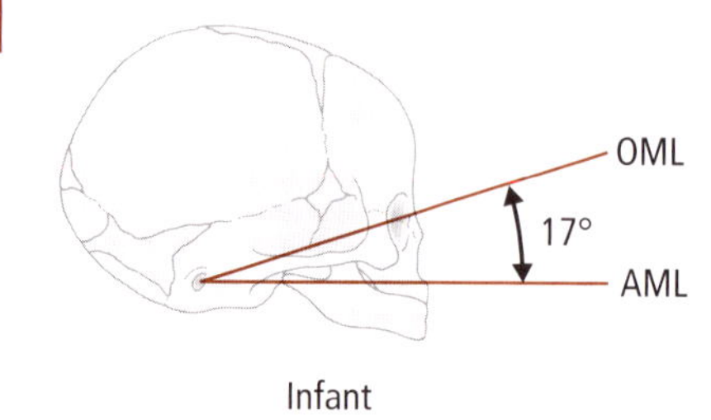

FIGURE 9-46

The angles formed between the orbitomeatal line and the acanthiomeatal line for **A**, an adult, **B**, a 1-year old toddler, and **C**, a newborn infant. For angled frontal projections of the head on infants, on average, reduce the adult CR angles *by* about one-third.

For example, to obtain a Townes projection on an infant, the recommended angle would be about 20°, that is, 30° minus one-third. What would be the angle for a Caldwell projection? The answer is about 10°–11° (15° minus one-third). For older toddlers (1 year of age), increase the angle used beyond the rule. For children 3 or more years old, use the adult angle.

Be careful in applying this rule for the Waters projection. Remember, as explained earlier in this chapter, that the actual amount of head extension for the Waters is 53°, not 37°, so this rule is applied by taking off one-third of 53°. Remember, too, that if the head extension were reduced by one-third, the 37° angle formed between the OML and the plate would *increase*, not decrease. Because this is somewhat tricky, it is presented as one of the following Critical Thinking Challenges (after the Summary).

On all pediatric procedures, remember the importance of proper, tight collimation, safe and secure immobilization, and gonadal shielding as appropriate.

SUMMARY

1. In adapting skull positions, whenever a compensating angle would be greater than 45°, an alternative general approach to positioning should be used rather than such excessive angulation. These include reversing the position and angles, and changing between recumbent, standing, and seated positions.
2. From the OML, the average degrees of arc for the various skull landmark lines should be memorized. They are: IOML = 7°, NML = 17°, AML = 27°, GML = 10°, and MML = 53°. Using these figures, compensating angles for various degrees of head flexion and extension can be very accurately estimated.
3. For the Waters position, extension of the head is 53°, not 37°.
4. To get tilt out of a lateral head position, keep the elbow off the table, and use sponges or angulation as needed to ensure the CR passes parallel to the interpupillary line.
5. On average, the patient lying supine will have his head dropped back into 12°–15° of extension.
6. For angled frontal projections of the skull on infants, reduce angles by about one-third, with a lesser reduction for toddlers.
7. Recommendations for specific procedures such as the zygomatic arches and the mandible are presented throughout the chapter.

CRITICAL THINKING CHALLENGE 9.1

ADAPTING A REVERSED CALDWELL (#1)

Observe Figure 9-47. Note the line indicating the vertical.

For this patient position, what tube angle (degrees and direction) would be needed to obtain a proper reverse* Caldwell *projection?

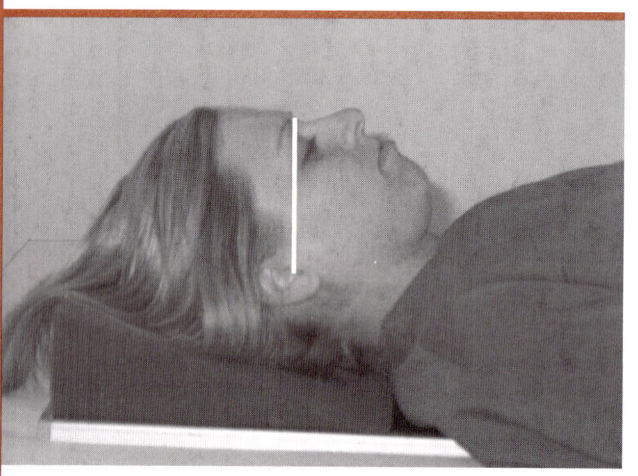
Courtesy of Quinn B. Carroll

FIGURE 9-47
Critical Thinking Challenge 9.1 for a reverse Caldwell projection.

CRITICAL THINKING CHALLENGE 9.2

ADAPTING A REVERSED CALDWELL (#2)

On an average patient lying supine, you estimate that the vertical is about two-thirds of the way from the *IOML* to the *AML*, shown in Figure 9-48.

What is the correct tube angle (degrees and direction) for a reverse Caldwell projection?

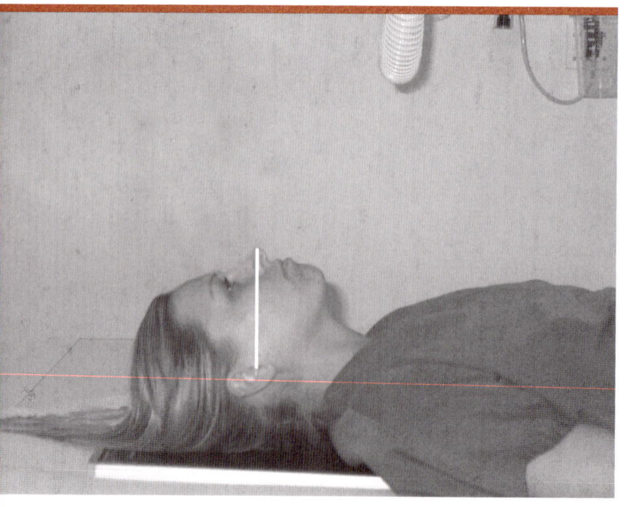
Courtesy of Quinn B. Carroll

FIGURE 9-48
Critical Thinking Challenge 9.2 for a reverse Caldwell projection.

ADAPTING A REVERSED WATERS

CRITICAL THINKING CHALLENGE 9.3

On an average patient lying supine, you estimate that the vertical is about one-third of the way from the *AML* to the *MML*, shown in Figure 9-49.

For this patient position, what tube angle (degrees and direction) would be needed to obtain a proper reverse Waters projection?

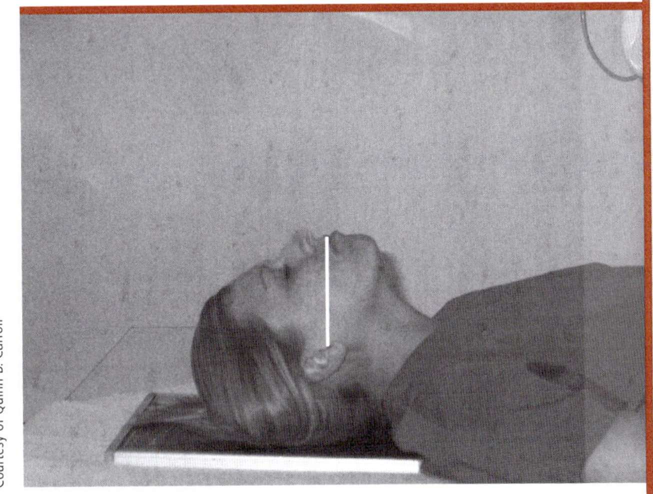

Courtesy of Quinn B. Carroll

FIGURE 9-49
Critical Thinking Challenge 9.3 for a reverse Waters projection.

MODIFIED WATERS FOR INFANT

CRITICAL THINKING CHALLENGE 9.4

Adapting the degree of head extension for a proper Waters position on a 4-month-old infant, what would be the angle measure between the OML and the plate?

MODIFIED TOWNES

CRITICAL THINKING CHALLENGE 9.5

On an average patient lying supine, you estimate that the vertical is about two-thirds of the way from the *OML* to the *GBL*, shown in Figure 9-50.

For this patient position, what tube angle (degrees and direction) would be needed to obtain a proper* Townes *projection?

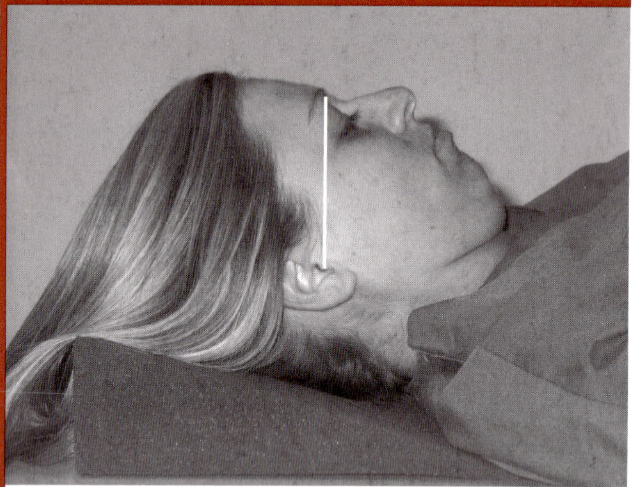

FIGURE 9-50
Critical Thinking Challenge 9.4 for a modified Townes projection.

(Answers to Critical Thinking Challenges are found in the Appendix.)

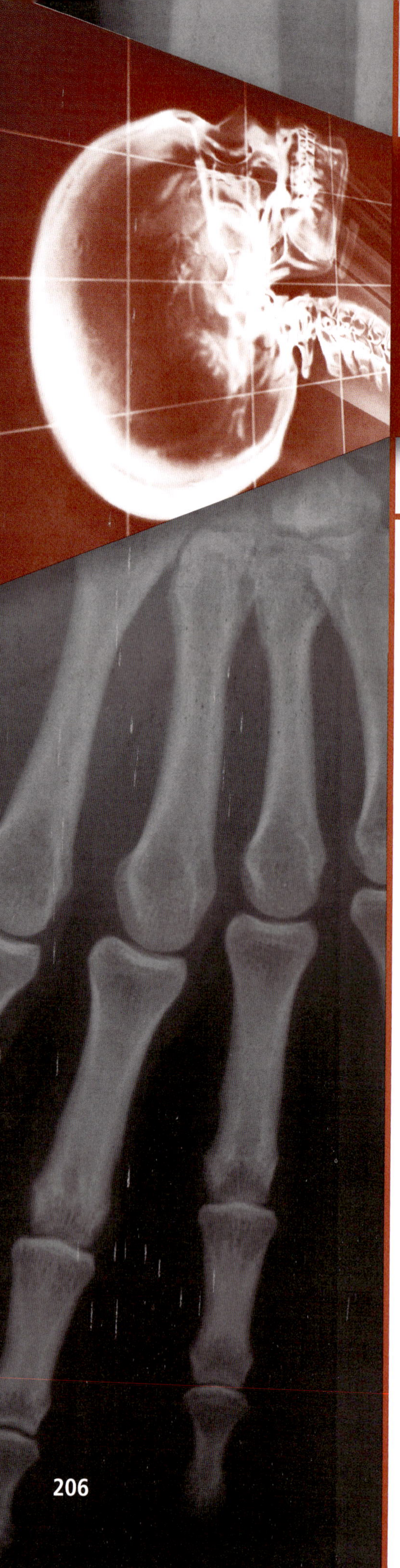

CHAPTER 10

Simplified Centering and Tips for Routine Positions

OUTLINE

Continues

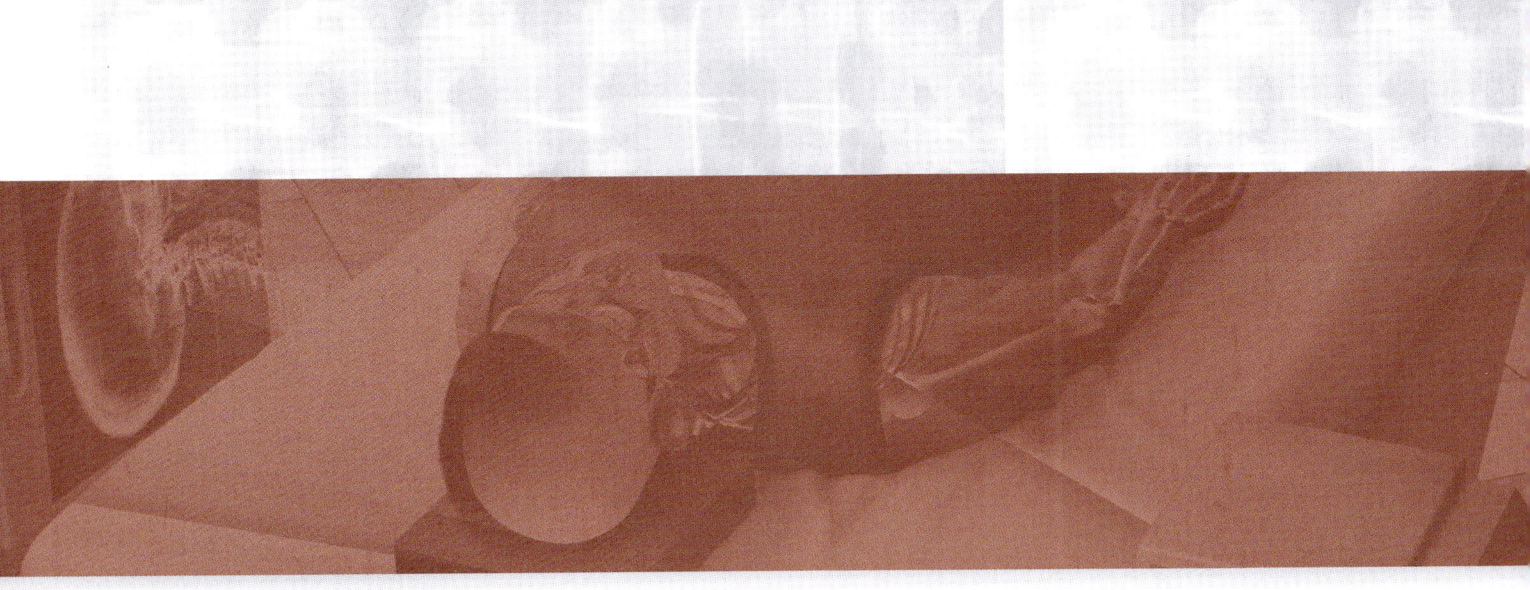

OUTLINE *continued*

OBJECTIVES

Upon completion of this chapter, you should be able to:

1. For each radiographic projection, state specific recommendations for simplified centering that ensure the inclusion of all anatomy of interest rather than focusing on the CR location alone.
2. Recite the collimation rule for distal extremities.
3. State and explain the value of each of the six guidelines for good centering rules.
4. Describe how the "universal landmark," the ASIS, can be used to avoid palpation of the symphysis pubis and still achieve good centering for various pelvic and abdominal studies.

5. Explain the value of *palpation* of bony landmarks in determining the correct angle and centering of the CR. For the lateral "spot" projection of L5–S1, specify three sets of landmarks that can be used.
6. Describe the critical effects of SID upon beam divergence in demonstrating the anatomy of interest. For the odontoid projections, specify these effects and how to use them to advantage.
7. Describe the critical effects of CR centering and angling in opening anatomical joint spaces and foramina. For lateral projections of the knee, specify these effects and how to use them to advantage.
8. For both "cross-table" and "frog" lateral hip projections, explain those fine points of positioning that result in placing the femoral neck truly perpendicular to the CR for proper demonstration and best desuperimpose obstructing anatomy.

INTRODUCTION

This chapter will present specific recommendations for centering each position. However, a very different approach will be used from that which is found in the typical positioning atlas.

The theme stated at the outset of this book was to find common patterns and generic rules that make it possible to adapt systematic ways that produce much more consistent results, whatever the situation. Such guiding principles also serve to simplify routine radiographic positions. We will begin with some of these.

DEFINING COLLIMATED EDGES

With the exception of specific joints or foramina that must be "opened up," the ideal collimation and centering for most radiographic projections are determined by the anatomy that is *included within the view* rather than by the specific location of the central ray. For example, on a skull series or a hand series, where the *edges of the collimated field* fall is actually more critical than the exact centering point for the CR.

In the case of the facial bones and associated skull anatomy, one must ask whether it is even realistic to try to identify a *single centering point* for many projections in the first place. This is the one part of the human body that may be said to vary *dramatically* in morphology from one patient to the next. To make this point, experienced radiographers need to only consider what they have witnessed in the various shapes of the human jaw, the two extremes of which might be described as a very "square" jaw and the very "pointed, slanting" jaw. The angle at which the side body of the mandible extends downward from the gonion (the "angle" of the jaw) varies across an impressive range, as much as 30°, wreaking havoc with any rule for head extension on the AP cervical spine projection. Variations in the length of the chin versus that of the alveolar process of the maxilla cause challenges with odontoid positioning. The prominence and shape of the nose alters the appearance of many frontal skull and facial bone positions.

Anthropologically, skulls are divided into dolichocephalic, mesocephalic, and brachycephalic categories because of substantial differences in the width-to-length ratio of the cranium. Some have unusually prominent arches above the eyes; some have unusually large mastoid processes. All of these variations affect not only the appropriate degree of flexion/extension and of beam angulation, they also alter centering points.

As an example, consider the lateral projection for the sinuses. Two of the most popular positioning atlases disagree on the ideal centering point: One says it is "midway along a line from the outer canthus of the eye to the EAM," while the other lists it as "½ inch to 1 inch posterior to the outer canthus of the eye," substantially more anterior. Interestingly, the authors of the first textbook essentially "cheat" by providing a sample radiograph that does not strictly follow their own instructions. When a cylinder "cone" is used or the field is well collimated, it can be shown that this "midway" guideline risks clipping the frontal or maxillary sinuses anteriorly, while allowing excess light field behind the ear. Two examples are presented in Figure 10-1. Note also that the degree of chin flexion, which can vary substantially, will alter the superior-to-inferior centering of the field even though one follows the textbook rule (such as "1 inch posterior to the outer canthus").

These issues complicate and argue against using a single centering point rule for the lateral sinus projection. The final criterion for proper centering and collimation is simply that *all groups of sinuses be included* within the view. Landmarks for properly locating the edges of the field can be easily defined on this basis, as follows: To include the *frontal* sinuses, the upper edge of the field should extend *at least halfway up the forehead*. To include the *maxillary* sinuses, the lower edge of the field must extend downward at least to the junction of the lips. And, to include the *sphenoid* sinuses, the posterior edge of the field should extend back at least to the external auditory meatus (EAM), as shown in Figures 10-2 and 10-3.

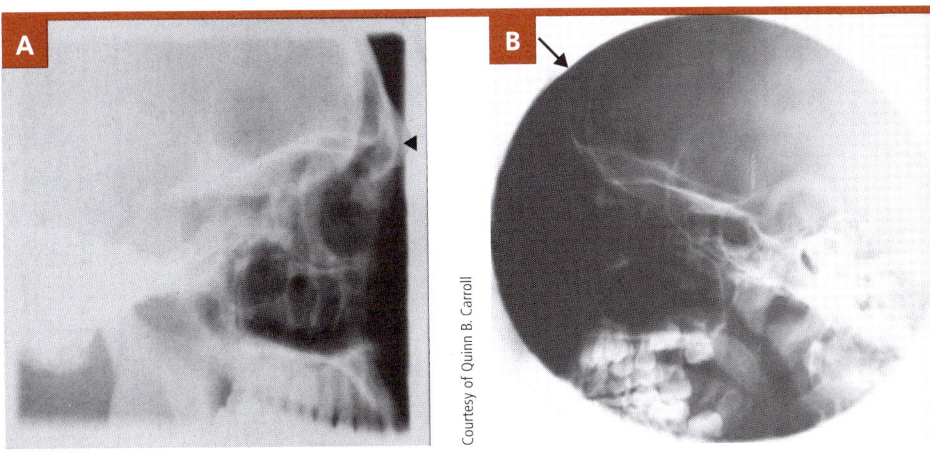

FIGURE 10-1

Lateral "coned" views for sinuses centered midway from the outer canthus to the *external auditory meatus* (EAM). Both include an excess amount of skull posterior to the ear; In **A**, a square field was used and the glabella was clipped off (arrow). In **B**, a circular field was used—the frontal sinuses (arrow) were clipped and the maxillary sinuses were nearly clipped off anteriorly.

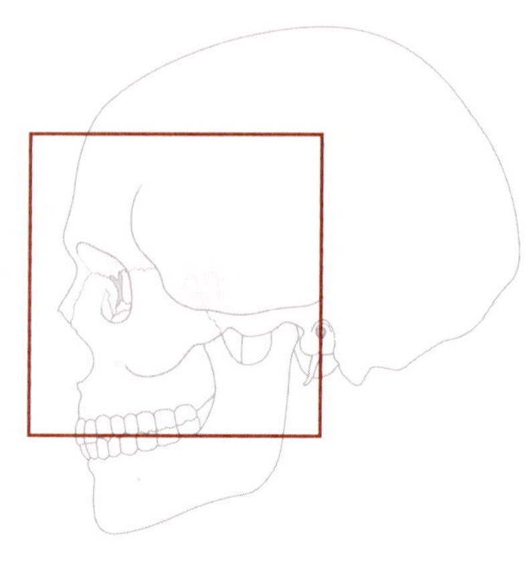

FIGURE 10-2

Alternative approach to centering a lateral sinus view using borders rather than the CR location: *Center to include the EAM posteriorly, the junction of the lips inferiorly, and the lower half of the forehead superiorly.* See Figure 8-3.

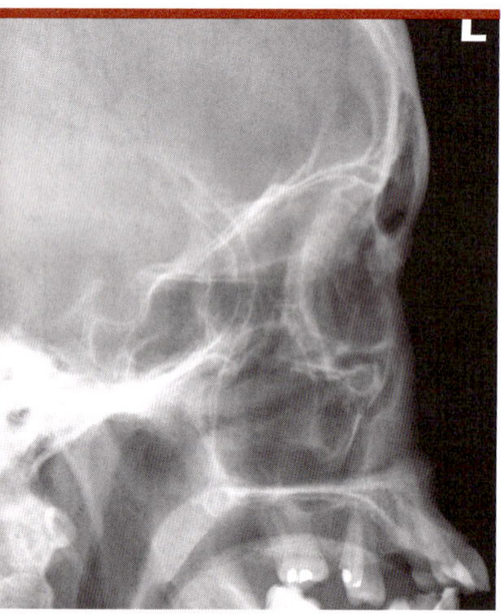

FIGURE 10-3

Lateral sinus view using "border" centering as explained in Figure 8-2. This method *adapts* for different skull shapes to always include all four sets of sinuses.

Courtesy of Community Hospital of the Monterey Peninsula, Diagnostic and Interventional Radiology.

These three simple rules are absolutely *generic*: They automatically adapt the actual centering point for different shapes of skulls, so they are *applicable to all patients*. Wherever appropriate, such helpful rules will be presented in this chapter.

Now consider the terminal extremities. Radiographic projections of the fingers, hands, calcanei, or feet are done with a light border around three sides of the anatomy. Clipping off the tip of the thumb will result in a repeated exposure, whereas "misdirecting" the CR ½-inch away from the third metacarpophalangeal joint will not. Again, the important criterion is the *inclusion of all anatomy of interest* within the collimated field.

For nearly all positions, the inclusion of all anatomy of interest is more important than the specific location of the CR. (The only exceptions are specific single joints such as the knee, ankle, and elbow.)

This rule overrides any exact centering point for the CR, unless there is specific interest in opening a designated joint.

The reliability of the light field in locating edges is an issue. It is not uncommon for the designated field edge, indicated by the light field, to be as much as ½-inch off from the actual edge of the x-ray beam. It must further be appreciated that this is entirely within the acceptable limits of quality control. (Two percent of 40-inch SID = 0.8 inch of acceptable deviation for each edge of the light field.) For example, the student must remember that in routine practice, if there is less than ½-inch of light field extending beyond the tip of the finger, it is possible that the tip of the finger will be cut off on the actual x-ray exposure when it is made, as in Figure 10-4. The following rule must be observed:

For distal extremities, always allow a minimum of ½ inch of light around every side of the anatomy.

BEST PRACTICE TIP

For nearly all positions, the inclusion of all anatomy of interest is more important than the specific location of the CR. (The only exceptions are specific single joints such as the knee, ankle, and elbow.)

BEST PRACTICE TIP

For distal extremities, always allow a minimum of ½ inch of light around every side of the anatomy.

A similar rule can be stated for both PA and lateral skull projections: The ½-inch rule can generally be applied for PA and lateral skull projections when the collimator accuracy is within guidelines (Figure 10-5). However, angled projections, such as the Townes, the obscuring effect of thick hair on the field light, incorrect calibration of some equipment, and the importance of not re-exposing the eye lens unnecessarily all converge to require a little more leeway. *Always allow an even amount, about 1 inch, of light around every side of the skull* (Figure 10-5). This will nearly fill up a 10- × 12-inch cassette. The precise location of the CR is a secondary consideration for these projections.

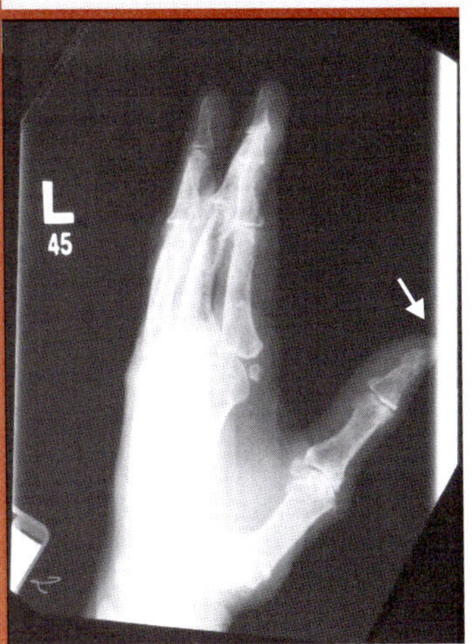

Courtesy of Quinn B. Carroll

FIGURE 10-4
On this radiograph, the soft tissue at the tip of the thumb was included within the edge of the *light* field, but was clipped off by the actual x-ray field (arrow), which lay ½ inch *inside* the indicated light edge.

WHAT MAKES A GOOD CENTERING RULE?

Students are often confused by the many different centering tips they hear—there seem to be as many methods as there are individual radiographers! All one can do is be selective. A good centering rule *can* be distinguished from a poor one. This is done by putting each recommendation to the following tests, which will each be discussed:

1. Does the rule seem to make good *anatomical* sense? Does it use stable, reliable *bony* landmarks?
2. Does the rule tend to *automatically compensate* for larger or smaller patients? Is it *self-correcting* for normal variations in anatomy?
3. Is the rule *independent* of the radiographer's own body size, large or small?
4. Is the rule *simple*, and can it be applied *easily* without special equipment?
5. Is the rule easy on the *patient* and quick to use?
6. Does the rule *consistently* produce the desired results in the image, so that *repeat rates are actually reduced*?

1. Does the rule seem to make good anatomical sense? Does it use stable, reliable bony landmarks?

For example, centering for the gallbladder by referring to the level of the elbow may seem to "work," in that the sides of obese patients push the arm out and up, thus pulling the centering point higher. But of course, there is no direct anatomical connection between the gallbladder and the elbow! A rule using the curvature of the ribs or other bony anatomy close to the actual gallbladder makes more sense.

As another example, one textbook recommends centering for the PA chest by palpating for the vertebra prominens (C7), and then "going one handbreadth down" from it. Because this rule is based on the breadth of the *radiographer's hand*, it does not guarantee consistent centering over T7 from patient to patient, *whereas simply counting down by palpating the spinous processes from C7 to T7 does.* Why estimate where T7 is when you can feel it? This is simple common sense.

(The radiographer's handbreadth can be useful in measuring distances from specific palpated landmarks, *provided* the radiographer has actually *measured* his or her hand with a ruler to establish a reasonably accurate basis for this method.)

Unfortunately, counting spinous processes by palpation is not as easy as one might expect, especially when surrounding ligaments and tendons are tight. (In this book, we advocate using the inferior angles of the scapulae.) Nevertheless, counting down the vertebrae is still more reliable than the "handbreadth" approach.

As discussed in Chapter 1, bony landmarks, especially immovable ones, are generally more reliable than soft tissue landmarks. Also, *palpation* of bony landmarks is more reliable than "eyeballing" the anatomy.

2. Does the rule tend to automatically compensate for larger or smaller patients? Is it self-correcting for normal variations in anatomy?

Some rules will pull the centering point up higher when applied to a taller patient, or appropriately down for a shorter patient. For soft-tissue organs such as the stomach and gallbladder, an ideal rule would automatically pull the centering point up for obese patients or down on thin patients, where the organ is expected to lie according to the habitus of the body.

A "fixed" rule fails to do this. For example, always centering a PA chest by placing the top of the light field 1 inch above the shoulder is a "fixed" rule. It does not take into account that on very short patients, this will result in an excessive amount of field extending down into the abdomen, effectively placing the CR at T9 or T10 rather than at T7. If the field is collimated to and centered to the typical 14- × 17-inch cassette or IR plate, this results in a radiograph that includes an excessive amount of the abdomen within the field. On small female patients, it is possible that even the ovaries may be exposed within the direct beam. Furthermore, this is a common cause of automatic exposure control (AEC) exposures extending too long, because the detector cells are placed partly over abdominal tissue below the diaphragms. Even though such practices may not result in unacceptable image quality, especially with digital equipment, these are important issues in overexposing the patient to radiation.

Another example of a "fixed" rule was cited in the previous section: "For the PA chest, center one handbreadth down from the palpated vertebra prominens (C7)." Note that this rule provides no correction based upon the body size of the patient. For a particular radiographer, it will always result in the same distance from C7 regardless of how big or small the patient is. Imagine a rather large radiographer using this method on a small, slight patient: The resulting centering will be much too far down the patient's back, perhaps over T9 or T10.

Here is an example of a rule that *does* automatically adjust for body habitus: "For the AP projection of the stomach, center to a level midway from the iliac crest to the xiphoid tip." Note that using this rule, if a patient has an unusually long waist, the distance from the iliac crest to the sternum will be longer and the centering point will be automatically pulled up higher. For a patient with a short waistline, this method will pull the centering point down lower just as the stomach is expected to lie.

Another example of a self-correcting rule is: "For the AP chest, center to a point midway between the sternal notch and the xiphoid tip." This method adjusts for patient size, because smaller patients will have smaller sternums.

3. Is the rule independent of the radiographer's own body size, large or small?

The rule now cited twice, "For PA chests, center one handbreadth down from the palpated vertebra prominens," is *also* an example of a centering rule being inappropriately dependent upon the radiographer's own body size. Note that this rule is based upon the breadth of the *radiographer's hand*, not the patient's body size. In fact (except for the starting point), it has nothing at all to do with the patient! Applying it can therefore only yield inconsistent results from one patient to the next.

4. Is the rule simple, and can it be applied easily without special equipment?

This guideline is based upon the philosophy of Occam's razor, a longstanding principle of science that, to paraphrase, states: "The simplest explanation is most likely to be the true explanation." In practical application, we might restate Occam's razor as: "The simplest approach is most likely to be the best approach." If a particular method for centering is overburdened with exceptions and qualifications, then perhaps a simpler, more universally applicable rule should be sought out.

For example, let us turn once again (for the fourth time) to the proverbial "one handbreadth below C7" centering for the PA chest: The textbook that espouses this method provides a footnote stating that, "If the radiographer is a male, subtract 1 inch from the handbreadth." The original rule is thus corrected for the radiographer's gender. (Of course, there *is* an expected difference in average body size based on gender.) If there were only this one correction, the general approach might be tolerable. However, as one begins to ponder this, one soon realizes that if the gender of the radiographer makes enough difference to warrant a correcting factor, then the gender of the *patient* might also make enough difference for another correction. What if the patient is a large male, and the radiographer is a smaller female? Should she then *add* an inch to the "handbreadth"? From a rule that appears to assume female gender for both the radiographer and the patient, we soon end up with three corrections to one rule in order to account for four possible scenarios.

Some rules also require a special device to apply. These will obviously find more limited application in practice than those that do not require access to particular equipment. Even the need for a protractor or a ruler makes a rule less handy and useful in daily practice.

5. Is the rule easy on the patient and quick to use?

This concept is also based upon Occam's razor mentioned earlier. The utility of any rule is partly dependent on its ease and speed of application. Here in particular, however, we ask the separate question of how much commotion and discomfort it might bring to the patient, who is our first concern.

6. Does the rule consistently produce the desired results in the image, so that repeat rates are actually reduced?

This is the ultimate criterion for *any* adopted practice or procedure in radiography. It should be stressed that repeat rates can be objectively measured even for specific isolated causes such as "AP C-spine with overflexed chin," and therefore provide a *scientific* approach to actually documenting what "works" and what does not. This is in contrast to the frequent comment, "It works for me," which is completely subjective.

Radiography is a medical field in which the code of ethics includes the application of *scientific method*. While it may require some time investment (weeks or months), it is not difficult to pick any particular notion in radiography and subject it to *proof* by monitoring the actual repeat rates when it is used versus the repeat rates when it is not used. Some care must be taken to provide a large enough sample (more than one radiographer in each group, those using the method and those not), and to avoid contamination of results by accidently measuring other causes than the one in question.

Unfortunately, the advent of digital imaging has made it easy for individual radiographers to discard unsatisfactory images without a trace, and has thus complicated the tracking of repeat rates. Some manufacturers are beginning to include automatic tracking software within their systems to help address this important need. But any student (not to mention any quality control technologist), can still conduct a reasonably valid and objective study of the radiographic images to which he or she has access.

Choosing a Rule

Needless to say, any rule you might adopt will not likely satisfy *all* of these six criteria for a good rule. *We might expect every rule to have advantages and disadvantages.* You must weigh these in choosing which rule to use. Adopt any rule that violates one of the criteria but meets several.

You may have noted repeated reference to the rule for the PA chest, "center one handbreadth below C7." This rule violates at least *four* of the listed criteria (#1 through #4). It is a *terrible* rule! It demonstrates how these criteria can be used to identify ideas that should absolutely be discarded. Considerable grief and repeated exposures could be saved if all of the tips and tricks of the trade were subjected to these six questions.

AVOIDING THE SYMPHYSIS PUBIS

Many of the centering rules presented in positioning texts require the radiographer to palpate or feel for the patient's symphysis pubis. Remarkably, other guidelines refer to the ischial tuberosities, as if one would ever palpate for this landmark on a patient! While experienced radiographers may be comfortable with palpation of the symphysis pubis, this does not mean that the *patient* is comfortable with it. Most radiography students would prefer to develop some alternative centering rules.

It is a simple matter to adjust all rules referring to the symphysis pubis so that the landmark used is the anterior superior iliac spine (ASIS) or the greater trochanter of the femur, for example. The diagram in Figure 10-5 shows the average distances between the iliac crest, ASIS, tip of the sacrum, and greater trochanter of the femur in relation to the symphysis pubis. Using this scale, alternative centering methods will be presented in the next section for the urinary system, sacrum, coccyx, and any other anatomy to which the pubic symphysis is often referred.

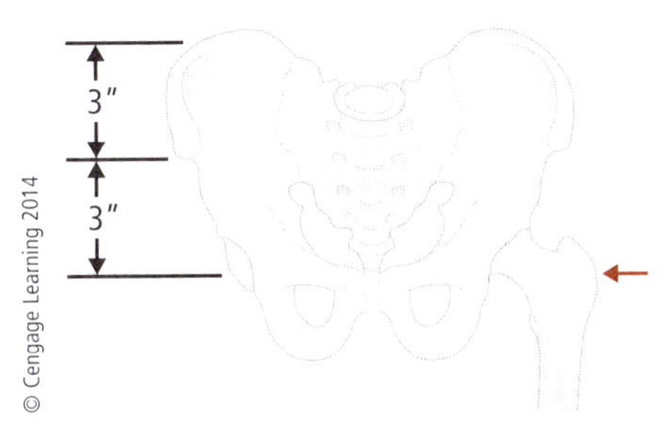

FIGURE 10-5

Diagram showing the mid-way position of the anterior superior iliac spine (ASIS) between the symphysic pubis and the iliac crests, lying 3 inches from each on the average male, slightly less on the average female. The palpable *sides* of the greater trochanters are approximately in line with the top of the symphysis pubis (arrow) and the tip of the sacrum about 1 inch above it. All these provide alternatives to palpating the symphysis pubis.

The key relationship is that *the ASIS lies 3 inches above the upper edge of the pubic bones, on average* (Figure 10-5). For female patients, this distance is somewhat less, and on small females may only be 2 inches. (It thus violates *one* of our six criteria for a good rule.) Using the AP coccyx as an example, many textbooks recommend centering "2 inches above the symphysis pubis." Simply subtract this amount from 3 inches and center that amount *below* the palpated ASIS. For the average male patient, centering for the AP coccyx will be 1 inch below the ASIS. On small female patients, only come down ½ inch from the ASIS, because there is less distance to the pubic symphysis. A few other examples are as follows: Centering for the AP sacrum will be 1½ inches below the ASIS; for the cystogram, 2 inches below the ASIS; and, for the male cystourethrogram, 3 inches below the ASIS. In this chapter, all centering points that traditionally refer to the symphysis pubis will be given using the ASIS as a reference.

THE ASIS: THE "UNIVERSAL LANDMARK"

There are times when even the iliac crest, so widely used, cannot be easily located on hypersthenic patients in the midaxillary line. Yet, even on very large patients one can almost always locate the ASIS by feeling for the "front corner" of the crest. This point seems to accumulate very little fat over it and does not lie adjacent to hard ligaments or tendons. *The top of the iliac crest lies about 3 inches above the palpated ASIS on nearly all patients.* This is also shown in Figure 10-5. (Note that for the male pelvis, the ASIS marks the midpoint between the iliac crests and the symphysis pubis, being equidistant from both. On the female, it is slightly *below* this center point.)

To take advantage of these last two rules of thumb, it is critical that you accurately locate the ASIS and not guess at it. Having found any portion of the crest of the ilium by palpation, slide your fingers downward along the anterior ridge, continuing until you literally lose the bone where it drops off. *Then*, back up to the last point where the bone can be felt. This is the ASIS.

Do NOT simply feel for the anterior portion of the iliac crest—this will place you too high. You must accurately pinpoint the anterior spine itself. You *cannot* do this without going through the entire exercise: You must follow the anterior crest down to its most inferior point. And, it is impossible to know the inferiormost point without following the bone until it "drops off."

COMPENSATION FOR BEAM ANGLES

Remember the principles discussed in Chapter 2. All of the centering points recommended in this chapter assume a vertical x-ray beam, or specify the x-ray beam angle in connection with the centering point under discussion. Remember that from this recommended point, any increase in caudal angulation requires that you adjust the centering point more cephalic, and accompany any increase in cephalic angle with recentering more caudally.

LEFT VERSUS RIGHT LATERAL SPINES

Almost all x-ray rooms are arranged such that when the radiographer approaches the table, the patient's head lies to the radiographer's left. This is because you will be able to utilize *the anode heel effect* properly. The x-ray tube is always installed with the anode to the *left*, so the x-ray beam is less intense toward the left. For the torso in AP projection with the patient supine, the thinner shoulder area is also to the left. From this position, the patient is normally rolled onto her left side for lateral projections. The left lateral is easier to position than a right lateral because, with the patient facing away, the posterior side is exposed so that you can both see and palpate the spine as needed.

When spine positions are done at the upright Bucky (chest board), it does not make any diagnostic difference whether the left or right lateral is performed. So, the radiographer should just set the patient up the easiest way to be able to see the posterior side. Many radiographers still position the patient in the left lateral position even if it is more difficult to do it this way. Diagnostically, a right lateral spine view is just as good as a left lateral spine view. Be sure, however, to accurately mark the view provided for the radiologist.

Using Long SID

For rib series, spines, and abdominal procedures, the use of a 72-inch (180-cm) SID rather than 40 inches (100 cm) allows more anatomy to be demonstrated on any given projection due to reduced magnification effects. As demonstrated in Chapter 3, Figure 3-5, this can be very effective indeed, adding a total of 3 inches more anatomy to a 17-inch long field.

MOVING A STANDING PATIENT 1–2 INCHES ONLY

When the radiographer instructs patients to move just 1 or 2 inches to the side on their own, patients almost always shuffle both feet and move too far. To get a patient to move laterally just 1 inch, have him move *one foot* 2 inches over in the desired direction of shift, while keeping the opposite foot planted at its original position. This will shift the body midline 1 inch in that direction. Sliding a single foot over only 1 inch will shift the midline of the body by ½ inch in that direction. The shift distance for the midline of the body will always be half of the distance that one foot is moved.

THE CENTERING GUIDELINES

This section is designed to be concise and to the point. Wherever you can adopt centering rules in accordance with any of the guiding principles previously presented, we will fully discuss them. Where there is agreement with standard positioning atlases, we will not belabor the discussion nor include illustrations. We include in each section centering points typically given in standard positioning atlases.

Note that we give many of these guidelines in the form of locating the *edges* of the field, or what anatomical landmarks you must include within the field, rather than giving a specific point for the CR. These are based on paradigm #6 in Chapter 1, and have the added advantage that it becomes unnecessary to designate whether the imaging plate is placed *crosswise* or *lengthwise*. Orientation of the IR plate is implicit in the guidelines for what anatomical landmarks to include.

Each entry in this chapter consists of recommended guidelines followed by "Comments on Other Methods." We subject each method to the six guidelines for good rules, and we make an honest attempt to openly discuss the primary advantages and disadvantages of each approach. We strategically place important additional concerns regarding angles, distances, technique, and so on, and flag them with the boldfaced designation of "**NOTE**."

CHEST

PA

Center to the Level of the Palpated Inferior Angles of the Scapulae (Level of T7).

This method automatically adjusts itself for larger or smaller body sizes. Larger patients tend to have longer scapulae, adjusting the centering point appropriately downward (and leaving less of the IR or cassette above the shoulders). Shorter patients have smaller scapulae and centering is appropriately pulled upward. One must beware, however, of how the scapulae move with different arm positions. The method assumes that the arms are alongside the body.

Comments on Other Methods

Counting Vertebrae from C7

It would seem that the most accurate way to locate the centering point at T7 would be to simply feel for the spinous processes and count down starting from C7, the vertebra prominens.

This *is* accurate, but ironically, on many patients, especially highly muscular patients, these upper spinous processes are not easy to count down by palpation. It is recommended as a secondary approach.

"Hand-Spread" from C7

This method consists of spreading the thumb and little finger as far out as possible, placing one of them on C7 and centering at the bottom end of this "hand's" breadth.

This approach is not only subject to variation between male and female patients, but also to significant variation between *male and female radiographers*, whose hands are of very different sizes. All the required adjustments make it overcomplicated as well as inaccurate.

Level of the Top of the IR Plate

This method consists of always placing the upper edge of the IR plate or cassette above the patient's shoulders by a set amount, most commonly 1½ inches. Some radiographers designate this amount as 1 inch and some only ½ inch.

If used, this method *must* be adjusted for different sizes of patients to allow more of the plate above the shoulders on shorter patients, and less of the plate above the shoulders on large patients. When a single "blanket rule" is used for all patients, there will be an extraordinary amount of abdomen included on the PA chest on short patients, throwing off the AEC exposure times and resulting in unnecessary patient exposure. On very large patients, if the top of the plate is not brought down lower (closer to the shoulders), there is a high risk of clipping the costophrenic angles of the lungs from the view. In the past, this has been a common approach to chest centering, but it is not recommended here, especially in an age when the use of AEC is predominant.

Averaged Distance (7–8 Inches) Below the Vertebra Prominens

Centering the same distance down from C7 on *all* patients will result in the same problems listed earlier for "Level of Top of IR plate." This is an averaged distance (7 inches for female patients and 8 inches for male patients) and does not allow for the full range of adjustments as does the scapula method. It does not automatically adjust for actual patient size, but effectively presents one blanket rule for females and another for males. It is not recommended.

Adjustments for Body Habitus

One of the advantages of the "scapula" centering method is that it does a good job of adjusting automatically for different patient's habitus. As a reminder, refer to the diagrams in Figure 3-3, Chapter 3, illustrating how the edges of the light field should appear for large and muscular patients and for obese patients.

AP (Sitting or Supine)

Center to a point midway between the palpated manubrial notch and the palpated xiphoid tip. Larger patients have longer sternums, so this rule has the advantage of being self-correcting for different patient sizes.

Angle perpendicular to the *sternum*, 5° *caudal* in relation to the IR plate or cassette. This compensates the upward divergence of the shoulder shadows at shorter distances and also prevents lordotic views.

Comments on Other Methods

At 3–4 Inches Below the Jugular Notch

This is not self-correcting for larger and smaller patients. On very large patients, it places the centering point too high; on very small patients, it places the centering point too low.

Level of the Top of the IR Plate

As more fully discussed in the previous section on PA chests, this method is not self-correcting for different body sizes. For large patients, the radiographer must adjust the top of the plate lower, closer to the shoulders, to avoid clipping the bottom of the lungs. For small patients, the radiographer must adjust the top of the plate higher to avoid excessive abdominal exposure. It is not generally recommended.

Lateral

Center to the level of the bottom of the scapulae, palpated *prior to raising the arms.*

As for the PA described earlier, the bottom angles of the scapula can be used if they are palpated *prior to raising the arms over the head*, or one can count down vertebrae from C7 to T7.

A favorite tip is to always lower the chest board by about *1 inch* from the PA projection just taken (regardless of whether it was done crosswise or lengthwise). This is primarily based upon the effect of the patient "rolling" his shoulders forward on the PA projection, which tends to pull the entire chest a bit higher. Since this is not done on the lateral position, the torso is relaxed into a slightly lower position.

(A common misconception is that this is done because the right hemidiaphragm, which is now at some distance from the IR in the lateral position, is subjected to substantial downward divergence within the x-ray beam. This concept is true, but it is cancelled out by the fact that the right hemidiaphragm already sits anatomically higher than the left because of the size of the liver.)

Comments on Other Methods

See comments under Chest: PA. Also see Figure 3-3 in Chapter 3 for extremely large patients.

Value of Apical Lordotic and Lateral Projections: Lung Fissures and Lobes

Figure 10-6 illustrates the shape and position of the fissures separating the lobes of each lung: two fissures for the right lung, and one for the left. On both sides, the entire length of the *inferior* lobe lies posterior to the other lobes. Note that on both sides, the *major fissures,* which separate the inferior lobes, slant downward toward the front. Due to pathology (or sometimes trauma), fluid can accumulate within these potential spaces, just as with a pleural effusion—this condition is called an *interlobar effusion.*

Fluid accumulation in the *minor fissure* of the right lung is usually apparent on a routine PA or AP image of the chest, because this fissure lies close to horizontal for a standing patient. But, because the *major fissures* on both sides lie at an angle, small amounts of

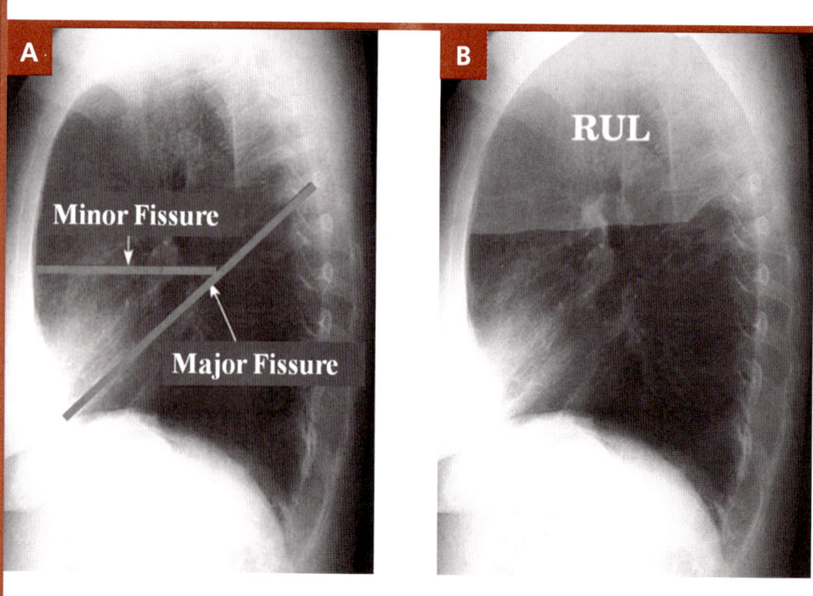

FIGURE 10-6

The downward slant of lung fissures is demonstrated for the right lung **A** and the left lung **E**. This points up the value of the apical lordotic position in demonstrating interlobar effusions. The pulmonary lobes separated by these fissures are then shaded in as follows: **B** right upper lobe; **C** right middle lobe; **D** right lower lobe; **F** left upper lobe; and **G** left lower lobe. Note the great extent to which these lobes will overlap each other when seen on a single AP or PA view. This underscores the value of the lateral projection.

Radiograph courtesy of Community Hospital of the Monterey Peninsula, Diagnostic and Interventional Radiology

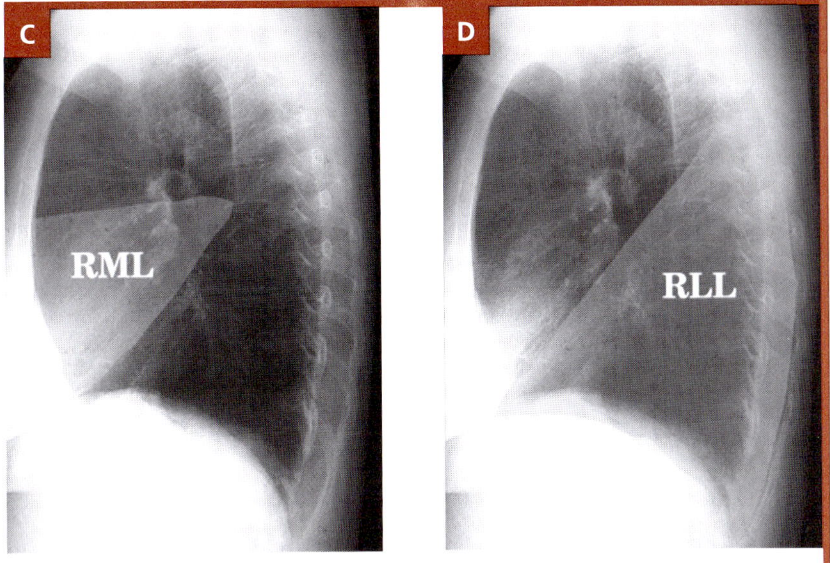

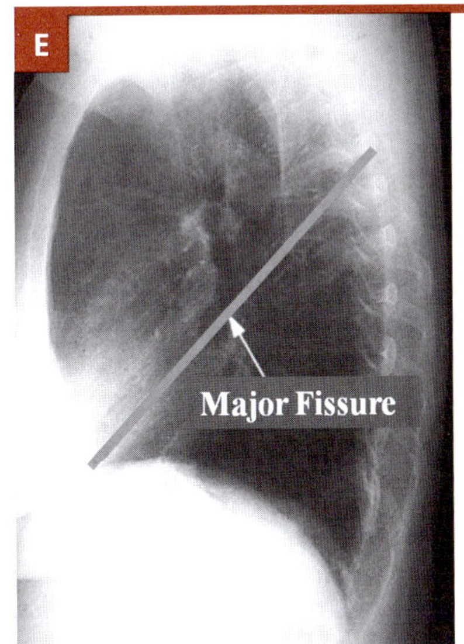

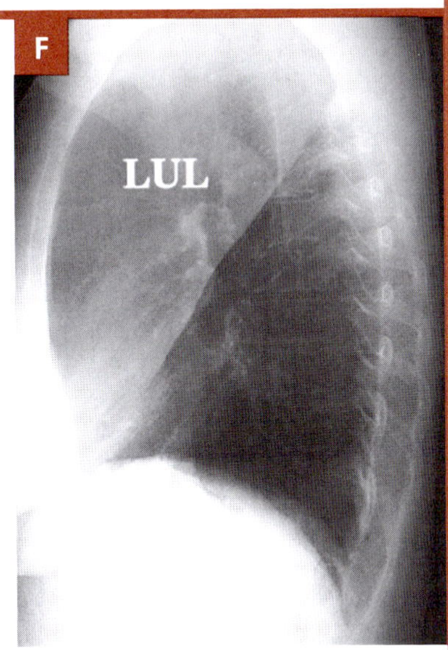

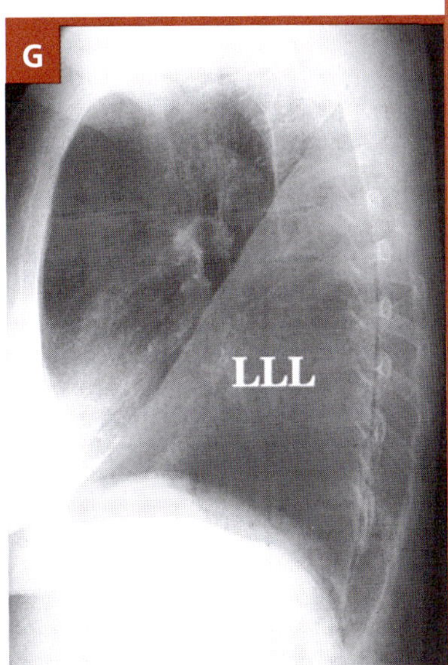

FIGURE 10-6 (*Continued*)

The downward slant of lung fissures is demonstrated for the right lung **A** and the left lung **E**. This points up the value of the apical lordotic position in demonstrating interlobar effusions. The pulmonary lobes separated by these fissures are then shaded in as follows: **B** right upper lobe; **C** right middle lobe; **D** right lower lobe; **F** left upper lobe; and **G** left lower lobe. Note the great extent to which these lobes will overlap each other when seen on a single AP or PA view. This underscores the value of the lateral projection.

Radiograph courtesy of Community Hospital of the Monterey Peninsula, Diagnostic and Interventional Radiology

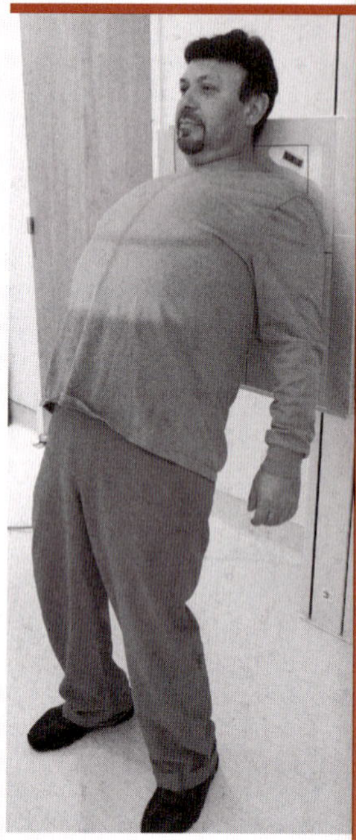

FIGURE 10-7
Proper apical lordotic position for demonstrating fluid levels including interlobar effusions, with the patient leaning back 15°–20°.

fluid within these spaces can escape detection on any frontal view. Sometimes the radiologist may see a suspicious light density on the frontal view, and have a hard time distinguishing with full confidence the same area on a lateral view from vessel markings within the lung. In such a situation, the radiologist may request an *apical lordotic* projection of the chest (Figure 10-7). By leaning the patient back, the major fissures are positioned closer to the horizontal plane so that whatever fluid may be present will form a more visible density as a semi-"fluid level."

Certain types of tumors and other pathology tend to locate in the apices of the lungs, and the apical lordotic projection is indicated to demonstrate the entire apex area without superimposition of the clavicle. Indeed, displacement of the clavicle upward *completely* out of the lung field, above the first rib, is the criterion for sufficient angle (or leaning of the patient) on this projection (Figure 10-8). However, this projection is *also* very useful in demonstrating interlobar effusions accumulating within the major fissures, as also shown in Figure 10-8. Note that for this purpose, a *modified* apical lordotic position using angulation of the x-ray beam rather than leaning of the patient *will not do*. The position must be accomplished by leaning the patient back.

These anatomical relationships also underscore the importance of the *lateral* projection for chest pathology: Note that on both sides, the lower lobe lies *entirely behind* the upper lobe(s). Lesions or abnormal densities seen on the PA view cannot always be isolated to a particular lobe unless the lateral view is included for the diagnosis.

Decubitus Chest

The primary reason for ordering a decubitus chest is to visualize fluid in the pleural cavity. For this reason, it is critical to get the entire lateral rib margin of the side that is down. Because a patient could easily sink into a pad, the preferred method to make sure the patient is on something solid is to put a plastic slider board (a "smooth mover," Figure 10-9, identified by an arrow) on top of any pad or bedding.

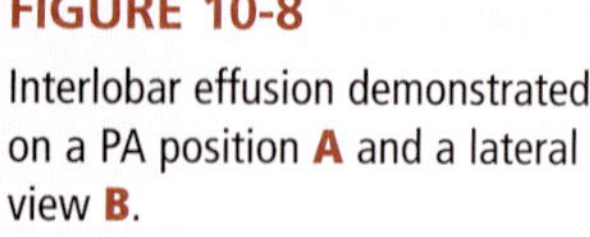
FIGURE 10-8
Interlobar effusion demonstrated on a PA position **A** and a lateral view **B**.

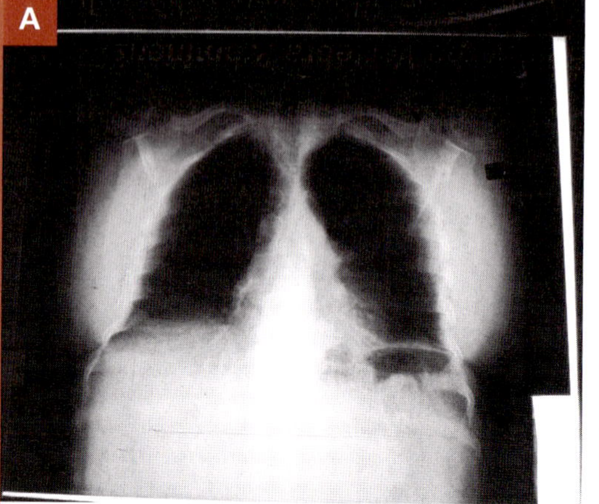

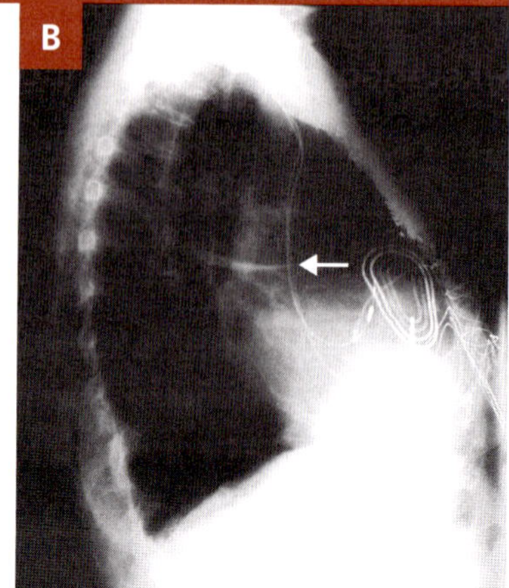

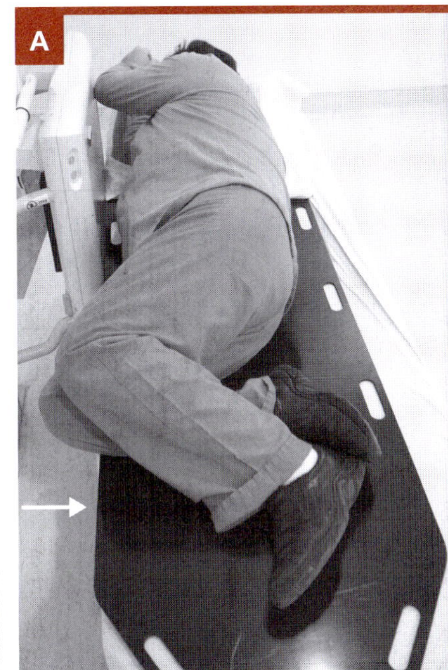

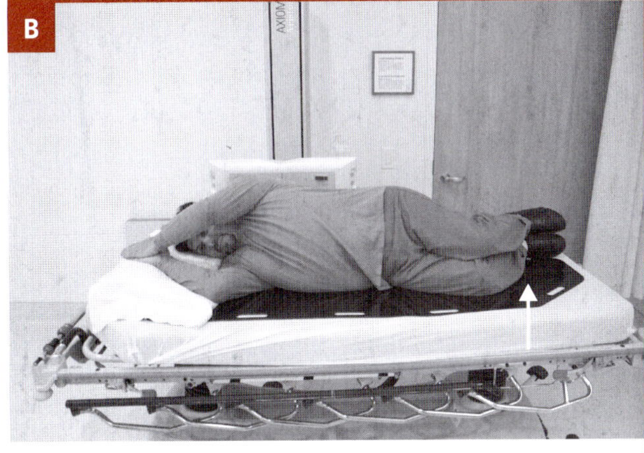

FIGURE 10-9

A *smooth mover* (arrow in images A and B) slider board prevents superimposition of a pad or bedding from the patient sinking down into it, greatly facilitating successful decubitus projections.

As soon as possible, roll the patient into the lateral position with the affected side down. The patient should ideally remain in this position for 5 minutes before making the exposure. During this time, set up the x-ray tube and IR. Make sure that the bottom of the IR plate or cassette is 1 full inch lower than the slider board so there is no chance of clipping the downside lungs.

Remember that for a decubitus chest, either the right or left side may be down depending on what lung has suspected pleural fluid, while a decubitus abdomen should always have the left side down.

Note that it is **always** easier to position a patient for a decubitus in AP projection rather than PA. In the PA projection, the elbows and bent knees are often in the way and the abdomen cannot be positioned as close to the IR. Placing the patient's knees off the edge of the table or gurney also can make the patient nervous about falling.

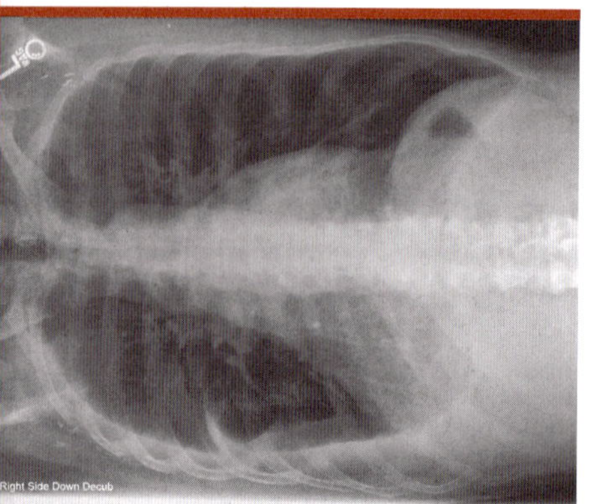

FIGURE 10-10

Conventional lead side markers must never be used for any other purpose than anatomical labeling. For a decubitus chest, this side marker is correctly placed on the upside, while the *decubitus* annotation is later added in shoulder tissue on the downside to avoid confusion between the markers.

Courtesy of Community Hospital of the Monterey Peninsula, Diagnostic and Interventional Radiology

Marking any decubitus position (chest or abdomen) correctly is very important. Many radiographers place all markers along the upside of the IR for ease of visibility. However, this side of the patient is opposite to the actual name of the decubitus position, and placing the side marker and the position marker close together can create confusion. The leaded right *side* marker is considered a legal document and must not be used for any other purpose than denoting the anatomical right or left side of the patient. This marker should not be "combined" in any way to create a marker denoting a *position* rather than the anatomy.

With digital imaging equipment, the best approach is use the leaded side marker correctly, anatomically. Then use the electronic *annotation* feature after the image has been processed to denote the decubitus position as shown in Figure 10-10, on the downside but in the upper portion of the anatomy where it will lie over shoulder tissue, well away from the lungs.

Ribs

Determining Anterior versus Posterior Positioning

As with all procedural routines, the specific projections required in any department for a rib series will ultimately depend on the preference of the radiologists. Rib series are unique in that the radiographer must decide whether to place the patient in AP or PA projection based on the location of the injury. The frontal projections are straightforward—an AP should be taken for posterior injury, and a PA should be taken for anterior injury. If lateral views are taken, a right lateral projection is taken for a right-sided injury and vice versa. For posterior injuries, it comes naturally for the radiographer to place the side of the injury closest to the IR. An LPO will be done for a left posterior injury and an RPO for a right posterior injury, in order to "lay out" this portion of the ribs parallel to the IR. However, the *oblique projections for anterior injuries* are complicated by superimposition of the spine, and many departments use incorrect positioning for these obliques.

Obliques for Anterior Injuries

Most routines in radiography place the patient so that the area of interest is closest to the image receptor for the oblique projections. However, for *anterior injuries to the ribs,* regardless of whether an anterior oblique or posterior oblique position is being used, *the spine is always rotated **away** from the injury site*. The correct oblique position for an anterior injury is counterintuitive: In order to avoid having the spine superimpose the area of the injury, a right anterior oblique (RAO) must be done for a left anterior injury and a left anterior oblique (LAO) for a right anterior injury. This means that the unilaterally collimated light field will be centered *to the upside* of the obliqued body, with a rather unusual appearance. Even though the area of the injury is not placed parallel to the IR, this is nonetheless the correct position, because it keeps the spine from superimposing this area, which is the larger issue.

Some departments have resorted to simply taking *both* oblique positions and including the full chest on each, regardless of whether the injury is right or left. This provides several benefits:

- Avoids having to sort out which position to do
- Guarantees that the correct view is included in the series
- Provides the radiologist more overall information

An ethical argument may be raised because of the additional area of exposed tissue, including a relative *doubling* of exposure to the female breasts. However, chest and rib techniques are so low in comparison with most radiographic procedures to begin with that in the context of radiobiology this is a fairly minor issue.

It should be emphasized that if a department chooses to require properly collimated *unilateral views* for the oblique ribs, the *correct* anterior oblique, with the injured side *up* off of the IR or table, should be routine. The light field must cover an area from the spine to the lateral rib cage on the injured side. The lateral border of the light field is easy to position, but the spine is on the backside and difficult to see. The edge of the medial light field should be *halfway between the sternum and unaffected lateral rib border*.

One tool that can help visualize whether the ribs have the spine superimposing them or not is to use your hands as shown in Figure 10-13 to simulate the spine and rib cage. Turn your hands sideways, bend your fingers, and then touch your thumbs and fingertips. The touching thumbnails represent the spine and the rest of the thumbs are the posterior ribs. The fingers are the anterior ribs. Now just imagine which way the CR is pointing and you can see if the spine is superimposing those ribs or not. For example, in Figure 10-11 the arrow represents the CR and imagine that the IR is placed in front of the fingers, so the projection is PA and the right hand (with the sweater) represents is the right ribs. This represents an RAO position, and shows that the spine is superimposing the right anterior ribs. From the previous discussion, recall that this position would be used for a *left* anterior injury.

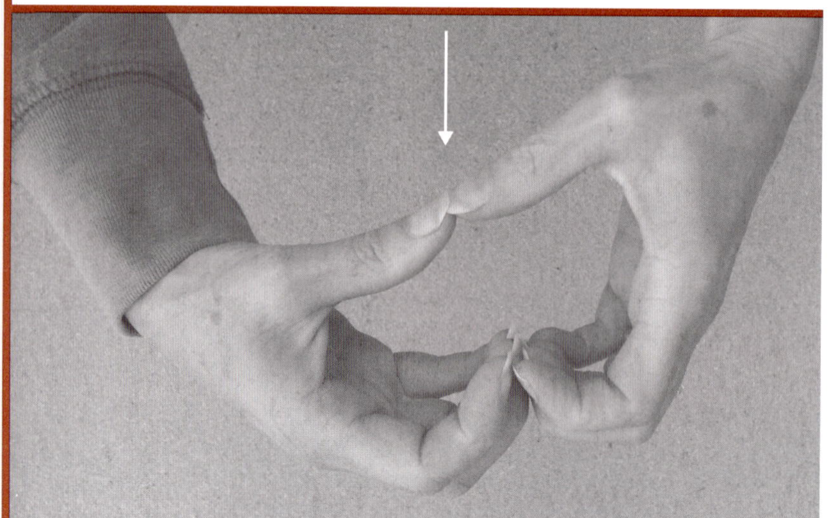

FIGURE 10-11
Simulation of the chest in which the touching thumbs represent the spine and the fingers represent the anterior ribs helps visualize how rotation of the chest positions the spine and rib anatomy relative to each other.

Unilateral AP, PA, and Oblique

With a 10- × 17-inch lengthwise *field*, place the top edge of the *field* 1 inch above the acromion. Center side to side to include the length of the *downside* ribs.

On a good inspiration, 10 posterior ribs should be visualized above the middle of the diaphragm.

Comments on Other Methods

At 3–4 Inches Below the Jugular Notch

This is roughly equivalent to the rule presented here.

Unilateral Below the Diaphragm

Place the *bottom* edge of a 10- × 12-inch lengthwise *field* at the level of the iliac crest.

This places the bottom of the *image receptor plate* about 1 inch *below* the iliac crest.

Despite where the site of injury or pain is located, most facilities will include a "below-the-diaphragm" projection. This spares the radiographer from having to diagnose if the injury is above or below the diaphragm. Because the technical factors needed for above-the-diaphragm and below-the-diaphragm ribs are so different, a complete rib series must include both. (The above-the-diaphragm technique is essentially a "chest" technique, while the below-the-diaphragm technique must penetrate the abdominal organs.)

Breathing suspended on *expiration* should be used for the below-the-diaphragm projection. On a good expiration, the bottom four to five ribs should be seen below the diaphragm, as shown in Figure 10-12. The diaphragm moves close to 3 inches between a good inspiration and expiration.

Comments on Other Methods

Midway Xiphoid to the Lower Rib

This is roughly equivalent to the previous rule.

Bilateral

Position as for a chest (see the previous section).

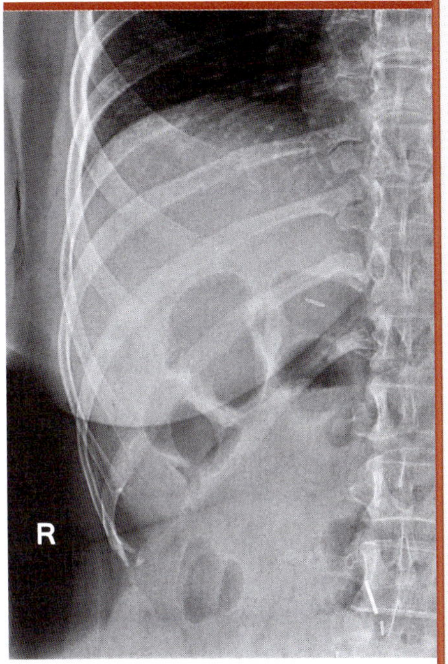

STERNUM

All Projections

Allow 1 inch of light *field* above the palpated jugular notch and 1 inch below the palpated xiphoid process, using a 5-inch-wide field.

FIGURE 10-12

For a rib series, good *expiration* for the below-the-diaphragm projection demonstrates 4 to 5 posterior ribs below the diaphragm (4½ ribs here).

Courtesy of Community Hospital of the Monterey Peninsula, Diagnostic and Interventional Radiology

Comments on Other Methods

Midway Jugular Notch to Xiphoid

This is roughly equivalent but does not address which anatomy or landmarks should be included.

Easy Method for Positioning the Sternum

Start with the patient in the *AP* position. Use the previously discussed method of centering and collimation. The average light field should not be larger than 12 inches × 5 inches. With the patient in AP position, it is very easy to both center the CR and collimate as shown in Figure 10-13*A*. Next, with the patient out of the way, center the IR (Bucky) to the CR, and place the side marker on the IR in the top right or left corner of the field (Figure 10-13***B***). Now position the patient facing the IR in a shallow RAO, 15°–20° off of PA. Center the midsternum to the vertical midline built into the image receptor, x-ray table, or chest board (Figure 10-13**C**). This will ensure that the sternum is perfectly centered. The collimated light field on the patient's back surface may appear incorrect or unusual (Figure 10-13***D***), but do not change collimation or centering because this method ensures that both will be correct.

Use of Shortened SID

A 30-inch SID can be used to advantage for the PA oblique sternum or for the SC joints in order to magnify and blur the obscuring upside spine and ribs. The use of short SID, including its implications for radiation exposure to the patient, is fully discussed in Chapter 4.

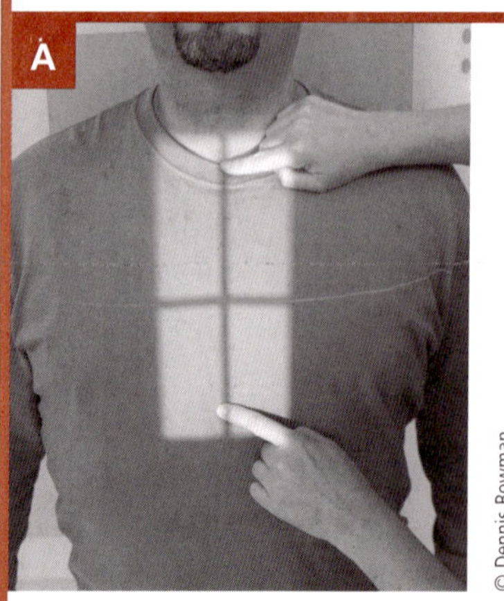

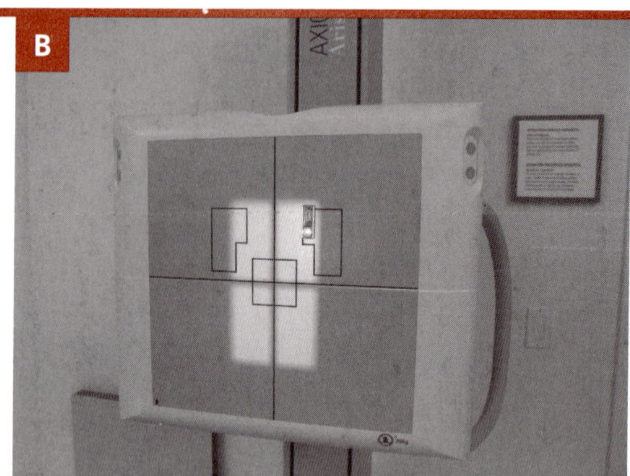

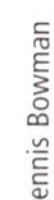

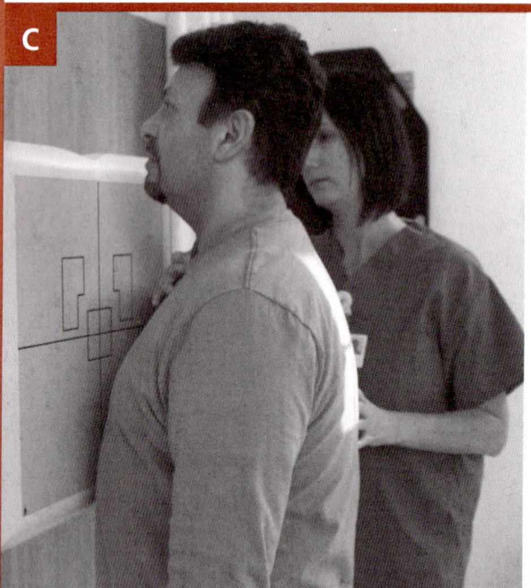

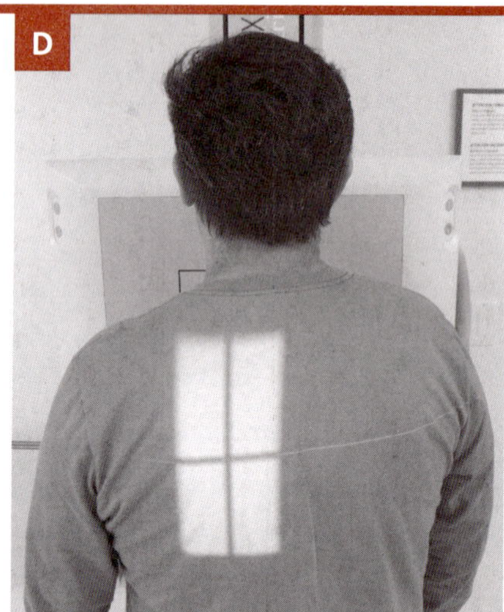

FIGURE 10-13

Easy method for positioning the oblique sternum: **A** center and collimate the field with the patient in *AP position;* **B** remove the patient to center the Bucky to the field and place the marker; **C** center the patient to the table midline in 15°–20° RAO for the final position **D**.

Use of Breathing Technique

Breathing technique also improves the demonstration of the sternum through the ribs, and to *maximize* visualization of the sternum, breathing technique may be combined with the shortened SID method discussed earlier. As with the lateral T-spine projection, the objective is to blur the overlying ribs and prominent lung markings. This allows the sternum to be better seen *through* these structures that cannot be desuperimposed by positioning alone. Because there is some risk of moving the sternum itself during the breathing, it is important to have the patient breath normally and not exaggerate his breaths.

ABDOMEN

AP

After centering the central ray to the iliac crest as a *starting point*, check that the bottom edge of the light field includes the *top* of the symphysis pubis (3 inches below the ASIS).

Then check that, if possible, the top edge of the light field includes the xiphoid process.

This rule ensures two things. First, the floor of the bladder is included within the field of view. Second, it ensures that the field of view includes the upper poles of the kidneys and as much as possible of the abdominal organs that lie just below the diaphragms. These are just the priorities for abdominal views, and there is an easy landmark for each.

Remember from Chapter 3 that the light field appears smaller on the surface of a large patient, so the top edge will be lower and the bottom edge higher than normal. On a thick patient, this may give the appearance that both the xiphoid and the symphysis pubis are being clipped off. "Split the difference" between these two, giving slight priority to the bladder at the bottom edge, and on the vast majority of patients the deeper organs of interest will be included within the view.

Comments on Other Methods

Center to the Iliac Crest

This is a great starting point and an easy landmark, but it simply does not take into account the anatomy that must be included within the view, nor the variation in shapes of the pelvis. When you apply the earlier recommended rule to be sure the anatomy of interest is included, you will find that on different patients the CR may fall somewhat below or above the iliac crest. Since priority is generally given to include the lower pelvic anatomy and symphysis pubis, it is better to err on the side of centering a bit lower than the crest. Especially with *male* patients, whose iliac bones are consistently taller, adopt a centering point ½ inch below the iliac crest as a routine procedure.

Large Abdomens Requiring Two Exposures

When a patient is too large to properly fit the entire abdomen within one exposure, it is common practice to turn the IR plates crosswise and position for both a lower and an upper abdomen as shown in Figure 10-14.

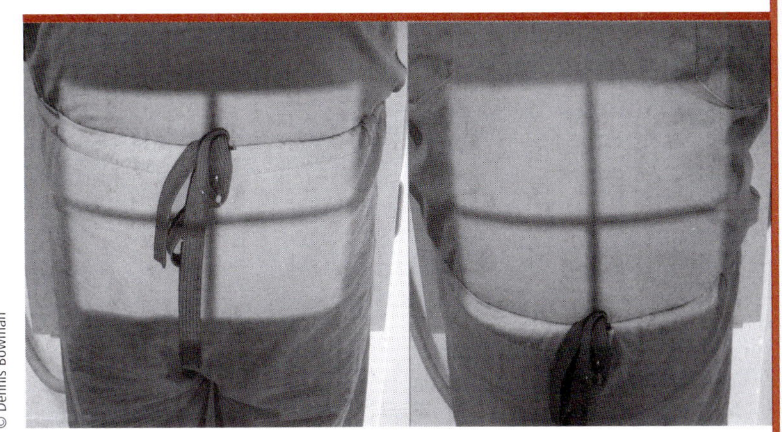

FIGURE 10-14

Abdomen projections for a very large patient: centering and collimation for crosswise IR placement.

This method works as long as the patient is less than 45 centimeters wide and over 6 feet tall (Figure 10-15). Of course, with any excess of the image receptor plate protruding from the sides of the patient, use collimation such that the entire plate is not covered.

If the patient is shorter than 6 feet tall and wider than 45 centimeters, a far better method is to put the IR lengthwise and position a right and left side abdomen (Figure 10-16). Figure 10-17 demonstrates a BE scout on a patient who was close to 60 centimeters wide. The entire abdomen is clearly demonstrated side to side, with appropriate overlap in the middle. Using this method allows the radiographer to get an extra 7 inches (17 cm) of width on the abdomen image.

Patients falling in between these measurements are of average body habitus and should fit on a 14- × 17-inch IR plate placed lengthwise as is the routine. For patients that are *both* taller than 6 feet and wider than 45 centimeters, some anatomy will be clipped using either of the methods and you must decide what anatomy takes precedence.

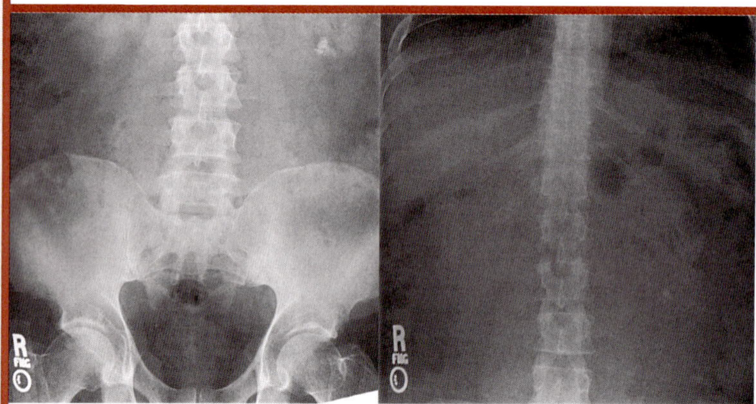

FIGURE 10-15

Resulting views for crosswise IR placement on a very large abdomen.

Courtesy of Community Hospital of the Monterey Peninsula, Diagnostic and Interventional Radiology

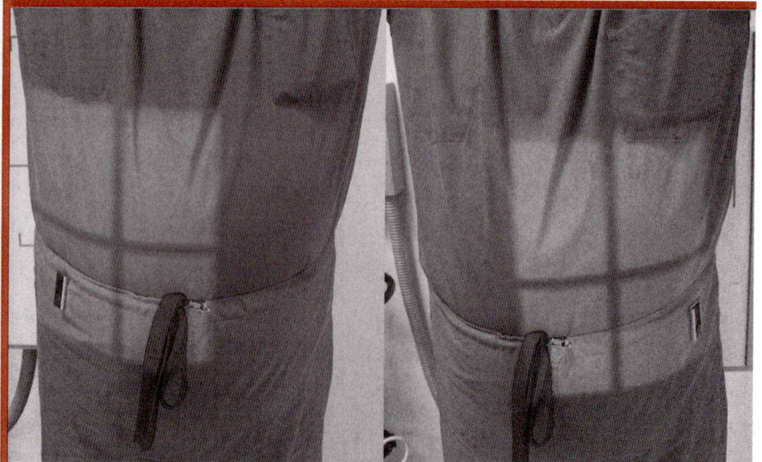

FIGURE 10-16

Abdomen projections for a very large patient: centering and collimation for lengthwise IR placement.

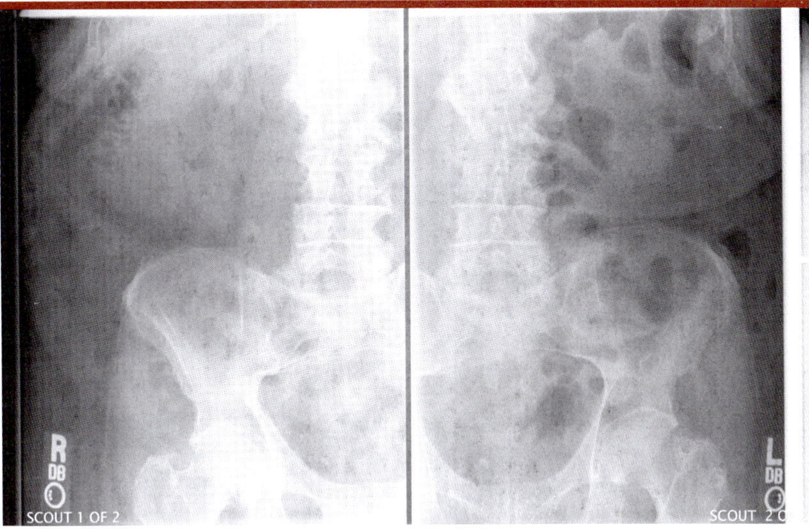

FIGURE 10-17

Resulting views for lengthwise IR placement on a very large abdomen.

Courtesy of Community Hospital of the Monterey Peninsula, Diagnostic and Interventional Radiology

Decubitus Abdomen

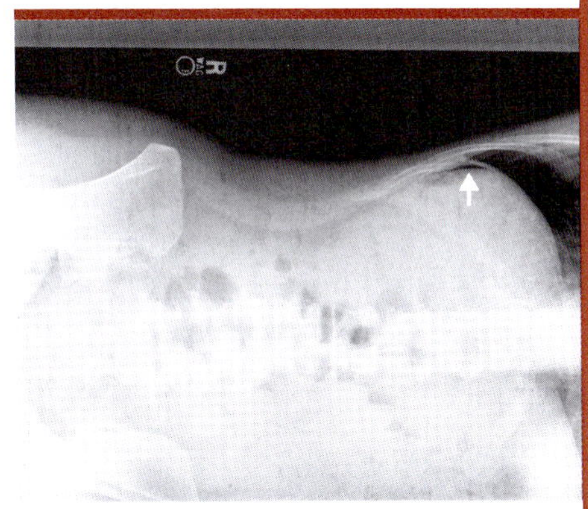

FIGURE 10-18

A decubitus abdomen view must include both entire hemidiaphragms and the upside rib margin. Note free abdominal air under upper ribs (arrow).

Courtesy of Community Hospital of the Monterey Peninsula, Diagnostic and Interventional Radiology

A decubitus abdomen projection always needs to be positioned with the left side down in order to demonstrate any free peritoneal air underneath it rather than over the stomach, which normally has gas in it. Unlike the decubitus chest projection, the priority here is to include the *upside* rib margin where free air will rise. The whole dome of the upside hemidiaphragm must be demonstrated (Figure 10-18), so it is important to center 2–3 inches above the iliac crest.

Other pertinent pathology for decubitus abdomen views includes air/fluid levels due to small bowel obstruction.

Abdomen/Chest for Feeding Tube

The abdomen projection to include a feeding tube is very different from all other abdomen views. The goal is to center over the domes of the diaphragm (Figure 10-19). An excellent landmark to use is to simply center to the level of the palpated xiphoid tip.

Do not collimate lengthwise smaller than the IR plate, because the end of the feeding tube might be anywhere within the mid- to lower chest or upper abdomen (the reason for ordering the view). There will be a good deal of lung field included within the upper half of the view. This projection is taken to make sure that the end of the feeding tube is in the stomach as shown in Figure 10-20*A*, and not still in the midesophagus, coiled at the esophagogastric junction, or worse,

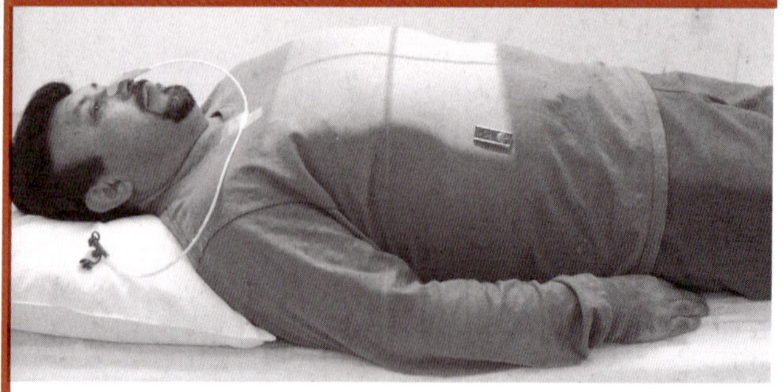

FIGURE 10-19

Proper torso centering for feeding tube placement is directly over the diaphragms (xiphoid tip).

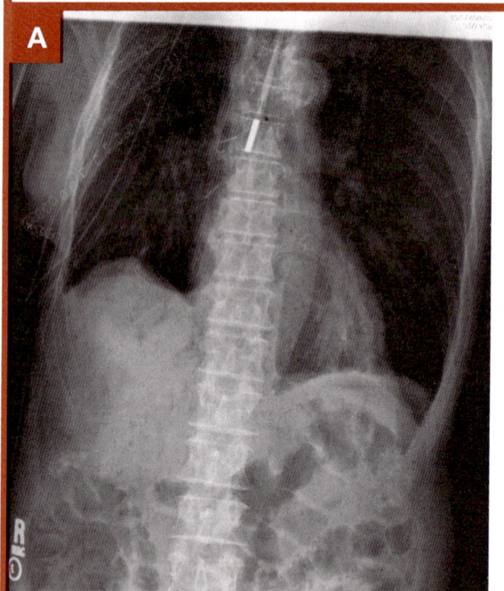

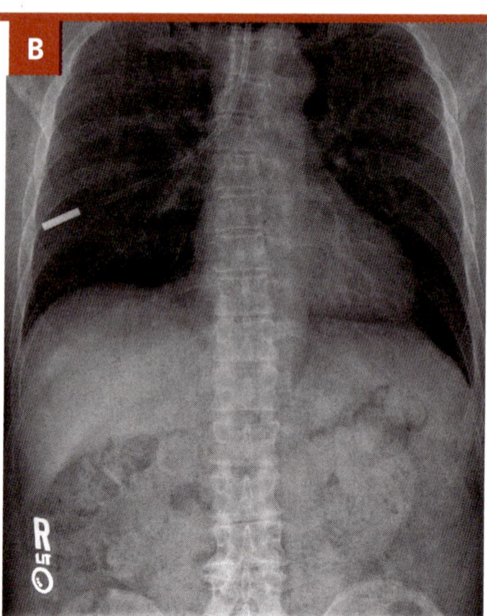

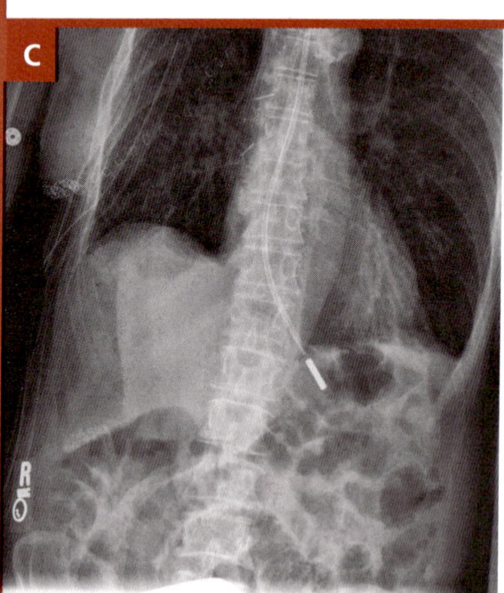

FIGURE 10-20

View **A** demonstrates the feeding tube still within the esophagus; **B** shows the tube accidentally inserted into a branch of the right bronchus; and **C** shows the end of the tube properly positioned within the stomach.

Courtesy of Community Hospital of the Monterey Peninsula, Diagnostic and Interventional Radiology

in the lungs. If the feeding tube has been accidentally inserted into the lungs, it could be found within either bronchus (Figure 10-20***B***). Figure 10-20***C*** demonstrates both perfect positioning and a perfectly positioned feeding tube.

URINARY SYSTEM

AP Survey Views

Less than 5 minutes post injection: Upper edge of light field to include xiphoid process. Five minutes or more postinjection: Lower edge of light field to include upper edge of symphysis pubis (3 inches below the ASIS).

Center as for an abdomen. However, views taken up to 5 minutes postinjection should include the xiphoid tip as a priority (whether a large or small IR plate and collimated field is used) to ensure the kidneys are included in their entirety. Views taken after 5 minutes should include the symphysis pubis as a priority, to ensure that the floor of the bladder is included.

Posterior Oblique

Center the superior-to-inferior level the same as for an AP projection (see previous discussion). Adjust the side-to-side centering upside (3 inches on average) from midline, such that the CR exits the palpated spine.

This shift follows paradigms #7 through #9 in Chapter 1 (1 inch for every 10°), and the guidelines in Chapter 5. With the body rotated 25°–30°, for the average patient the CR will be shifted upside 3 inches from the anterior midline. (Some texts recommend only 2 inches of upside shift, but use very thin models who are certainly *not* average, to illustrate.) For every 5 centimeters of additional body thickness beyond average, add another inch to the upside shift. To double check, the CR should exit at the palpated spinous processes.

"Coned-Down" Kidneys

Center at a level midway between the *lowest* rib margin and the xiphoid process, to the midline of the body.

The lowest rib margin must be palpated in the midaxillary line above the iliac crest, and is in fact the lateralmost aspect of rib #10. This is a self-adjusting rule, which automatically pulls the centering point up on patients with longer waists, and down on those with short torsos.

Comments on Other Methods

Midway Crest to Xiphoid

Nearly identical to the rule presented, this rule is also self-correcting for different body types, but turns out a little low.

"Coned-Down" Bladder

Center in the midline 1 inch below the palpated ASIS.

This is effectively identical to centering 2 inches above the symphysis pubis, but avoids palpation of the pubic bone. For female patients, center only ½ inch below the ASIS. For obliques of the bladder, also shift the CR upside but only by 2 inches (because the bladder lies anterior.)

STOMACH

AP

Using palpation, center at a level midway between the *lowest* rib in the midlateral plane and the xiphoid process. Center side to side to include *most* of the left side and *one-half* of the right side of the torso (Figure 10-21).

FIGURE 10-21

Top-down view of centering for AP stomach; side to side, center to include *all* of the patient's left side and *one-half* of the patient's right side.

A centering point midway between the lowest rib margin (rib #10 in the midcoronal plane) and the xiphoid process is somewhat self-correcting for patients with a longer or steeper rib cage. Using a point midway from the *iliac crest* to the xiphoid is more sensitive in self-correcting for longer or shorter *abdomens*, but tends to be somewhat low.

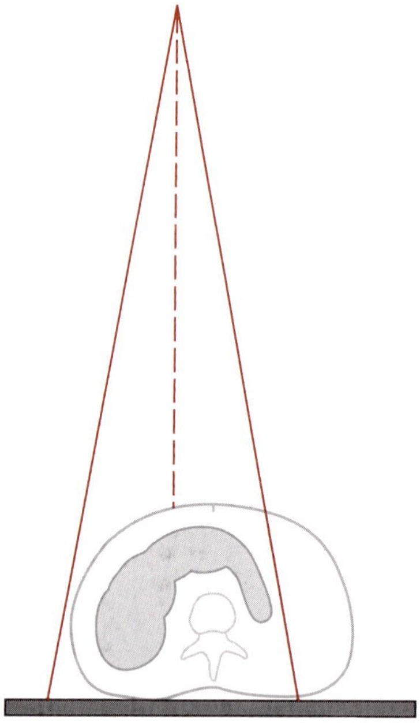

Comments on Other Methods

Mid-left Side

For side-to-side centering, this is much too far to the left and risks clipping off the duodenal C-loop, which extends halfway across the *right* side of the body.

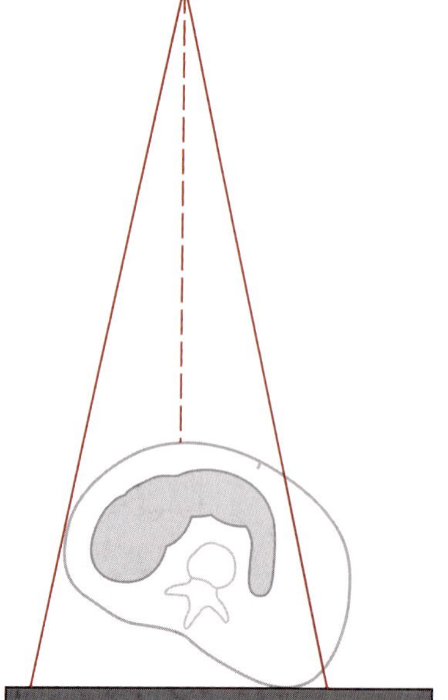

FIGURE 10-22

Top-down view of centering for RPO stomach; side to side, center to include *most* of the patient's left side and *one-half* of the patient's right side.

RPO

Center superior-to-inferior *level* as for the AP (discussed earlier). Center side to side to include *most* of the left side and *one-half* of the right side of the torso (Figure 10-22).

LPO

Center *level* as for the AP. Center side to side to exit the spine.

This will appear on the patient's surface to "cut off" a roughly equal amount of the right and left side, as you sight directly down from the head of the table (Figure 10-23).

Comments on Other Methods

Midway to the Upside

For side-to-side centering, this is much too far to the right (the upside) and risks clipping off the fundus of the stomach, which extends to the left rib margins.

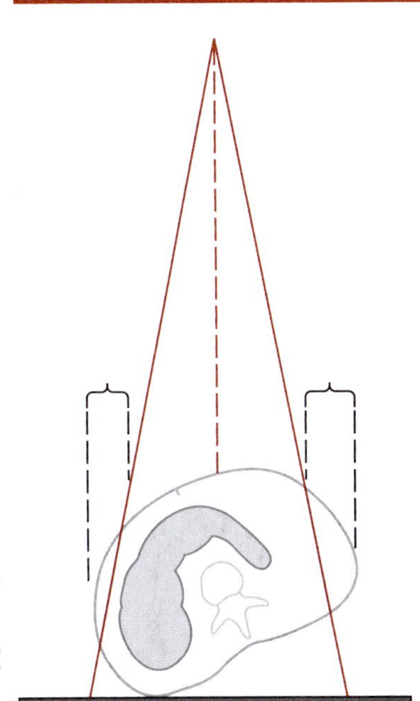

FIGURE 10-23

Top-down view of centering for LPO stomach; side to side, from *directly above the patient* it will appear that the light field is "clipping" roughly equal amounts of the torso to either side (brackets).

RAO

The centering *level* is as for the AP. Center side to side to include *all* of the left side and 2 *inches* to the right of the spinous processes.

Comments on Other Methods

Midway to the Upside

For side-to-side centering, this will be close to the same rule, but will be slightly too far to the left on some patients. Unless 2 inches of light are allowed to the right of the spinous processes, the duodenal C-loop may be clipped off.

Lateral

The centering *level* is as for the AP. Center midway from the patient's back to the front surface of the *belly* as it lies.

Both rules are self-correcting. For example, on an obese patient the second (front-to-back centering) rule will pull the centering point more anterior to include the more mobile lower portion of the stomach within the belly.

Comments on Other Methods

At 1–2 Inches Above the Lower Rib Margin

This rule is not self-correcting for patients with a longer or steeper rib cage. As discussed under the AP stomach, centering midway from the rib margin to the xiphoid process does correct somewhat for this, and centering midway from the iliac crest to the xiphoid further corrects for longer or shorter waistlines.

COLON

AP

Bottom edge of light field to include the top edge of the symphysis pubis (3 inches below the ASIS); then, if possible, top edge of light field to include the xiphoid process.

Comments on Other Methods

Center to the Iliac Crest

On most patients, the recommended rule discussed earlier will be roughly equivalent to centering to the iliac crest, but it is more adaptable to variations in the torso. For patients with a very long torso, inclusion of the lower rectum takes precedence here, because the upper flexures of the colon can be included on the oblique positions to follow (or a crosswise projection of the upper abdomen may be included within the series).

LPO

Center the superior-to-inferior *level* as for AP Colon. Shift side-to-side centering 3 inches upside from the midline on average, and add an inch for every 5 centimeters of additional body thickness.

Paradigms #8 and #9 indicate 1 inch of shift in centering for every 10° of body rotation; therefore, a 30° oblique will require 3 inches of upside shift for the average patient. Add an inch of shift for every 5 centimeters (2 inches) of additional body thickness (paradigm #10).

Since the hepatic flexure of the colon is depressed by the liver, there is never a problem with including it within these views along with the distal rectum, so the same *level* of centering for the AP projection can be used.

Comments on Other Methods

At 1–2 Inches Upside, at the Level of the Crest

This is insufficient upside centering for oblique positions at a true 25°–30° of rotation. The crest rule is not self-correcting.

RPO

Center the top edge of the light field 2 inches above the xiphoid process. Center 3 inches upside from the midline on average, and add an inch for every 5 centimeters of additional body thickness.

This is the only view specifically designed to demonstrate the splenic flexure of the colon, so it is essential to include it. The splenic flexure lies very high up under the left diaphragm. When breathing is properly suspended on expiration, the raised left hemidiaphragm pulls the flexure up higher still. Centering 2 inches higher than the other views ensures that the splenic flexure will be fully demonstrated on at least one image in the series.

The upside shift here is based upon paradigms #8 through #10 from Chapter 1. See the discussion in this chapter under Colon LPO for side-to-side centering.

Sigmoid

Center the CR in the midline at a level 2 inches below the ASIS.

Given the distorted field for a 35° beam angle, this typical textbook rule is as reliable as alternative methods. The resulting view should include the rectum from the anal sphincter up to the rectosigmoid curve in its entirety.

The sigmoid projection can also be done in PA projection with the patient prone. For a large (14- × 17-inches) IR, center the CR to enter at the level of the *posterior* superior iliac spines (PSIS), which can be palpated by following the iliac crest down and medially to its end point. (The "dimples of Venus," two indentations in the skin at the "small" of the back, usually lie right over the PSISs.) For a small (10- × 12-inches) IR, center 2 inches (5 cm) below the level of the palpated PSISs.

Use of Shortened SID

A 30-inch SID can be used to advantage for the angled projection of the sigmoid colon, taking advantage of beam divergence to desuperimpose loops of colon. The use of short SID, including its implications for radiation exposure to the patient, is fully discussed in Chapter 4.

GALLBLADDER

AP and Oblique

For the average patient, center at a level midway from the right iliac crest to the xiphoid process, and 2 inches to the right of midline. For hypersthenic patients, shift up and right by 1 inch each. For asthenic patients, shift down and medial by 1 inch each.

Comments on Other Methods

Level of the Lowest Rib

This rule is not self-correcting, and is somewhat lower than the rule suggested. The adjustments for different body types are fairly consistent between textbooks.

SACRUM

AP

With a 15° cephalic angle, center 1 inch below the palpated ASIS, in the midline.

This method avoids palpation of the symphysis pubis.

Comments on Other Methods

Midway of the Symphysis Pubis to the ASIS

This method has the advantage of being self-correcting for different shapes of pelves. But, for accuracy, it requires palpation of the symphysis pubis.

At 2 Inches Above the Symphysis Pubis

This method is not self-correcting for different shapes of pelves. It also requires palpation of the symphysis pubis for accuracy.

Lateral

Place top edge of a 10- × 12-inch cassette at the level of the iliac crest. Center 1–2 inches posterior to the midcoronal plane.

For a patient with a relatively straight back, center 1 inch posterior to the midcoronal line. When there is substantial lordotic curvature in the lumbar spine (swayback), center 2 inches posterior to the midcoronal line.

Comments on Other Methods

At 3–4 Inches Posterior to the ASIS

This is similar to the guideline discussed earlier, and neither one is self-correcting. The exact posterior centering must be evaluated by the degree of lordotic curvature in the lumbar spine.

COCCYX

AP

With a 10° caudal angle, center in the midline to a level 1 inch below the palpated ASIS.

This method avoids palpation of the symphysis pubis.

Comments on Other Methods

At 2 Inches Above the Symphysis Pubis

This method is not self-correcting for different shapes of pelves. It also requires palpation of the symphysis pubis for accuracy.

Lateral

Center 2–3 inches posterior to the midcoronal plane. The centering *level* is to the easily observed or palpated apex (bottom tip) of the sacrum.

For a patient with a relatively straight back, center 2 inches posterior to the midcoronal line. When there is substantial lordotic curvature in the lumbar spine (swayback), center 3 inches posterior to the midcoronal line. Observation or palpation of the actual anatomy of interest is, by definition, self-correcting and the most accurate approach.

Comments on Other Methods

At 3–4 Inches Posterior to and 2 Inches Inferior to the ASIS

This is a cumbersome and inaccurate guideline. It is not self-correcting. The apex of the sacrum (level of the top of the coccyx) is easily observed or palpated and can be centered accordingly without using any other landmarks. Center 1–2 inches *anterior* to the actual bone, to avoid excess light field striking the table behind the patient.

LUMBAR SPINE

AP

Center in the midline at a level 1½ inches above the iliac crest for the lumbar spine, or at the level of the crest for the lumbosacral spine.

This is in agreement with most positioning atlases.

AP Oblique

Center the superior-to-inferior *level* as for the AP. Adjust side-to-side centering upside (4 inches on average) from the midline, such that the CR exits the palpated spine.

This shift follows paradigms #8 and #9 in Chapter 1 (1 inch for every 10°), and the guidelines in Chapter 5. With the body rotated 35°–45°, for the average patient the CR will be shifted upside 4 inches from the anterior midline. For every 5 centimeters of additional body thickness beyond average, add another inch to the upside shift (paradigm #10). To double check, the CR should exit at the palpated spinous processes. This approach is self-correcting not only for body habitus, but also for the amount of obliquity used in the position.

PA Oblique

Center the superior-to-inferior *level* as for the AP. Adjust side-to-side centering upside (3 inches on average for the PA oblique) from the palpated spinous processes.

Comments on Other Methods

At 2 Inches Medial to the Upside ASIS

This guideline is not self-correcting for body habitus or for obliquity of rotation. It well approximates the side-to-side centering for the *average* patient, but it offers no correction for different thicknesses of the abdomen. Furthermore, *no portion of the human body presents more variations than the abdomen.* Therefore, a self-correcting method is strongly needed here.

Lateral

Center the *level* as for the AP. For anterior-to-posterior centering, center to the *skeletal* midcoronal plane, regardless of body habitus.

This is in agreement with most positioning atlases.

Lateral L5–S1 "Spot"

Center at a level 3 fingerbreadths (1½ inches) below the iliac crest, and up to 1 inch posterior to the midcoronal plane. Determine the angle needed by *palpation*.

For a patient with a relatively straight back, center in the midcoronal line. When there is substantial lordotic curvature in the lumbar spine (swayback), center 1 inch posterior to the midcoronal line.

See the following section for various methods of determining the proper tube angle by palpation. Use the guidelines from Chapter 2 and paradigms #7 through #9 from Chapter 1 to compensate centering for beam angles.

Comments on Other Methods

At 2 Inches Posterior to the ASIS

This point is much too far anterior, and is not self-correcting.

Angle 5°–8° Caudal

This is a "blanket rule" even if applied to only one gender of patient. Such a rule only guarantees a certain repeat rate, because there are male patients who require a caudal angle as well as female patients who need no angle. Proper beam angulation should be determined *objectively* by palpation and observation of bony anatomy as described in the following section.

Determining Beam Angle for the Lateral L5–S1 "Spot" Projection

In all normal conditions, the L5–S1 disk space is "locked" into place by the firmly fixed pelvic bones around it. Palpation of these extremely reliable bony landmarks allows the angle of the x-ray beam to be adjusted so that it passes right through the open space of the joint. As noted in Chapter 2, scoliosis can present an exception to this rule. (See Critical Thinking Challenge 10.4 at the end of this chapter.)

There are at least three methods by which this angle can be accurately determined by palpation. Whichever method you find preferable, the essential thing is that you use *direct palpation of bony anatomy* and become adept at accurately locating that specific anatomy.

Method #1

While squatting or kneeling at the level of the patient, use your left hand to carefully locate the spinous process of L5 (or L4). Keep your finger on this point. With your right hand, place a finger on the apex

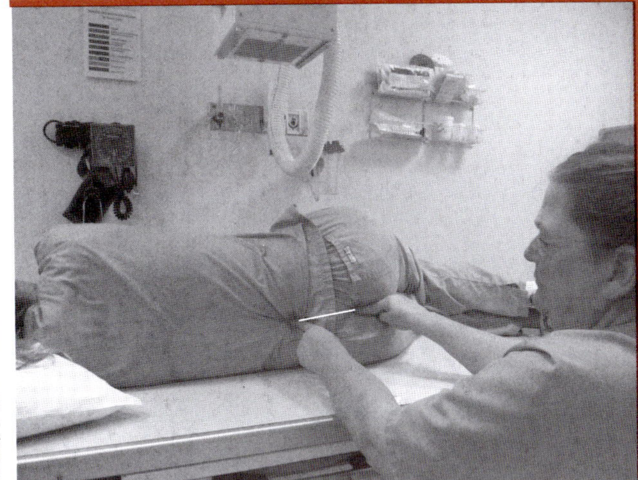

Courtesy of Quinn B. Carroll

FIGURE 10-24

L5–S5 palpation method for determining the CR angle on a spot lateral projection of L5–S1.

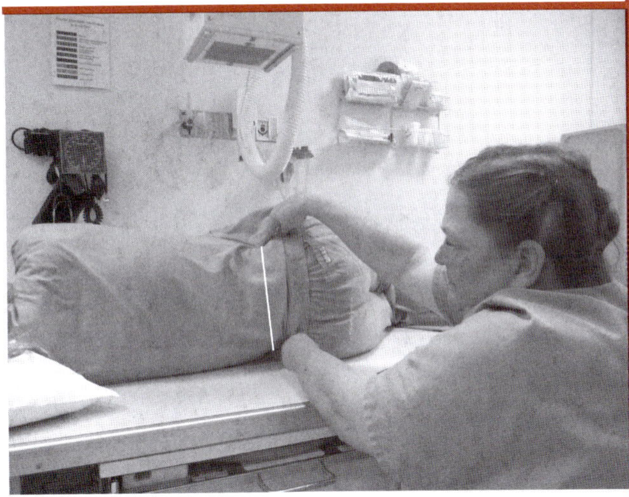

Courtesy of Quinn B. Carroll

FIGURE 10-25

Iliac crests palpation method for determining the CR angle on a spot lateral projection of L5–S1.

(lower tip) of the sacrum (Figure 10-24). The x-ray beam must be angled *perpendicular* to the line formed between your fingers.

Disadvantage: Palpation of the apex of the sacrum is required, so be certain that you inform the patient you will be feeling for his "tail bone." Since this is a *very* accurate method, it is well worth the effort.

Method #2

While squatting or kneeling at the level of the patient, place a finger on each of the iliac crests, upper and lower. Fully extend your arms so you can observe the line formed between your fingers from as great a distance as possible (Figure 10-25). The x-ray beam must be angled *parallel* to this line.

Disadvantage: The downside crest can be difficult to palpate correctly, and the long line between the iliac crests can be difficult to see from this close proximity.

Method #3

While squatting or kneeling at the level of the patient, place a finger on each of the posterior superior iliac spines (PSISs) (Figure 10-26).

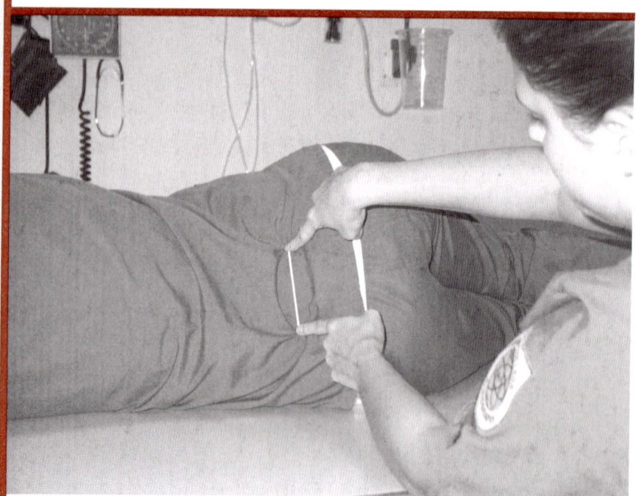

FIGURE 10-26

Posterior superior iliac spine (PSIS) palpation method for determining the CR angle on a spot lateral projection of L5–S1.

These are bony prominences at the most posterior end of the iliac crests where they join the sacrum to form the sacroiliac joints. They can also be distinguished by palpable and observable "dimples" on most patients, about 4 inches apart in the sacroiliac area. The x-ray beam must be angled *parallel* to the line formed between these points (and may also be *centered* in this way).

Disadvantage: Locating the PSISs by palpation requires some practice for accuracy.

These methods are far more reliable than any method merely observing the patient's body or any "blanket rule." They are so self-correcting that even for patients with severe scoliosis, the correct angle can be determined on the first exposure made. Repeats will be avoided if the radiographer will trust to objective palpation rather than subjective impressions about the patient.

Using the Lateral Image as a Guide, or to Preclude the L5–S1 Exposure with Digital Imaging

In the digital imaging world, images come up on the console within seconds after making an exposure. Therefore, the lateral lumbar spine view can always be visually checked first before making the actual exposure for the L5–S1 "spot" view.

As was fully described in Chapter 4 (see Figures 4-8 and 4-9), when the L5–S1 junction is adequately opened on the routine lateral image, with CR centering over L3, it means that there was a caudally diverging angle of about 5°–7° passed right through the L5–S1 joint, and this indicates that 5°–7° of caudal angle on the CR itself will best open the joint for the spot projection. If the joint is closed on the routine lateral view, the most likely indication is that *less or no* angle should be used for the spot projection. See Chapter 4 for a more complete discussion.

Another advantage afforded by digital imaging technology over conventional radiography is the vast improvement in the balance of image brightness (density) and contrast across the entire image. In the case of the lateral L5–S1 disk space, the obstructive effect of the thick iliac crests overlying the disk space is largely marginalized. With conventional radiography, this was actually the *main* reason for separating this view from the routine lateral lumbar spine projection—with the overlying iliac bones, this one joint was usually much too light for proper demonstration. Digital imaging has effectively rendered this whole issue moot, *except where the L5–S1 disk space is at an unusual angle such that an angled projection is required to open the space, such as for* positioning *purposes.*

Therefore, some departments no longer add the spot view to the routine series as long as the L5–S1 joint is adequately opened up on the routine lateral view. This is sound practice, and strongly recommended, especially in light of the fact that the lateral lumbar projections produce the highest entrance skin exposure to the patient of *all* "bone" procedures performed in the imaging department. (Elimination of this one view can reduce the cumulative "distributed" skin exposure for the lumbar spine series from approximately 5R [5,000 mR] to less than 3R.)

THORACOLUMBAR SPINE

AP

CR centering for a thoracolumbar spine is to the T12–L1 interspace. The xiphoid tip is at the T9–T10 interspace, and the lower costal margin (lowest palpable rib *laterally* in the midcoronal plane) is at the L2–L3 intervertebral disc space. This places the T12–L1 interspace exactly between them. Using both hands, center midway between the palpated xiphoid tip and the palpated lower costal margin as shown in Figure 10-27A. (An alternative is to center 2–2½ inches below the xiphoid tip, depending on patient size.)

Field size varies between different imaging departments, and may be anywhere between 8 and 17 inches of length with the IR to match.

Lateral

Since it is difficult to palpate the xiphoid process when the patient is lateral and facing away, the lower costal margin can be used alone as the starting point. Center 2–2½ inches superior (depending on patient size), shown in Figure 10-27*B*. As with the frontal view, the field may be from 8 to 17 inches in length.

THORACIC SPINE

AP

The top edge of the light field must fall at least 2 inches above the jugular notch. The bottom edge of the light field must be at least 2½ inches below the xiphoid tip.

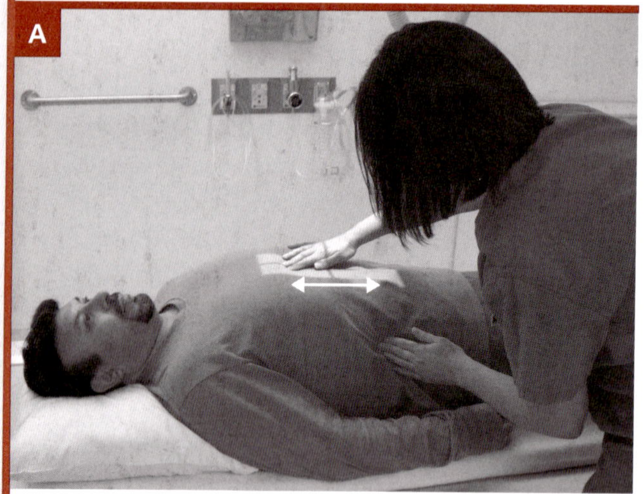

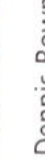

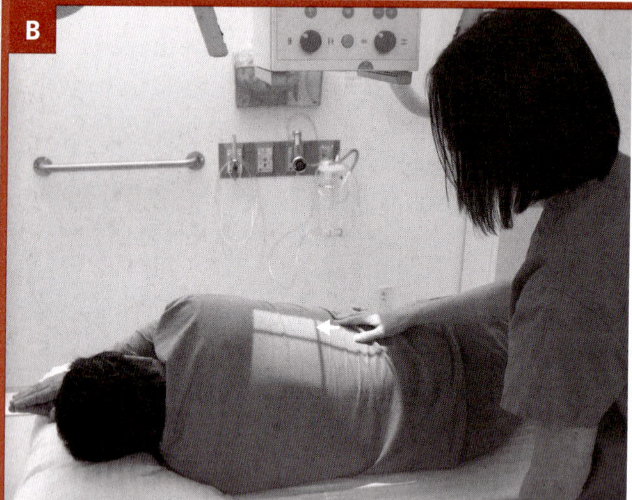

FIGURE 10-27

Centering for the thoracolumbar spine is midway between the palpated xiphoid tip and the palpated lower costal margin for the AP projection **A** and for the lateral projection it is 2–2½ inches above the palpated lower rib margin **B**.

Comments on Other Methods

At 3–4 Inches Below the Jugular Notch

This guideline is a good average, but is not self-correcting for larger or small torsos (while the rule of centering midway from the jugular notch to the xiphoid process *is* self-correcting). The recommendation described earlier allows even for some lengthwise collimation on very small patients.

Collimation

Unless the patient has somewhat severe scoliosis, the side-to-side collimation can always be 6 inches (14 cm). To check for scoliosis, have the patient bend slightly forward so that his spinous processes can be gently felt from C7 to the upper lumbar vertebrae (Figure 10-28). If the patient does have scoliosis, a wider field size may be needed. As previously stated, *the best way to collimate is to already know the size of the light field and use the collimator readout to determine exactly how much you have collimated*. Precollimating is always a great way to make sure you are collimated tightly, because the light field looks different on the surface of patients with different body habitus, as discussed in Chapter 3.

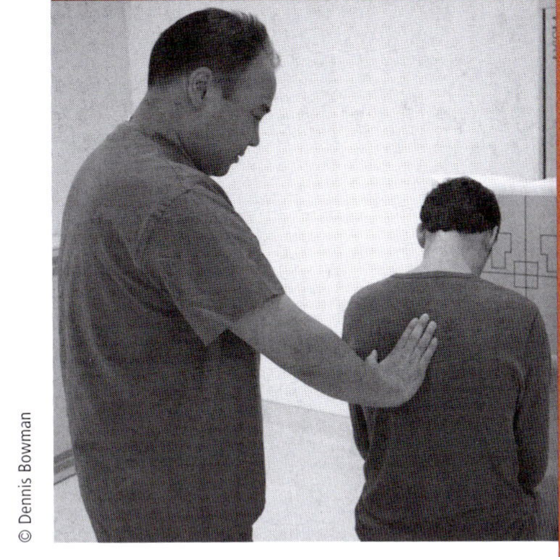

FIGURE 10-28
Checking for scoliosis by palpation of the spinous processes with the patient bending forward. The collimated field will be opened wider for patients with scoliosis.

Lateral

Center the superior-to-inferior *level* as for the AP, and 1 inch posterior to the midcoronal plane (see the following notes).

Inclusion of T1 can be ensured by placing the patient's upside arm *down* alongside the body for a moment and checking for at least ½ inch of light clearing the upside shoulder above. When the arm is placed back into position, 1–2 inches of the upside shoulder will appear to be "clipping" the upper edge of the field, but this is misleading. As patients become more and more kyphotic in their thoracic curvature, centering must be shifted more posterior.

CERVICAL SPINE

AP

Place the top of the image plate 1½ inches above the top of the ear. (Beam angled 15° cephalic.)

This is in agreement with most positioning atlases, placing the CR through the thyroid cartilage.

NOTE: It is essential for the AP C-spine projection to raise the patient's chin until the bottom surface of the mandible is projected directly over the base of the skull as shown in Figure 10-29. The bottom surface of the occipital bone can be palpated with one finger and the chin observed, allowing for slight downward divergence of the x-ray beam (i.e., the chin can be slightly higher than the occiput). This view *must* clearly demonstrate *all* of C3, which is obscured on the open-mouth projection by the mandible. Note that in Figure 10-29, not only is all of C3 visible, but the entire body portion of C2 as well.

Lateral

Place the top of the imaging plate at the top of the ear (Figure 10-30A).

This is in agreement with most positioning atlases, placing the CR through the thyroid cartilage.

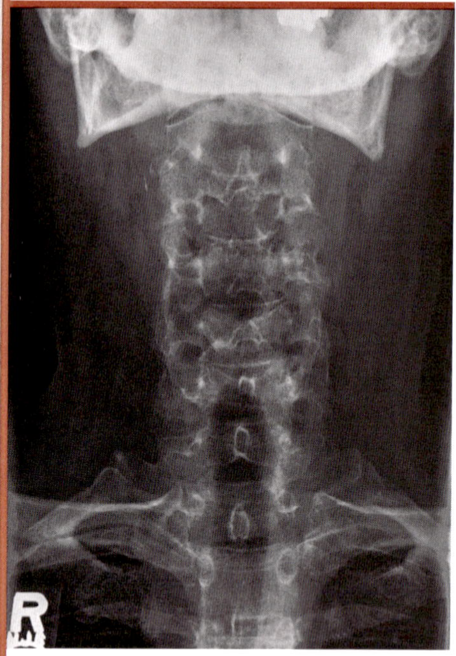

FIGURE 10-29
For the AP projection of the C-spine, raising the chin until the bottom of the mentum just superimposes the base of the occipital bone behind ensures maximum visualization of C3 through C7 (here, even the body of C2 is demonstrated in its entirety).
Courtesy of Community Hospital of the Monterey Peninsula, Diagnostic and Interventional Radiology

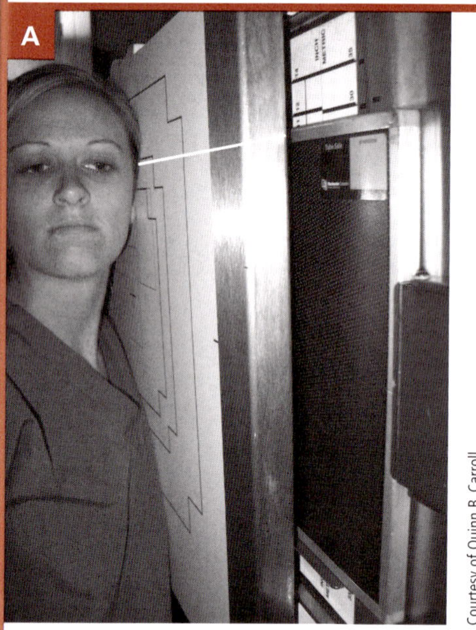

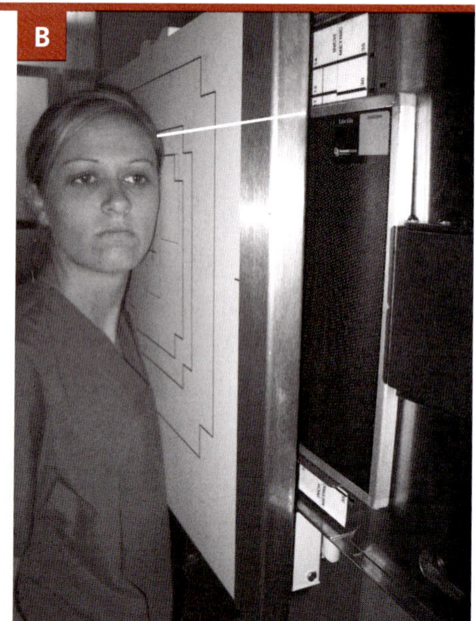

FIGURE 10-30
When using 10- × 12-inch IR plates for a cervical spine series, simply place the top of the plate level with the top of the patient's ear **A** for lateral and anterior oblique positions, and 1½ inches above the top of the ear **B** for posterior oblique projections.

Anterior Oblique

Place the top of the imaging plate at the top of the ear (using a 15° caudal angle), as shown in Figure 10-30*A*.

This is in agreement with most positioning atlases, placing the CR through the thyroid cartilage.

Posterior Oblique

Place the top of the imaging plate 1½ inches above the top of the ear (using a 15° cephalic angle), as shown in Figure 10-30*B*.

This is in agreement with most positioning atlases, placing the CR through the thyroid cartilage.

Odontoid

Center through the mid–open mouth.

See the following note on chin flexion. This is in agreement with most positioning atlases.

Proper Reference Line for Head Flexion

The recommended referral line to adjust flexion/extension is from the bottom of the upper incisor teeth to the *base of the occipital bone*, palpated with the broad side of the finger as it is slid up behind the neck. The mastoid tips vary greatly in size and shape, and a line drawn through these is not reliable.

Criticality of the SID for the Open-Mouth Odontoid Projection

The open-mouth projection should *never* be taken with a 72-inch SID. Figure 10-31*A* diagrams how a longer SID actually demagnifies the open mouth, so that the teeth obscure more of C1 and C2 including the odontoid process. It is just as if the mouth had been partially closed. At a reduced distance as shown in Figure 10-31*B*, normal beam

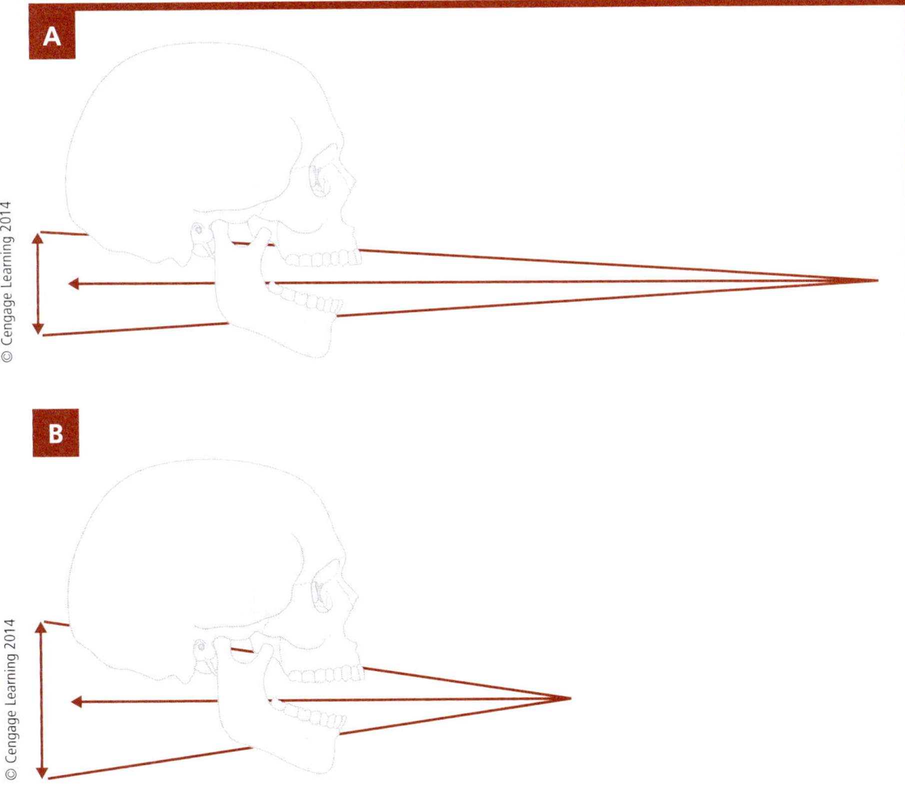

FIGURE 10-31

Diagrams of the open-mouth odontoid projection placing the divergent lines of the beam precisely through the upper and lower teeth to indicate where they are projected on the plate (left). When a 72-inch SID is used **A** the open mouth is effectively demagnified as if it were partially closed. In **B**, the use of a short SID (40 inches or less) projects the teeth farther apart, opening more of the upper cervical vertebrae and dens to an unobscured view.

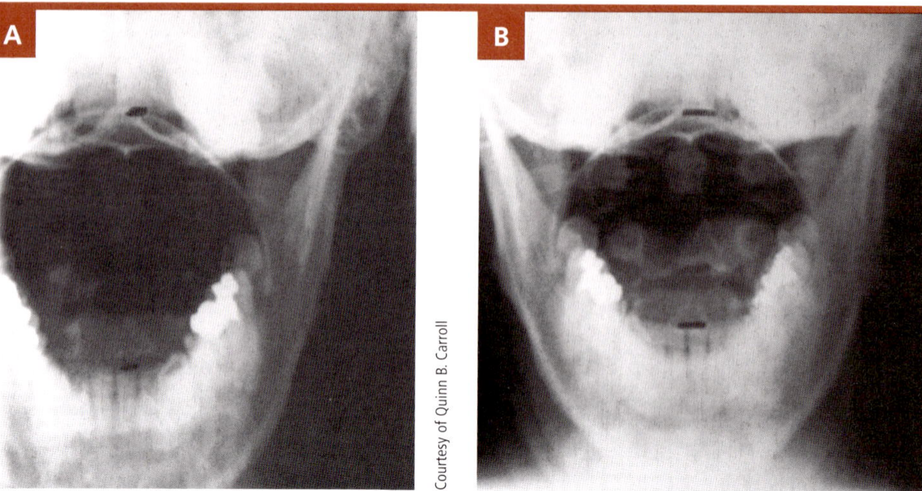

FIGURE 10-32
Radiographs of the open-mouth odontoid projection, proving the significant difference between a short and a long SID. In **A**, a 72-inch SID was used. In **B**, 40-inch SID was used and the teeth are projected almost 1 centimeter farther apart vertically, so more of C1 and C2 can be seen.

divergence, as it magnifies the open mouth, projects the upper teeth more upward and the lower teeth more downward.

This effect is both measurable and significant, as proven by the experiment shown in Figure 10-32. The artifact visible in these two radiographs is a glass placed in the subject's mouth to prevent any variation in the degree to which the mouth was actually opened between the two projections (to prevent any "cheating"). The teeth were carefully and precisely closed onto the circular glass, and both projections were taken upright using the chest board. The only change made between the two projections was the SID, with Radiograph **A** taken at 40 inches, and Radiograph **B** exposed at 72 inches. On the resulting views, the distance between the upper and lower incisor teeth was measured (indicated by the black marks). At the 40-inch SID, the mouth was opened 0.8 centimeter or approximately ⅓ inch *more* than at 72 inches. This is a substantial and visible difference, with the shorter SID desuperimposing nearly 1 centimeter more of the vertebrae and dens to an open view for diagnosis.

To save time and trouble, some radiographers prefer to take all five cervical views, including the AP and the odontoid views, upright at the chest board. There is nothing at all inherently wrong with taking the odontoid projection standing, except that *it must not be done at 72-inch SID*. The tube should be moved in to 40 inches for a proper view.

With many DR machines, the grid must be changed out when switching SID between 72 and 40 inches. Radiographers will be tempted to leave the SID at 72 for the odontoid projection. But, this is an important consideration in properly demonstrating the anatomy of C1 and C2. It would be better to just do the entire series at 40 inches, even if this means performing it recumbent on the x-ray table rather than using the upright chest board.

Now if reducing the SID to 40 inches is good, it might be argued that a 30-inch SID would be even better. Indeed, some radiographers routinely use 30 inches for the odontoid projection. In fact, there are several instances in which the magnification effects of shorter distances can actually be used to advantage, whenever they magnify unwanted anatomy *more* than the anatomy of interest. This concept is thoroughly discussed, including its implications for radiation exposure to the patient, in Chapter 4.

HAND AND DIGITS

General Digits

Centering roughly to the PIP joint, allow at least ½ inch of light field on each side and beyond the tips of the fingers, and 1 inch into the palm proximally.

This is in agreement with most positioning atlases.

Alternative Positioning for the AP or PA Thumb

The standard positioning for an AP thumb is to have the patient internally rotate the arm until the thumb is in a true AP position as illustrated in Figure 10-33*A*. Most patients can do this, but not without the metacarpals superimposing the proximal phalanx as shown in Figure 10-33*B*. This occurs because the thick "pad" of soft tissue over the fourth and fifth metacarpals gets in the way when the palm is folded as shown in Figure 10-34*A*. The additional internal

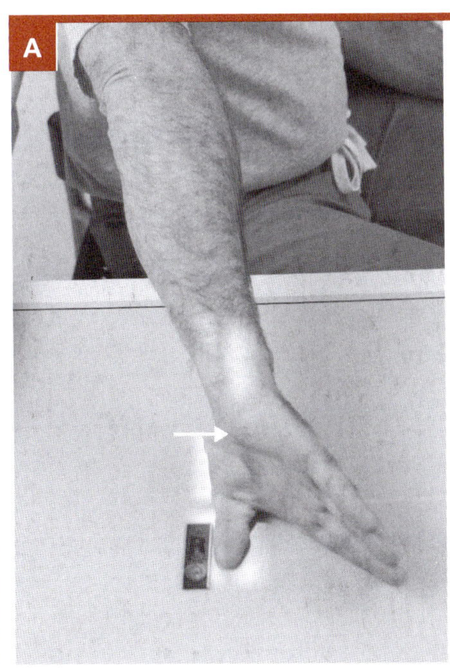

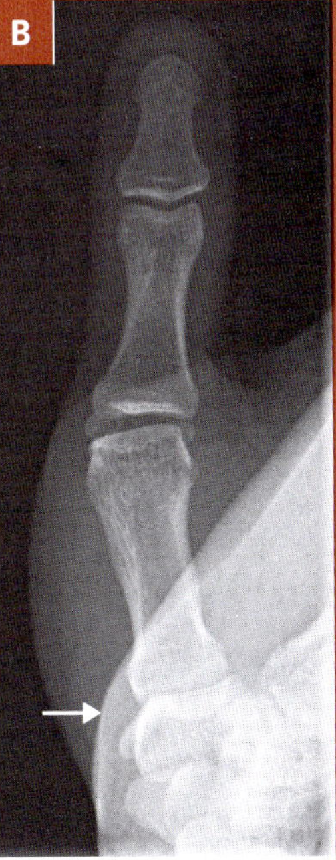

FIGURE 10-33 Conventional positioning of the AP thumb risks getting the tissue "pad" over the 4th and 5th metacarpals in the way **A** superimposing metacarpals over the 1st proximal phalanx **B**.

Part B is Courtesy of Community Hospital of the Monterey Peninsula, Diagnostic and Interventional Radiology

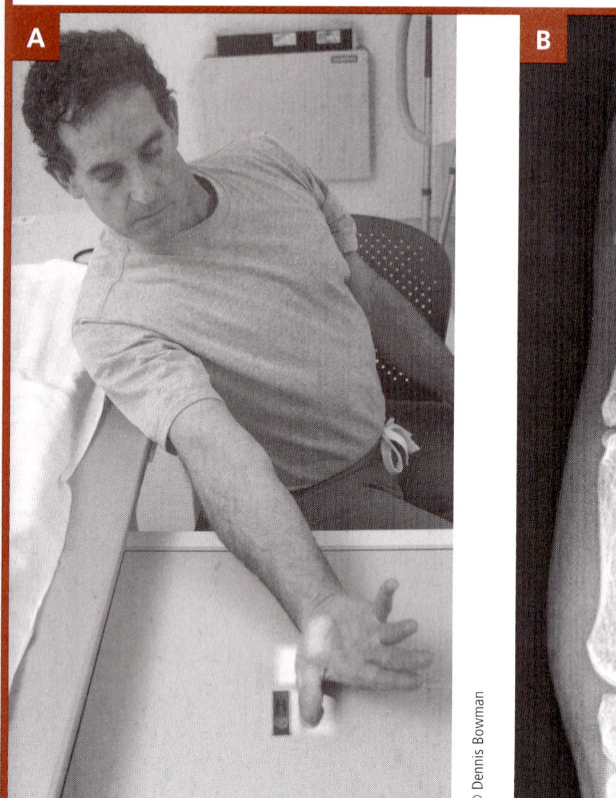

FIGURE 10-34
External rotation of the arm until the thumb in true AP position is no more uncomfortable than the conventional method **A** and avoids the problem of superimposing the metacarpals over the 1st proximal phalanx **B**.

rotation required to get this soft tissue out of the way usually results in rolling the thumb itself into a rotated position from the proper AP projection.

For many patients, an easier way to position the AP thumb is to have the patient *externally* rotate the arm out until the thumb is in the true AP position, shown in Figure 10-34*A*. The patient will have to lean his entire body toward the affected side in order to get the proper external rotation, but this is no more difficult than the extreme internal rotation method. This approach completely eliminates the problem of getting the metacarpals superimposed over the phalanx, shown in Figure 10-34*B*.

Some patients may be unable to perform either of these two positions. In this case, a *PA* thumb should be performed. Because there is only slight rotation of the arm, almost all patients can get into this position, but a 1–2-inch OID "gap" will be created, causing some magnification and slight loss of sharpness. Since the thumb is suspended, there is also a possibility of motion.

Have the patient lay the hand flat and then slowly lift the thumb off the IR until it is in the true PA position. This can be done without lifting any of the fingertips off of the IR plate. Make sure that the entire phalanx is parallel with the IR as shown in Figure 10-35*A*. The resulting image is always free from any soft tissue superimposition (Figure 10-35*B*).

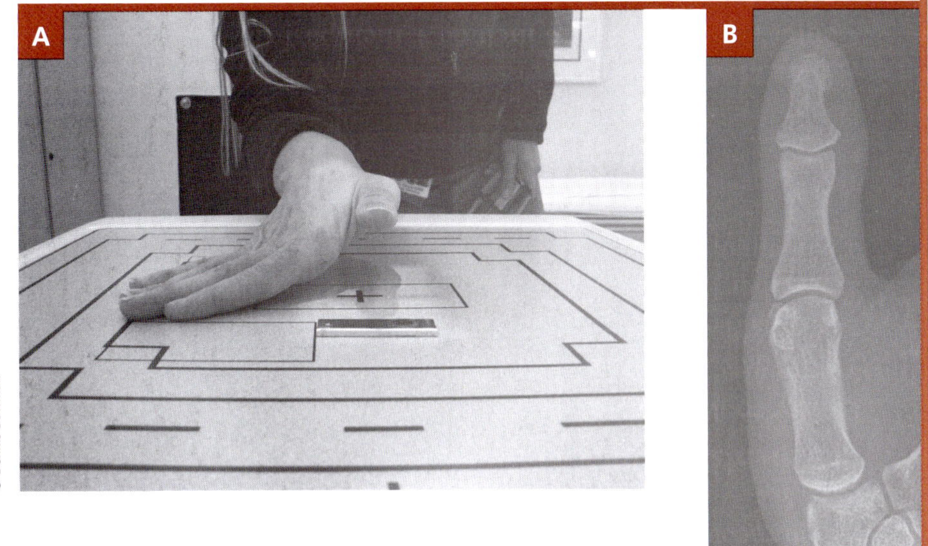

FIGURE 10-35

From the PA hand position, the thumb side can be gently lifted until the thumb is in true *PA* position **A**. The resulting view has only very slight magnification and demonstrates the thumb without any superimposed tissues **B**.

Part B is Courtesy of Community Hospital of the Monterey Peninsula, Diagnostic and Interventional Radiology

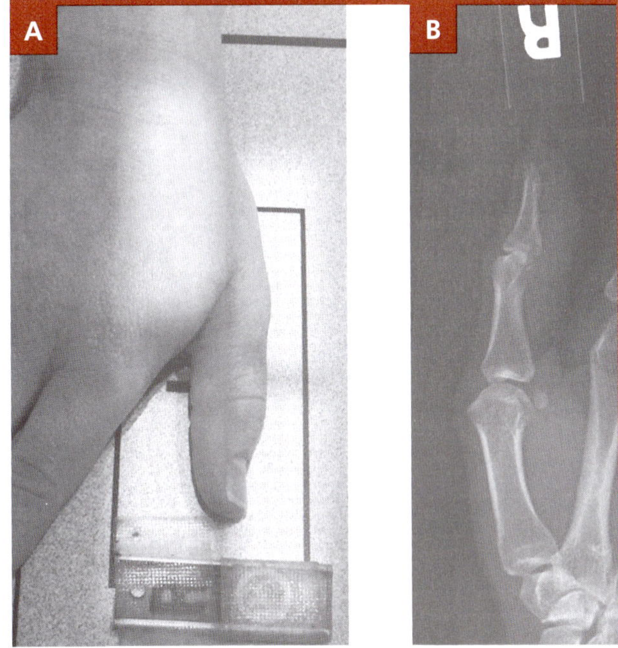

FIGURE 10-36

The oblique thumb is often positioned with the knuckles of the hand still bent **A**. resulting in too steep obliquity of the thumb **B**.

Part B is Courtesy of Community Hospital of the Monterey Peninsula, Diagnostic and Interventional Radiology

Oblique Thumb

The oblique seems like an easy projection, but is often improperly positioned. Often, the patient's hand is just placed in a relaxed prone position. With the knuckles slightly bent, this often places the obliquity of the thumb itself too steep as shown in Figure 10-36. Most often, the only correction needed is to fully flatten the hand as shown in Figure 10-37. In all cases, the obliquity of the thumb itself should be carefully positioned to make sure it lies in a true 45° plane.

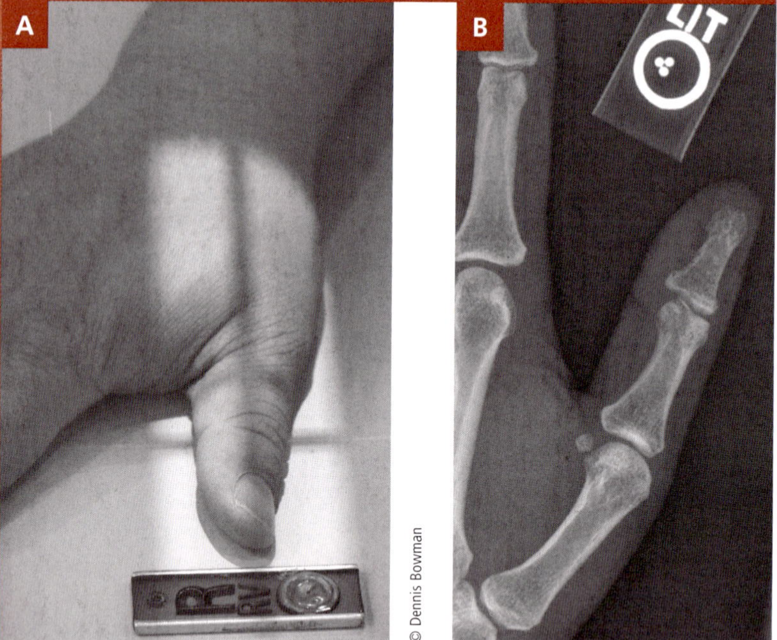

FIGURE 10-37

By completely flattening the hand **A**, the thumb can be brought down to the correct 45° obliquity **B**.

Part B is Courtesy of Community Hospital of the Monterey Peninsula, Diagnostic and Interventional Radiology

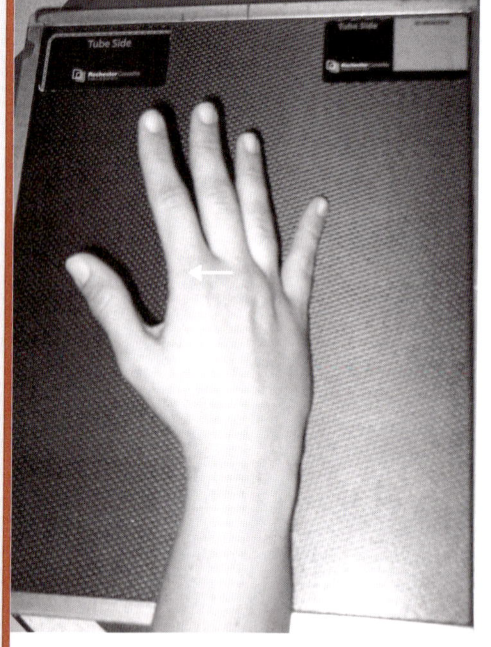

FIGURE 10-38

Centering for the oblique hand is to the *second metacarpophalangeal* (MCP) joint (arrow), *not to the third MCP*, allowing about a 1-inch light field around every side.

PA Hand

Centering to the third metacarpal (MCP) joint, allow about 1 inch of light field around every side, and 1 inch past the crease of the wrist proximally.

This is in agreement with most positioning atlases.

Oblique Hand

Centering to the *second* MCP joint as shown in Figure 10-38 (*not* the third MCP as described in many positioning texts), allow about

1 inch of light field around every side, and 1 inch past the crease of the wrist proximally.

Comments on Other Methods

Center to the Third MCP

This rule, given in most positioning atlases, actually creates a problem keeping the thumb within the light field. Note that it is unchanged from the centering for the PA hand and ignores the fact that rotating any body part shifts the centering point. Centering to the *second* MCP joint allows an even amount of light field around every side.

Note on Lateral Hand Positioning

Nearly all positioning textbooks indicate that for the hand, *both* the metacarpals and the distal bones of the forearm should be superimposed for a true lateral position. Looking at the back of your wrists, you can palpate and usually *see* the head of your own ulna *protruding* posteriorly on the medial (little finger) side. This means that it lies somewhat posterior to the base of the radius, and is "crooked" relative to the plane of the metacarpals of the hand. Radiographs proving this point are illustrated in Chapter 12. *Wrist anatomy should not be used as criteria for a true lateral position of the hand.* The only criterion is that the metacarpal area or palm of the hand is placed perpendicular to the image receptor.

"Stacked" Lateral Hand

Centering to the second MCP joint, allow 1 inch of light on every side, and 1 inch past the crease of the wrist proximally.

This is in agreement with most positioning atlases.

"Fanned" Lateral Hand

Center to a point in space midway between the second MCP joint and the thumb, as shown in Figure 10-39. Allow 1 inch of light on every side and past the crease of the wrist proximally.

Comments on Other Methods

Center to the Second MCP

This rule, given in most positioning atlases, creates a problem keeping the thumb within the light field. Note that it is unchanged from the "stacked" lateral, and does not account for the change of fanning of the hand and thus extending the thumb farther to the side.

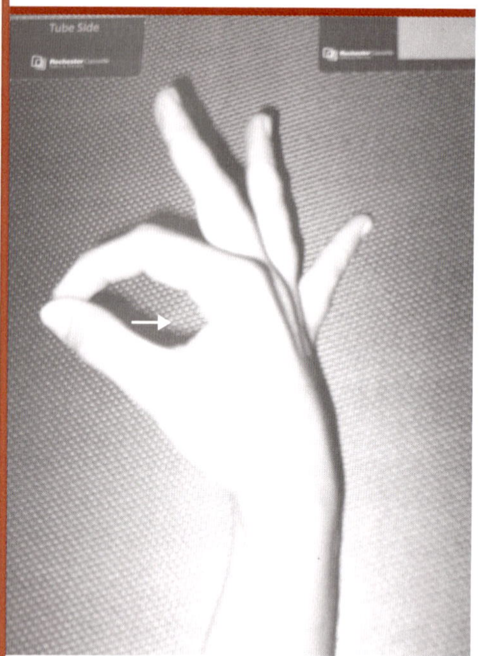

Courtesy of Quinn B. Carroll

FIGURE 10-39

Centering for the "fanned" lateral hand is to a point in space midway between the second MCP joint and the thumb (arrow), *not to the second MCP,* allowing 1 inch of light on every side.

WRIST

All Projections

Center ½ to 1 inch proximal to the crease of the wrist, to include at least the distal one-third of the forearm.

Bear in mind that *"wrist" series most often ordered to rule out fractures of the distal forearm bones* rather than fractures of the carpals. By centering 1 inch proximal to the wrist and opening the light field so that it extends to the knuckles, the distal half of the forearm can be included in the view. This is recommended. Even when centering at the crease of the wrist, always include *at least* one-third of the forearm within the view.

Comments on Other Methods

Center to Midcarpals

This is only slightly more distal and includes less of the forearm. Most "wrist" series are actually ordered to see the bones of the distal forearm rather than the joint space. Including one-third of these bones is a *minimum*.

FOREARM

All Projections

Center and collimate to include 1 inch past the wrist joint distally and 2 inches past the "crease" of the elbow proximally.

CASE STUDY

Case Study #10.1: Why at Least One-Third of the Forearm Must Be Included for a Wrist Series

A 15-year-old male was seen in the emergency department (ED) after a skateboarding fall. Although he had tenderness in the wrist, he was easily able to move the wrist in all positions. Because of this ease of movement, the radiographer assumed that the patient did not have a wrist fracture. The ED physician noticed something abnormal at the very bottom of the lateral view (arrow in Figure 10-40***A***), so he ordered a forearm series. In Figure 10-40***B***, it can be seen that this abnormality was the very edge (arrow) of a radius fracture. The fracture was almost missed on this patient, who was hurting perhaps less than he would have been from a sprained joint. Note if the original wrist series had been centered and collimated to include the distal one-third of the forearm, rather than centered directly over the wrist joint, the fracture would have been included.

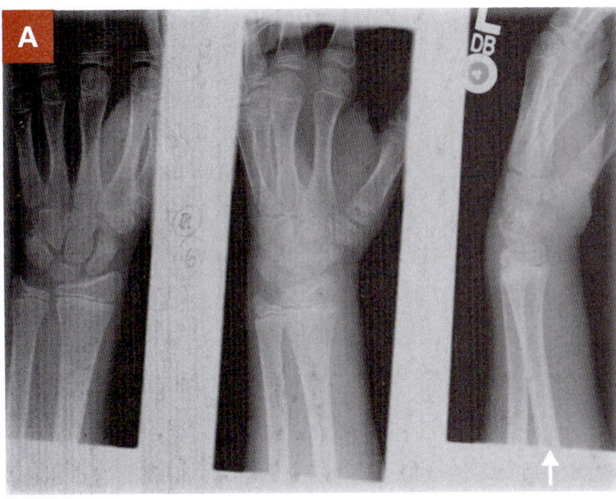

FIGURE 10-40

Wrist series should generally be centered 1 inch proximal to the wrist joint proper, to include at least one-third of the forearm. Here, an ED physician just noticed the abnormality shown by the arrow in **A** and ordered a repeated exam to include more of the forearm. The second set **B** showed a serious fracture that would have been missed with conventional centering and collimation.

Courtesy of Community Hospital of the Monterey Peninsula, Diagnostic and Interventional Radiology

Comments on Other Methods

Center to Midforearm

This generalized statement does not address the crucial question of what anatomy or landmarks should be included within the field.

ELBOW

AP and Oblique

Center and collimate to include the proximal 4 inches of the forearm and the distal 4 inches of the humerus.

Hand Position for the Internal Elbow Oblique

Because rotating an elbow internally is so easy for the patient to perform, it is often overrotated through carelessness. Positioning textbooks generally recommend placing the hand palm down, completely *pronated*, in order to bring the elbow into a 45° obliquity. In reality, the elbow can be maneuvered from nearly AP position (Figure 10-41*A*) all the way into a lateral position (Figure 10-41*B*) while the hand is maintained in a prone position. Place your hand palm down and maneuver your elbow—you will find that the key to the position of the elbow is in the movement of the *shoulder*, not the hand. When a patient pronates the hand, the elbow naturally falls into a position that varies from patient to patient and may range from a shallow oblique to a very steep oblique.

To position the elbow into a true 45° internal oblique, have the patient begin *from an AP position* and internally rotate the hand until the carefully observed anterior surface of the elbow lies at 45°. This may

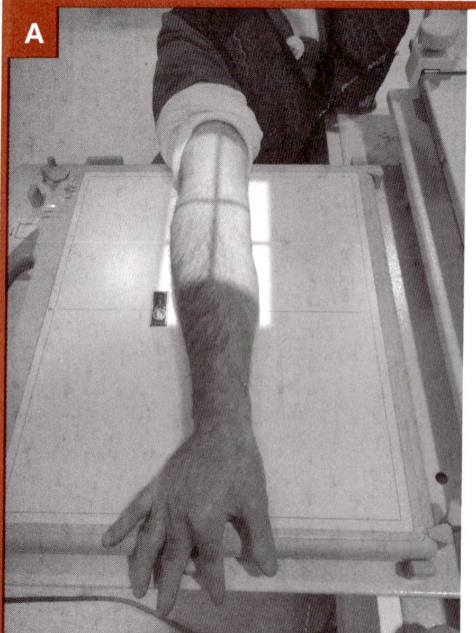

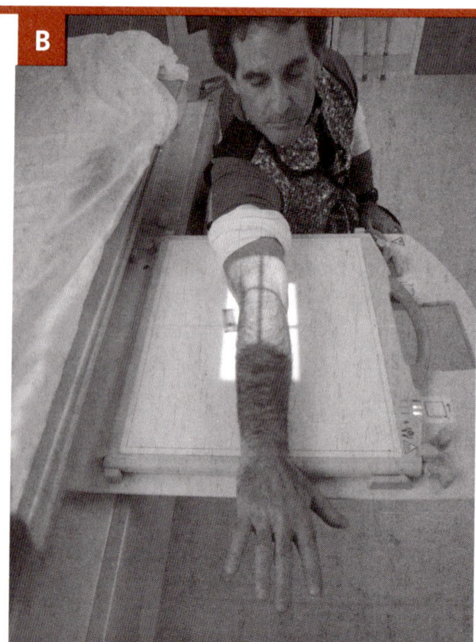

FIGURE 10-41
Because the elbow can be maneuvered from nearly AP position **A** to lateral position **B** with the hand maintained prone, the key to a proper oblique position of the elbow lies in the degree of shoulder, not wrist, rotation.

require stopping *before the hand is even lateral* on some patients, as shown in Figure 10-42. (Note that when the patient is standing and the hand is internally rotated, it may have to be hyperrotated *beyond the prone position* before it brings the shoulder rotation with it to the point where the elbow lies truly at 45°.) The position the hand ends up in is irrelevant. The correctly positioned image should have the radius completely superimposed over the ulna.

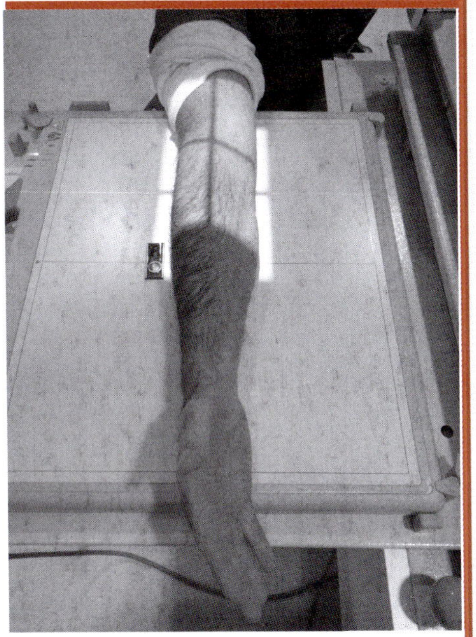

© Dennis Bowman

FIGURE 10-42

On some patients, the proper rotation for the oblique elbow is attained before the hand is even lateral (not to mention completely pronated).

Comments on Other Methods

Center to Midelbow

This does not address the crucial question of what anatomy or landmarks should be included within the field.

Lateral

Center 3 inches anteromedial to the tip of the olecranon process, on a diagonal that places the CR into the soft tissue crease of the elbow (Figure 10-43). Then collimate a square field to include 1 inch of light field below the forearm and 1 inch of light behind the humerus.

Use of Lead Sheets with Digital Imaging

Prior to the advent of digital radiography, some radiographers centered the CR to the elbow joint, then used leaded rubber sheets or a lead apron to "collimate" the edge of the light field. For digital imaging, the presence of this lead within the exposure field frequently causes errors in histogram analysis and exposure indicator values, so it must be

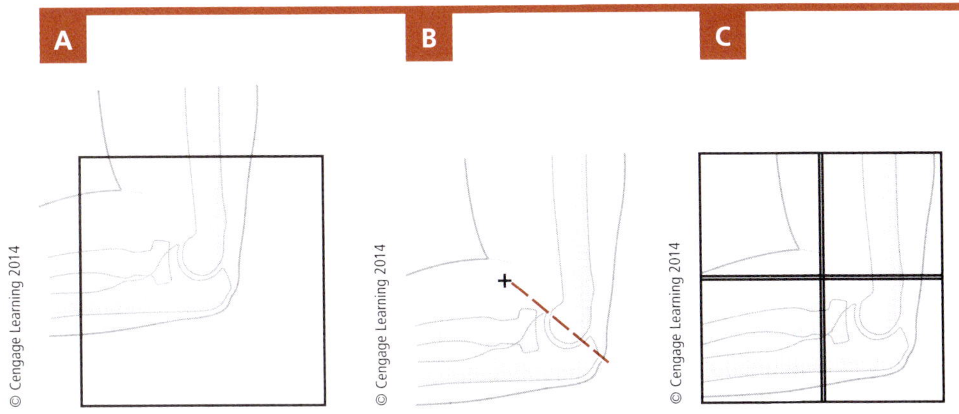

FIGURE 10-43

Centering for the lateral elbow is not to the bony joint **A**, but 3 inches anteromedial to the olecranon process, on a diagonal **B** that places the CR into the soft-tissue crease of the elbow. This way, more of the humerus, ulna, and radius bones are included **C** with only slight distortion in the joint spaces.

avoided. The centering and collimation described earlier are strongly recommended for digital imaging systems.

Comments on Other Methods

Center to Bony Joint

This creates the problem that, if collimated tightly, an insufficient few inches of the forearm and humerus bones are included within the view, and if collimation is opened, an inordinate amount of (scatter-producing) light field extends below and behind the elbow on the table. (See Figure 10-43). This centering is recommended if interest is specifically in the joint *space*. But, most elbows are done to screen for trauma, so it is desirable to include as much of the long bones as possible at the expense of very slight distortion in the joint spaces.

At 1½ Inches Medial to the Olecranon Process

This is along the same line as the recommended rule. It is more vague and does not address what anatomy should be included.

HUMERUS

All Projections

Center to include 1 inch past the elbow joint and 1 inch of light above the acromion (top of shoulder).

Comments on Other Methods

Center to Midhumerus

This generalized statement does not address the crucial question of what anatomy or landmarks should be included within the field.

NOTE: For the transthoracic and several other trauma positions for the humerus, see Chapter 6.

Externally Rotated "Arm-to-the-Square" Lateral Humerus

When the patient is supine but still able to move the arm, it is often very difficult to have the patient perform the conventional lateral position with the elbow bent at 90°, and the back of the hand against the crest and the shoulder and elbow down against the tabletop. In this instance, the patient might better tolerate abducting the humerus about 90° from the body, with the elbow flexed to 90° and the wrist externally rotated until it is in a lateral position with the thumb pointing toward the floor, as demonstrated in Figure 10-44. Chapter 8 further

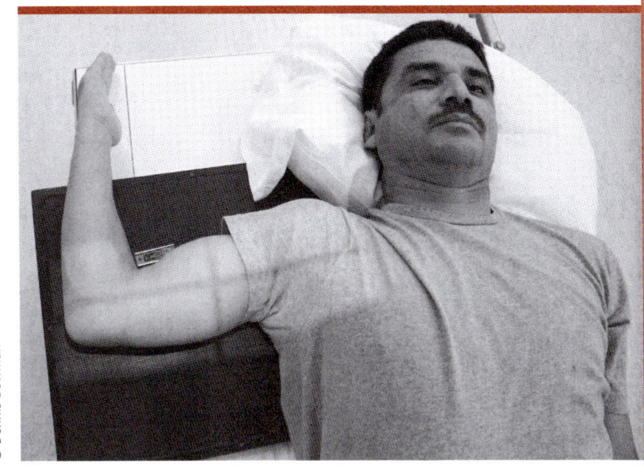

FIGURE 10-44

For a lateral humerus on a non-trauma patient, a mediolateral projection using this "arm-to-the-square" position is much more tolerable than placing the hand on the hip and trying to force the humerus into a lateromedial projection.

elaborates upon this projection. The resulting image is practically guaranteed to demonstrate the humerus in true lateral position.

Trauma Humerus Positions

Note that several different methods for positioning the humerus are presented in Chapter 8.

SHOULDER

All Projections

Center 1 inch inferior to the coracoid process to include 1 inch of light lateral to the arm and 1 inch above the shoulder.

This is in agreement with most positioning atlases. Many departments prefer to include the entire clavicle within the shoulder views. In this case, center to the midclavicle to include ½ inch medial to the sternoclavicular joint, ½ inch of light lateral to the arm, and 1 inch above the distal acromion.

Walker Method Axillary Shoulder for DR Equipment

The conventional axillary lateral position of the shoulder cannot be performed on DR equipment with the image receptor built into the table. A method for obtaining an axillary projection with DR equipment has been developed. See Chapter 6 for a full description of this projection.

PA Scapular Y

Like the lateral scapula, this position demonstrates the scapula in the true lateral position. The difference is that we are not trying to keep the humerus from superimposing the body of the scapula. Rather, the humerus can and should hang straight down while positioning for the scapular Y, because this brings the average scapula to a 45° angle, halfway to the desired position. Depending on the size of the patient's chest and arms, the elbow might need to be moved laterally or medially until the humerus is perpendicular to the floor, as shown in Figure 10-45A.

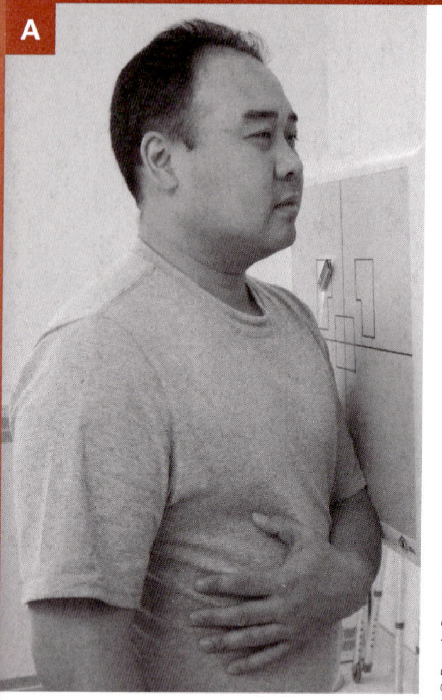

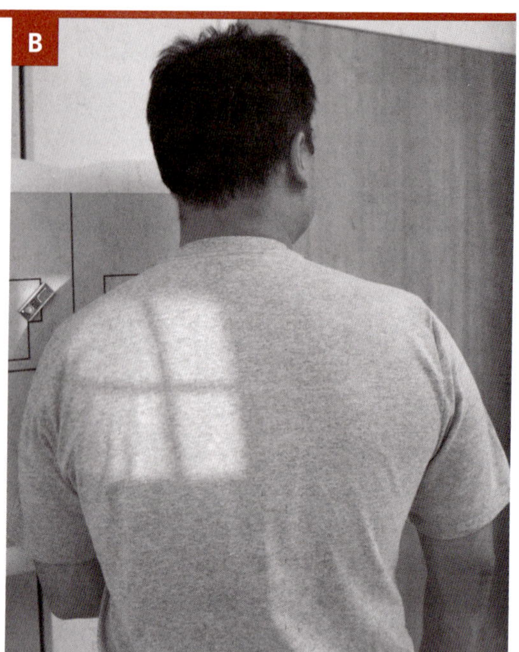

FIGURE 10-45

For the standing PA scapular "Y" position, adjust the elbow until the humerus is vertical **A**, then rotate the body into a 45° anterior oblique, leaving 1 inch of light above the acromion **B**.

The forearm and hand can be placed across the abdomen if that is more comfortable. At this point, rotate the patient's body 45° with the affected side closest to the IR (LAO for the left scapula). Center side to side to the midhumerus with the proper collimation (8 × 5 inches) and the top of the light field ½ inch above the acromion (Figure 10-45***B***).

AP Scapular Y ("Mercedes View")

The AP scapular Y positioning criteria is really identical to that of the PA, so the positions mirror each other. Rotate the patient 45° using an angled sponge with the affected side away from the IR. Ensure that the humerus is parallel with the spine. Again, the patient's elbow might need to be moved laterally or medially and the forearm and hand can be rested on the abdomen. Center side to side to the midhumerus with collimation to an 8- × 5-inch field, and with the top of the light field ½ inch above the acromion (Figure 10-46).

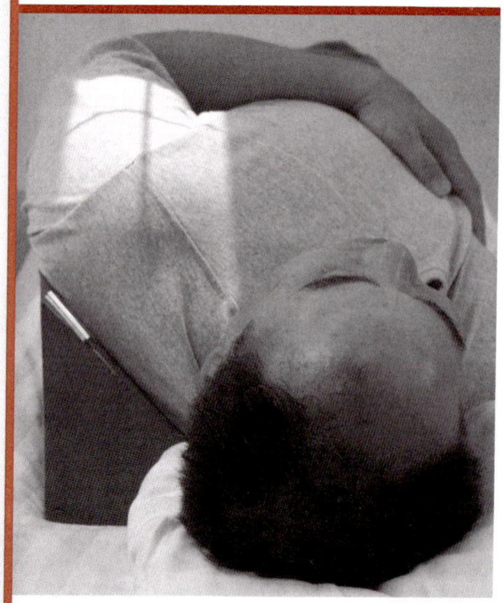

FIGURE 10-46

The AP "Mercedes view" of the scapular "Y" mirrors the PA method in Figure 10-45, with a 5- × 8-inch field centered to the midhumerus allowing about ½ inch of light above the acromion.

© Dennis Bowman

For both the PA and AP scapular Y projections, the image should demonstrate a true lateral scapula (lateral and medial borders of the scapula superimposed) with the humerus overlying the scapula. The acromion, coracoid process, and scapular body should combine to form a "Y." In addition, the acromion and lateral clavicle should make one continuous arc. The superior scapular angle is superimposed over the clavicle (Figure 10-47).

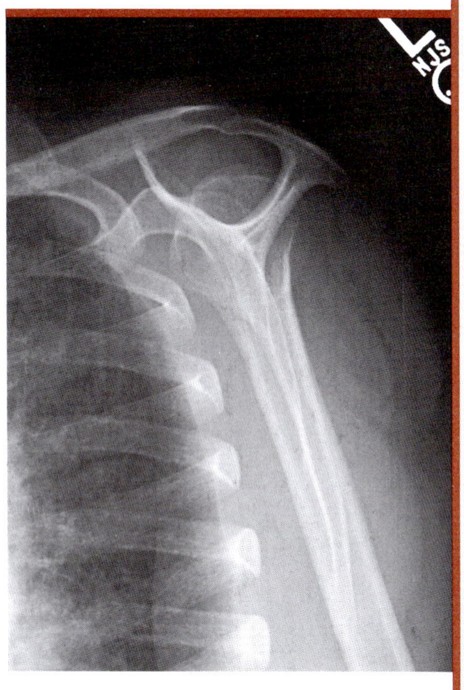

FIGURE 10-47

A properly positioned "Y" view, whether AP or PA, shows the scapular body in true lateral, joining the coracoid and acromion processes to form a symmetrical "Y," the lateral clavicle and acromion forming a continuous arch.

Courtesy of Community Hospital of the Monterey Peninsula, Diagnostic and Interventional Radiology

Notes for the Lateral Scapula

The degree to which the scapula rotates when the affected arm is brought across the chest depends on how flexible a patient's shoulder and upper back are. The most common error in positioning a lateral scapula is to overrotate the scapula past the true lateral position, by rotating the patient's body too much. The following points will help avoid this.

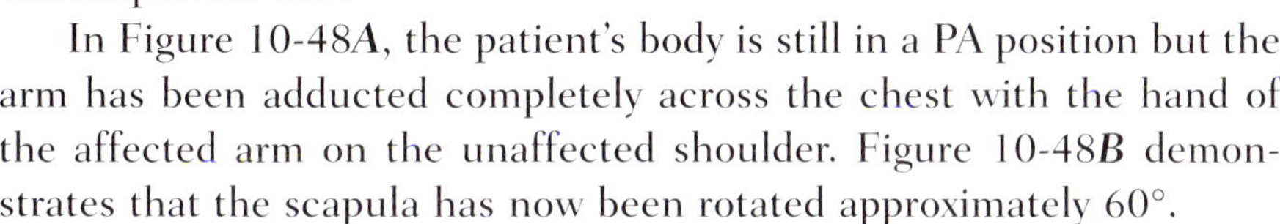

In Figure 10-48*A*, the patient's body is still in a PA position but the arm has been adducted completely across the chest with the hand of the affected arm on the unaffected shoulder. Figure 10-48*B* demonstrates that the scapula has now been rotated approximately 60°.

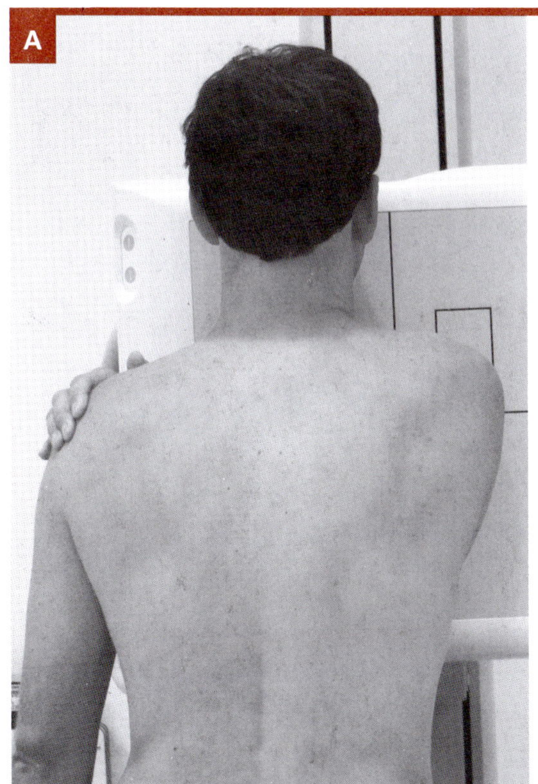

© Dennis Bowman

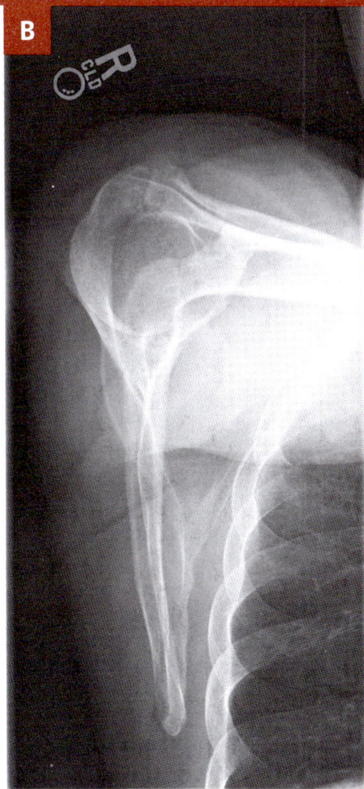

Courtesy of Community Hospital of the Monterey Peninsula, Diagnostic and Interventional Radiology

FIGURE 10-48

For the mediolateral projection of the scapula, note that with the patient's body still in PA position **A** the scapula can be rotated 60° toward lateral **B** just by adducting the arm across in front of the patient.

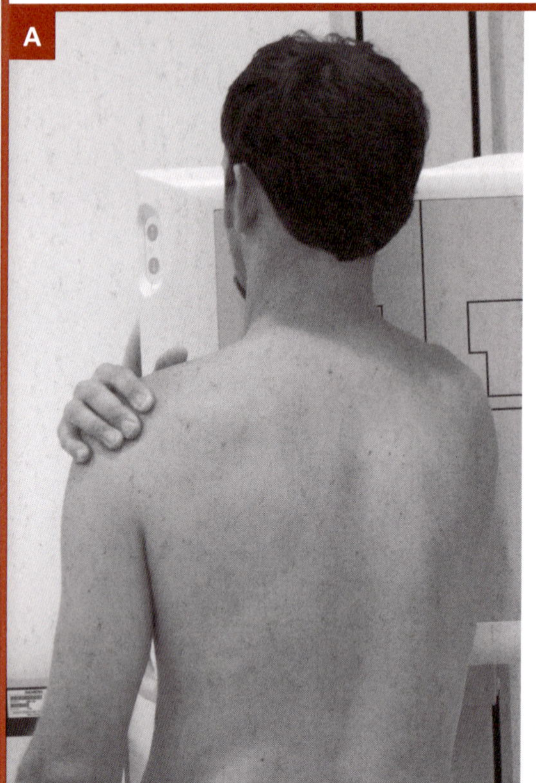

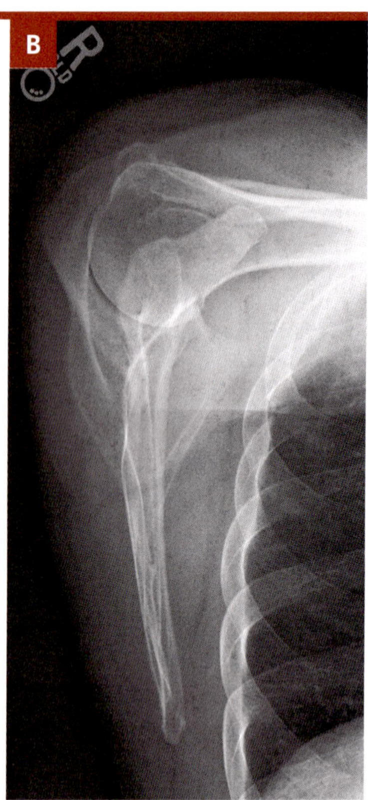

FIGURE 10-49

For the mediolateral projection of the scapula, only 20°–30° of body rotation **A** is needed to get the body of the scapula into true lateral position **B**. A very common mistake is to overrotate the body bringing the scapula past lateral.

This means that the patient's body only needs to be rotated an additional 30° (Figure 10-49*A*) for the scapula to be placed into true lateral position as shown in Figure 10-49*B*. If the patient is more limber, only 20° of rotation may be necessary. More than 30° of rotation will be needed for the less agile patient. Because of the difference in body habitus and flexibility, always palpate the borders of the scapula to check if the blade is perpendicular to the IR. A large muscle overlies the lateral border of the scapula, and with the patient's arm adducted it is still more difficult to palpate, so you will need to "dig" somewhat to accurately locate the edge of this bone.

FOOT

AP and Oblique

Center to the base of the third metatarsal and collimate to include at least ½ inch of light on the sides and beyond the toes.

This is in agreement with most positioning atlases.

Lateral

Center to the base of the third metatarsal and collimate to include the medial malleolus above, and at least ½ inch of light beneath and beyond the toes.

This is in agreement with most positioning atlases.

Toes

Preferred Method for Separating the Lateral Toes

Compared to gauze or tongue blades, tape is the preferred method for separating toes because it leaves the least artifacts in the image. It is best to use 1-inch pliable tape (never paper tape because it is not stretchy). Using the middle toe as an example, begin by taping up the first and second toes in such a way that the triangle of the loop around the toes meets in the middle as shown in Figure 10-50*A* (arrow). Leave a long tail on the tape to be stuck down later. Now do the same thing for the fourth and fifth toes. The patient does not need to be in the lateral position for this.

Place the patient into the lateral position and center the affected toe to the IR. Slowly pull both pieces of tape in opposite directions (Figure 10-50*B*). When the taped toes have been pulled out as much as possible, bring the tape down and stick it to the IR or tabletop. If done correctly, all of the affected toe should be free of superimposition from any of the other toes, except the head of the proximal phalanx as shown in Figure 10-50*C*. Figure 10-51 illustrates a radiograph with the resulting maximized degree of separation between the toes.

ANKLE

AP and Oblique

Center midway between the malleoli, or slightly above, to include at least 4 inches of the distal leg.

This is in general agreement with most positioning atlases.

Lateral

Center to the medial malleolus, or slightly above, to include at least 4 inches of the distal leg.

This is in general agreement with most positioning atlases.

LEG

All Projections

Center to include at least the apex of the patella above and ½ inch past the *lateral* malleolus below.

Comments on Other Methods

Center to the Midleg

This generalized statement does not address the crucial question of what anatomy or landmarks should be included within the field.

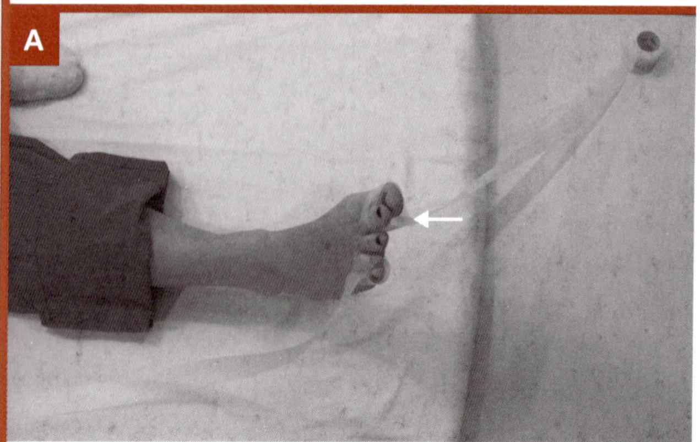

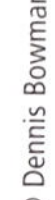

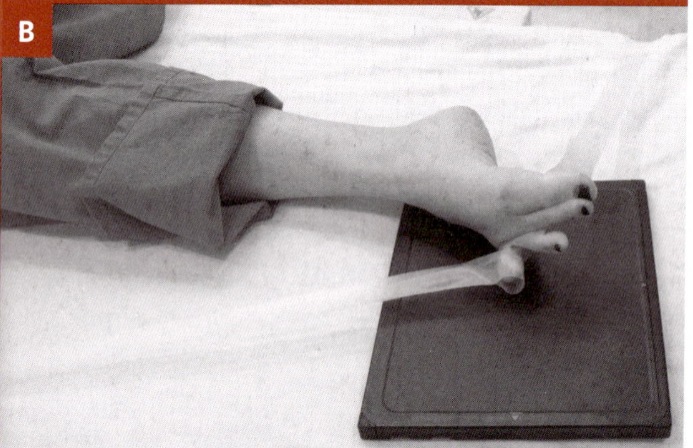

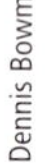

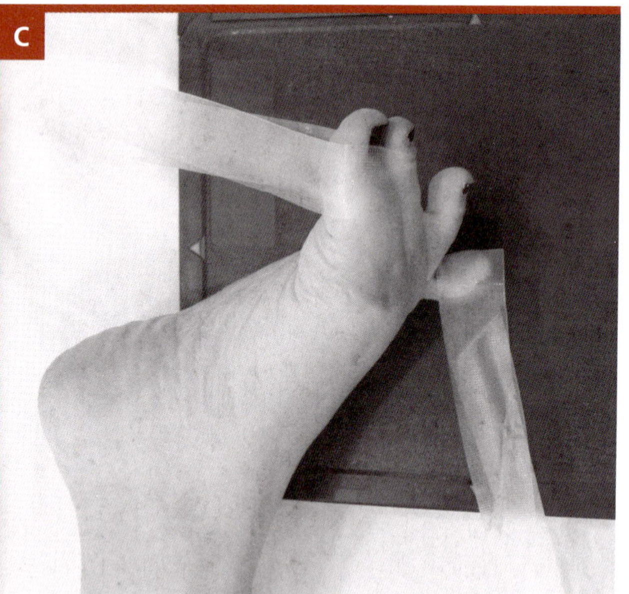

© Dennis Bowman

FIGURE 10-50

Using tape to separate the toes for a lateral projection of the third toe **A**. Triangular loop formed around the first two toes, and another around the fourth and fifth toes **B**. Long tails of tape stuck to tabletop to achieve maximum fanning **C**.

Adapting for DR Equipment

With the image receptor built into the table for DR units, for very tall patients it will not be possible to fit the entire leg within the 17-inch length of receptor plate available. It will often be necessary to take two views, upper and lower, for each position in this series. Include about 2 inches past the nearest joint space in each view.

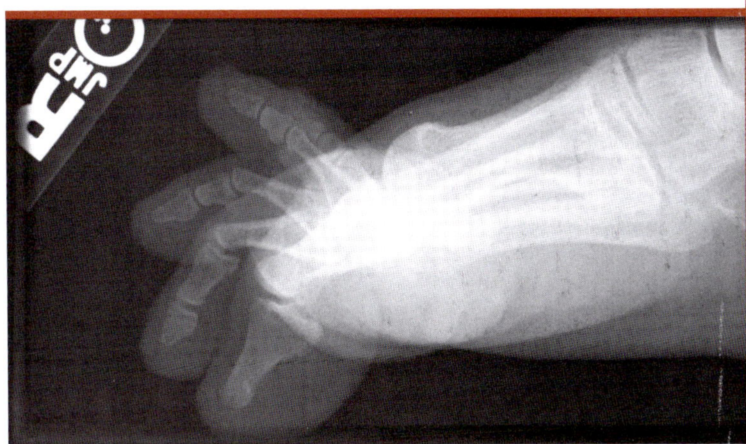

FIGURE 10-51

Radiograph showing excellent separation of the toes from the third toe using the method in Figure 10-50.

Courtesy of Community Hospital of the Monterey Peninsula, Diagnostic and Interventional Radiology

For mobile DR units, the IR plate can still be arranged diagonally, as used to be done with conventional film cassettes, in order to fit larger legs within a single view.

KNEE

AP

Center 1 centimeter below the apex of the patella and collimate to include at least 5 inches above and below this point.

This is in agreement with most positioning atlases.

Lateral

Center 1 inch below the palpated medial epicondyle and collimate to include at least 5 inches above and below this point.

This is in agreement with most positioning atlases.

Criticality of Proper Centering and Beam Angle for the Lateral Knee

The knee joint is *not* horizontal but is tilted slightly because the medial condyle is larger and extends below the lateral condyle. This necessitates a 5° cephalic angle. There is a tendency among radiographers to "eyeball" lateral knees and center roughly at the crease of the knee. As shown in Figure 10-52, this places the knee joint in a divergent beam that cancels out much of the cephalic angle, defeating the purpose of the angle and closing the knee joint.

Note that centering high *without angling the CR cephalic* is even worse, placing the joint in a *caudally diverging* beam when the joint space opens in a *cephalic* direction.

To better open the joint space on lateral projections, remember to use the angle and *center 1½ inches below the crease of the knee, over the upper tibia.*

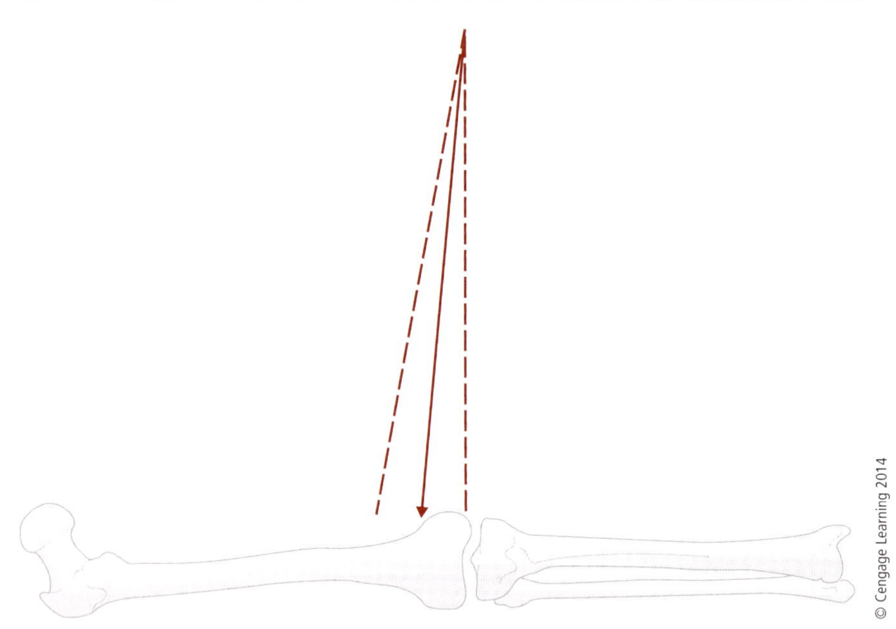

FIGURE 10-52

Centering high for a lateral knee projection places the joint in a diverging beam that cancels out the recommended cephalic angle and closes the tilted joint space. (Centering high *without* the CR angle is even worse, placing the joint in a caudally divergent beam.)

Axial Patella: Hughston Method

A "reverse Hughston" type of approach to obtaining axial views of the patella with the patient sitting in a wheelchair, which also is adaptable for fixed DR equipment, is presented in Chapter 6.

The Hughston method of obtaining an axial view of the patella is very easy to position and can be done either bilaterally or for a single knee. Start with the patient prone and place a 40°–44° cephalic angle on the x-ray tube. Have the patient bend his knees past 45° and then move the table or the tube until the patient can gently bring his pointed toes down onto the collimator. Collimator boxes can become very hot from the light bulb inside, so it is important to insulate with a small folded towel beneath the patient's feet, or to have the patient keep his socks on as shown in Figure 10-53*A*.

Some textbooks show the knee bent and being held in place with tape. It is more comfortable for the patient to just rest his feet against the collimator box as shown in Figure 10-53*A*. So the feet can reach the collimator, it will usually require an SID somewhat less than 40 inches. Center the CR to the apex of the patella(s), shown in Figure 10-53*B* for a bilateral projection. Make sure the knee(s) are not rotated. The resulting image should demonstrate the entire patella free from superimposition of the tibia, with the subpatellar space open as shown in Figure 10-54.

FEMUR

All Projections

Center a 17-inch-long field with the bottom light edge at the apex of the patella.

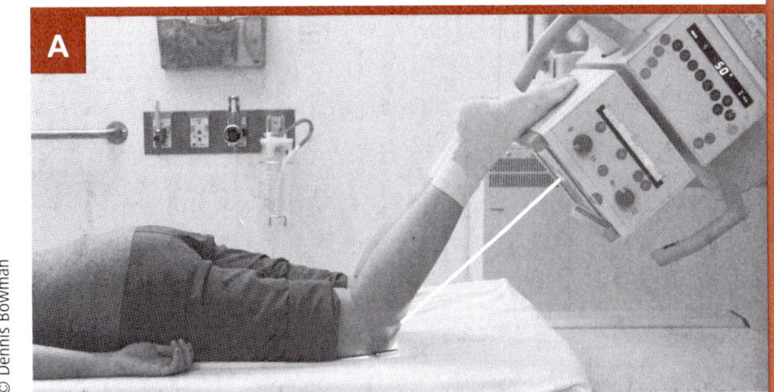

© Dennis Bowman

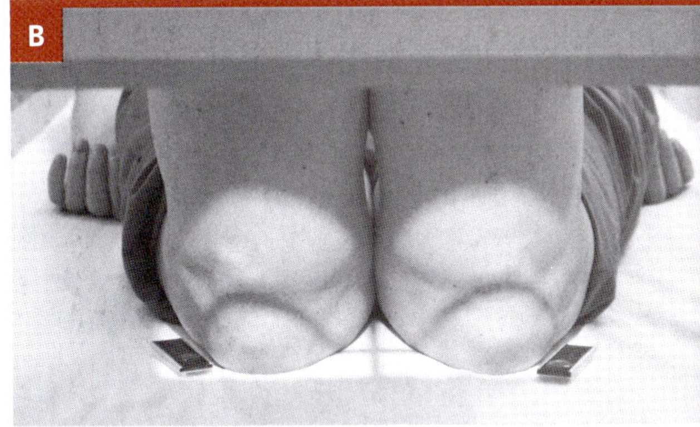

© Dennis Bowman

FIGURE 10-53

The Hughston method for axial patellas, with the x-ray tube at 40° and the pointed toes, insulated from collimator heat by wearing socks, resting on the collimator to form a 45° angle of the tibias **A**. Centering for a bilateral projection of the axial patellae is shown in **B**.

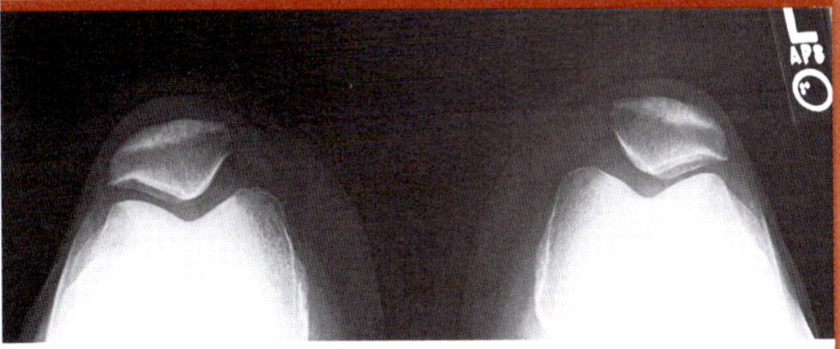

FIGURE 10-54

A bilateral Hughston view showing good opening of the subpatellar spaces.

Courtesy of Community Hospital of the Monterey Peninsula, Diagnostic and Interventional Radiology

Comments on Other Methods

Center to the Midfemur

This generalized statement does not address the crucial question of what anatomy or landmarks should be included within the field. Remember that at least one full joint space should be included on all extremity views. Centering to the midfemur on large patients risks clipping *both* joint spaces at the same time.

Adapting for DR Equipment

When using a cassette system such as CR, the entire femur can often be fit onto a 14- × 17-inch (35- × 43-cm) cassette by placing it *diagonally* under the patient's thigh. This method does not include much of the iliac bone above the acetabulum, nor of the tibial plateau beneath the knee joint. Many radiology departments now define their femur routine as not including the hip joint, and require the referring physician to order a separate hip series to see this area properly. For those departments that prefer to at least make the attempt to include the entire femur within a femur series, positioning the anatomy diagonally across the IR is often the only way to achieve this on adult patients.

With the image receptor built into the table for DR units, for very tall patients it will not be possible to use this kind of diagonal placement to fit the entire femur within the 17-inch length of IR available. It may be necessary to take two views, upper and lower, for each position in this series. Include about 2 inches past the nearest joint space in each view.

For mobile DR units, the IR plate can still be arranged diagonally in order to fit larger legs within a single view.

HIPS

AP and "Frog" Lateral

Place the *top* of the light field at the level of the ASIS. This can be done regardless of the field size or IR plate size used.

The longer the IR, the more femur is demonstrated. This positioning will always demonstrate approximately 2½–3 inches of the pelvic bones *above* the acetabulum and hip joint (Figure 10-55).

Comments on Other Methods

Center the CR to a Point 3 Inches Below and 1 Inch Medial to the Palpated ASIS

This avoids palpation of the pubic bone, and arrives at the same point as the conventional method.

At 2½ Inches Distal to the Midpoint ASIS to SP

This is an accurate rule. However, the earlier recommendation is equivalent and avoids palpation of the pubic bone.

Body Position for the "Frog" Lateral Hip

Many radiographers attempt the lateral hip position with the patient supine, effectively mixing it up with the pediatric "Cleaves" method for bilateral hips. Typically, an AP of the pelvis has already been obtained, so *there is no reason the body cannot be obliqued* to obtain a true lateral of the femoral neck, as shown in Figure 10-56.

On the other hand, it is *not* necessary to rotate the knee all the way down to the tabletop. The following note discusses this.

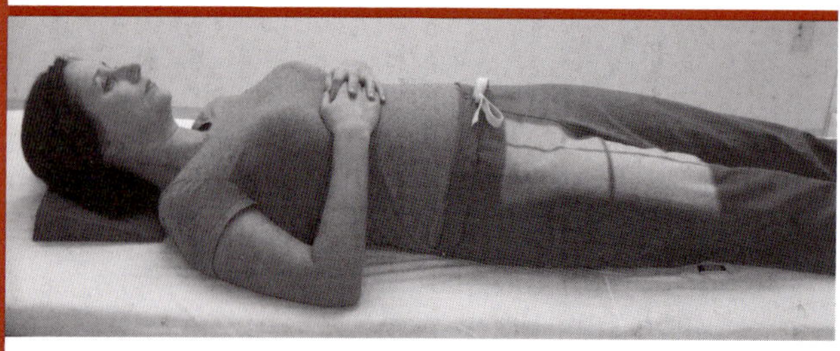

FIGURE 10-55

For either AP or "frog" lateral projections of the hip, regardless of the length of the image receptor or amount of femur included within the view, always place the top of the light field at the level of the ASIS.

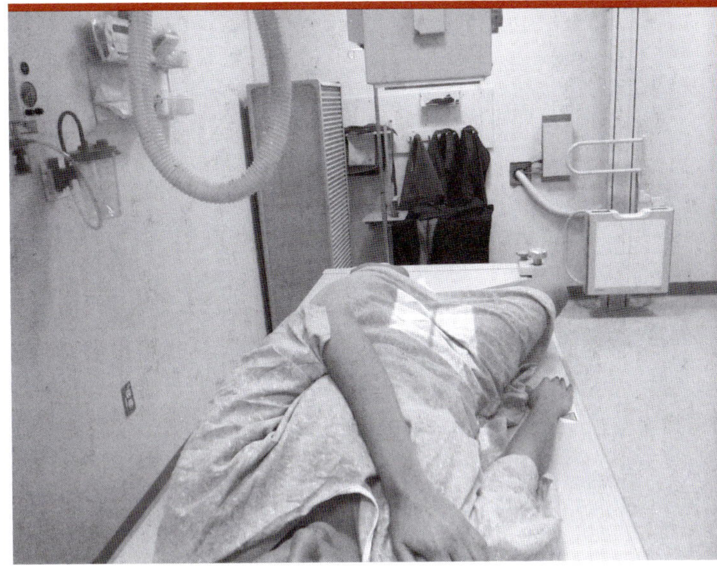

Courtesy of Quinn B. Carroll

FIGURE 10-56

For a unilateral hip projection, oblique the torso as needed to bring the femoral neck down to a parallel position. (But, stop 15° short of bringing the knee all the way down to the table.)

How to Obtain a True Lateral "Frog" Hip

To place the femoral neck in perfectly true lateral position, do *not* rotate the thigh all the way down such that the knee is close to the tabletop. Rather, stop 15° short of this with the knee itself up off the table 3 or 4 inches. (Remember that for a true *AP* hip, the leg is internally rotated 15° in order to position the femoral neck parallel to the plate. This *also* applies to true lateral projections, where the femoral neck should be placed *perpendicular* to the plate.)

Cross-Table Lateral (Danelius-Miller Method)

Center to pass through a point 3 inches below and 1 inch medial to the palpated ASIS.

This should put the top of the IR into the bottom ribs. If the top of IR is just at the top of the crest, there is a good chance that the acetabulum will be clipped from the view. See additional comments for AP.

Proper Abduction of the Contrary Thigh

Be sure to *abduct* the contrary thigh in addition to hyperflexing it (Figure 10-57). This ensures that the gluteal soft tissue of the contrary leg, especially on larger patients, will not obscure the view of the hip joint and femoral neck as shown in the radiographs in Figure 10-58.

For patients who have any trouble abducting the thigh, the anchor leg stabilizer shown in Chapter 8, Figure 8-52, comes highly recommended in conjunction with the *Ferlic* hip filter.

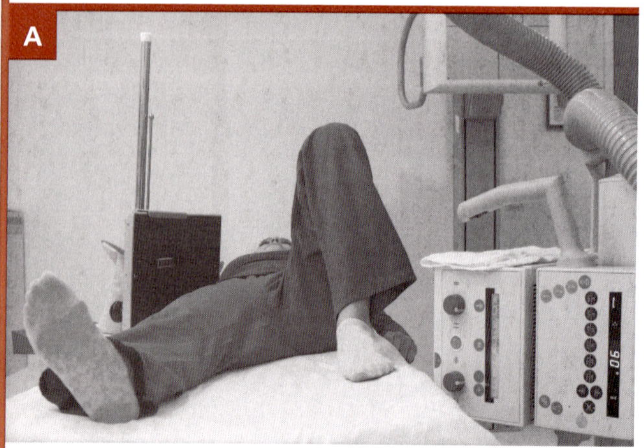

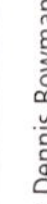

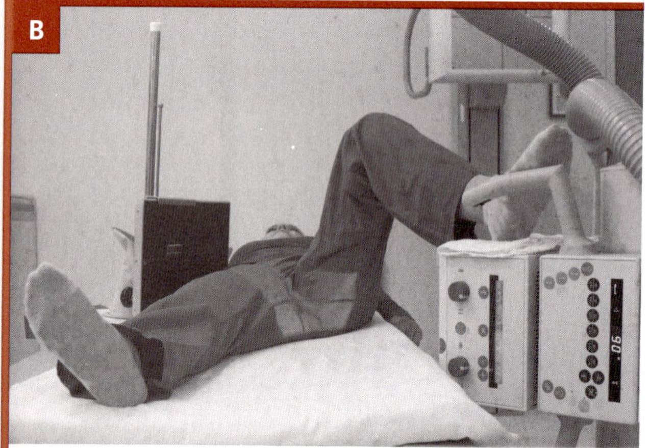

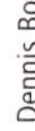

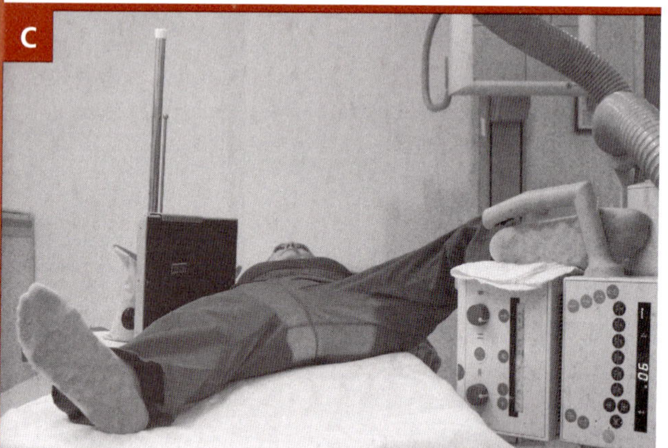

FIGURE 10-57

For a cross-table lateral hip projection, be sure to abduct the contrary leg **B** in addition to hyper-flexing it **A** in order to ensure that the contrary gluteal tissue is not superimposed over the femoral neck area. Better still, rest the contrary foot on its side on the collimator as in **C** for even better abduction. Be sure to protect the foot from a hot collimator with towels and/or socks.

How to Obtain a True Lateral "Groin" Hip

To place the femoral neck perfectly parallel, *if the patient is capable of doing it by himself without harm*, rotate the affected leg internally 15°. (Remember that for a true *AP* hip, the leg is internally rotated 15° in order to position the femoral neck parallel to the plate. This *also* applies to true lateral projections, where the femoral neck should be placed *perpendicular* to the plate.) This must *not* be done on a trauma patient with a suspected hip fracture.

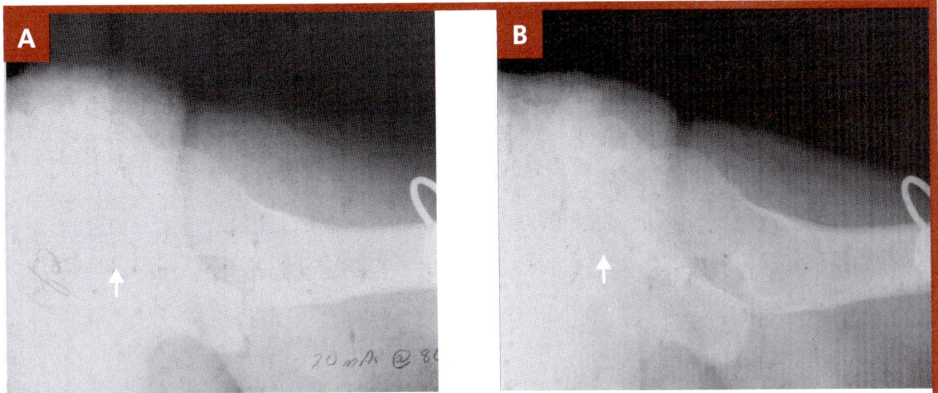

FIGURE 10-58

Radiograph **B** shows the difference in getting the gluteal tissue out of the way when abducting the contrary leg, as demonstrated in Figure 8-18. Compare the visibility of the area of the acetabulum (arrow), which is obscured in **A**.

Carroll, Q. Evaluating Radiographs, 1993, Figure 167, Courtesy of Charles C Thomas, Publisher, Ltd., Springfield, Illinois.

PELVIS

AP

Place the top edge of a 14- × 17-inch crosswise light field 4 inches above the easily palpated ASIS (or 1 inch above the iliac crest), centered to the midline.

Comments on Other Methods

Midway ASIS to the SP

This is roughly equivalent, but the earlier recommendation avoids palpation of the pubic bone.

SI JOINTS

Oblique

Center 1 inch medial to the ASIS with a 5- × 8-inch lengthwise field. This is in agreement with most positioning atlases.

SKULL

NOTE: See Chapter 9 for a full discussion of skull positioning notes other than centering, with full illustrations.

PA

Center a 10- × 12-inch lengthwise field to allow 1 inch of light off both sides and above the skull (above the scalp, discounting the hair.)

Comments on Other Methods

Exit Glabella

This does not address what anatomy to include. It is equivalent, just not as descriptive.

Lateral

Center a 10- × 12-inch crosswise field to allow 1 inch of light off the front, the back, and above the skull.

Comments on Other Methods

At 2 Inches Above the EAM

This is not self-correcting for different types of skulls and does not address what anatomy to include. Following this recommended rule, you will find that placing an even amount of light all around will result in the CR falling anterior or posterior to this point for different types of skulls.

Townes

Center a 10- × 12-inch lengthwise field to allow just ½ inch of light above the shadow of the top of the scalp (compressing the hair).

Comments on Other Methods

At 2½ Inches Above the Glabella

For this position, small changes in chin flexion cause substantial changes in the entrance centering point farther down the forehead or sometimes above the hairline. (This is why many positioning atlases *also* recommend adjusting the CR so that it "passes through the EAM.") It is difficult for patients lying on their back to flex the chin to the point where the OML is perpendicular, and this causes the correct centering point to fall farther down the forehead than usual. By using this recommended rule, the CR will always *exit* the occipital bone at back of the head correctly. The EAM rule is helpful. *Entrance* point rules are all unreliable and not recommended for use.

Sinuses or Facial Bone Series with Collimation or "Cone"

Collimating First for Caldwell or Waters

For both the Caldwell or Waters projections, always collimate and mark the IR first (Figure 10-59). All patients' sinuses will fit into a

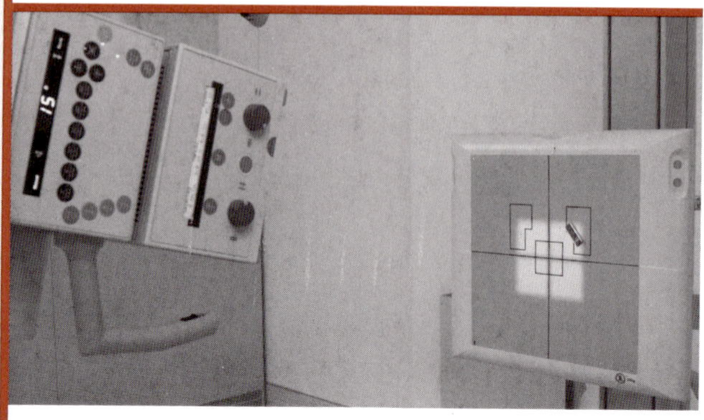

FIGURE 10-59

For either the Caldwell or the Waters projection, collimate the field and place markers before placing the patient into position. This provides proper and consistent field size regardless of hair style or patient condition.

collimated 6- × 6-inch square light field with plenty of room in any of the four corners for the marker. When collimation is done after the patient is against the IR, the tendency is to open the field wider than is needed because the light field appears small on the back of the patient's head, and the effect of thick hair making it more difficult to visualize the skull.

Including the Entire Mandible on Facial Bone Projections

There are two schools of thought on what anatomy to include on a facial bone series, with some departments preferring to include the mandible on all views in a facial bone series as shown in Figure 10-60*A*. Since the upper landmark for the facial bones is the supraorbital ridge and the bottom is the mentum, the centering point will be lower than the nasion. The recommended centering point for this view is to exit the acanthion (Figure 10-60*B*).

Caldwell

Center and collimate to include from the midforehead down to the junction of the lips.

Comments on Other Methods

Exit Nasion

This is roughly equivalent, but does not address what anatomy or landmarks to include.

Waters

Center and collimate to include from the midforehead down to the junction of the lips.

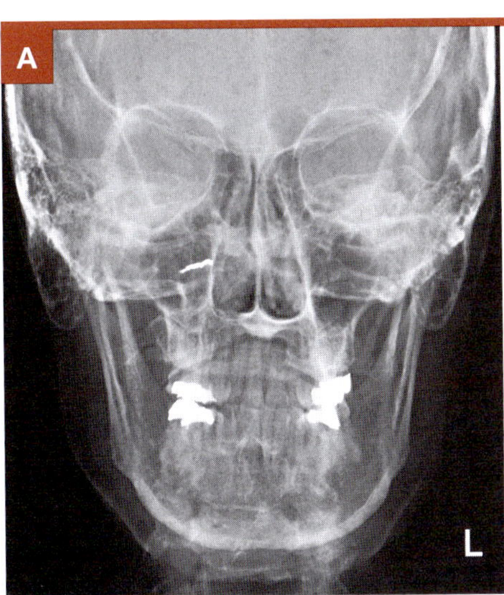

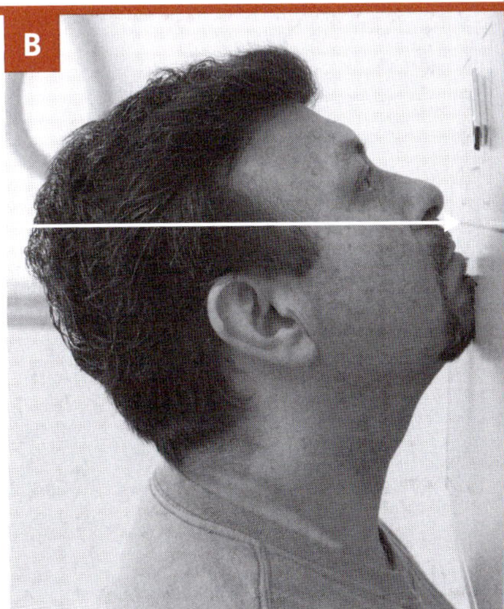

FIGURE 10-60

When the preferred routine for a facial bone series is to include the mandible **A**, center to exit the acanthion **B**.

Part A is Courtesy of Community Hospital of the Monterey Peninsula, Diagnostic and Interventional Radiology

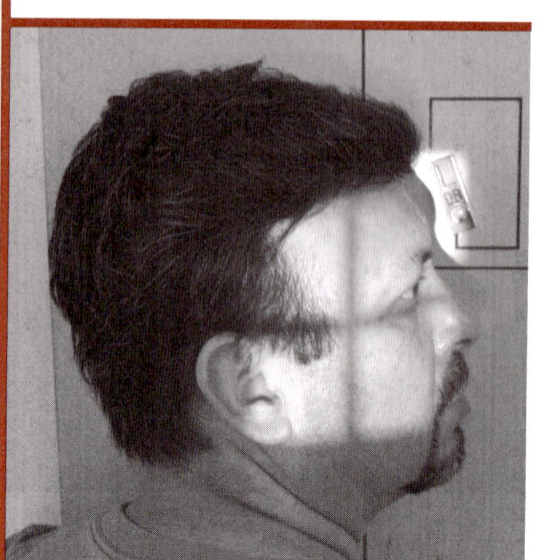

© Dennis Bowman

FIGURE 10-61

On the lateral projection for either facial bones or a sinus series, collimate and center to include up to at least the mid-forehead, down to the junction of the lips, and posteriorly to the EAM.

Comments on Other Methods

Exit Acanthion

This is equivalent, but does not address what anatomy or landmarks to include.

Lateral

Center and collimate to include up to the midforehead, down to the junction of the lips, and posteriorly to the EAM (Figure 10-61).

Comments on Other Methods

Midway from the Outer Canthus to the EAM

This point is too far posterior on many patients. It is not self-correcting for changes in flexion or extension, and does not address what anatomy or landmarks to include.

At ½–1 Inch Posterior to the Outer Canthus

This is roughly equivalent, but does not address what anatomy or landmarks to include.

Submentovertex

Center and collimate to include from the mental point (chin) to the gonions (angles of the mandible).

Comments on Other Methods

At 1½ Inches Below the Chin

This is roughly equivalent, but does not address what anatomy or landmarks to include.

Pass ¾ Inch Anterior EAM

This is also roughly equivalent, but does not address what anatomy or landmarks to include.

NOTE: See Chapter 9 on skull positioning for additional notes and illustrations.

MANDIBLE

PA

Center to exit the junction of the lips, to include from the top of the ear to 1 inch below the chin.

This agrees with most positioning atlases.

Lateral Oblique

Center just below and just anterior to the *upside* gonion (mandibular angle).

Comments on Other Methods

Center to the "Region of Interest"

This is nonspecific.

Townes for the Mandible

It is common to confuse the Townes projection for a *skull* with the Townes projection for a *mandible*. Some facilities include the Townes mandible projection within their routine for a facial bones series. The Townes for a mandible does not need to include the skull. The head extension and position are the same, but the centering is completely different. Some departments want the entire mandible included (Figure 10-62*A*) while others only want the upper "half," the proximal body and ramus, since the distal portion of the ramus and the mentum are superimposed over the spine (Figure 10-62*B*). This collimated view is sometimes called

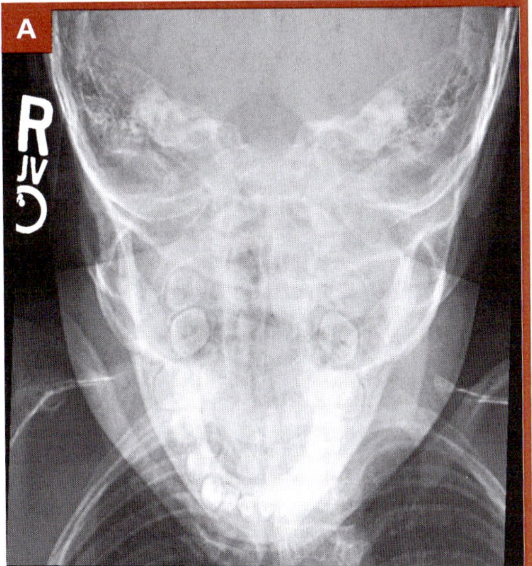

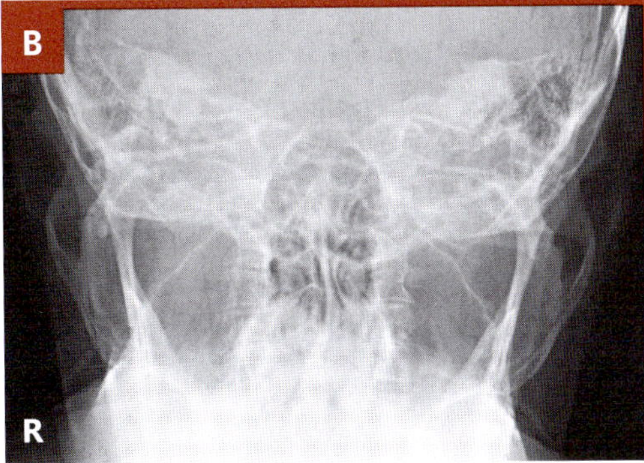

FIGURE 10-62

Townes views to include the mandible **A**, or only the rami of the mandible **B**.

Courtesy of Community Hospital of the Monterey Peninsula, Diagnostic and Interventional Radiology

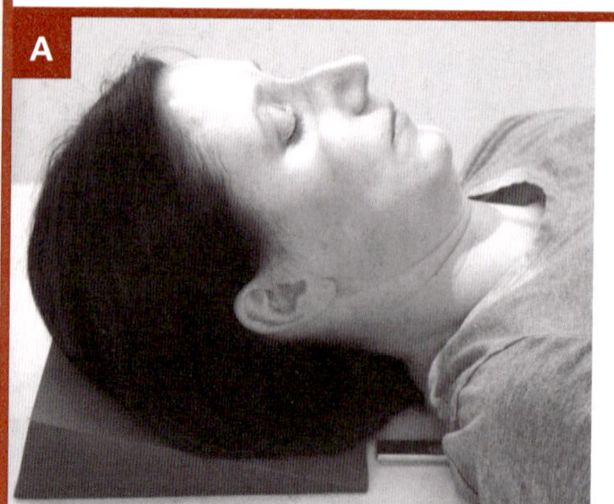

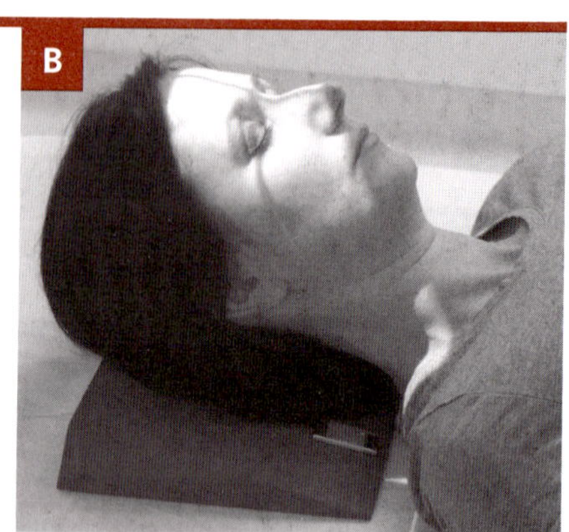

FIGURE 10-63

Centering for the Townes projections is 1-inch inferior to the nasion to include the mandible **A**, and to the glabella for the "slit" view without the lower jaw included **B**.

a "slit Townes," which is helpful because the name is indicative that this is not a Townes for the skull.

To include the entire mandible, the CR should enter at the bridge of the nose about 1 inch inferior to the nasion. Make sure that the TMJs are included at the top of the light field, and the mentum at the bottom (Figure 10-63*A*). The "slit Townes" is centered higher with the CR entering at the glabella (Figure 10-63*B*).

NOTE: See Chapter 9 on skulls for additional positioning notes and illustrations.

TEMPOROMANDIBULAR JOINTS (TMJS) OR MASTOIDS

Townes

Center to pass through the TMJ, 1 inch anterior to the EAM.

Comments on Other Methods

At 3 Inches Above the Nasion

This is misleading because it is not self-correcting for flexion/extension of the chin, as is any other landmark using facial features. The recommended rule can be easily visualized and is independent of head flexion or extension.

Law

Center 1½ inches above and 1½ inches posterior to the corresponding *upside* TMJ or EAM. For mastoid air cells, collimate to include at least a 3-inch diameter field around this point.

This follows paradigms #8 and #9 in Chapter 1, making exact compensation for both tube angle and head rotation. See Figure 5-11 in Chapter 5.

Comments on Other Methods

At 1½ Inches Above the Upside EAM

This rule fails to adequately shift the CR posteriorly to fully compensate for 15° of head rotation.

See paradigms #7 through #9 in Chapter 1.

At 2 Inches Above and 2 Inches Posterior to the EAM

This is along the same line of reasoning for the rule recommended earlier, but overcompensates the amount of shift. See paradigms #7 through #9 in Chapter 1.

Schuller

Center 2½ inches above the corresponding *upside* TMJ or EAM. For mastoid air cells, collimate to include at least a 3-inch diameter field around this point.

This follows paradigms #7 through #9 in Chapter 1, making exact compensation for both tube angles.

Comments on Other Methods

At 2 Inches Above the Upside EAM

This is along the same line of reasoning for the rule recommended earlier, but undercompensates the amount of shift. See paradigms #7 through #9 in Chapter 1.

Use of Shortened SID

A 30-inch SID can be used to advantage for the Law or Schuller projections in order to magnify and blur the obscuring upside skull anatomy. The use of short SID, including its implications for radiation exposure to the patient, is fully discussed in Chapter 4.

PETROUS PORTION

Stenvers

Center 3–4 inches posterior to and ½ inch inferior to the *upside* EAM. Collimate to include at least a 3-inch diameter field around this point.

This is in agreement with most positioning atlases, but also addresses what anatomy or landmarks to include.

Arcelin

Center 1 inch anterior and ¾ inch superior to the *upside* EAM. Collimate to include at least a 3-inch diameter field around this point.

This is in agreement with most positioning atlases, but also addresses what anatomy or landmarks to include.

Law

Refer to section under "TMJs."

Schuller

Refer to section under "Temporomandibular Joints or Mastoids."

ORBITS/OPTIC FORAMINA

Rhese

Center to exit the midorbit, which is easily seen when positioned correctly with the forehead and eyebrow *off* of the table (or for reverse position, *enter* midorbit).

This is in agreement with most positioning atlases.

NOTE: See Chapter 9 on skull positioning for additional notes and illustrations.

Waters

Refer to section under "Sinuses."

ZYGOMATIC ARCHES

All Projections

Center to pass through the level of the TMJ, ½ inch anterior to the EAM.

NOTE: See the simplified alternative methods for positioning the zygomatic arches in Chapter 9.

NASAL BONES

Lateral

Center ½ inch below the nasion with a tightly collimated field. This is in agreement with most positioning atlases.

Superoinferior

Center a tightly collimated field to skim the glabella. This is equivalent to the rules in most positioning atlases.

SUMMARY

1. For most positions, the inclusion of all anatomy of interest is more important than the specific location of the CR. With this in mind, specific recommendations for simplified centering are made for each body part throughout this chapter.
2. For distal extremities, always allow a minimum of ½ inch of light around every side of the anatomy.
3. Good centering rules are those that make good *anatomical* sense and use reliable bony landmarks; they will *automatically compensate* for larger or smaller patients, *self-correcting* for normal variations in anatomy; they will be *independent* of the radiographer's own body size; they will be *simple*, and able to be applied *easily* without special equipment; they will be easy on the *patient* and quick to use; and they will *consistently* produce the desired results in the image, so that *repeat rates are actually reduced*.
4. Palpation of the symphysis pubis can be avoided by using the "universal landmark," the ASIS. The ASIS lies 3 inches above the upper edge of the pubic bones, on average, somewhat less on females (and 3 inches below the iliac crest.) With this in mind, reformulate *all* positions referring to the symphysis pubis using the ASIS as a starting point for palpation.
5. To determine the correct angle of the CR for the lateral "spot" projection of L5–S1, always use *palpation* of bony landmarks. These landmarks include the spinous processes of L5 and S5, the iliac crests, or the posterior superior iliac spines (PSISs).
6. For the open-mouth odontoid projection, the recommended referral line to adjust flexion or extension is from the bottom of the upper incisor teeth to the *base of the occipital bone*. Never use a long 72-inch SID for the open-mouth odontoid projection.

7. To better open the joint space on lateral projections of the knee, remember to use a slight cephalic angle and center 1½ inches *below* the crease of the knee, over the upper tibia. Centering too high cancels out the beam angle and closes the joint space.

8. For any lateral hip projection, to place the femoral neck perfectly parallel, rotate the affected leg back internally 15° from where a lateral knee would be positioned. This applies to both the "frog" and the "groin" lateral methods, but should only be used on the groin lateral *if patients are capable of doing it by themselves without harm.*

9. For the "frog" lateral hip, the body may be obliqued as needed to get the femoral neck into true lateral position. For a "groin" lateral hip, be sure to *abduct* the contrary thigh as well as hyperflexing it.

CRITICAL THINKING CHALLENGE 10.1

CENTERING RULE FOR PA CHEST

Analyze the following rule according to each of the *Criteria for Good Centering Rules* presented at the beginning of this chapter: "For the PA chest, center the CR to the level of the inferior angle of the scapulae."

Which of the criteria does this rule meet? Is it self-correcting for different body habitus?

Which (if any) of the criteria might this rule conflict with? Explain why.

CRITICAL THINKING CHALLENGE 10.2

HEAD POSITION FOR THE LATERAL (OBLIQUE) MANDIBLE

Some textbooks recommend that, for the lateral (oblique) projection of the mandible, to demonstrate the ramus, the face must be rotated 15° toward the tabletop. This is designed to place the ramus portion of the mandible parallel with the tabletop.

Explain how this might* prevent *the proper visualization of the entire ramus area.

CORRECTING HEAD ROTATION FOR THE RHESE POSITION

CRITICAL THINKING CHALLENGE 10.3

For the Rhese position for the optic foramen and orbit, the head should be rotated such that the midsagittal plane lies 53° from the tabletop to demonstrate the downside orbit. You have the patient prone and are attempting to demonstrate the right orbit. But, the patient is unable to rotate his head much at all toward his left. You decide to leave his head in the straight PA position and use an angle on the CR.

How many degrees of CR angle must you use, and in which direction, to obtain this position? What must you do with the x-ray tube to allow this type of angulation? Can you use this angle with the CR cassette placed in the Bucky, or with a built-in DR detector? What are your options for using or not using a grid?

ANGULATION ADJUSTMENT FOR NORMAL LATERAL L5–S1 "SPOT"

CRITICAL THINKING CHALLENGE 10.4

Suppose you are performing a lateral L5–S1 "spot" projection on a normal patient with some "sagging" of the lumbar spine, and you decide to use a caudal angle on the CR to better open the joint space. As noted in this chapter, for normal patients without scoliosis, the L5–S1 joint is "locked into place" within the pelvic girdle.

Review the centering shift rule for beam angles discussed in paradigm #8 in Chapter 1 and in Chapter 2. Why might this cancel out the need to apply this rule, as long as your centering rule is based upon the iliac crest?

(Answers to Critical Thinking Challenges are found in the Appendix.)

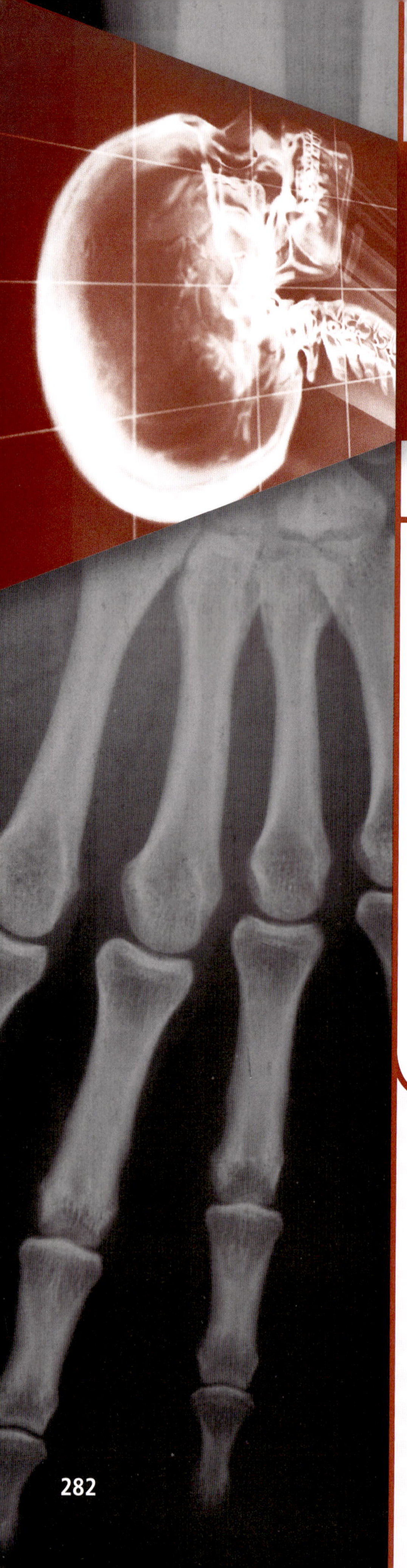

CHAPTER 11

Determining Exact Corrections from Image Evaluation

OUTLINE

OBJECTIVES

Upon completion of this chapter, you should be able to:

1. Memorize the number of degrees that warrant a repeated exposure for off-angle, off-rotation, incorrect tilt, flexion, or extension.
2. In the evaluation of radiographs taken of torso or skull anatomy, state the rule for observed shift between anatomical landmarks for beam angulation, body rotation, tilt, flexion, or extension.
3. In the evaluation of radiographs taken of the spines or extremities, state the rule for observed shift between anatomical landmarks for beam angulation, body rotation, tilt, flexion, or extension.

Continues

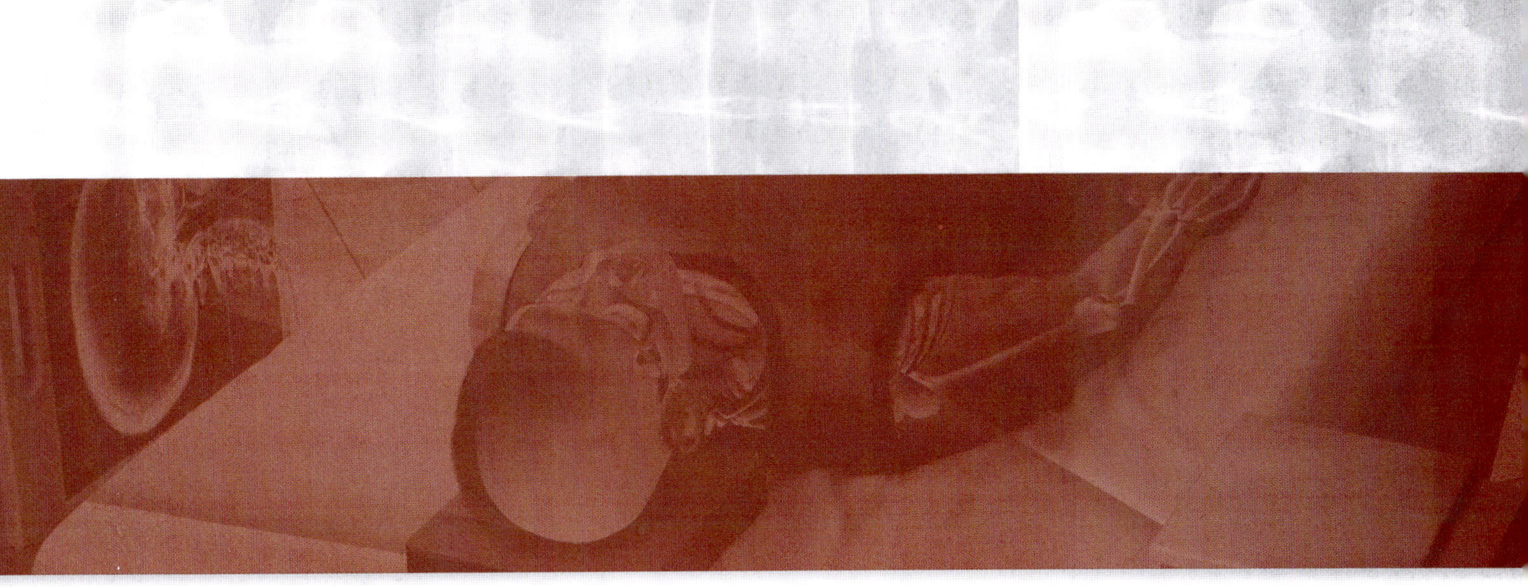

OBJECTIVES *continued*

4. In the evaluation of the lateral chest radiograph, state the rule of observed shift between landmarks for beam angulation, body rotation, tilt, flexion, or extension.
5. In critiquing a position on a radiograph, explain the three guidelines that determine the best anatomical parts to observe for shift to evaluate beam angulation, body rotation, tilt, flexion, or extension.

INTRODUCTION

Historically, radiography education has failed to even attempt to *quantify* the criteria by which we judge a radiographic position. One result, for example, is that most radiographers can state that a particular position was "rotated," but *not by how much*. This information is both extremely useful and important to have at one's command. It allows us to make clear and precise positioning corrections. For example, "Turn the patient's head to the right about 5°," rather than merely stating, "Turn the patient's head more to the right." It empowers us to establish a universal rule for *what constitutes a repeatable error*, as stated in paradigm #20 in Chapter 1. For radiographers, nothing could be more pertinent.

One might ask what specific type of expertise radiographers should possess to an even greater degree than a radiologist? The fine points of evaluating positions would certainly be at the top of that list. These skills are at the heart of radiography.

Paradigm #19 in Chapter 1 states that it is indeed *possible* to quantify the rules for evaluating positions, and to establish a kind of universal norm for what is repeatable. Perhaps one reason it has not been previously done is that these types of rules are, by their nature, dependent upon the thickness of body parts, which varies across a wide range. So, the task might seem insurmountable at first. But a few rules can be established for *ranges* of body part thickness that have broad application, and that is what this chapter sets out to do. Such rules based on ranges of thickness are by necessity "rounded out," and so they must be expected to take the form of *estimations* or "rules of thumb," which will suffer some minor inaccuracies. Yet, the benefits of having a few condensed, simple, practical rules that can be applied on a daily basis are so great as to make the attempt well worthwhile.

As described in Chapter 1, images throughout this book are smaller than the original radiographs, and CR or DR images on a display monitor are smaller than the original field used when the exposures were made. References to all distances, both measured (such as "1 inch of shift"), and relative (such as "2 fingerbreadths"), must be taken in the context of the typical field sizes originally projected when the exposures were made. The reader must use his or her imagination to visualize the actual distances in the context of the original projected field size, or relative to the *patient* in the image.

RULES FOR SHIFT IN THE IMAGE

General Shift Rule for Angling, Rotation, Tilt, and Flexion/Extension in the Torso and Skull

The same rule presented in Chapter 2 for recentering the CR to compensate for beam angles, and presented in Chapter 5 for recentering the CR to compensate for rotation of the torso or skull, can also be applied in critiquing radiographs for proper positioning of nearly all procedures involving the torso or skull. It might be phrased as follows:

> Generally, for the evaluation of radiographs taken of torso or skull anatomy, every *1 inch* of shift observed between landmarks represents about *10°* of beam angulation, body rotation, tilt, flexion, or extension.

BEST PRACTICE TIP

Generally, for the evaluation of radiographs taken of torso or skull anatomy, every *1 inch* of shift observed between landmarks represents about *10°* of beam angulation, body rotation, tilt, flexion, or extension.

How Much is Repeatable?

The decision whether or not to retake a projection because of poor positioning is, of course, somewhat dependent upon the individual standards of different radiologists and radiographers. The benefit must also be weighed against the degree of discomfort a repeated procedure might cause the patient on a case-by-case basis. Sometimes a better view is just not worth the trouble.

Nonetheless, it *is* possible to establish an *average* criterion by surveying what most radiographers do in practice. Thus, for example, a general rule for how much off-rotation warrants a repeated exposure can be determined, and this *should* be done for the benefit of new students, if not for all students.

Just such a survey of radiographers was conducted, noting the degree of shift they identified on various radiographs as "repeatable." A protractor device was then constructed allowing two objects to be placed at various distances from the pivot point (simulating the *depth* of anatomy within the patient for different procedures). This was radiographed longitudinally at both 40-inch and 72-inch SID to determine the actual degree of rotation causing the amount of shift identified by the radiographers. The experiment was repeated extensively for a reliable result. This resulting principle may be stated in the following:

> Generally, the amount of off-angle, off-rotation, incorrect tilt, flexion, or extension that is considered to warrant a repeated exposure is *more than* 3°.

BEST PRACTICE TIP

Generally, the amount of off-angle, off-rotation, incorrect tilt, flexion, or extension that is considered to warrant a repeated exposure is *more than 3°*.

For example, a cervical spine requiring 15° of angulation should be repeated if the actual angle was more than 18° or less than 12°. A 45° oblique lumbar spine is repeatable if the body rotation was more than 48° or less than 42°. A lateral skull is repeatable if the head was tilted more than 3° either way. A Waters projection for sinuses is repeatable if the orbitomeatal line, which should lie at a 37° angle from the tabletop, is more than 40° or less than 34°. And, a Holmblad projection (with the patient "on all fours") for the intercondylar fossa of the femur, in which the femur should lie at a 70° angle from the tabletop, should not be flexed from the hip so that it is more than 73°, nor extended so that it is less than 67°. These several examples were selected to make the point that this is a wonderfully universal rule in that it applies not only to angulation of the beam, but to *all* body part movements as well.

By stating the rule in degrees (rather than amounts of shift), only one universal rule is needed. All amounts of apparent shift of anatomy on a radiograph resulting for various thicknesses of anatomy can then be extrapolated from it. Because 72-inch projections cause *less* shift than 40-inch projections, the rule is based on a 40-inch SID such as is used for most routine projections. In this way, a "repeatable shift" rule applied to a 72-inch projection will indicate even *more* than 3° of rotation, denoting all the more that a retake is indicated.

Practical Application Examples of the Shift Rule

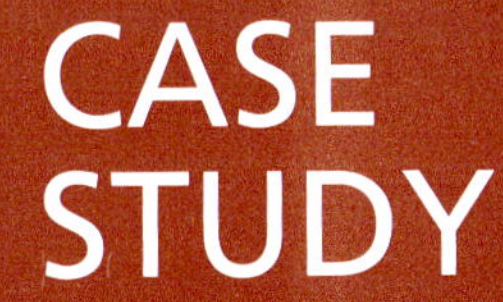

Case Study #1: Evaluation of Tilt for the Lateral-Oblique Mandible View

Figure 11-1 presents two lateral-oblique views of the mandible that demonstrate the vertical shift between the right and left gonions. Radiograph **A** shows about 2½ inches of up-and-down shift. Radiograph **B** shows about 3½ inches of up-and-down shift. How many degrees of combined head tilt and cephalic beam angle do these represent, which radiograph needs to be corrected, and by how much?

ANSWER: *Using the shift rule of thumb, you may surmise that any combination of head tilt and cephalic beam angle used in radiograph* **A** *totaled about 25° (10° for each inch of shift). For ideal demonstration of this anatomy, the head tilt and/or tube angle must be close to 35°, an additional 10° as shown in radiograph* **B**, *with 3½ inches of vertical shift apparent. When you*

(continues)

*examine radiograph **A**, using this rule, you can easily estimate that the correction needed is an additional 10° of cephalic tube angle or head tilt toward the tabletop.*

CASE STUDY

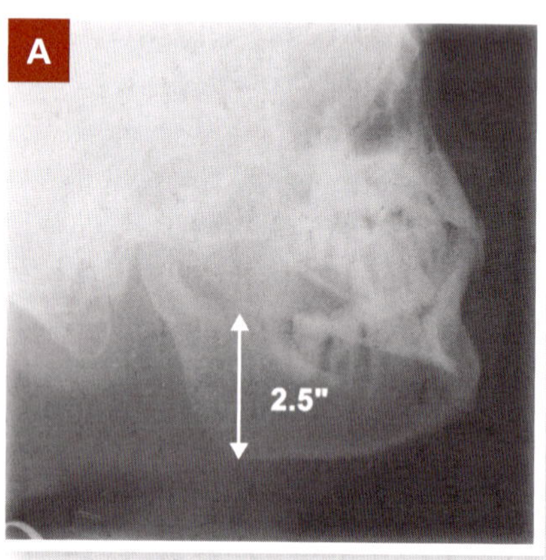

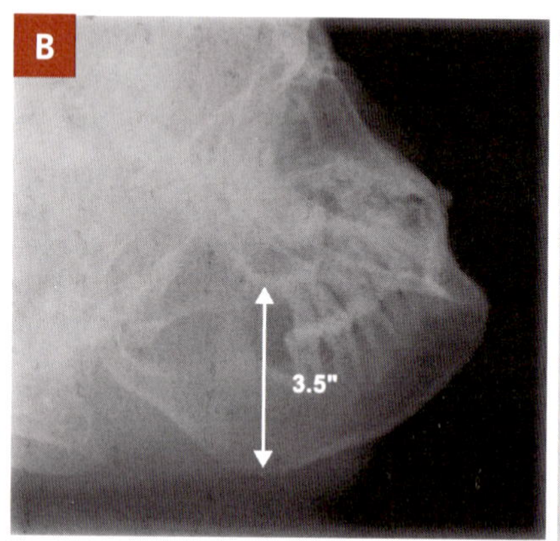

FIGURE 11-1

Views of a lateral (oblique) phantom mandible to interpret vertical shift of the gonions (arrows). In **A**, 2½ inches of shift = 25° of CR angle and/or head tilt. In **B**, 3½ inches of shift = 35° of angle and/or tilt.

Carroll, Q. Evaluating Radiographs, 1993, Figures 196 & 197, Courtesy of Charles C Thomas, Publisher, Ltd., Springfield, Illinois.

Case Study #2: Evaluation of Rotation for a PA Chest

The radiograph in Figure 11-2 is from a standard PA projection of the chest. A common landmark to use in evaluating rotation on this view is the symmetry of the sternoclavicular joints relative to the posterior midline as indicated by the spinous processes. Note that for this particular patient there is about 2 inches of distance between the two SC joints (arrows). Were the position perfectly straight, the SC joints would lie symmetrically 1 inch to either side of the midline spinous processes (line).

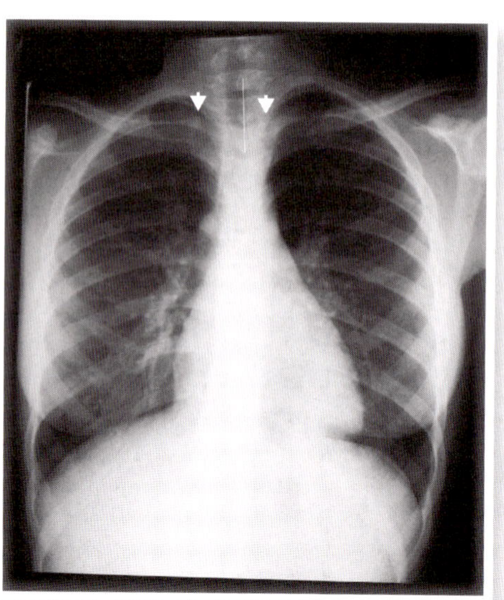

Courtesy of Quinn B. Carroll

FIGURE 11-2

PA chest view showing the right SC joint 1½ inches away from the midline spinous processes (line), and the left SC joint ½ inch away from the mid-line (arrows). There is ½ inch of shift to the patient's right, equal to 5° of rotation.

But, in Figure 11-2, the patient's *right* SC joint appears to be about 1½ inches away from the midline of the spine, while the *left* SC joint is only about ½ inch away. How much rotation does this represent? Is it repeatable? And, how should you correct the position?

ANSWER: *The amount of actual shift* present *is about ½ inch (from*

CASE STUDY

where the SC joints would be *symmetrically positioned). Rotation is to the patient's right. That is, both SC joints have been shifted to the right about ½ inch from where they should be. By the shift rule of thumb, it comes out to about 5° of body rotation. While this may not sound like much, it is repeatable. It exceeds the 3° limit discussed in the previous section.*

Case Study #3: Evaluation of Flexion/Extension for the Odontoid View

A "coned-down" projection for the odontoid is presented in Figure 11-3. The bottom edge of the upper incisor teeth is seen about ½ inch above the bottom edge of the occipital bone. Is the patient's head overflexed or overextended, and by how much? What options are available for correcting this position?

ANSWER: *Using the shift rule of thumb, this indicates about 5° of overextension of the head with the chin pulled up too much. To correct this problem on the repeated radiograph, two options are available: 1) Use a narrow-triangle sponge slid under the upper part of the head to help flex the chin back down 5°, or 2) Angle the x-ray beam 5°* caudally.

This is a great demonstration of the usefulness of the shift rule of thumb. Without it, most radiographers will know that the chin must be flexed or the tube angled caudally, but they have no guide as to how much *to flex the chin or angle the tube. The shift rule of thumb gives us the* amount *by which these corrections should be made.*

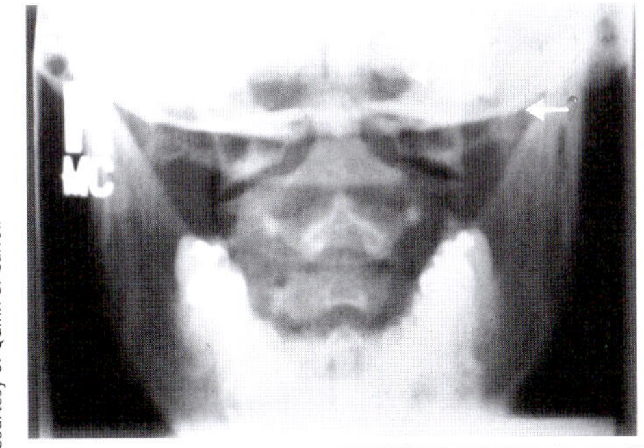

Courtesy of Quinn B. Carroll

FIGURE 11-3
Odontoid view showing the lower edge of the upper incisors ½ inch above the bottom edge of the occipital bone (arrows). This represents 5° of head extension.

Corollary Rule for the General Extremities and Spine

The shift rule presented earlier is based on the assumption that the thickness of the body part being radiographed is in an average range for the torso or the PA skull (in the 18–24 centimeters range.) As discussed in Chapter 1, when the body part is much thinner, the expected amount

BEST PRACTICE TIP

For the evaluation of radiographs taken of the spines or the extremities, every ½ inch of shift observed between landmarks represents *10°* of beam angulation, body rotation, tilt, flexion, or extension.

NOTE: This is one-half of the shift for the general rule.

of shift will decrease. This is true for angulation, rotation, tilt, flexion/extension, and abduction/adduction. A useful corollary rule of thumb can be stated for extremities in general, and also for the spine. The adult lumbar spine (measured from the anterior surface of the vertebral body to the posterior tip of the spinous process), the elbow, and the ankle all fall within a thickness range from 7 to 10 centimeters. Simply divide the general shift rule into *one-half*, as described in the following:

> For the evaluation of radiographs taken of the spines or the extremities, every ½ inch of shift observed between landmarks represents *10°* of beam angulation, body rotation, tilt, flexion, or extension.

NOTE: This is one-half of the shift for the general rule.

Practical Application Examples for the Extremities and the Spine

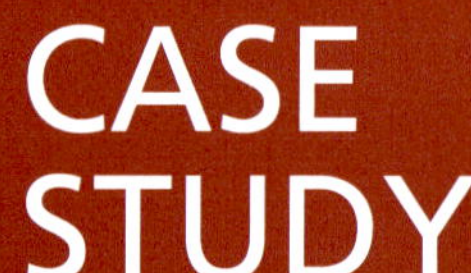

Case Study #4: Rotated Lateral Knee

A lateral view of the knee, Figure 11-4, shows the posterior aspect of the medial condyle shifted ½ inch behind the lateral condyle. Is this a repeatable amount of rotation? In correcting this position for a repeated exposure, how many degrees must the knee be further rotated downward toward the tabletop?

ANSWER: *Using the corollary rule, the answer is about 10° (definitely repeatable). This is likely more than one would have rotated the knee to correct it without any rule for guidance, and indeed there is a tendency to underestimate these types of corrections. This rule, by quantifying the corrective rotation needed, reduces the probability of further repeated exposures.*

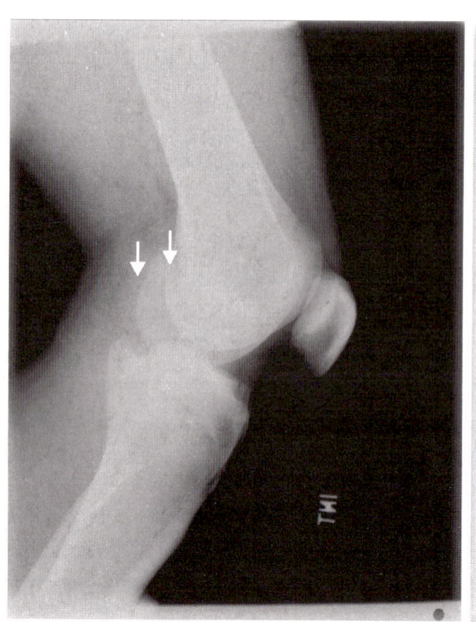

FIGURE 11-4
Lateral knee with the posterior aspect of medial condyle shifted ½ inch behind the lateral condyle. Using the corollary rule for thinner body parts, this represents about 10° of medial rotation in the knee.
Carroll, Q. Evaluating Radiographs, 1993, Figure 158, Courtesy of Charles C Thomas, Publisher, Ltd., Springfield, Illinois.

CASE STUDY

Case Study #5: Rotated Lateral Lumbar Spines

Rotation in lateral views of the lumbar spine is indicated by double lines at the posterior surfaces of the vertebral bodies, shown in magnified views in Figure 11-5. The shift between these posterior surfaces is about ⅛ inch for radiograph **A**, more than ¼ inch for radiograph **B**. How rotated is the spine in each case? Is either radiograph repeatable?

ANSWER: *Using the corollary rule, ¼ inch of shift would indicate approximately 5° of rotation. Radiograph **A** is rotated only about 2°–3° and is not repeatable. Radiograph **B** is rotated more than 5° and is definitely repeatable.*

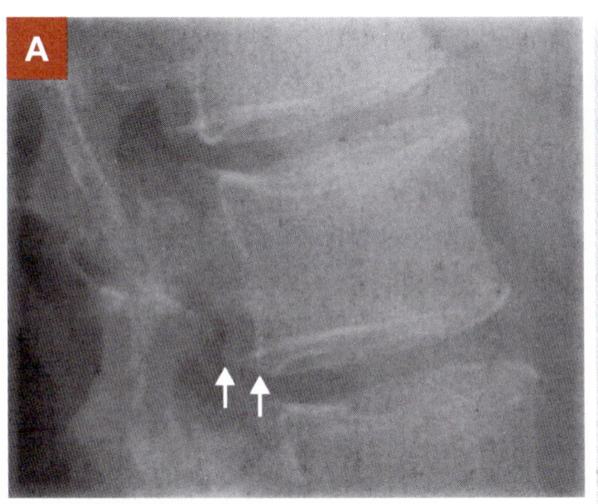

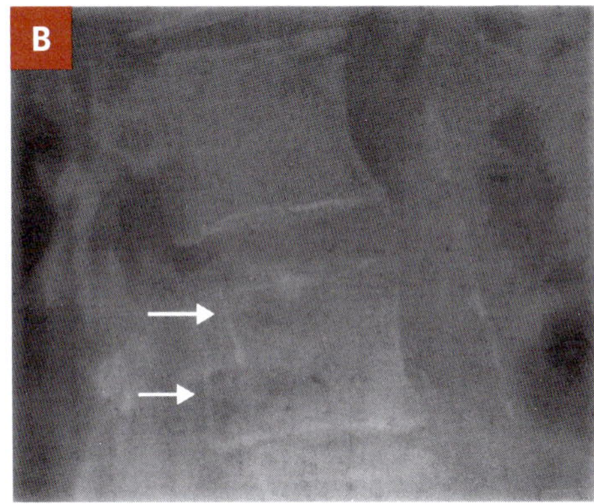

FIGURE 11-5
Magnified views of rotated lateral L-spines. Radiograph **A** shows about ⅛ inch of shift between the posterior surfaces of vertebral bodies (arrows). Using the corollary rule, this indicates only 2°–3° rotation. Radiograph **B** presents more than ¼ inch of shift representing more than 5° of rotation, and should be repeated.

Carroll, Q. Evaluating Radiographs, 1993, Figure 104, Courtesy of Charles C Thomas, Publisher, Ltd., Springfield, Illinois.

Corollary Rule for the Lateral Chest View

The lateral chest view presents a case in which the body part is much thicker than the PA torso, a difference of 8–10 centimeters. Therefore, as discussed in Chapter 1, the amount of shift increases significantly. A useful corollary rule can be stated for the lateral chest (or pelvis), by simply *doubling* the general shift rule, as described in the following:

> For the evaluation of the lateral chest radiograph, every *2 inches* of shift observed between landmarks represents *10°* of beam angulation, body rotation, tilt, flexion, or extension.

NOTE: This is double the shift for the general rule.

BEST PRACTICE TIP

For the evaluation of the lateral chest radiograph, every *2 inches* of shift observed between landmarks represents *10°* of beam angulation, body rotation, tilt, flexion, or extension.

NOTE: This is double the shift for the general rule.

CASE STUDY

Case Study #6: Rotated Lateral Chest View

Figure 11-6 is a lateral view of the chest that shows the posterior costophrenic angles and the posterior right and left ribs shifted side to side by about 1 inch (arrows). How rotated is the chest and should it be repeated?

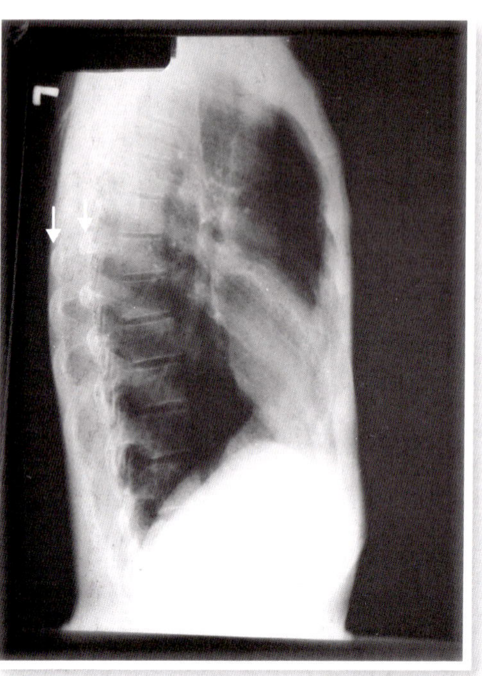

FIGURE 11-6
This lateral chest view demonstrates about 1 inch of shift between the posterior right and left ribs (arrows). Using the corollary rule, this indicates a repeatable 5° of rotation.
Carroll, Q. Evaluating Radiographs, 1993, Figure 82, Courtesy of Charles C Thomas, Publisher, Ltd., Springfield, Illinois.

ANSWER: *Using the corollary rule, 1 inch of shift would indicate about 5° of rotation. We have defined the cut-off point for repeatable errors at about 3°. Even though 5° may seem a minor amount, it does result in a bit more than the frequently used "2 fingerbreadths" of shift between the posterior ribs, and most radiographers would wish to attempt a corrected view.* ■

To this point, we have presented only three rules to memorize. These are the *general* shift rule for torsos and skulls (1 inch of shift = 10° of angle, rotation, etc.), the corollary rule for extremities and spines that cuts the amount of shift in half, and the corollary rule for lateral chests that doubles the amount of shift. The intent has been to reduce the concept of shift to as few rules as possible, with reasonable accuracy but broad enough application to cover the entire human body.

Special Rules for the Skull

Note that in the foregoing discussion, for the sake of simplification, skulls were grouped together with the torso under the *general* rule for shift. Indeed, this rule is adequate to be *roughly* applied to head anatomy, and can be used with confidence. For some skull positions, however, a high degree of accuracy is needed. Since, in fact, the skull is slightly smaller than the torso (22 centimeters average for the AP torso, and 19 centimeters average for the PA skull), a smaller amount of shift in the skull will indicate a slightly larger change in degrees. More exact rules governing this relationship are presented in the next chapter under the section on *Skull, Sinus, and Facial Bone Surveys*.

Computed Radiography (CR) and Digital Radiography (DR) Images

All of the preceding exercises—the general rule for shift in the image, and its two corollary rules—refer to distances for *conventional* radiographs in which the final presentation of the image, for example on a 14- × 17-inch cassette, corresponds not only to the size of the actual cassette used, but also closely corresponds to the actual size of the real anatomy. This was one advantage of conventional radiography, because the radiologist could take measurements directly off of the cassettes.

CR and DR present electronic images on cathode ray tubes (CRTs) that vary in size and are often much smaller than the original cassette used as an image receptor. With a little imagination, one can visualize the relative distances indicated and mentally compensate for the smaller image size.

Let us use the "2 fingerbreadths" rule for rotation on a lateral chest as an example: You may be examining a CR image of a lateral chest on a small LCD screen. You cannot literally put two fingers up against the screen to determine if the chest is repeatably rotated or not, as you might with a 14- × 17-inch cassette. But you may imagine 2 fingerbreadths *to scale* within the image, or the *patient's* fingerbreadths, being placed against the posterior ribs in the image. In the PA chest image, the distance between the top of any posterior rib and the *bottom* of the next lower rib will be roughly equivalent to 2 fingerbreadths, and may be used as a gauge. Many other anatomical comparisons are available, and you may be inventive in using them.

Thus, all of the shift distances referred to throughout this book might simply be considered as relative to the *patient* in the image rather than the radiographer evaluating the image: It is "2 of the *patient's* fingerbreadths," or, "1 inch of shift relative to the *patient*" in the image. All such distances are to be taken in this context. Experienced radiographers can make this leap of imagination intuitively and at will. Students new to the field only need a little practice to develop the skill.

SELECTING GOOD ANATOMICAL CRITERIA

(From Carroll, Q. *Evaluating Radiographs*, 1993, Charles C Thomas, Publisher. Reproduced with permission.)

To accurately evaluate the positioning in a radiographic image, the particular anatomical parts one chooses to observe must be selected carefully. There are definite criteria by which to judge which anatomy will work best. You should always select a *pair* of identical structures that are relatively fixed in place. The best anatomy will be very sensitive to part rotation, flexion, extension, or tilt, so that only slight rotation or other movement will cause the anatomy to shift *a lot* across the image, making it easy to detect. On the other hand, it must *not* be subject to very much shift due to normal x-ray beam divergence, which might mimic rotation or other movement of the body part. Generally, do *not*

BEST PRACTICE TIP

In evaluating a radiograph for positioning, observe only anatomical structures that:

1. Comprise a pair of identical anatomical parts distant from each other and from the midline of the body.
2. Have a long axis perpendicular to the expected direction of shift.
3. Are close to the central ray in the direction of expected shift.

use anatomy that does not satisfy the following three rules—these will each be fully explained.

In evaluating a radiograph for positioning, observe only anatomical structures that:

1. Comprise a pair of identical anatomical parts distant from each other and from the midline of the body.
2. Have a long axis perpendicular to the expected direction of shift.
3. Are close to the central ray in the direction of expected shift.

1. Distant from Each Other and from the Midline

Observed anatomy must be a pair of landmarks *distant* from each other and from the midline of the body part, which is the axis of rotation. Figure 11-7 shows how 20° of rotation affects the projected images of objects at different distances. The *squares*, far from each other and from the midline, are projected well apart on the imaging plate, whereas the projected images of the *circles* are only slightly shifted. The circles are both closer together and closer to the midline of the body.

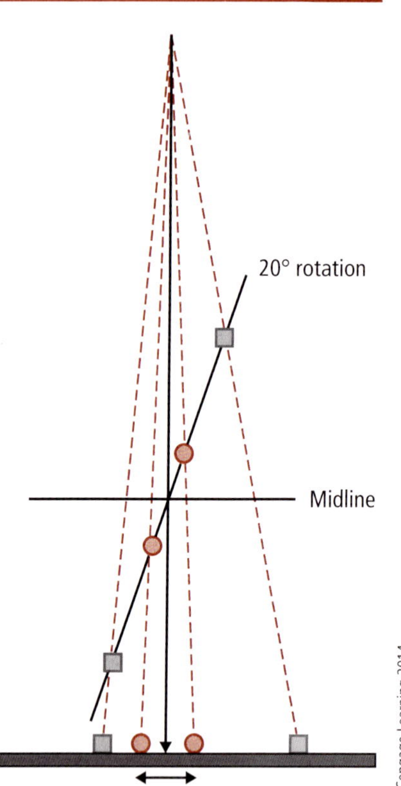

FIGURE 11-7

Observed anatomy must be a pair of landmarks *distant* from each other and from the mid-line. Here 20° of rotation results in the projected images of the *squares* being shifted well apart on the imaging plate below, whereas the projected images of the *circles* are only slightly shifted. The circles are both closer together and closer to the midline of the body.

An example of this principle is found in a traditional method of judging rotation on a lateral skull view, in which the *posterior clinoid processes* are observed to see if they have shifted off of each other horizontally. Note that the clinoid processes are only a half-inch away from each other, and only a quarter-inch from the midline of the skull! This means that a lot of skull rotation must be present to see them shift off of each other in an obvious way on the radiograph. They are too close together to be sensitive as an indicator of skull rotation. There are several other anatomical structures in the skull that better serve this purpose. These will be discussed later.

2. Perpendicular to Expected Shift

Figure 11-8 shows two pairs of lines that are shifted an *equal* amount laterally (side-to-side). Note that the vertical line pair **A** *appears* to be farther apart than the diagonal line pair **B**. This is a subjective, optical illusion, yet it has a real effect upon our judgment. The more

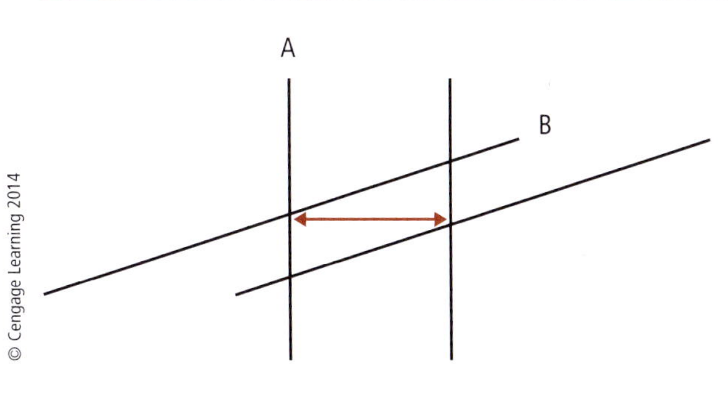

FIGURE 11-8

Observed anatomy must be perpendicular to the expected direction of shift. Note that with the same amount of lateral rotation, the diagonal lines B *appear* to shift less than the vertical lines A. (Furthermore, *tilt* can cause a similar appearance for the diagonal lines.)

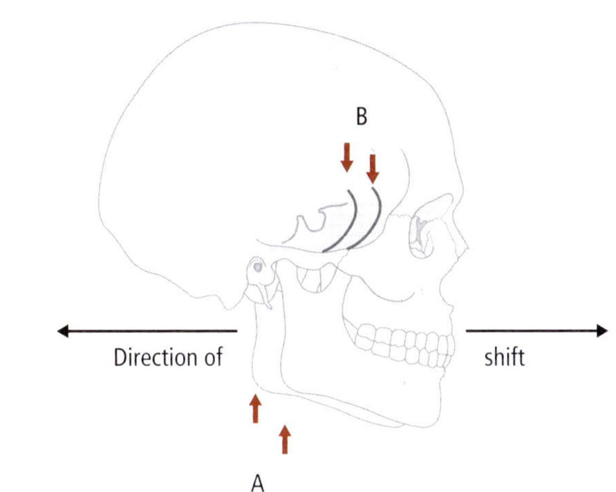

FIGURE 11-9

Examples of perpendicular lines in the lateral skull view to judge rotation by including: A, the posterior edges of the two mandibular rami, and B, the *vertical portions* of the greater wings of the sphenoid bone.

Image redrawn from Carroll, Q. Evaluating Radiographs, 1993, Figure 72, Courtesy of Charles C Thomas, Publisher, Ltd., Springfield, Illinois.

perpendicular lines are to the direction of shift, the easier it is to see the separation.

There is a second reason for this rule: Note that the middle portion of the diagonal lines in Figure 11-8 would look identical if the actual shift had been *vertical* rather than *horizontal*, that is, *tilt* could have caused this appearance just as well as rotation. To be certain that you are checking rotation (not tilt), the lines observed must be close to vertical—that is, perpendicular to the shift. Figure 11-9 diagrams two examples of lines that run vertically in the lateral skull view: the posterior edges of the mandibular rami, and the vertical portions of the greater wings of the sphenoid bone. These both work very well in judging rotation on the lateral view.

Figure 11-10 is a radiograph of the lateral knee applying the principle of perpendicularity. The edges of the femoral condyles can be used to evaluate this view. But, note that you should observe only the posterior, *vertical* portions of the femoral condyles to judge rotation (arrows). The horizontal bottom portions of the condyles (lines) indicate *tilt*, or *cephalic or caudal angulation*, not rotation. To evaluate *tilt* in the skull, you must use lines close to the *horizontal*. The only lines suitable

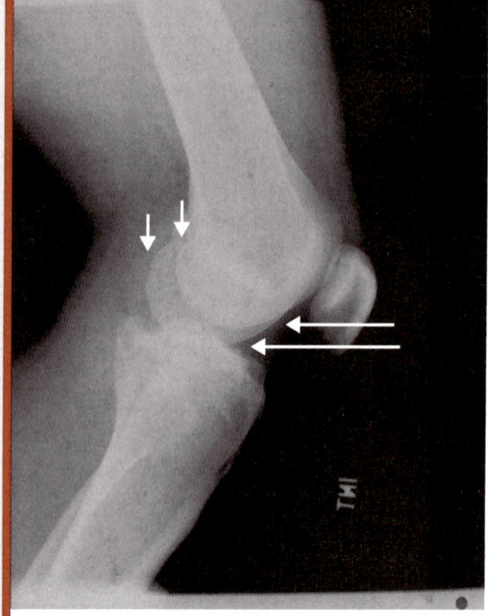

FIGURE 11-10

Radiograph of the knee applying the principle of perpendicularity. Note that only the posterior, vertical portions of the femoral condyles should be observed to judge rotation (arrows). The horizontal bottom portions of the condyles (lines) indicate *tilt*, or *cephalic or caudal angulation*, not rotation.

Carroll, Q. Evaluating Radiographs, 1993, Figure 158, Courtesy of Charles C Thomas, Publisher, Ltd., Springfield, Illinois.

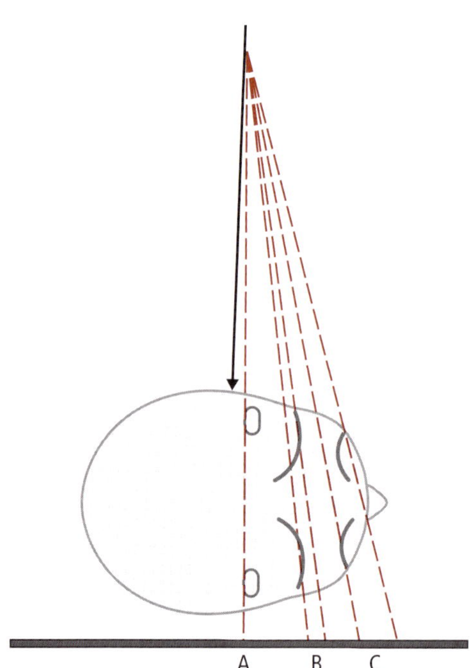

FIGURE 11-11

Observed anatomy must be as close to the central ray as possible, in the direction of expected shift. For a lateral skull, note that the midlateral rims of the two orbits C are *expected* to be projected off each other due to normal beam divergence, even though this skull is *not* rotated. The images of the greater wings of the sphenoid bone B are shifted less because they lie closer to the CR. The TMJs or mandibular condyles A are close to the CR and can realistically be expected to superimpose each other on a straight lateral view. Therefore, of the three, only the TMJs are good indicators of skull rotation for the lateral projection.

Image redrawn from Carroll, Q. Evaluating Radiographs, 1993, Figure 74, Courtesy of Charles C Thomas, Publisher, Ltd., Springfield, Illinois.

for this purpose are the orbital plates of the frontal bone (the "roofs" of the orbits). This is more fully discussed in the next chapter.

3. Close to the CR in the Direction of Expected Shift

Figure 11-11 is an axial diagram of a lateral skull projection, showing normal beam divergence. Note that the midlateral rims of the two

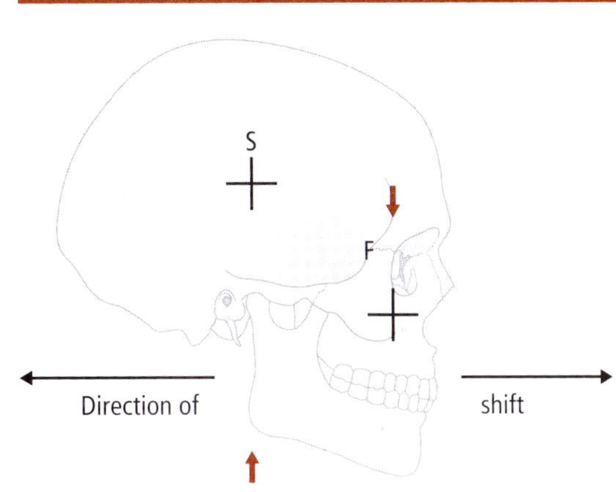

FIGURE 11-12

Centering points for the lateral skull S and the coned-down lateral facial bone (or sinus) projection F. For the facial bone or sinus lateral, the midlateral rims of the orbits (top arrow) lie close to the CR and *can* be used to judge rotation. However, for the lateral *skull,* they lie too far away *side-to-side* from the CR location. For the lateral skull, the posterior edges of the mandibular rami (bottom arrow) are most recommended, because they lie directly beneath the CR.

Image redrawn from Carroll, Q. Evaluating Radiographs, 1993, Figure 180, Courtesy of Charles C Thomas, Publisher, Ltd., Springfield, Illinois.

orbits (**C**) are *expected* to be projected off of each other due to normal beam divergence, even though this skull is *not* rotated. (The orbital rims have been recommended in some textbooks for judging rotation on a lateral skull view. This is incorrect.) The images of the greater wings of the sphenoid bone (**B**) are shifted less because they lie closer to the CR—in less divergent beams. The mandibular condyles (**A**) are close to the CR and can realistically be expected to be projected on top of each other, and thus superimpose each other on a straight lateral view. Of the three, only the mandibular condyles (or TMJs) are good indicators of skull rotation for the lateral projection.

Figure 11-12 diagrams the centering points for the lateral skull and the coned-down lateral facial bone (or sinus) projection. For the facial bone or sinus lateral, the midlateral rims of the orbits lie close to the CR and *can* be used to judge rotation. However, for the lateral *skull*, they lie too far away *side-to-side* from the CR location. For the lateral skull, the posterior edges of the mandibular rami are most recommended, because they lie directly beneath the CR.

Note that the anatomy need only be close to the CR *in the direction of expected shift*. In Figure 11-12, the mandibular rami lie at some distance *below* the CR, but this is irrelevant for checking *rotation*—they need only be in line in a side-to-side dimension, the direction of expected shift. If you were evaluating *tilt* of the head, then the anatomy must be close to the CR in the "vertical" dimension.

Particularly with regard to radiographs of the head, many different recommendations have been made regarding which anatomy to observe in determining whether a position was correctly performed. By applying these three basic rules, radiographers can narrow down these choices to those criteria that are most accurate and useful.

SUMMARY

1. Generally, for the evaluation of radiographs taken of torso or skull anatomy, every *1 inch* of shift observed between landmarks represents *10°* of beam angulation, body rotation, tilt, flexion, or extension.

2. Generally, the amount of off-angle, off-rotation, incorrect tilt, flexion, or extension that is considered to warrant a repeated exposure is *more than 3°*.

3. For the evaluation of radiographs taken of the spines or the extremities, every *½ inch* of shift observed between landmarks represents *10°* of beam angulation, body rotation, tilt, flexion, or extension. This is one-half of the shift for the general rule.

4. For the evaluation of the lateral chest radiograph, every *2 inches* of shift observed between landmarks represents *10°* of beam angulation, body rotation, tilt, flexion, or extension. This is double the shift for the general rule.

5. All of the shift distances referred to throughout this book should be considered as relative to the *patient* in the image. This is adapted for different sizes of images presented in CR and DR.

6. For critiquing a position on a radiograph, the best anatomical parts to observe will always be a pair of stable, bony anatomical parts that are distant from each other *and* from the midline of the body, have a long axis perpendicular to the expected direction of shift, and lie close to the central ray in the direction of expected shift.

CRITICAL THINKING CHALLENGE 11.1

CORRECTION FOR AN AP CERVICAL SPINE PROJECTION

On an AP view of the C-spine, the base of the skull is seen to lie 1½ inches higher than the mentum of the mandible (chin). The base of the skull and the mentum should be superimposed on this projection.

Describe the exact error in the position of the patient's head, which way it must be moved and by how many inches to correct this projection.

PRECISE CASSETTE CRITIQUE FOR TMJS/MASTOIDS

CRITICAL THINKING CHALLENGE 11.2

Observe the radiograph of TMJs and mastoids in Figure 11-13. Carefully compare the posterior edges of the mandibular rami at the arrows for sharpness: Determine which one is the upside and which one is the downside anatomy. Following these lines upward, find the two TMJs and note the two external auditory meatus (EAMs) that are posterior to them.

By observing the distance and direction between the two TMJs or EAMs, state the angle and direction of the CR that was used to produce this radiograph, assuming the head was in a true lateral position.

For this position, the head should be in true lateral position. Is there any rotation present? If so, how much?

Finally, find the traditional name for this method.

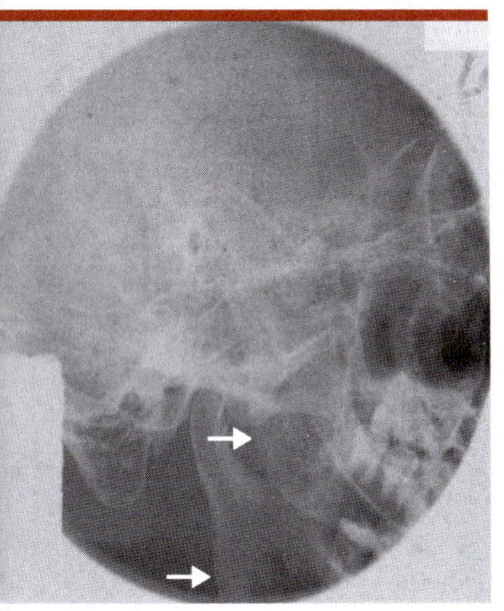

Courtesy of Quinn B. Carroll

FIGURE 11-13

Radiograph for Critical Thinking Challenge 11.1.

CORRECTING HEAD EXTENSION FOR THE RHESE POSITION

CRITICAL THINKING CHALLENGE 11.3

For the Rhese position for the optic foramen and orbit, extend the head until the acanthiomeatal line (AML) is perpendicular to the tabletop. The patient was able to get her head into the proper amount of rotation. But, although she has raised her chin as far as she can, it is not extended enough to get the AML perpendicular. Having memorized the landmark lines taught in Chapter 9 (Figure 9-2), you estimate that her head is extended about 20°.

How many degrees of CR angle must be used, and in which direction, to correct for this position?

(Answers to Critical Thinking Challenges are found in the Appendix.)

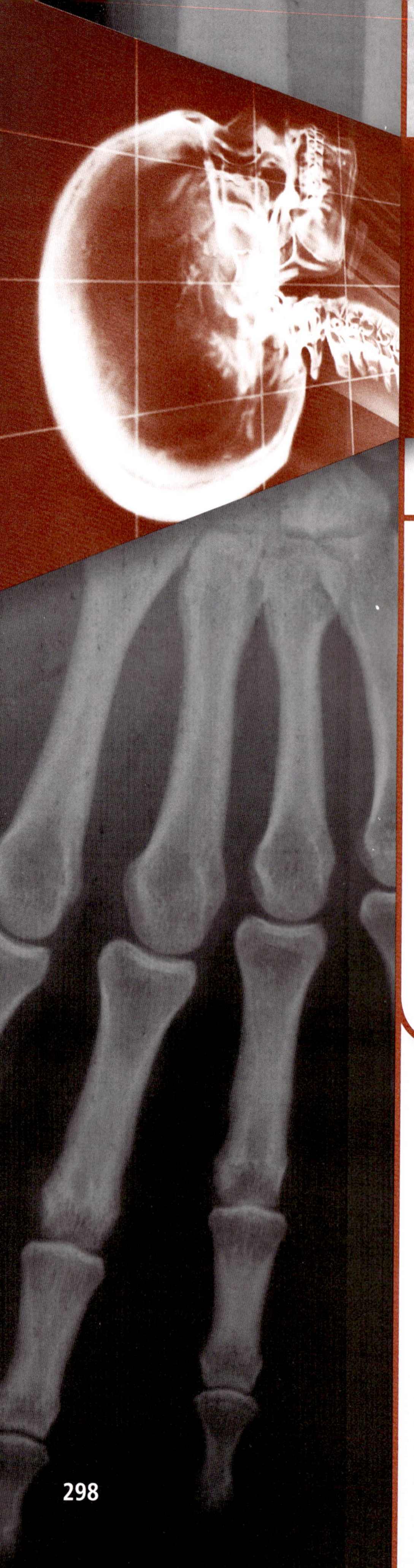

CHAPTER 12

Specific Corrections from Image Evaluation

OUTLINE

OBJECTIVES

Upon completion of this chapter, you should be able to:

1. Distinguish between downside and upside anatomy on radiographs for all parts of the body.
2. Combine this information with skills from the previous chapter to not only quantify errors in positioning, but also to identify the *direction* of the body movement or beam angulation.
3. State the specific shift rule for skull radiographs for quantifying the degrees of rotation, tilt, flexion, extension, or beam angle.
4. List specific recommendations for positioning each body part.

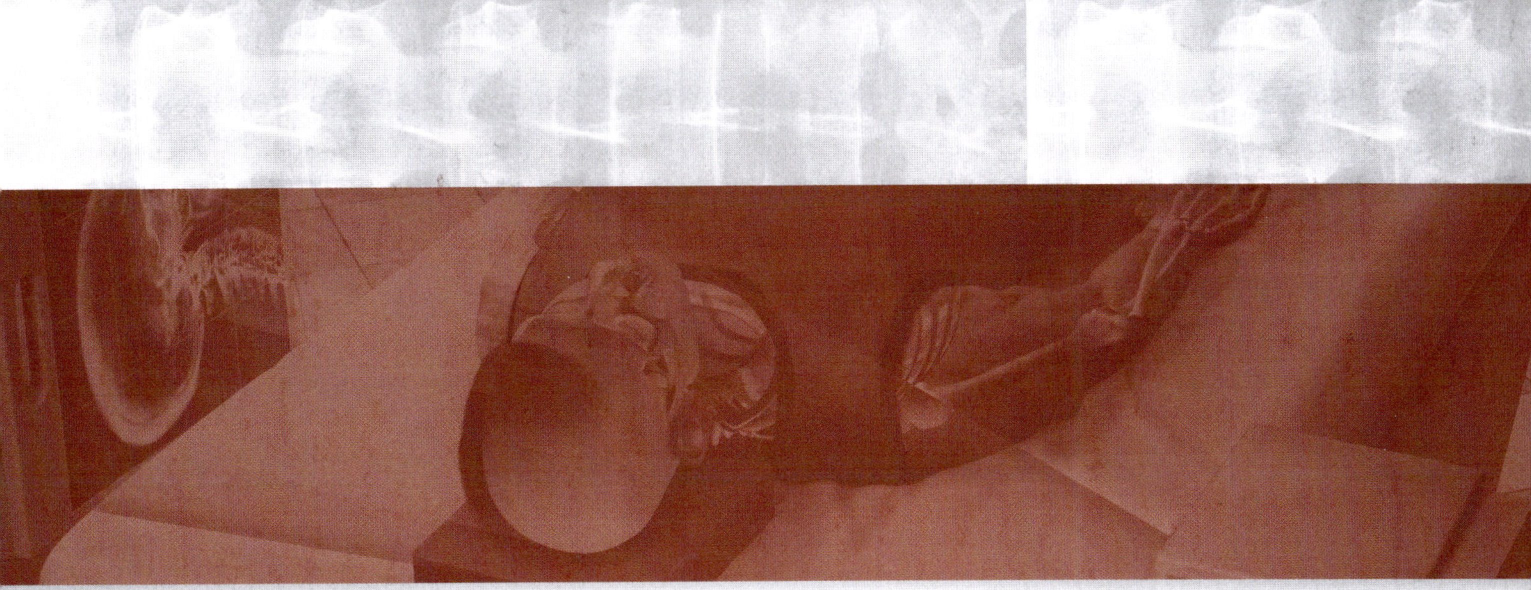

INTRODUCTION

Having discussed the various rules to interpret the shift observed in radiographs and quantify it into degrees of rotation, beam angulation and so forth, it can still be difficult with some anatomy to evaluate *which way* the part is rotated or the beam angled. For example, with a radiograph of the lateral knee in which one femoral condyle lies posterior to the other, such as in Figure 12-1, it may be obvious that rotation is present and, from previous chapters, that the amount is approximately 10°. However, it is unclear whether the knee was *over*rotated downward toward the table or *under*rotated. You must first be able to identify the lateral condyle versus the medial condyle.

An intimate knowledge of the anatomy itself is required for this, and it is not always easy. This chapter will address helpful methods for identifying the specific right and left, medial and lateral, and anterior and posterior anatomy. This will give you confidence in evaluating the *direction* as well as the amount of correction needed for every specific case.

Identification by Magnification and Blur

It would seem at first glance that you could identify on a radiographic image which set of ribs, which TMJ, or which condyle is the *upside* and which is the *downside* by the appearance of magnification and blur. We know that, in principle, the upside anatomy, farthest from the image receptor plate, will always be more blurry at its edges and larger in size. In practice, however, at least three problems complicate this observation.

First, many body parts are of such small thickness to begin with that the *degree* of difference between the upside and downside is just not obvious. Second, differences in size can be *anatomical* rather than geometrical: Some diseases result in the bones on one side of the body being physically larger than the opposite side. Further, *normal* anatomical differences can even be misinterpreted as magnification. An example is the left lung being naturally longer than the right

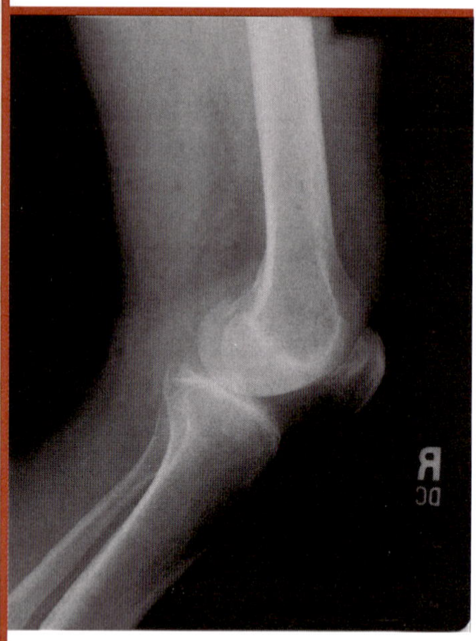

FIGURE 12-1

This lateral view of the knee shows obvious rotation, but it is more difficult to determine *which way* it is rotated, medially or laterally based on the appearance of the condyles alone. In this case, knowledge of the normal position of the proximal *fibula* can help.

Carroll, Q. Evaluating Radiographs, 1993, Figure 158, Courtesy of Charles C Thomas, Publisher, Ltd., Springfield, Illinois.

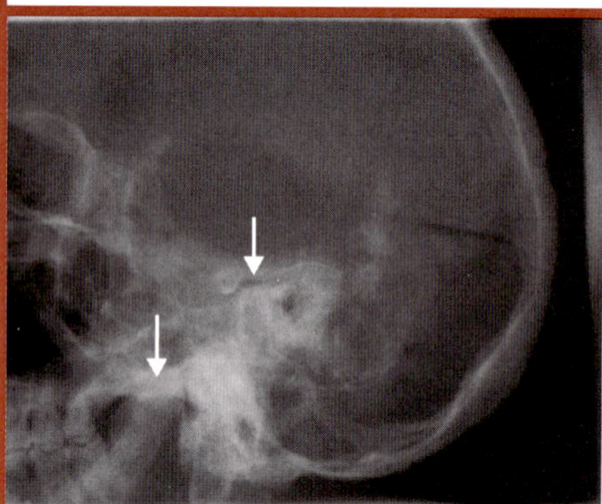

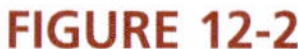

FIGURE 12-2

Laws view in which the *upside* TMJ is easily identified by its obvious magnification (large arrow). For many radiographs, the magnification of the upside anatomy is not so apparent.

Carroll, Q. Evaluating Radiographs, 1993, Figure 199, Courtesy of Charles C Thomas, Publisher, Ltd., Springfield, Illinois.

lung. In the case of the lateral chest view, the resulting higher anatomical position of the right hemidiaphragm actually cancels out the geometrical projection of the right diaphragm downward by the diverging x-ray beam, enough so that the two diaphragms often cross over each other in the image. This renders it impossible to simply "pick the lower diaphragm as the left." You must learn the anatomy, the shape of each hemidiaphragm, more intimately.

Finally, some anatomy (such as the rib cage) has very low inherent radiographic contrast. Visually, this low contrast can be easily misinterpreted as blur. High-contrast bones subjectively seem to have sharp edges, and low-contrast bones, whose edges are less apparent, mimic blur that is in fact not present.

In practical application, there are many positions where the differences in magnification and blur are obvious on the image, and these will be used. Figure 12-2 demonstrates the use of obvious magnification and blur in evaluating a radiograph of the temporomandibular joint. But, given the limitations described earlier, it is often necessary to also use other anatomical clues to confirm your assessment of the image.

CHEST

PA/AP

For the PA or AP view, the symmetry of the sternoclavicular joints in relation to the midline of the spine, as discussed in most positioning texts, is recommended. Generally, the projection should be repeated if the SC joints are shifted more than 1 centimeter (the width of the small fingernail) to either side. In AP torso projections, 1 centimeter of shift translates to approximately 3° of body rotation.

It is possible for the patient to have his hips twisted, rotating only the lower chest. While the SC joints will be aligned indicating that the upper chest is straight, the distance from the two costophrenic angles to the midline of the thoracolumbar spine will be uneven. You must ignore the heart shadow in making this evaluation and strictly use the midline of the spine, measuring to the lateral ribs at the costophrenic angles.

The xiphoid process can be difficult to see, but when it can be identified, it works well in evaluating abdominal or chest rotation. It should be centered over the midline of the spine. Each inch of shift to the left or right indicates 10° of body rotation.

Lateral

For the lateral view, the superimposition of the posterior right and left ribs discussed in most positioning texts generally works well, but can be confusing. The two sets of shifted ribs are set against spinous processes, laminae, and pedicles. And, on some patients with flattened ribs, the normal space between the posterior vertebral bodies and ribs can mimic the space between the two sets of ribs. Also, it helps to examine the superimposition of the **right and left *posterior costophrenic angles* of the** lungs. These are often much easier to identify than the ribs.

Generally, you should repeat the projection if the posterior costophrenic angles or posterior ribs are shifted more than 2 centimeters, or 2 fingerbreadths.

On a lateral view, as shown in Figure 12-3, the *lower* posterior costophrenic angle is nearly always the *right* costophrenic angle, regardless of the position of the anterior halves of the two hemidiaphragms.

Having identified which posterior costophrenic angle is right and which is left, use the concepts and rules discussed in Chapters 1 and 6 to determine which way and how much the chest is rotated.

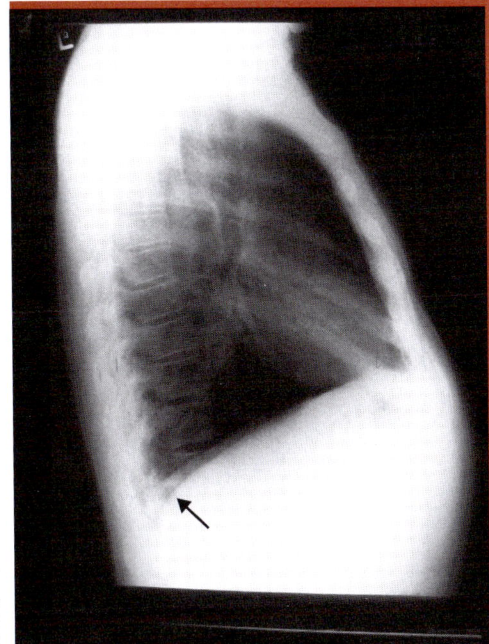

Courtesy of Quinn B. Carroll

FIGURE 12-3
On this lateral chest view, the lower *posterior* costophrenic angle (arrow) is the *right* diaphragm.

Oblique

For a true 45° oblique position of the chest, the bases of the lungs on one side will be foreshortened to appear *one-half* as wide as the opposite side. The ribs and the diaphragm appear one-half as long. If this foreshortened side is *less* than one-half as wide, then the body rotation is too *steep*. If it is *more* than one-half as wide, the position is too shallow.

ABDOMEN, URINARY AND GI SYSTEMS, AND PELVIS

AP

For all abdominal studies, including those with contrast agents, you can use the following reliable *bony* landmarks for evaluation of frontal positions.

When the symphysis pubis is included on the radiograph, it should be aligned with the midline of the sacrum and spine at the spinous processes. While there is some normal side-to-side deviation in these processes, you can draw an "average" line through them collectively to accurately locate the posterior midline. Generally, the symphysis should not be shifted more than ½ inch to either side of this midline, or the projection should be repeated (Figure 12-4). The concepts in Chapters 1 and 6 apply. Every inch of shift translates to about 10° of rotation.

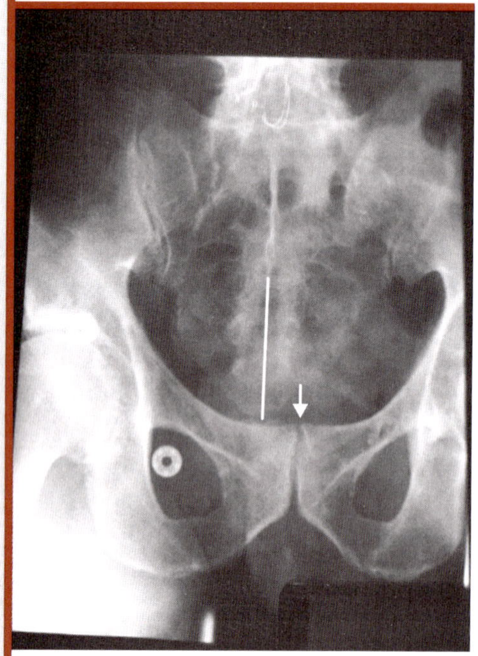

FIGURE 12-4

Closeup of an AP pelvis showing the symphysis pubis (arrow) shifted more than ½ inch from the sacral midline (line), indicating a repeatable amount of rotation to the patient's left.

Carroll, Q. Evaluating Radiographs, 1993, Figure 110, Courtesy of Charles C Thomas, Publisher, Ltd., Springfield, Illinois.

When the symphysis pubis is not included on the radiograph, you may examine spinal anatomy for rotation as described in the next section, *Spines*.

The xiphoid process can be difficult to see, but when you can identify it, it works as well as the symphysis pubis in evaluating abdominal or chest rotation. It should be centered over the midline of the spine. Each inch of shift to the left or right indicates 10° of body rotation.

For the supine pelvis, rotation will cause the *upside* iliac crest to foreshorten side to side, and the *downside* obturator foramen to begin to close off (Figure 12-5). Asymmetry of either the iliac crests or the obturator foramina easily identifies the presence and severity of rotation. Some rules of thumb can be derived for the *upside* iliac crest. As demonstrated in Figure 12-5*B*, 25° of rotation only foreshortens the crest, but a tight "looping" of the upside crest indicates rotation steeper than 30°. Oblique positions for the sacroiliac joints, and also for the urinary system, should be 25°–30°. Therefore, the degree of narrowing and tight looping of the crest as shown in Figure 12-5*B* would indicate *too steep* obliquity for these views. For reference, it takes a full 55° of rotation to bring the upside crest "end-on."

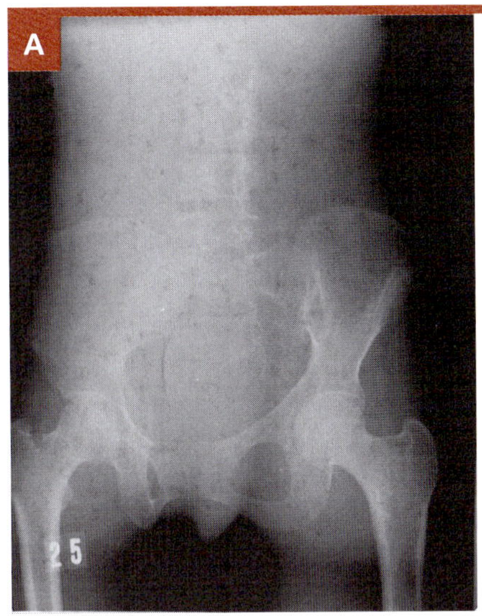

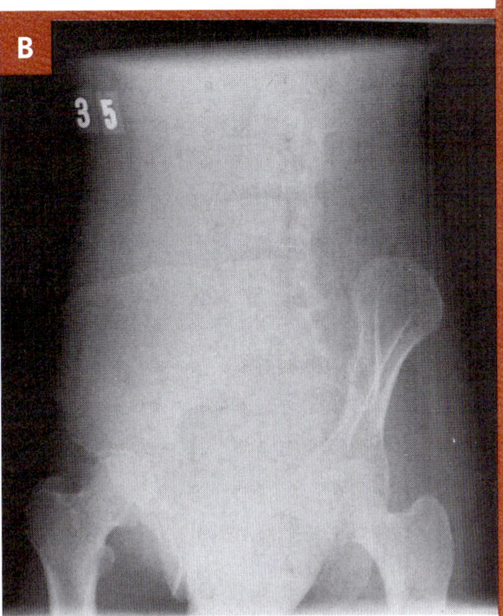

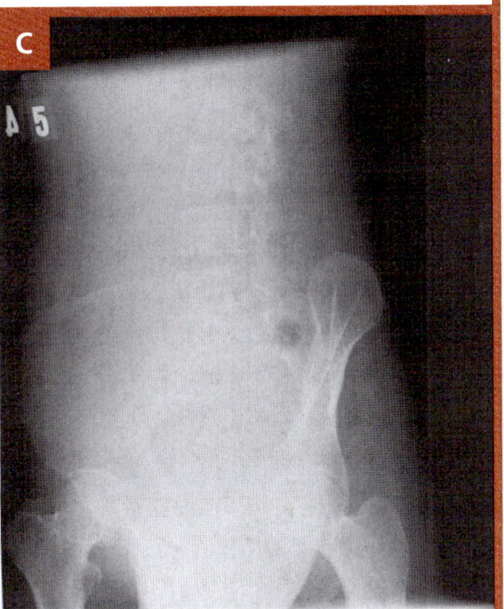

FIGURE 12-5

Series of abdomen phantom views demonstrating the appearance of the upside iliac crest and upside obturator foramen: **A** = 25°; **B** = 35°, too steep for the urinary system; **C** = 45°.

Carroll, Q. Evaluating Radiographs, 1993, Figure 90, Courtesy of Charles C Thomas, Publisher, Ltd., Springfield, Illinois.

SPINES

AP: Applicable to ALL Abdominal and Chest Procedures, L-Spine, T-Spine, and C-Spine

Evaluation of the spine is presented before continuing with the abdomen because the spine can be used not only for lumbar, thoracic, and cervical spine procedures, but also for any procedure within the abdomen and chest, including urinary and GI studies.

The spinous processes, seen end-on, appear as teardrop shapes positioned over the lower portion of each vertebral body and extending into the joint space below. They should be centered within the vertebral body when no rotation is present. Since they lie posterior to the vertebral body, they shift opposite to the direction in which the patient

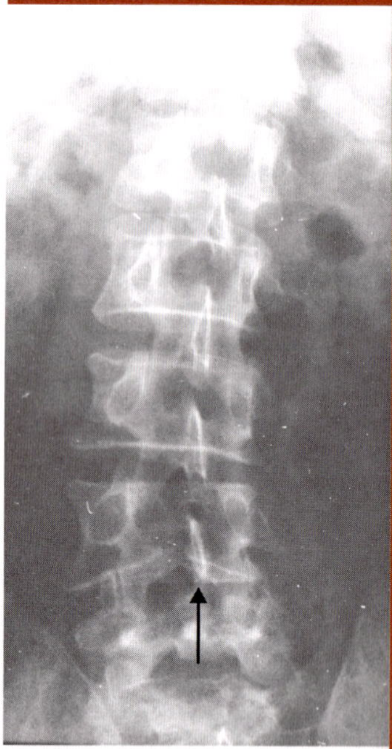

Courtesy of Quinn B. Carroll

FIGURE 12-6

AP lumbar spine view shows the spinous processes (arrow) shifted ¼ inch to the patient's left, indicating 5° of rotation to the *right*.

has turned. When they shift to the *patient's left* (not the *viewer's* left), as shown in Figure 12-6, the patient was turned toward his *right*, and vice versa.

As described in the last chapter, because the spinous process and vertebral body are so close together, the general shift rule must be cut in half. Therefore, every ½ inch of shift will represent 10° of rotation. In Figure 12-6, the spinous processes are shifted about ¼ inch to the left, yet this small amount indicates 5° or more of rotation to the patient's right.

In Chapter 1, we explained that the farther landmarks are away from each other, the more sensitive they are to rotation and the better they are for evaluation. Since the centering of the spinous processes is not as sensitive as anatomical landmarks that are farther away from each other, whenever better separated landmarks are included within the field of view, they should be used rather than the centering of the spinous processes.

Lateral Lumbar and Thoracic Spines

The body of each vertebra has a vertical groove or indentation along the back surface where the spinal cord runs against it. This results two back surfaces to the vertebral body, right and left of the spinal cord, that can be seen on a lateral view when the spine is rotated. These are shown as double lines on the lateral radiographs in Figure 12-7. If you can see only one line at the back surface of the vertebral body, no rotation is present. Every ¼ inch of shift indicates roughly 5° of rotation, and you should consider more than ¼ inch of shift as repeatable. In Figure 12-7, radiograph ***A*** is rotated but not repeatable, radiograph ***B*** is repeatably rotated.

Examine the intervertebral joint spaces for their openness. If the lower border of one vertebra overlaps the upper border of the next one below it, the joint is closed off as diagrammed in Figure 12-8. Sagging of the lumbar spine is important to understand, and is discussed in Chapter 4 (see Figures 4-1 and 4-4 in that chapter). If sagging is substantial, closing off the upper and lower joints, some building up of the waist with sponges will improve the alignment. If only the upper joints are closed off, a slight cephalic angle is in order.

When the joints are closed off on a lateral *thoracic* spine, it is usually due to the spine sloping upward toward the head due to the patient's broad shoulders or narrow waist. A cephalic angle will correct this—the amount can be estimated by palpating the spinous processes of T1 and T12.

Thoracic Spine Technique

Special technique considerations for both the AP and the lateral T-spine are presented in Chapter 13.

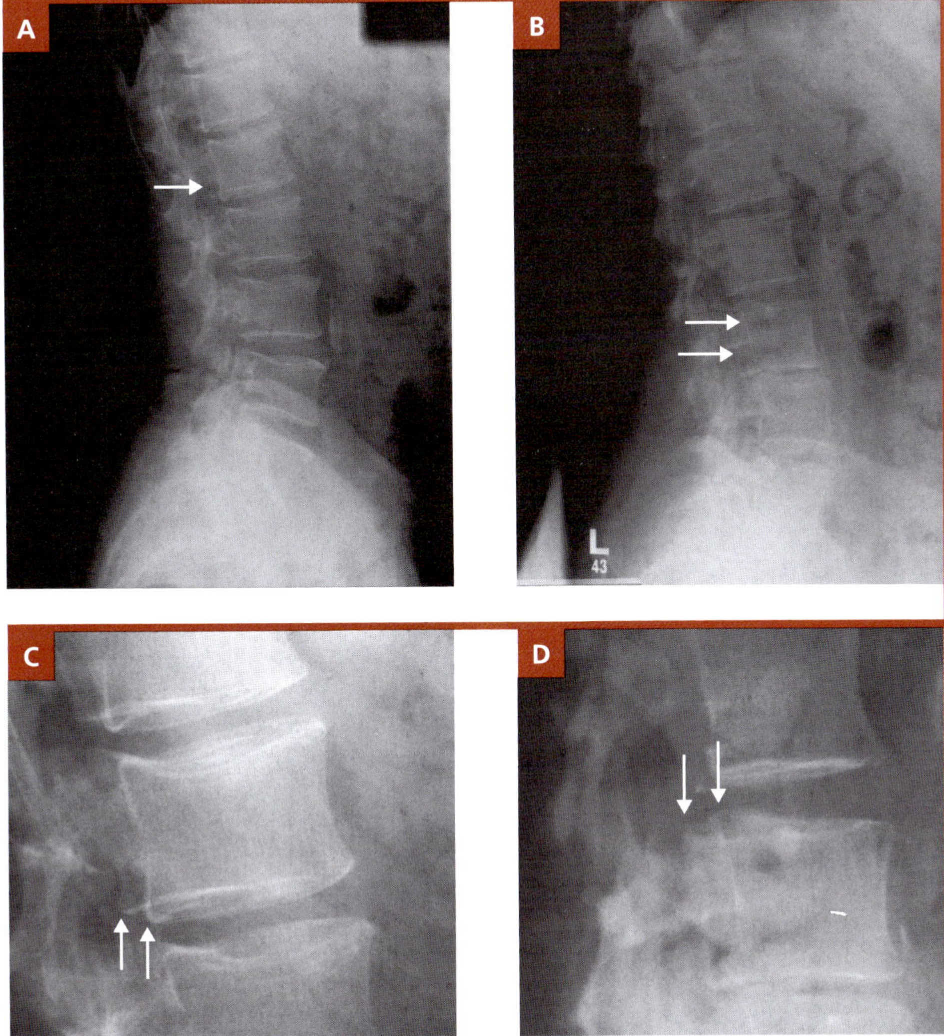

FIGURE 12-7

Lateral lumbar spine views showing double lines at the posterior surfaces of the vertebral bodies (arrows) from rotation. Radiograph **A** shows slight rotation. **B** shows ¼ inch of shift, indicating 5° of rotation, which is repeatable. **C** and **D** are magnified views to better see these lines.

Carroll, Q. Evaluating Radiographs, 1993, Figure 104, Courtesy of Charles C Thomas, Publisher, Ltd., Springfield, Illinois.

L5–S1 "Spot"

The greatest challenge when projecting the "coned-down" lateral view of the L5–S1 joint is opening the joint space up vertically (Figure 12-8), that is, determining the correct beam angle. This is demonstrated in the radiographs in Figure 12-9. Most corrections require *increasing caudal angulation*, which can be from 5° to as much as 15° or even 18° on some patients. However, some patients may be scoliotic and actually require a *cephalic* angle. It can be quite difficult to determine from the radiograph alone which way to angle on the repeat. Understanding the beam divergence geometry in Chapter 4 is important, and palpation of the spinous processes of L5 and the tip of the sacrum is essential to confirm your decision and avoid further repeats.

As discussed in Case Study #3 in Chapter 4, an examination of the routine lateral lumbar spine view is also very helpful. Take note of the *trend* of the joints becoming more closed off or opening more as they progress downward toward L5–S1. If they progressively open better, a

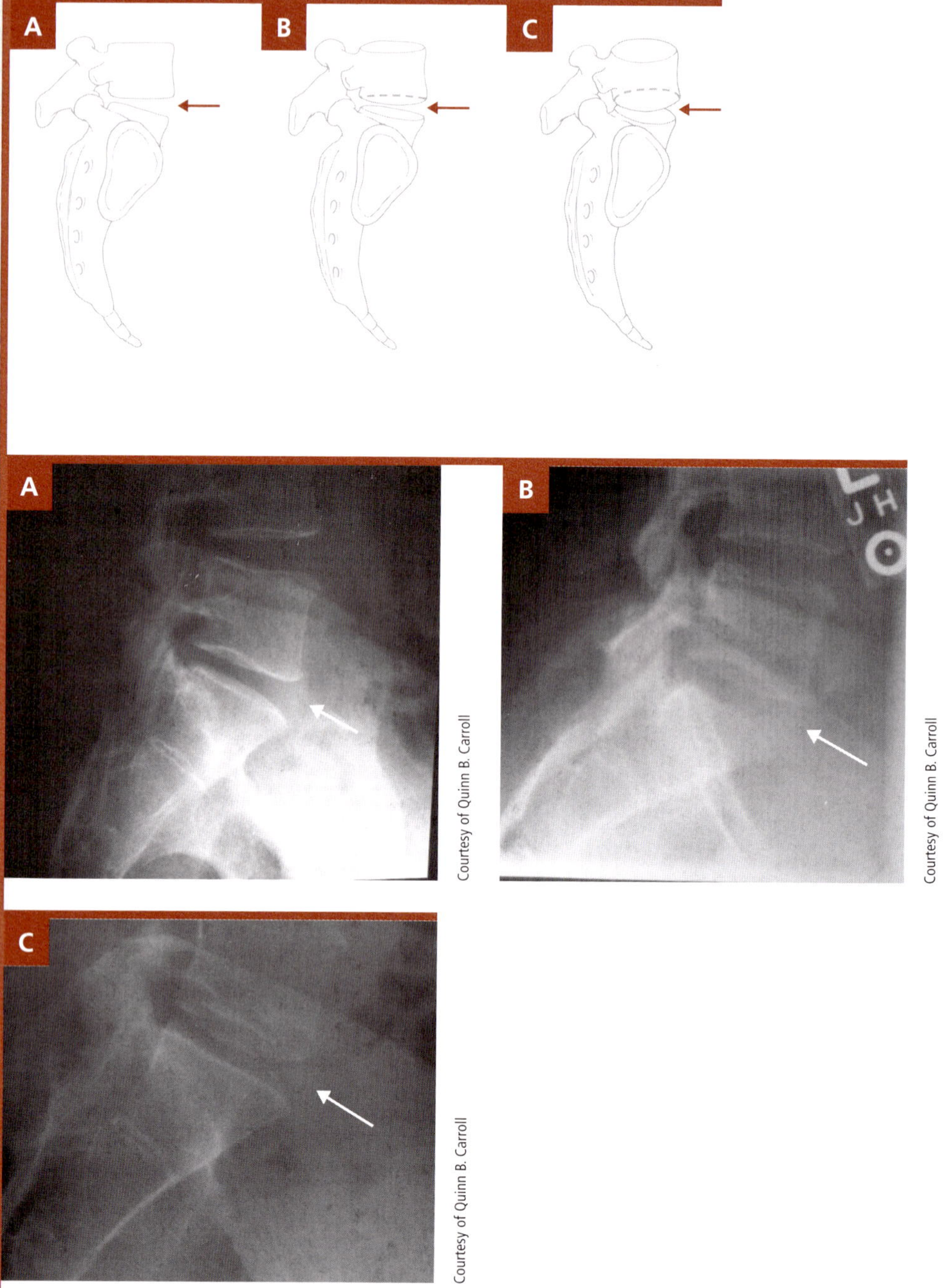

FIGURE 12-8

Diagram of progressive closing off of the lateral L5–S1 joint space due to improper CR angulation. **A** is ideal. **B** could be improved but is not repeatable as long as some space is visible across the joint—i.e., the vertebral bodies do not yet overlap. **C** is closed off and repeatable—The contours of the vertebral bodies form a sideways "V" (arrow).

Image redrawn from Carroll, Q. Evaluating Radiographs, 1993, Figure 105, Courtesy of Charles C Thomas, Publisher, Ltd., Springfield, Illinois.

FIGURE 12-9

Views of the lateral L5–S1 joint, following the diagrams in Figure 12-8, showing **A** a well-opened joint space; **B** barely acceptable opening of the joint space; and **C** a repeatable radiograph with the joint space closed off (arrow).

caudal angulation is indicated for L5–S1. If the lower ones progressively close off, a vertical beam is indicated. And sometimes, when severely closed, even a cephalic angle may be indicated. If the L5–S1 joint space is opened beautifully on the routine lateral view, the caudal angle for the L5–S1 projection should be 7°–8°, not just the popular "5°" (Figure 12-10*A*). (Also see Figure 4-9 in Chapter 4.) When the L5–S1 space is closed off by normal beam divergence on the routine lateral, it is likely that a CR close to perpendicular should be used for the *spot* projection (Figure 12-10***B***).

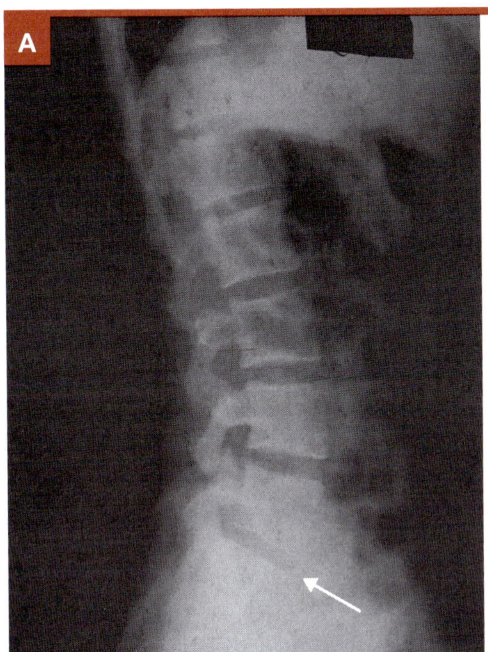

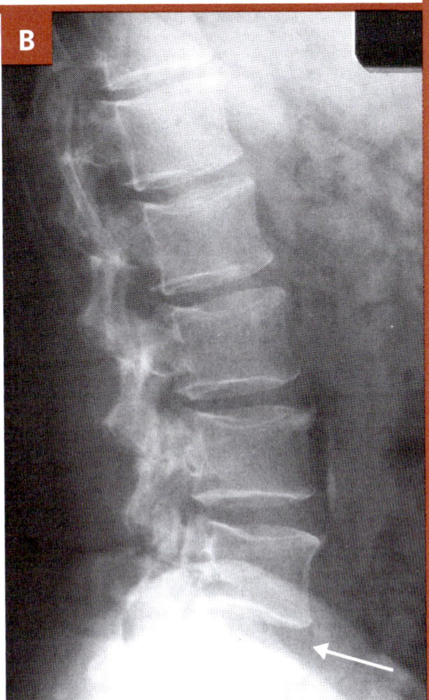

FIGURE 12-10

When the L5–S1 joint space is well-opened on the routine lateral L-spine view, as in **A**, a caudal angle of 7°–8° is indicated for the lateral L5–S1 *spot* projection (see Figure 4-9 in Chapter 4). When the L5–S1 space is closed off by normal beam divergence on the routine lateral **B**, it is likely that a CR close to perpendicular should be used on the *spot*.

Carroll, Q. Evaluating Radiographs, 1993, Figure 104, Courtesy of Charles C Thomas, Publisher, Ltd., Springfield, Illinois.

Oblique L-Spine

On projections of the spine, the posterior pedicles show up as ½-inch ovals overlapping the vertebral body. Observe these pedicles only in the *middle* three vertebrae, L2 through L4 (see Figure 12-11). At a true 45° obliquity, they will lie close to the exact center of the vertebral bodies (Figure 12-11*A*). When the rotation is too *shallow*, the pedicles move anterior to the midline of the vertebral bodies (Figure 12-11*B*). When rotation is too steep, the pedicles move posteriorly to the middle of the vertebral bodies as shown in Figure 12-11C.

AP C-Spine

The lordotic curvature of the cervical spine ranges from 15°–20° in the lower vertebrae, and is exaggerated in older patients or with degenerative disease. Although most radiographers are in the habit of using a fixed 15° cephalic angle on all patients, an *increase* in the angle is almost always indicated when the joint spaces are not well opened on the AP projection.

When C3 is overlapped *to any degree* by the chin, repeat the projection with the chin more extended. If the rounded occipital bone overlaps C3, flex the chin more and repeat the view. *The frontal view of the cervical spine is not adequate unless C3 through C7 are demonstrated in their entirety.*

Odontoid

Rotation of the head on the odontoid view is easily evaluated by checking the alignment of the middle of the chin with the odontoid process. If the middle of the chin is shifted to the *patient's right* in relation to

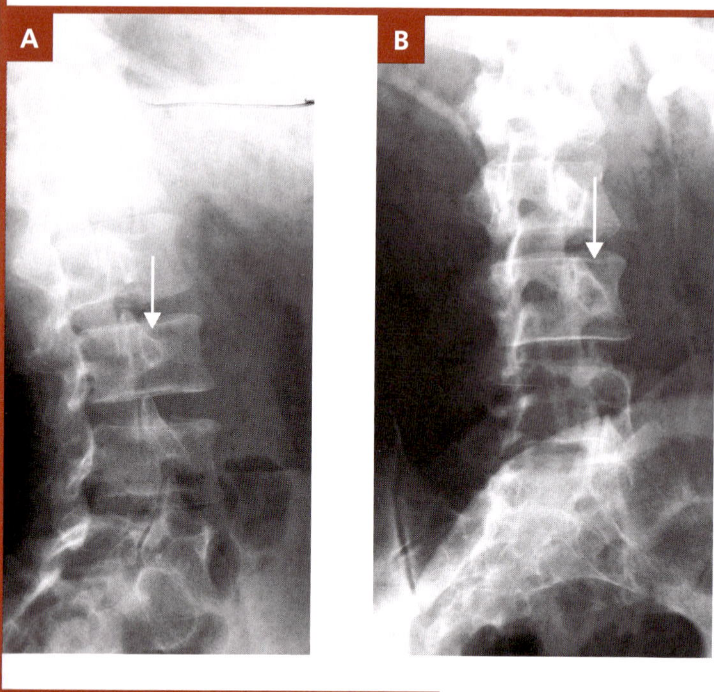

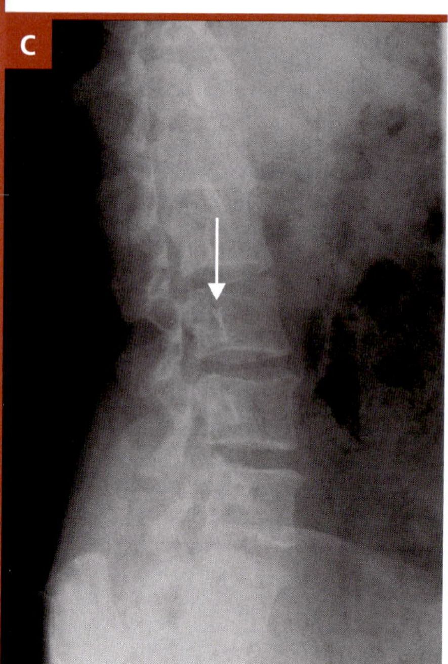

FIGURE 12-11

Oblique lumbar spine views showing the pedicles (arrows), close to the midvertebral body in **A** = proper 45° rotation; anterior to the midvertebral body in **B** = shallow rotation; and posterior to the midvertebral body in **C** = steep rotation.

Carroll, Q. Evaluating Radiographs, 1993, Figure 109, Courtesy of Charles C Thomas, Publisher, Ltd., Springfield, Illinois.

the odontoid process, the head is rotated *to* the right, and you will notice the left molar teeth encroaching upon the vertebrae, as shown in Figure 12-12. Every ½ inch of shift indicates 5° of rotation.

In Figure 12-12 you can also see that the bottom edge of the upper incisor teeth lies about ½ inch below the rounded line of the occipital bone. This represents 5° of overflexion of the chin. Perhaps more common is *overextension* of the head as seen in Figure 12-13, where the occipital bone lies ½ inch below the incisor teeth. This is

5° of overextension, often due to the patient having large shoulders that cause the head to fall back. A narrow-angle wedge sponge is recommended, slid well under the head, in order to flex the chin back down 5°.

Corrections in head flexion/extension on this view are often underestimated or overestimated. The shift rule of thumb, ½ inch for every 5°, is extremely helpful here. An additional odontoid view for practice is presented at the end of this chapter as Critical Thinking Challenge #1.

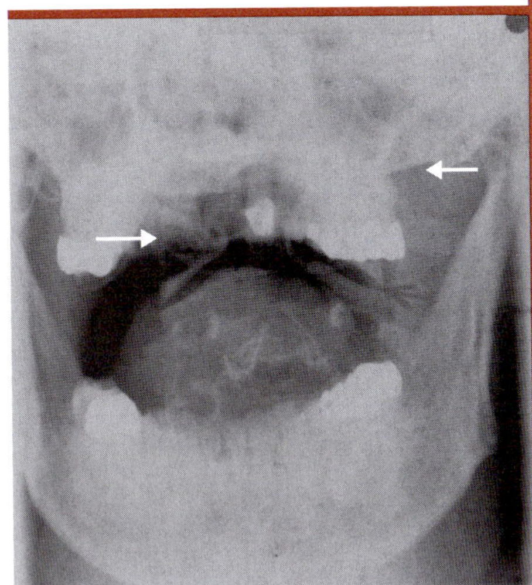

FIGURE 12-12

Odontoid view. The edges of the upper incisor teeth (lower arrow) lie ½ inch below the occipital bone, indicating 5° of hyperflexion. There is also rotation to the patient's right, causing the patient's left upper molar teeth to encroach upon the C1–C2 joint space.

Carroll, Q. Evaluating Radiographs, 1993, Figure 115, Courtesy of Charles C Thomas, Publisher, Ltd., Springfield, Illinois.

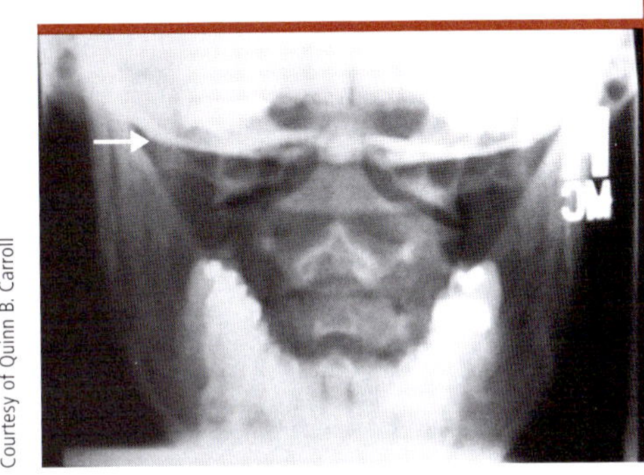

Courtesy of Quinn B. Carroll

FIGURE 12-13

Odontoid view showing the occipital bone ½ inch below the edge of the upper incisors (arrows), indicating 5° of hyperextension.

Oblique C-Spine

The main objective of this view is to open the intervertebral foramina as nicely rounded holes. When the shoulder rotation is either too steep or too shallow, these foramina begin to close off side to side, forming narrow ovals as shown in Figure 12-14. Observe the shoulders to determine if the body rotation was too steep or too shallow: If the ribs and other chest anatomy appear closer to a PA chest than to a lateral chest, the position is too shallow. If they look closer to a lateral chest than a PA, it is too steep.

NOTE: The gonions (posterior angles) of the mandible must clear the upper cervical vertebrae. Although some textbooks recommend keeping the head position in line with the 45° obliqued body, this will result in getting the posterior mandible in the way. Furthermore, the upper foramina actually open somewhat more laterally than 45°, which is the *average* angle at which the six foramina open. Turning the head almost into a lateral position, toward the tabletop, is recommended here.

Cervicothoracic Lateral

The cervicothoracic lateral is certainly one of the most challenging views to obtain, because the clavicles, the first pair of ribs, and the shoulders all superimpose the vertebrae of interest. There are two basic approaches to getting the shoulders out of the way: raising one arm and

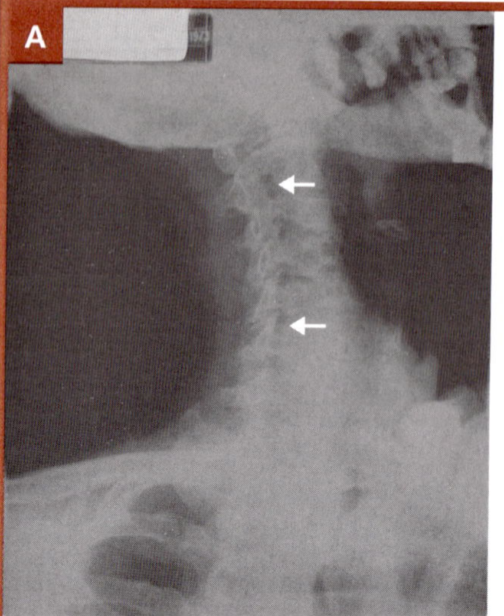

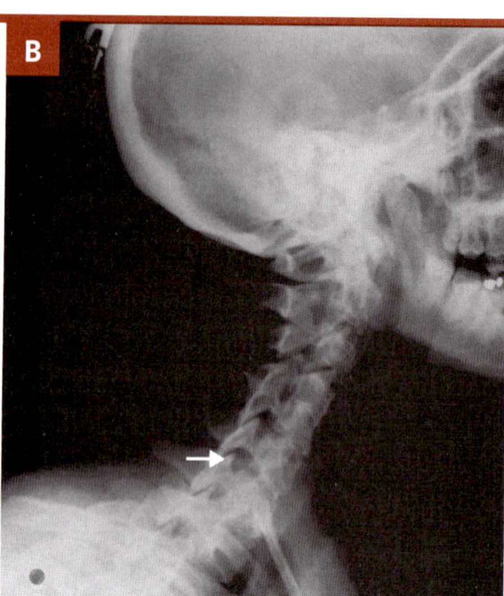

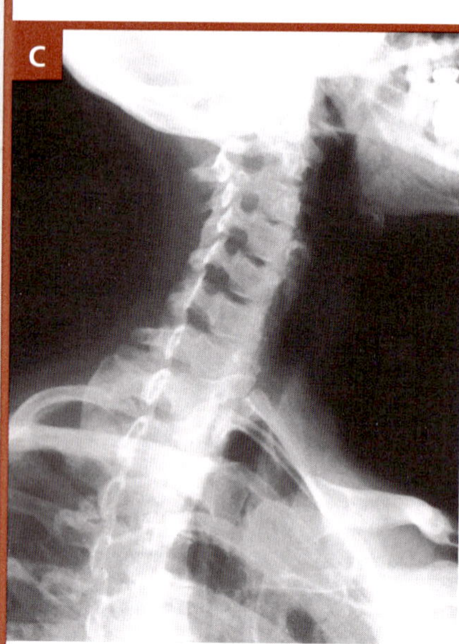

FIGURE 12-14

Oblique C-spines showing side-to-side narrowing of the intervertebral foramina (arrows), indicating significant rotation. Observe the patient's shoulders to determine whether the rotation is too steep or too shallow. In **A**, the body rotation is too shallow; in **B**, it is too steep. Proper opening of the intervertebral foramina is shown in **C** for comparison.

Carroll, Q. Evaluating Radiographs, 1993, Figure 119, Courtesy of Charles C Thomas, Publisher, Ltd., Springfield, Illinois.

lowering the other (the "swimmers" method), or pulling one arm back and the other forward (which we will here refer to as the "Twining" method). These two methods can also be combined. Which approach is best is controversial. Some textbooks do not even include the "pure" Twining method as it is presented here. We shall present radiographs of each, and let the reader judge which approach produces the best results.

In Figure 12-15, radiograph ***A*** is the pure "swimmer's" method and shows humeral head of the raised arm (arrow) superimposing the vertebral column. Radiograph ***B*** is a combined swimmer/twining method with the shoulders shifted forward and back (arrow) as well as up and down, better clearing C7, T1, and T2. The clavicles and the first pair of ribs cross over the vertebrae of interest, but you will note that this is true for *all* of these methods. At least the shoulders are completely removed from the vertebral column on this view.

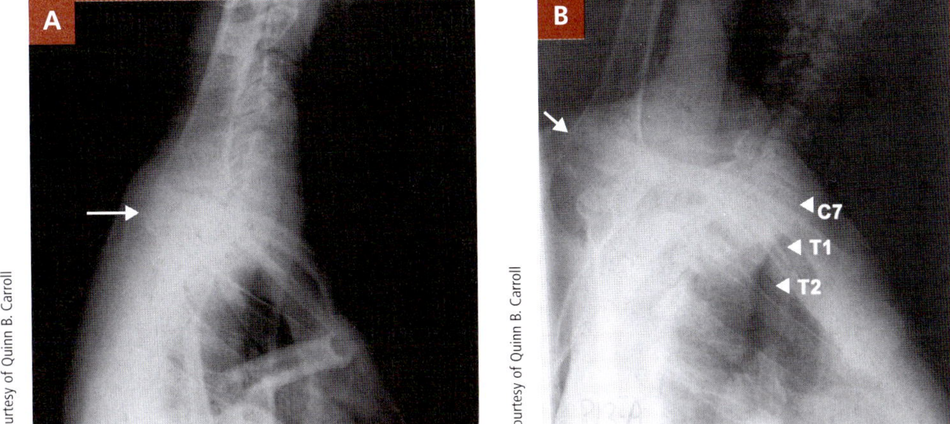

FIGURE 12-15

Cervicothoracic spine views: Radiograph **A** is the "swimmers" method with the raised arm (arrow) superimposing the vertebral column. Radiograph **B** is a combined swimmers/twining method with the shoulders shifted forward and back (arrow) as well as up and down, better clearing C7, T1, and T2.

Amazingly, the "Twining modification of the swimmers method" described in one textbook recommends pulling one shoulder forward, yet doing nothing with the opposite shoulder. Common sense would seem to indicate that if pulling one shoulder forward helps get it out of the way, pulling the other one *back* would also help!

The twining method is best done recumbent on the table, because the weight of the patient's body on the downside shoulder assists in pushing that shoulder up and forward. It is essential for this position that you begin with the patient in true lateral as if doing a lateral T-spine. Check the straightness of patient's back first. *Then* carefully, without rotating the patient out of lateral position, pull the downside arm straight forward, such that the shoulder *slips* forward. With practice, you will be surprised how far this shoulder can be displaced anteriorly without moving the torso out of lateral position. If the patient is able, have him place his upside hand on his hip and use the elbow for leverage. Finish by twisting the upside shoulder back as far as it will comfortably retract, again *without rotating the torso*. Center a 10- × 12-inch field to the upside coracoid process, in the "groove" directly anterior to the upside humeral head.

For patients who find protraction and retraction of the shoulders more difficult, *slight* rotation of the torso can be added to achieve the view, but with practice, you can radiograph most patients with the spine still in perfect lateral position as shown in Figure 12-16*A*.

Done correctly, on the twining view the heads of the two humeri (shoulders) will appear an inch or so to either side of the vertebrae, completely clearing them (Figure 12-16*A*). If the shoulders are shifted farther than this out to the sides, there is too much obliquity in the body. The key to this procedure is to place the body in true lateral position first, then twist the shoulders out of the way *without* rotating the body itself. If you skip this step, and the patient's shoulders are sloppily thrown into a steep oblique, the spine itself will not be lateral, as shown in Figure 12-16*B*.

Compare the combined swimmers/Twining view in Figure 12-15*B* with the "pure" twining view in Figure 12-16*A* and judge which best

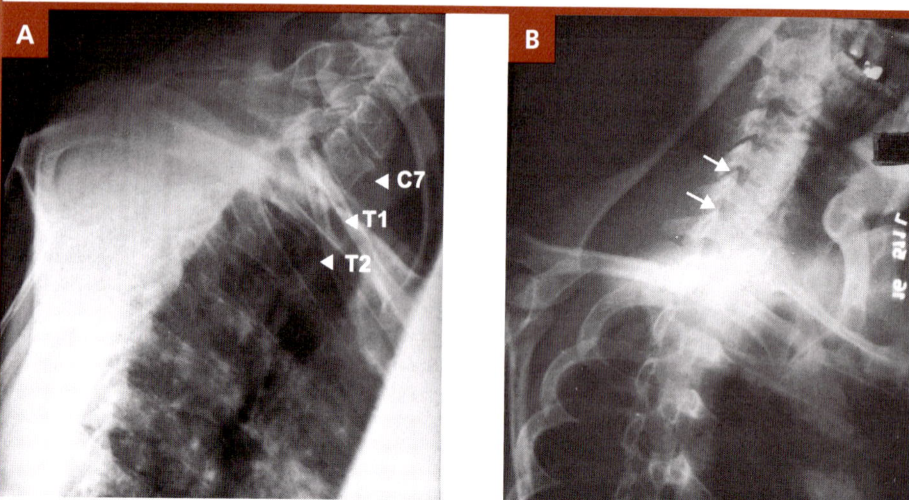

FIGURE 12-16

Cervicothoracic spine views: Radiograph **A** is a pure twining method in which the shoulders are only shifted forward and back, clearing C7, T1, and T2 well *without any rotation of the spine out of true lateral position.* Radiograph **B** was improperly positioned with the body so rotated that the cervical intervertebral foramina (arrows), normally seen only on oblique views, are opening up.

Carroll, Q. Evaluating Radiographs, 1993, Figure 121, Courtesy of Charles C Thomas, Publisher, Ltd., Springfield, Illinois.

demonstrates C7, T1, and T2. It does seem safe to conclude that whether the arms are raised and lowered or not, twisting the shoulders (protracting one and retracting the other) helps to better desuperimpose them from the vertebral column.

DIGITS, HAND, AND WRIST

PA and Oblique

Flexion of the fingers, on either the PA or the oblique view of the hand, closes the interphalangeal joints, as shown in Figure 12-17*A*. It is strongly recommended that obliques of the hand, whenever possible, be done with the patient's fingers fully extended. You can support them on a step-sponge or a 45° triangle sponge, in order to keep them parallel to the plate and open all interphalangeal joints as shown in Figure 12-17***B***.

With proper rotation for both the hand and the wrist, the oblique view will demonstrate the heads and the bases of the third, fourth, and fifth metacarpals overlapping each other, but *not* the shafts of these long bones. In Figure 12-17*A*, *the heads* of the metacarpals do not overlap each other, indicating very shallow (25°) rotation. On the other hand, when the *shafts* of the metacarpals overlap or come close to it, the rotation is too *steep* (Figure 12-17***B***).

The oblique wrist projection includes the bases and proximal shafts of these metacarpals, so they can also be used just as described here to determine whether the oblique wrist is rotated close to the required 45°, too shallow, or too steep.

Lateral

When the interphalangeal joints close off on lateral views, it is due to *tilt* of the respective fingers. For example, a common positioning mistake on the lateral view of the fourth digit, is to drop the tip of the

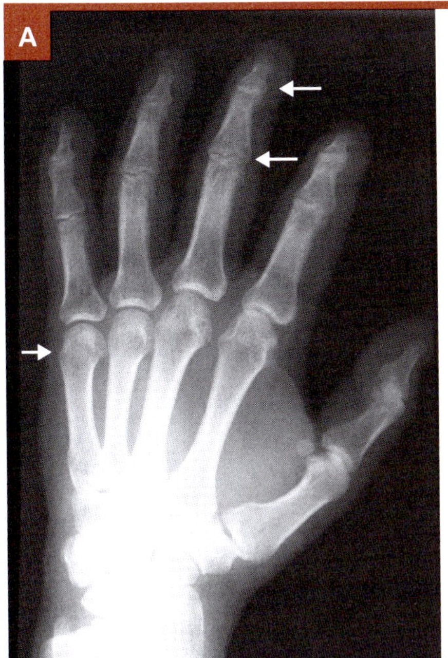

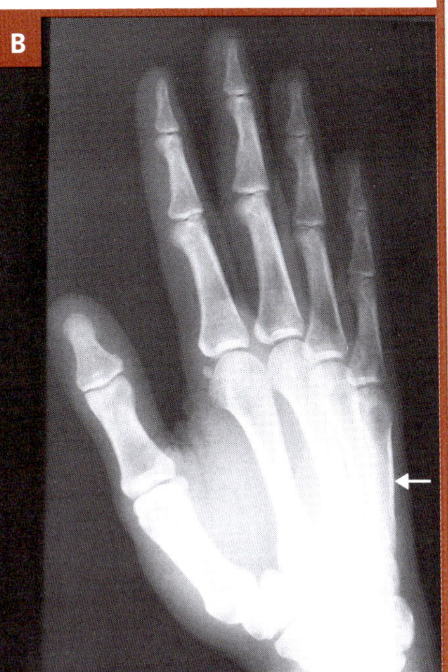

FIGURE 12-17

Oblique views of the hand showing **A**, improper flexion of the fingers with closed interphalangeal joints (upper two arrows). Radiograph **A** is also too shallow, because none of the heads (bottom arrow) of the third through fifth metacarpals overlap. **B** is too steep, because the shafts of the metacarpals begin to overlap (arrow).

Carroll, Q. Evaluating Radiographs, 1993, Figure 126, Courtesy of Charles C Thomas, Publisher, Ltd., Springfield, Illinois.

finger down onto the cassette in the interest of keeping the anatomy as close to the receptor as possible. As shown diagrammatically in Figure 12-18, this closes each interphalangeal joint by overlapping it with one of the condyles of the phalanx proximal to it. The proper position is to leave the fourth finger effectively "hanging" ½ inch or so above the film in order to keep it *parallel* to the film, so that the joints are kept open and there is no superimposition of the individual phalanges over one another.

Because the digits are of such small diameter, no shift rule of thumb presented in this book can be applied to quantify rotation and so on. Such quantification is not necessary in any practical sense. It is fairly simple to make corrections as described in the next section.

For lateral views of the hand or any of the fingers when the metacarpals are included within the visible field, you can easily identify the second metacarpal and digit by their proximity to the thumb, or the fifth metacarpal and digit because they are the smallest. Rotation with the second metacarpal approaching the thumb side is *pronation* rotation; with the fifth metacarpal approaching the thumbside, it is *supination* rotation.

Close examination of lateral hand and wrist radiographs will reveal that a true lateral position of the hand does *not* place the distal bones of the forearm directly over one another, as many technologists define a true lateral view of the wrist. That is, when the metacarpals of the hand are perfectly "stacked," the head of the ulna is found to lie somewhat posterior to the base of the radius, shown in Figure 12-19. To perfectly superimpose the distal radius and ulna for a lateral view of the

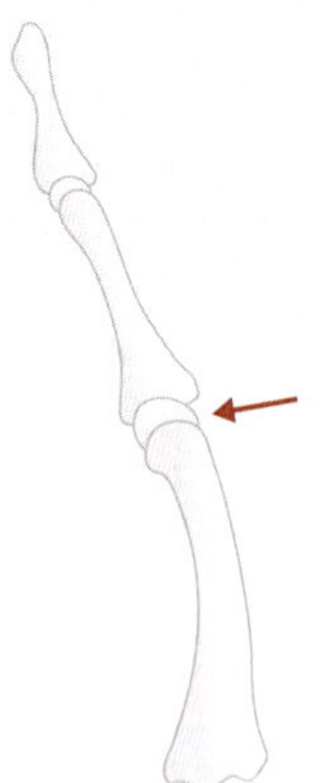

FIGURE 12-18

Diagram of the lateral fourth digit showing the appearance of improper tilt due to dropping the tip of the finger down to the IR plate. A phalangeal condyle (arrow) overlaps the joint space.

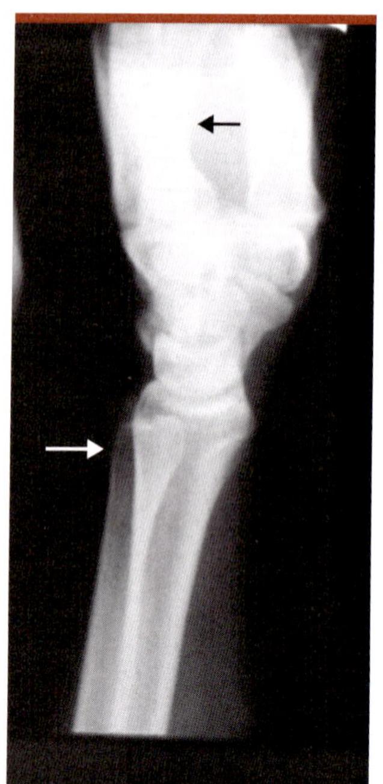

FIGURE 12-19

When the metacarpals of the lateral hand are superimposed (top arrow), note that the bones of the wrist are *not* (bottom arrow). Compare to Figure 12-18.

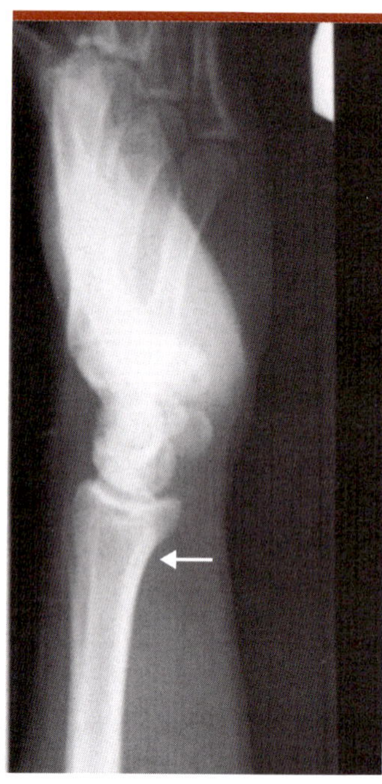

FIGURE 12-20

Slight 5° supination of the hand from lateral produces true lateral superimposition of the distal radius and ulna in the wrist (arrow).

Carroll, Q. Evaluating Radiographs, 1993, Figure 131, Courtesy of Charles C Thomas, Publisher, Ltd., Springfield, Illinois.

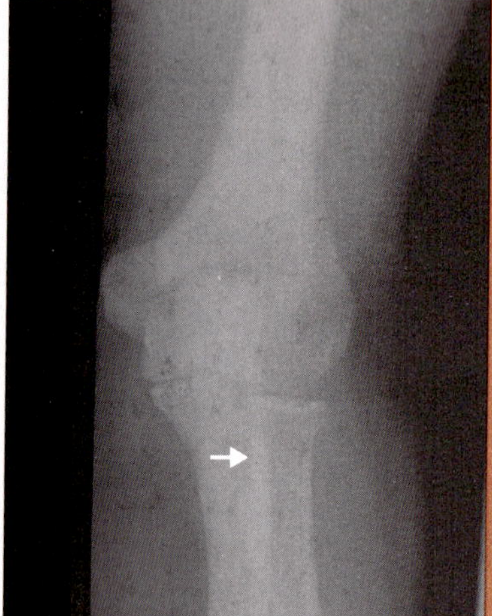

FIGURE 12-21

A true AP elbow shows one-quarter of the head of the radius overlapping the proximal ulna (arrow).

Carroll, Q. Evaluating Radiographs, 1993, Figure 134, Courtesy of Charles C Thomas, Publisher, Ltd., Springfield, Illinois.

wrist, the hand must be *supinated* 5° from its lateral position, shown in Figure 12-20. Thus, it is unrealistic to expect a lateral hand to also present the distal forearm in true lateral projection.

Lateral Hand and Digits

Like the obliques, you should perform projections of the lateral hand and digits with the digits all maintained parallel to the plate. This ensures the opening of all joints to rule out arthritis or other joint diseases, and it ensures that possible fractures at the distal or proximal ends of each phalanx are not obscured by superimposing bones.

ELBOW AND LONG BONES

AP and Obliques

In the elbow, there is no truly symmetrical anatomy that can be compared for evaluating rotation. The nonrotated AP shows a *fairly* symmetrical appearance to the condyles of the humerus, with about one-quarter of the head of the radius and radial tuberosity superimposing the proximal ulna (Figure 12-21). Internal rotation *increases* this overlap of the proximal radius and ulna, and external rotation *decreases* it.

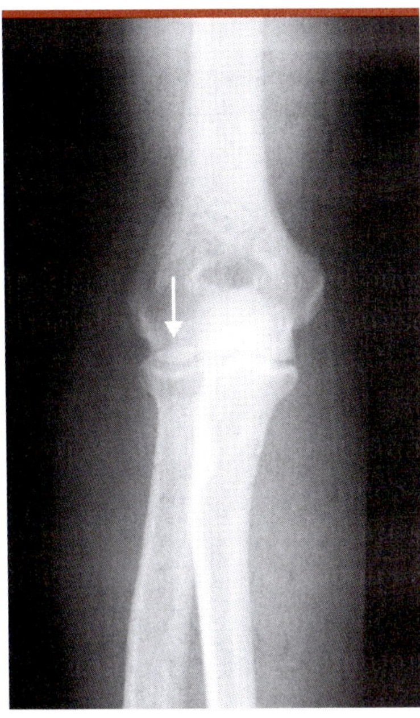

FIGURE 12-22

Flexion of the AP elbow overlaps the head of the radius and the capitellum (arrow).

Carroll, Q. Evaluating Radiographs, 1993, Figure 136, Courtesy of Charles C Thomas, Publisher, Ltd., Springfield, Illinois.

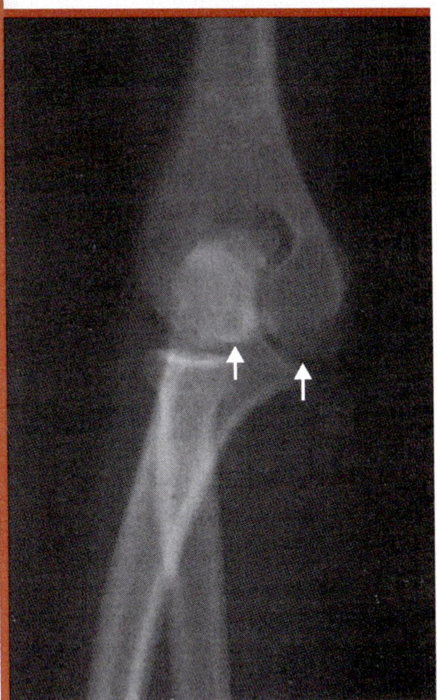

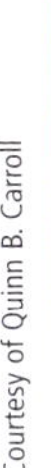

FIGURE 12-23

Proper internal rotation of the elbow shows ⅛-inch overlap of the two humeral condyles (arrows). This radiograph also shows how, on a rotated lateral elbow, the medial condyle of the humerus can be distinguished from the lateral condyle: The medial condyle (right arrow) is seen "locked into" the semilunar notch of the ulna.

Figure 12-21 also demonstrates the joint space between the head of the radius and the capitellum of the humerus opened as a narrow, but dark, space. Improper flexion of the elbow causes the head of the radius to overlap the capitellum of the humerus, shown in Figure 12-22.

A true 45° internal oblique of the elbow shows the two circular condyles of the humerus forming a nice "circle-eight" configuration with just ⅛ inch overlap of the two circles in the middle (Figure 12-23). The coronoid process of the ulna is in profile. A good *external* oblique of the elbow is judged by fully opening the proximal radioulnar joint as shown in Figure 12-24. This can often be achieved with 35° of external rotation, and it is not critical to twist the arm all the way outward to 45°.

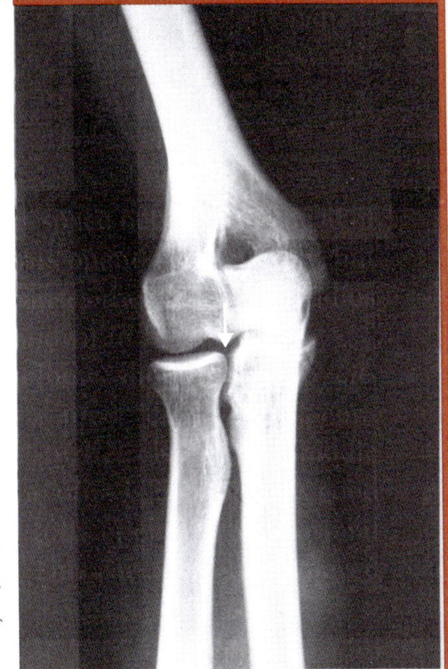

Courtesy of Quinn B. Carroll

FIGURE 12-24

Proper external rotation of the elbow shows full opening of the proximal radioulnar joint (arrow).

Lateral

When the elbow is bent such as for a lateral position, rotation is rarely a problem because the bending self-corrects any rotation as long as all of the arm is properly in contact with the tabletop or IR plate. This is true for the "sling" position or "arm-to-the-square" position of the humerus, as well as the routine lateral elbow. However, the internal rotation lateral position for the humerus with the elbow itself straightened is often difficult to achieve with no rotation. On this view, the two condyles of the distal humerus will show side-to-side shift instead of being superimposed, when rotation is present, as shown in Figure 12-23. You must identify which condyle is the lateral condyle and which is the medial in order to determine whether the arm was *over*rotated past lateral or *under*rotated. This is done as follows.

Determine which condyle lies directly above the disc-shaped head of the radius. The other condyle should appear "locked" into the semilunar notch of the ulna with its olecranon process wrapping right around it. See Figure 12-23 for example. The condyle associated with the head of the radius is the *lateral* condyle, and the one locked into the semilunar notch is the *medial* condyle. For the internal rotation position, on the radiograph, the two condyles should be directly on top of one another. If the *medial* condyle still lies medial to the lateral condyle to any degree, the arm has not been internally rotated enough. This is the most common rotation error for the internal rotation position. In rare cases, the *lateral* condyle will lie more medial, and this would indicate *over*rotation past lateral.

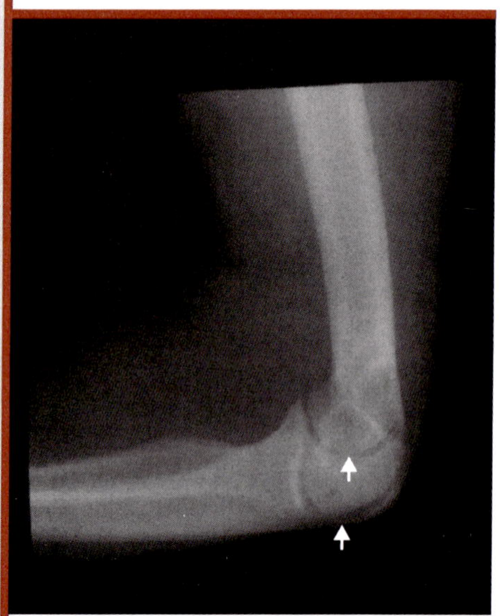

FIGURE 12-25

Lateral view of the elbow showing vertical desuperimposition of the humeral condyles (arrows). This tilt is indicative of not getting the patient's shoulder fully abducted (down to the level of the IR plate or tabletop.).

Carroll, Q. Evaluating Radiographs, 1993, Figure 139, Courtesy of Charles C Thomas, Publisher, Ltd., Springfield, Illinois.

For flexed-elbow laterals, as illustrated in Figure 12-25, by far the most common error is to leave the elbow *tilted* due to insufficient abduction at the shoulder. This is caused when the patient's shoulder is not brought down to the level of the table, so that the humerus slants downward to the table. This positioning error is diagnosed on the radiograph by *vertical* shifting of the two condyles. The solution is to bend the patient at the waist, or to raise the IR plate on a stack of sponges, until the humerus is horizontal along with the forearm.

SHOULDER GIRDLE

AP/PA Angled Clavicle

The purpose of an angle on any frontal projection of the clavicle is to project the entire clavicle above the scapula (or the scapula below the clavicle) for the clearest possible view. In Figure 12-26*A*, the superior angle of the scapula is still under part of the clavicle. Only a 15° angle was used, which is a common habit in spite of the recommendation by many textbooks to use 25°–30°, shown in Figure 12-26***B***. Follow the "textbook" method, especially if you have already obtained nonangled views as part of a routine.

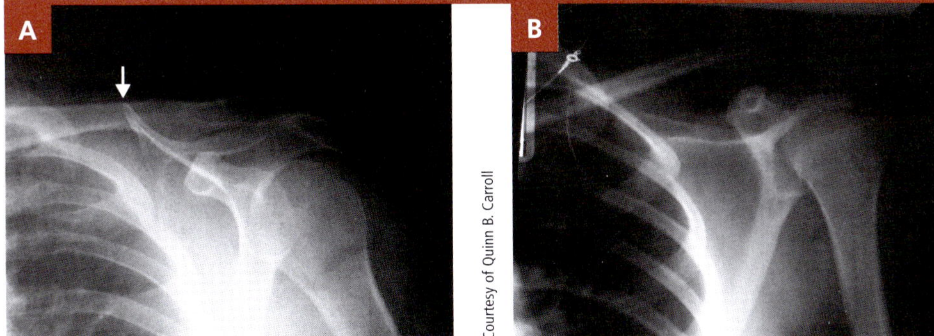

FIGURE 12-26

In Radiograph **A**, using a 15° cephalic angle, the superior angle of the scapula (arrow) still overlaps the clavicle. A 25°–30° cephalic angle is recommended for clavicles, shown in Radiograph **B**. (Both of these views are missing the sternal extremity and should be recentered.)

AP Shoulder/Humerus

As with the elbow, there is no bilaterally symmetrical anatomy that can be used to evaluate shoulder positions. We are reduced to identifying the ideal appearance of certain landmarks. The greater and lesser tuberosities are widely used. On the AP projection, the greater tuberosity should be in full profile on the outer corner of the humeral neck. There is also a distinct internal curvature only on the *medial* surface of the neck as it "turns" medially toward the scapula. There are rarely problems with this position.

Lateral Shoulder/Humerus

The traditional criterion for a good lateral view of the upper humerus has been to look for the *lesser* tuberosity to be in profile on the anterior surface of the bone. The lesser tuberosity can be very small and not always an obvious landmark. It is much easier to just examine the overall appearance of the neck area, which should appear to broaden symmetrically with the head of the humerus centered to it, as shown in Figure 12-27. This appearance is in opposition to the AP view, where the medial surface of the neck makes a distinct "turn" toward the body and the obvious greater tuberosity makes it nonsymmetrical. These criteria apply whether the lateral position was done by internal rotation, transaxillary, or transthoracic methods.

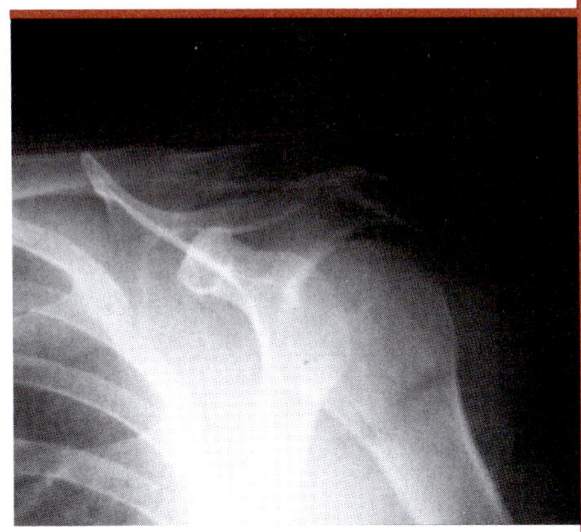

FIGURE 12-27

A true lateral of the head of the humerus shows a symmetrical appearance overall with the head centered relative to the shaft of the bone.

Lateral or "Y" Scapula

When the lateral scapula is correctly positioned perpendicular to the tabletop, a clear space can be seen on the radiograph between the rib cage and the scapula all the way along the blade of the scapula. This

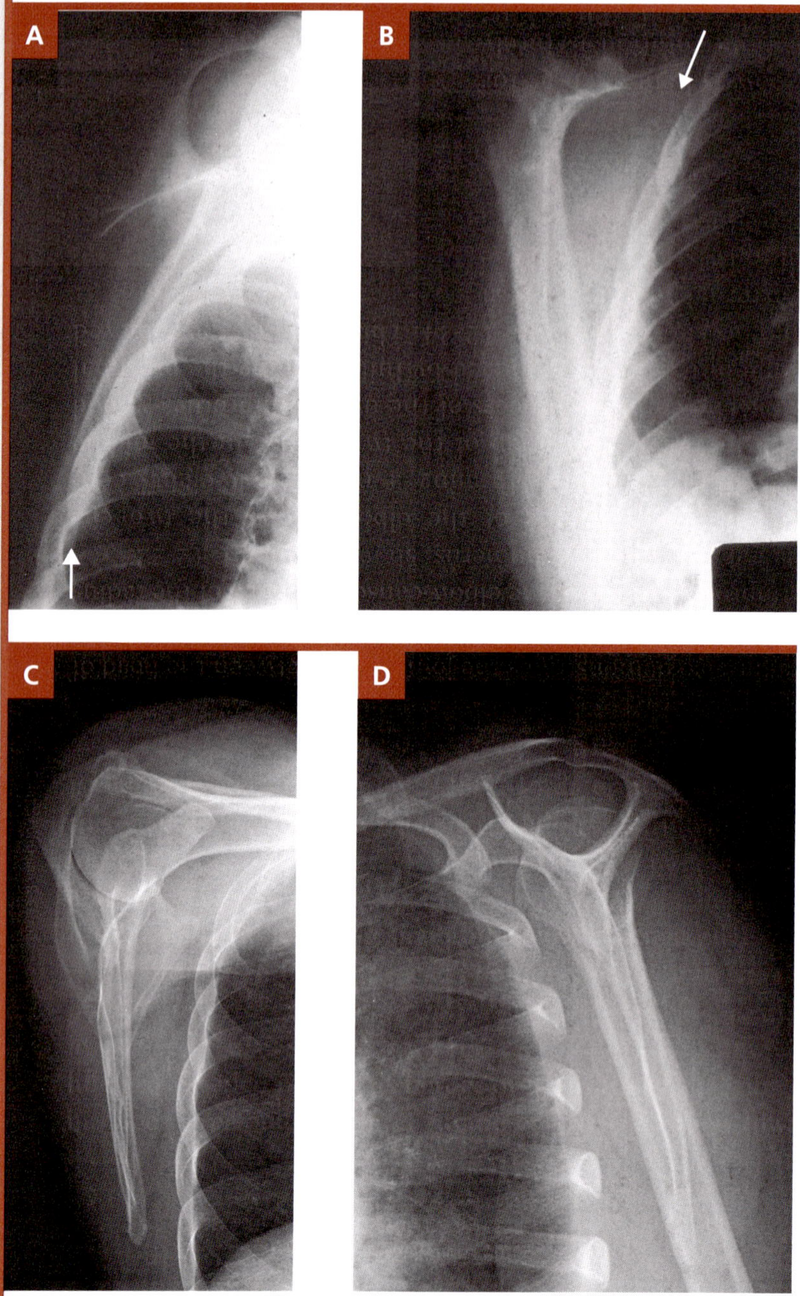

FIGURE 12-28

Lateral or "Y" views of the scapula showing **A**, the thicker lateral border (arrow) of the scapula running into the rib cage, indicating *over*rotation, and **B**, the thinner medial border (arrow) running into the rib cage, indicating *under*rotation. The lateral scapula in **C** and scapular "Y" view in **D** show the proper open subscapular space (arrow).

A & B: Carroll, Q. Evaluating Radiographs, 1993, Figure 144, Courtesy of Charles C Thomas, Publisher, Ltd., Springfield, Illinois.

C & D: Courtesy of Community Hospital of the Monterey Peninsula, Diagnostic and Interventional Radiology.

is demonstrated in Figure 12-28C. To determine whether rotation on this view is *over*rotation or *under*rotation, one must first identify the medial and lateral borders of the scapula. The lateral border is a thick and high-contrast ridge of bone, whereas the medial border is just a thin blade of bone with a smooth but low-contrast edge.

Figure 12-28 illustrates each border running into the rib cage from positioning errors: In radiograph A, the thicker lateral border is further identified by its association with the glenoid fossa and the head of the humerus nestled in it. This border overlaps the lateral ribs. The patient has been *over*rotated from a supine or prone position toward a lateral body position. That is, the body is too *steep*, having brought the lateral side of the scapula all the way up into a perpendicular position and then continuing to rotate on past that.

Radiograph **B** shows the thin, straight medial border that merges into the ribs at its lower half. This represents *under*rotation of the body. To correct it, roll the body into a slightly steeper obliquity. This will apply whether the anterior oblique or the posterior oblique position is used. Radiographs **C** and **D** demonstrate the proper degree of body rotation.

FOOT

AP

The purpose of the cephalic beam angle for the AP foot projection is to maximize desuperimposition of the tarsal bones as well as the phalanges by opening all of those joints that run *transversely* across the foot as shown in Figure 12-29. Even when an angle is utilized, it is frequently underestimated. The proper angle can range from 7°–15°, perpendicular to the arch of the foot, and when these joints are not open well, an *increased* angle is usually called for.

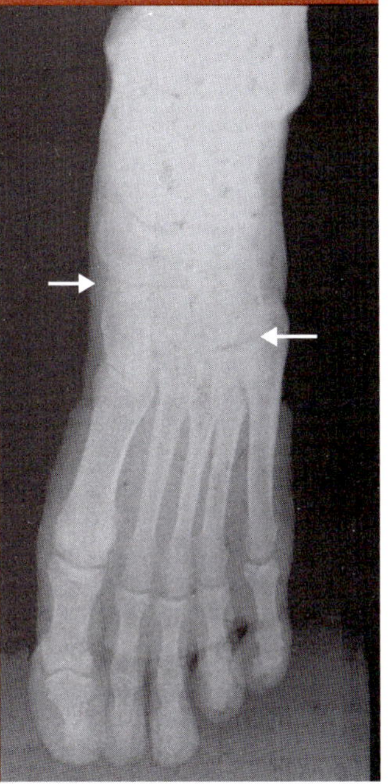

Courtesy of Quinn B. Carroll

FIGURE 12-29

On the AP foot, it is the transverse intertarsal joints (arrows) that a 7°–15° cephalic angle is designed to open.

Oblique

With the proper 30° of rotation, clear spaces should still exist between the *shafts* of the *second through the fifth* metatarsals (there will always be substantial overlapping of the first and second metatarsals). If none of the metatarsal *heads* overlap, the position is too shallow; if any of the second through the fifth metatarsal *shafts* overlap, the obliquity is too steep.

Lateral

The only reliable criterion for evaluating perfect rotation on the lateral view of the foot is evaluating the *heads* of the metatarsals, which should be stacked. In Figure 12-30A, the large head of the first metatarsal lies below the others, indicating *medial* rotation. To correct this, bring the

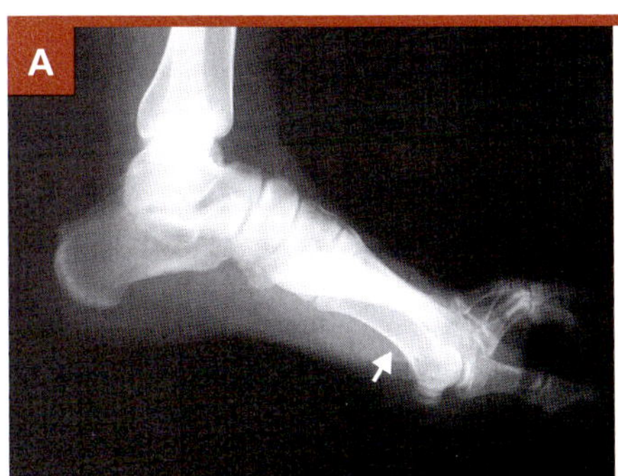

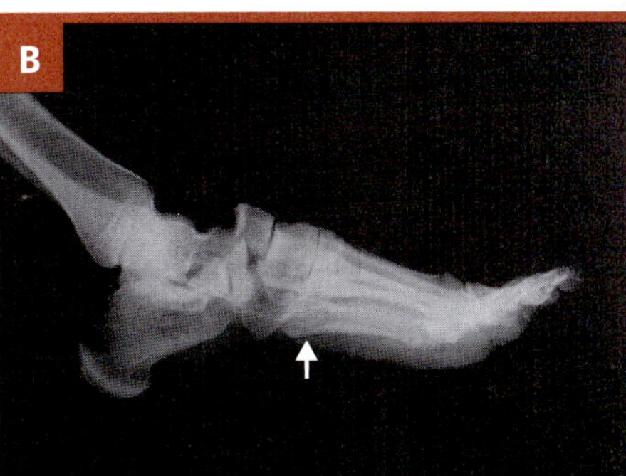

FIGURE 12-30

Lateral views of the foot showing **A**, *medial* rotation placing the thick first metatarsal lowest, and **B**, *lateral* rotation placing the fifth metatarsal lowest (this view also shows a subluxated talus from trauma).

Carroll, Q. Evaluating Radiographs, 1993, Figure 148B, Courtesy of Charles C Thomas, Publisher, Ltd., Springfield, Illinois.

knee down more toward the tabletop. When the fifth metatarsal, identifiable by the unique pointed "hook" at its base, lies below the others, *over*rotation past lateral is indicated (Figure 12-30*B*). Pull the knee up off of the table to correct it.

ANKLE

AP

The ankle is another joint, like the elbow and shoulder, that has no bilaterally symmetrical anatomy for comparison to determine rotation. But, a nonrotated position will demonstrate the joint space between the *medial malleolus* of the tibia and the *medial surface of the talus* opened up. (Do *not* confuse this joint with the talofibular joint, which lies laterally.) Approximately one-half of the width of the distal fibula will overlap the tibia. Lateral rotation is characterized by increasing overlap of the fibula and tibia, and medial rotation is characterized by decreasing overlap.

Oblique

Most routines designate the 15°–20° oblique position. This view is designed to open up the *distal tibiofibular joint* space as well as the space between the fibula and the talus, thus completely desuperimposing the distal fibula from the other bones. Either underrotation or overrotation will result in overlapping of the fibula and the tibia. However, these can be easily distinguished by observing the position of the *foot*, whether it continues almost straight downward (for *under*rotation) or veers off at an angle (for *over*rotation) medially.

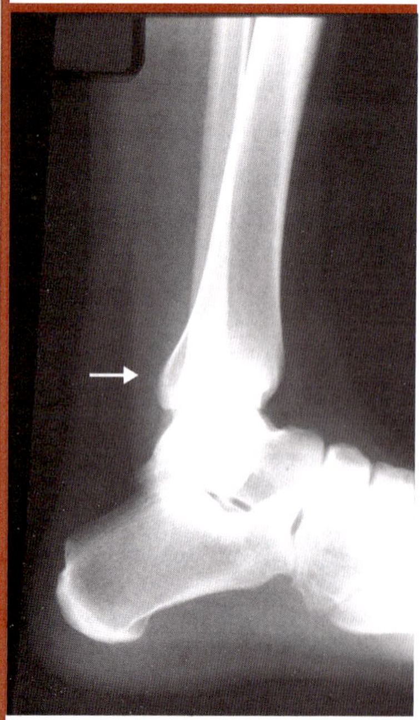

FIGURE 12-31

A proper lateral view of the ankle shows the distal fibula over the posterior one-half of the tibia (arrow). Anterior shift indicates *under*rotation of the leg, and posterior shift indicates *over*rotation.

Carroll, Q. Evaluating Radiographs, 1993, Figure 153, Courtesy of Charles C Thomas, Publisher, Ltd., Springfield, Illinois.

Lateral

In evaluating rotation on the lateral ankle view, observe only the distal-most portion of the fibula, (arrow on Figure 12-31), not the shaft. With proper rotation, the malleolus of the fibula should lie over the posterior *half* of the tibia, as shown in Figure 12-31. If *any* portion of the malleolus extends posterior to the tibia, *over*rotation is present. To correct it, twist the leg back medially so that the foot points slightly upward. Anterior shift of the distal fibula beyond the area shown in Figure 12-31 indicates *under*rotation of the leg downward toward the table.

KNEE AND LONG BONES

AP

On a nonrotated frontal view of the knee, the two tibial spines will appear nicely centered relative to the intercondylar groove of the femur above them, and the head of the fibula normally overlaps the tibia by ¼ to ⅜ inch. Medial rotation will move this overlapping portion of the head of the fibula (which lies *behind* the lateral tibia) laterally so there is less overlap. Lateral rotation will cause too much of the fibular head to overlap the tibia.

If the top surface of the medial tibial plateau overlaps the medial condyle of the *femur* to any degree, adjust the angle of the x-ray beam, most commonly by adding *cephalic* angulation. The best angle for the AP projection is controversial, and is highly dependent upon both the patient's body habitus (large torsos lift the femur up off the table, sloping the knee joint down more). It also depends upon whether the patient tends to force the knee down into a "locked" extended position or not. In some instances, a *caudal* angle is even indicated. Corrections in the beam angle are difficult to determine from the radiograph alone, and you must evaluate the result in the context of how the original position was performed. *However, most AP projections are improved with a 5° cephalic angle.*

Medial Oblique

This view is designed to desuperimpose the proximal fibula from the tibia, as indicated by a well-opened space at the proximal tibiofibular joint. Rotation either way will lead to superimposition of the fibula, but can be distinguished as insufficient rotation or overrotation by examining the relative position of the *patella* over the distal femur.

Lateral

To determine whether a poorly positioned lateral knee is rotated laterally or medially, there are three useful landmarks. *None* of these three landmarks is reliable for all cases, yet by using *all three* of them in combination, you can accurately assess rotation. The first is a small tubercle on the upper corner of the medial condyle of the femur (Figure 12-32). This positively identifies the condyle as the *medial* one. Unfortunately, the tubercle itself is only identifiable at certain degrees of knee rotation.

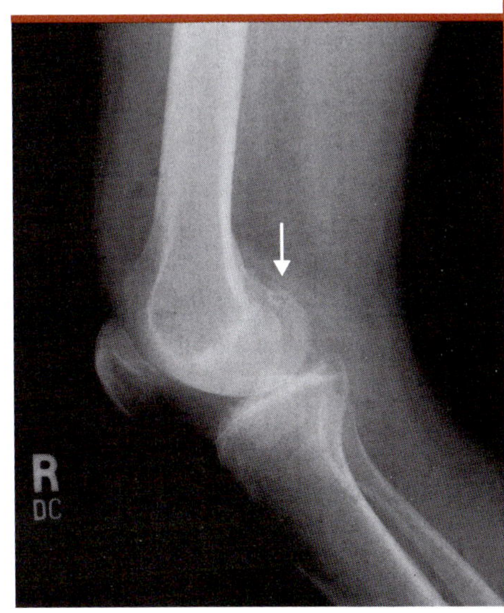

FIGURE 12-32

On a lateral knee view, the small tubercle (arrow) identifies the *medial* condyle, here lying posterior, which indicates *under*rotation. (Being the larger of the two, the *medial* condyle is also frequently projected as the *lower* of the two, but in this view a *proper* upward angle on the CR has cancelled out this effect.)

Carroll, Q. Evaluating Radiographs, 1993, Figure 158, Courtesy of Charles C Thomas, Publisher, Ltd., Springfield, Illinois.

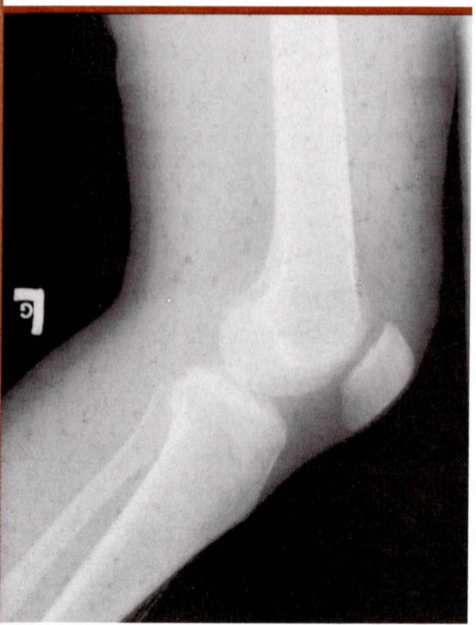

FIGURE 12-33

When the correct 5° cephalic angle is used to open the lateral knee joint, the medial condyle is projected up directly on top of the lateral condyle. Ironically, this makes it more difficult to distinguish which condyle is which. The angle should be used, nonetheless.

Carroll, Q. Evaluating Radiographs, 1993, Figure 158, Courtesy of Charles C Thomas, Publisher, Ltd., Springfield, Illinois.

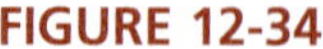

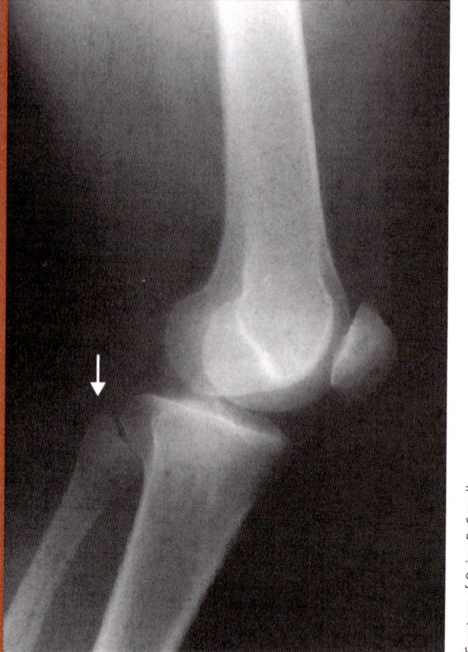

FIGURE 12-34

Overrotation of the lateral knee brings the head of the fibula (arrow) completely off the tibia posteriorly.

Courtesy of Quinn B. Carroll

Second, the femoral condyle that is projected *lower* is usually the *medial* condyle. The normal medial condyle is larger and anatomically extends lower than the lateral condyle. The 5° cephalic angle recommended by most textbooks for the lateral knee projection is designed to open the knee joint vertically as much as possible, by projecting the bottom surface of the medial condyle up in line with that of the lateral condyle (Figure 12-32). Ironically, when this is done perfectly, it then becomes impossible to determine which condyle *is* the medial one using this method. This is illustrated in Figure 12-33.

Once you identify the medial condyle using one of the preceding methods, if its posterior surface lies *behind* that of the lateral condyle, the knee is *medially* rotated. The correction for this is to roll the knee more downward toward the table. If the medial condyle lies *anterior* to the lateral condyle, the knee has been *over*-rotated past lateral, too far downward toward the table.

The third landmark that can be used is the amount of superimposition of the head of the fibula over the proximal tibia. The average amount of overlap for a nonrotated view is about ¼ to ⅜ inch. Overrotation laterally will bring the fibula completely off of the tibia, as shown in Figure 12-34. Enough medial rotation will bring the entire head of the fibula to overlap the tibia as in Figure 12-35.

As described earlier, to any degree that the medial condyle is seen *below* the lateral condyle, additional *cephalic* angle is needed to better open the knee joint. As discussed in Chapter 2, off-centering can cause the same effects as off-angling. For the lateral knee, this becomes an important consideration, because this projection is often centered *too high*. Radiographers tend to get into the habit of "eyeballing" the centering roughly at the crease of the knee or through the midpatella. The actual joint lies ½ inch or more below the lower edge of the patella. By centering 1–2 inches above the true joint, beam divergence projects the medial condyle back down over the joint. Therefore, centering high literally cancels out the 5° cephalic angle placed on the beam, defeating its purpose. Remember, for the cephalic angle to work, centering must be accurate and not too high.

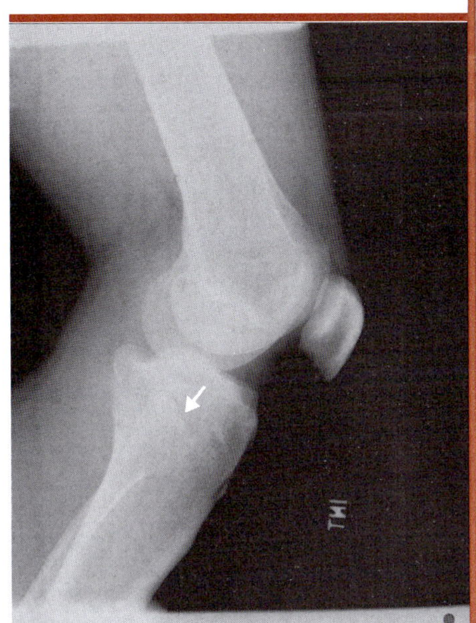

FIGURE 12-35

Underrotation of the lateral knee brings the *entire* head of the fibula (arrow) over the tibia. For most patients, only ¼ to ⅜ inch of the fibular head should overlap the tibia.

Carroll, Q. Evaluating Radiographs, 1993, Courtesy of Charles C Thomas, Publisher, Ltd., Springfield, Illinois.

Axial Patella

Figure 12-36, radiograph *A*, is an axial knee in which the rounded edge of the tibial plateau overlaps the patella and closes off the subpatellar joint space. If the Settegast ("sunrise") method was used for the projection, this would indicate that the beam was angled too much *upward* toward the ceiling (see Figure 12-37A), and therefore projected the tibia into the patella behind it. Radiograph ***B*** in Figure 12-36 shows the opposite effect when the beam is not angled upward enough (Figure 12-37*B*), so that it projects the patella into the femoral condyles behind it. The same type of reasoning can be applied to other axial methods including the Hughston method and the Merchant method. The key is to be able to identify which bone is superimposing the patella—the broadly rounded tibia, or the "M"-shaped condyles of the femur.

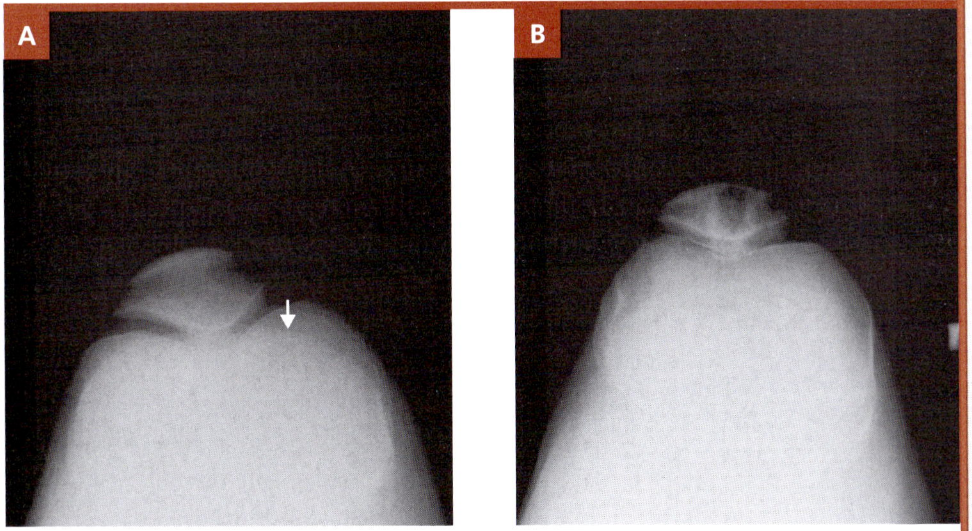

FIGURE 12-36

Axial views of the patella using the "sunrise" method shown in **A**, the tibial plateau (arrow) overlapping the patella, indicating overangulation upward, and **B**, the femoral condyles overlapping the patella, indicating underangulation.

Carroll, Q. Evaluating Radiographs, 1993, Figure 160, Courtesy of Charles C Thomas, Publisher, Ltd., Springfield, Illinois.

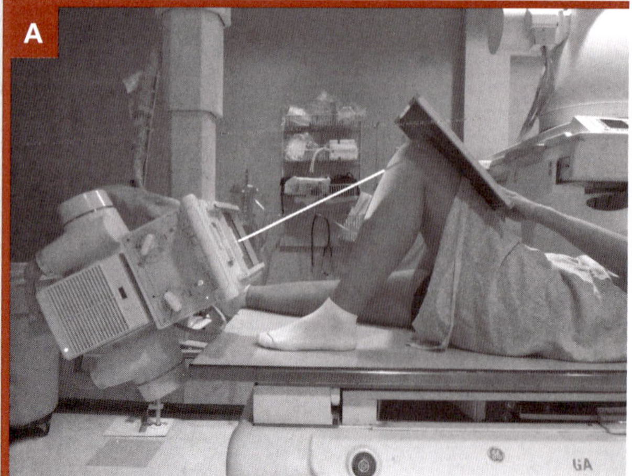

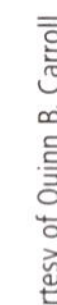

Courtesy of Quinn B. Carroll

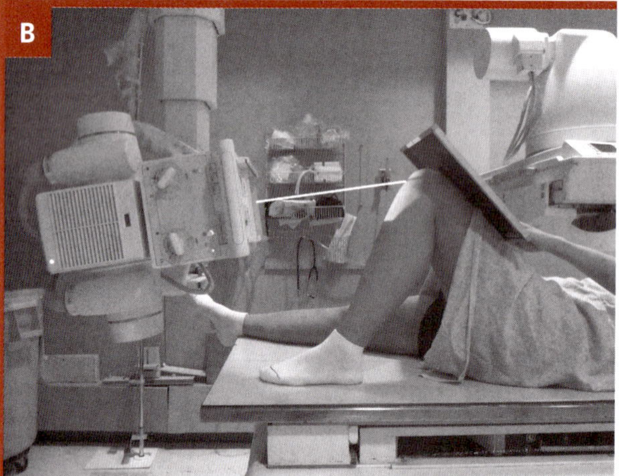

Courtesy of Quinn B. Carroll

FIGURE 12-37

Incorrect angles of the CR for the "sunrise" or Settegast method, resulting in the corresponding radiographs in Figure 12-36.

PELVIS AND HIPS

AP Pelvis

See the section on *Abdomen, Urinary and GI Systems, and Pelvis* near the beginning of this chapter.

AP Hips

The AP view of the hip with proper 15° internal rotation of the legs will demonstrate the lesser trochanter almost completely behind the shaft of the bone, and no portion of the greater trochanter overlaps the neck area. Failure to rotate the leg enough places the greater trochanter over the neck area, which is foreshortened as seen in Figure 12-38. The lesser trochanter is now protruding from the medial side of the upper shaft.

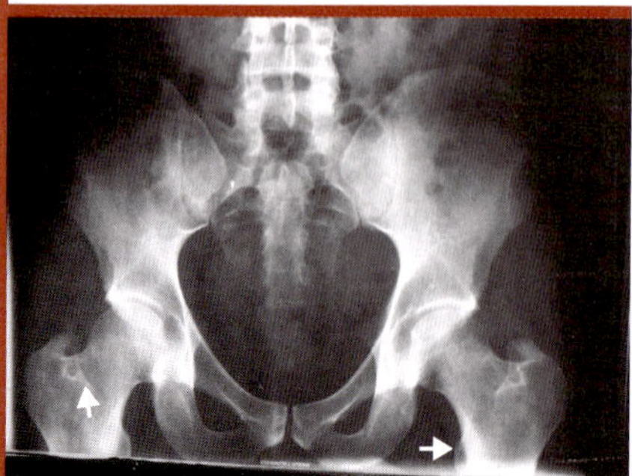

Courtesy of Quinn B. Carroll

FIGURE 12-38

On the AP pelvis, protrusion of the lesser trochanter (right arrow), and superimposition of the greater trochanter over the neck of the femur (left arrow), are indicative of failure to internally rotate the legs.

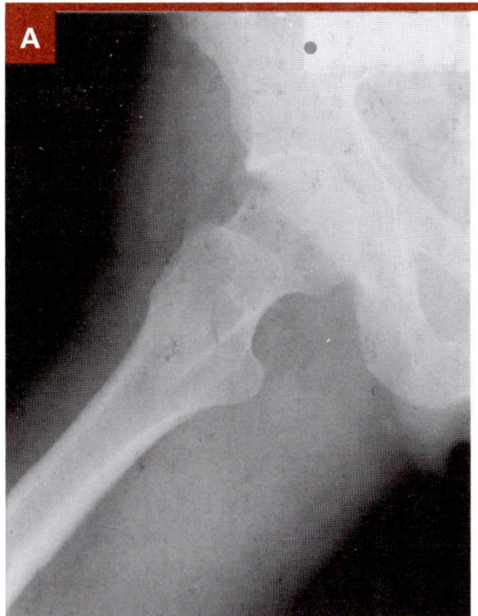

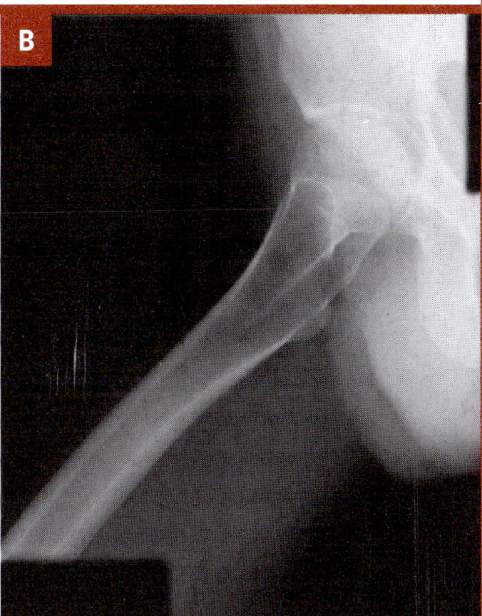

FIGURE 12-39

On a lateral view of the hip, a medially curved appearance to the femoral neck **A**, indicates insufficient lateral rotation. In true lateral **B**, there is a linear appearance with the greater trochanter centered over the femoral neck.

Carroll, Q. Evaluating Radiographs, 1993, Figure 165, Courtesy of Charles C Thomas, Publisher, Ltd., Springfield, Illinois.

Lateral

When the femur is rotated into a full, true lateral position, *whatever specific method is used*, the greater trochanter completely superimposes the femoral neck, centered along the shaft and over the head. The entire head, neck, and trochanter area appears linear (Figure 12-39*B*). With improper rotation, the neck area appears to curve toward the midline. In Figure 12-39*A*, there is insufficient lateral rotation of the thigh for a "frog"-type unilateral hip projection, and the neck appears to curve medially.

NOTE: Recall that on any AP projection of the hip, the leg must be internally rotated 15° in order to place the femoral neck parallel to the tabletop. *This principle should also apply to all* ***lateral*** *hip projections.* This means that for a groin lateral hip, *if* the leg can be rotated internally 15°, *it should be*. Of course, this will not be feasible when a hip fracture may be present. It also means that for the "frog" lateral hip, as the thigh is rolled out to the side, stop 15° *short* of bringing the knee all the way down into a lateral position. The knee should be 4 or 5 inches up off the tabletop.

Sacroiliac Joints

The objective of the oblique position for the SI joint is to open the joint, which lies at a 25°–30° obliquity, without superimposing the iliac crest over it (Figure 12-40*A*). Figure 12-40*B* shows a position that is too shallow, appearing nearly like an AP pelvis. With rotation too steep, the blade of the ilium comes over the joint as shown in Figure 12-40*C*.

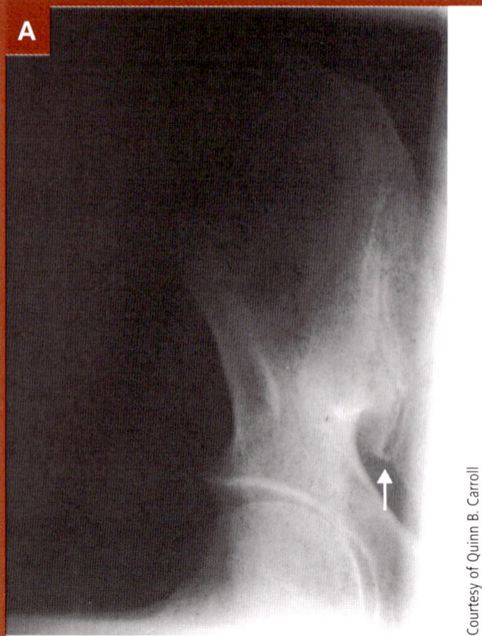

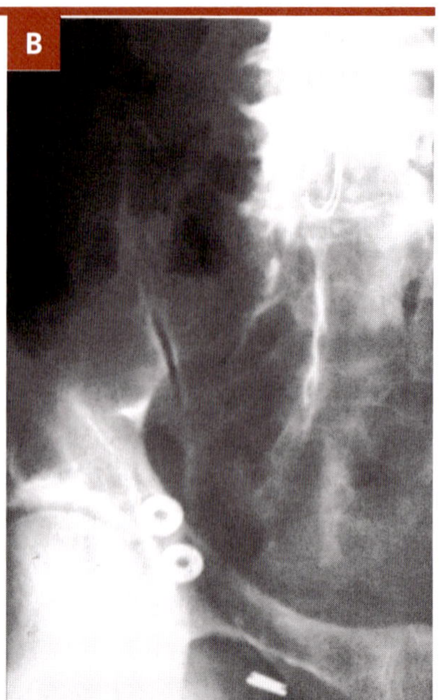

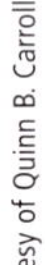

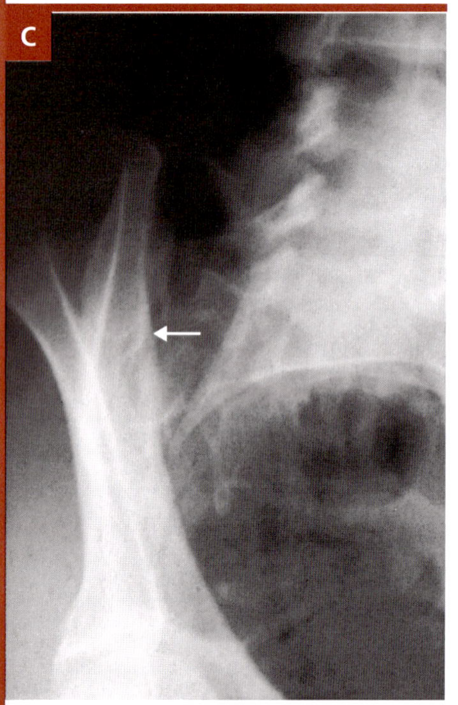

FIGURE 12-40

Oblique views for the sacroiliac joint showing **A**, correct opening of the joint (arrow) with a 25° oblique; **B**, shallow obliquity; and **C**, steep obliquity superimposing the blade of the ilium (arrow) over the joint.

BONY THORAX

Ribs

For a true 45° oblique position of the ribs above the diaphragm, the ribs on one side will be foreshortened to appear *one-half* as wide as the opposite side. If the foreshortened side is *less* than one-half as wide, then the body rotation is too *steep*. If it is *more* than one-half as wide, the position is too shallow.

Whether for anterior or posterior ribs, at least one view in the routine should show the rib without any portion overlapping the spine.

SKULL, SINUS, AND FACIAL BONE SURVEYS

Rules for Shift

You can *roughly* apply the general shift rule (every ½ inch of shift indicates about 5° of rotation, angle, etc.) to skull positions. We have discussed this elsewhere in this textbook. However, the average skull, measuring only 19 centimeters in AP, and only 15 cm in lateral, is somewhat smaller than the average torso (22 cm). This means that a smaller amount of shift will indicate a larger change in degrees. For the purpose of critiquing skull radiographs, high accuracy is needed. A more accurate version of the shift rule specific to skull positions is that *for skull radiographs, each* ***centimeter*** *of shift represents 6° of rotation, tilt, flexion, extension, or beam angle.* This rule will apply equally for frontal and lateral views of the skull. (It has been rounded between the 19-cm AP and the 15-cm lateral thicknesses for the skull.)

Now observe the diagram in Figure 12-41 illustrating these measurements as applied for flexion and extension (or equivalent angles) on *frontal* views of the skull. Note that the height of the orbit, indicated by the bracket, averages 4 centimeters. By then dividing the orbit into quarters, this gives us an extremely useful gauge by which to judge the degrees of movement or angle. *Each quarter of the orbit represents about 6° of rotation, tilt, flexion, extension, or beam angle.*

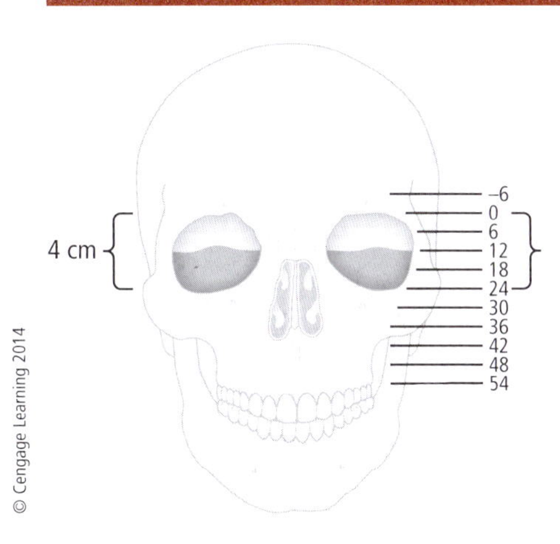

FIGURE 12-41

A scale for translating the position of the petrous ridges on frontal views of the skull into exact degrees of head flexion or extension, or CR angle. The orbits average 4 centimeters in height. Each "quarter orbit" or each centimeter of vertical shift in the petrous ridges represents 6° of movement or angle. These degrees of shift are measured from the roof of the orbit, where the petrous ridges are projected when the orbitomeatal line (OML) is at 0°, perpendicular to the tabletop. For PA projections, lower placement of the petrous ridges is due to head extension *or* to caudal angulation, and vice versa. This scale is applicable to Waters, Caldwell, and PA projections and all their modifications.

For skull radiographs, *each quarter of the orbit* (each centimeter of shift) represents 6° of rotation, tilt, flexion, extension, or beam angle.

The starting point for these measurements is the upper rim or "roof" of the orbit. Recall that for a PA skull projection, the petrous ridges should nearly "fill" the orbits, lying just under the orbital roofs. Correctly performed, this PA position places the orbitomeatal line (OML) *perpendicular* to the table, or at 0° of angle. This is then represented in Figure 12-41 by the "zero" mark placed at the level of the orbital roofs.

Note that in the same diagram in Figure 12-41 the petrous ridges have been sketched in at the level of the midorbits. This provides our first example in applying the skull shift rule: The petrous ridges lie halfway from the upper orbital rim to the lower rim; that is, *two-quarters* of the way, which translates into *12° of shift* (two sets of six). For a radiograph appearing this way, either the x-ray tube was angled 12° caudally, or the patient's chin was pulled up extending the orbitomeatal line 12°.

BEST PRACTICE TIP

For skull radiographs, *each quarter of the orbit* (each centimeter of shift) represents 6° of rotation, tilt, flexion, extension, or beam angle.

Let's practice a few other applications of Figure 12-41: When the petrous ridges are projected into the lower one-quarter of the orbit, they have been shifted "three-quarter orbits" downward, representing 18° of angle or extension. If they are projected right at the floor of the orbits, it represents 24° of angle or extension.

The exercise can be continued beyond the orbits themselves, using the "quarter-orbit" length as your gauge. If the petrous ridges are projected one "quarter orbit" *below* the floor of the orbits into the cheek bones, either the head was extended 30° (*five* sets of six), the CR was angled 30°, or some combination of the two (extension and angle) *totaled* 30°. Continue to the downward extreme on this scale in Figure 12-41, and note that it ends at 54° just above the upper teeth. This point is also just *below* the maxillary sinuses, and represents the position of the petrous ridges for a properly positioned *Waters* projection. Recall that the Waters position requires 53° of actual head extension (just 1° off from *nine* sets of six).

Finally, suppose the petrous ridges are projected 1 centimeter or one "quarter orbit" *above* the roofs of the orbits as shown in Figure 12-44, page 330. As indicated by the *minus* 6 on the scale in Figure 12-41, this would indicate 6° of head *flexion* or 6° of *cephalic* angulation.

You can also apply this scale, using "quarter orbits," to *rotation* on frontal skull views. For rotation, we have no "zero point" defined by where the petrous ridges or similar anatomy should lie relative to the orbits themselves. Nonetheless, the *scale* of measurement can still be used. For example, if the greater wings of the sphenoid bone lie one "quarter orbit" or 1 centimeter to the right of where they *should be*, it represents 6° of rotation to the right.

The scale can also be used for *lateral* skull views in a similar manner. For example, if, on a lateral skull view, the orbital plates of the frontal bone (roofs of the orbits) are shifted vertically off of each other by 1 centimeter, it represents 6° of *tilt*. Thus, in *all* of the criteria that follow in this unit for judging different skull positions, you can apply the rule of "*1 centimeter of shift (or one quarter orbit of shift), equals 6° of movement or angle*" for high-accuracy evaluation.

PA, Caldwell (PA Axial), and Waters (Parietoacanthial)

Chapter 9 explained how to select good anatomical criteria for evaluating positions on radiographs. We recommended that a pair of stable, bony landmarks be used that lie perpendicular to the direction of expected shift and are as far apart as possible from each other and from the midline. There are many pairs of bones in the skull that present bilaterally symmetrical landmarks, and you can be inventive. The following are just some examples.

Whenever the entire cranium is included in the view, a popular check for rotation is to observe the symmetry of the distances between the outer rims of the orbits and the sides of the cranial vault (Figure 12-42). The *foreshortened* side is the direction of rotation.

"Coned-down" views typically do not include the sides of the cranium, so you must find other criteria for evaluation of the position. The greater wings of the sphenoid, seen face-on within the orbits, form bony triangles that open downward and medially within each orbit. The lateral side of each triangle is actually the "temple" area on the side of the skull, the narrower portion just behind the orbits. It is formed by part of the greater sphenoid wing. Note in Figure 12-43 that this line combines with the lateral orbital rim to form a narrow "half-moon" or semilunar shape. A diagram is included to assist in identifying these "half-moon" shapes. The two "half-moons," right and left, should be symmetrical when no rotation is present, having an identical width side to side. When the head is rotated to the patient's right, the *right* half-moon expands in width, and the opposite one becomes more narrow. The direction of rotation is toward the half-moon that becomes wider. This method works extremely well on both Waters and Caldwell projections.

We can take this analysis of Figure 12-43 a bit further. The scale from Figure 12-41 allows us to quantify the rotation. The shift of the temples (greater wings of the sphenoid) is roughly ½ centimeter from where they should be if they were symmetrical. Using the scale of

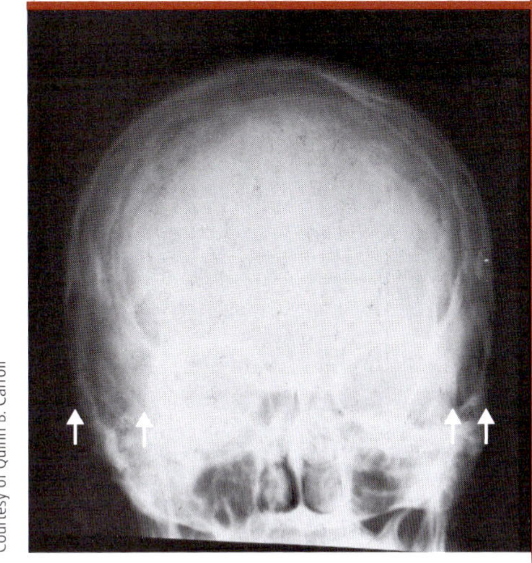
Courtesy of Quinn B. Carroll

FIGURE 12-42

On a frontal skull view, foreshortening of the distance between the outer rim of the orbit and the side of the cranial vault (arrows) indicates rotation *toward* that side.

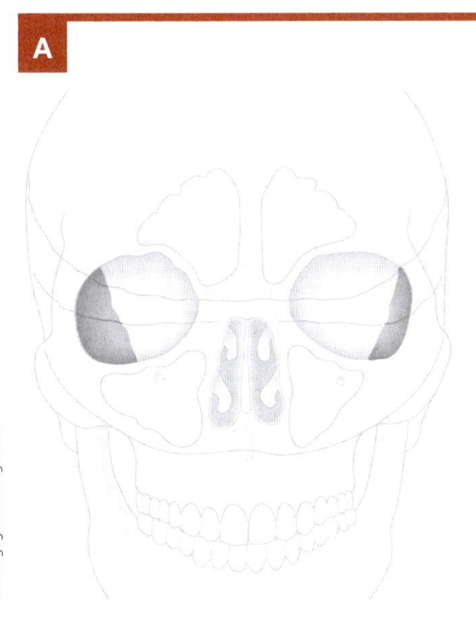

© Cengage Learning 2014

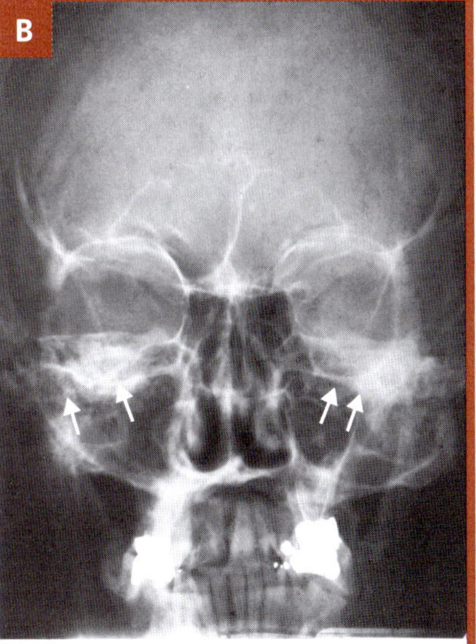

Courtesy of Quinn B. Carroll

FIGURE 12-43

On a "coned-down" frontal view in the skull, such as the Waters or Caldwell view, the "halfmoons" formed by the outer rims of the orbits and the temples (arrows) *expand* when the skull is rotated toward that side. The diagram **A** shows these "halfmoons" in bold for better identification in the radiograph **B**. The larger one, to the patient's right, indicates rotation to the right. Its shift is roughly ½ centimeter, indicating about 3° of rotation.

6° per centimeter, this indicates about 3° of rotation to the patient's right. By paradigm #20, were the shift any greater, the view would be repeatable—it is borderline.

An additional assessment for rotation is to observe the midline of the center of the chin or the nasal spine area (at the bottom of the nasal septum) to see if they are precisely centered in relation to the mandibular rami to either side. With rotation to the patient's right, these anterior midline landmarks will shift to the right, foreshortening the observed distance to the ramus of the mandible on the right side.

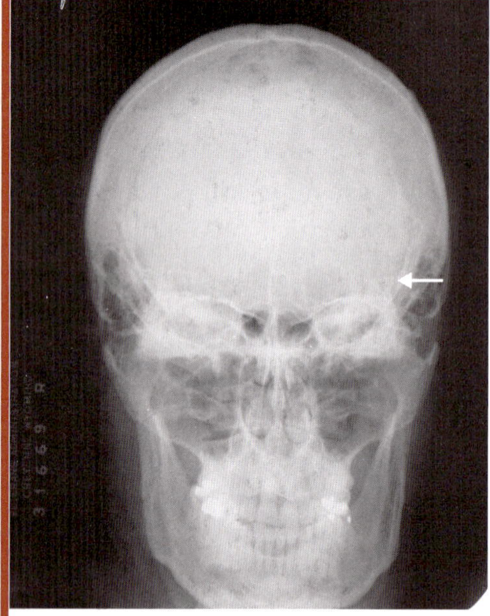

FIGURE 12-44

PA skull view showing petrous ridges (arrow) more than 1 centimeter above the orbits, indicating more than 6° of head flexion (or cephalic angulation).

Carroll, Q. Evaluating Radiographs, 1993, Figure 168, Courtesy of Charles C Thomas, Publisher, Ltd., Springfield, Illinois.

For the evaluation of proper flexion/extension of the skull, and of proper CR angulation, the vertical position of the petrous ridges can be universally used on all of these frontal views. For the PA skull, the petrous ridges should nearly "fill" the orbits, lying just under their superior rims. For the Caldwell projection, the ridges should fall in the lower one-third of the orbits. (Note that on the scale in Figure 12-41, this placement fits perfectly between 12° and 18°, which would fall in the midorbit and the lower one-quarter orbit, respectively.) For the Waters view, the petrous ridges should be projected just below the floors of the maxillary sinuses, passing through the maxillary molar teeth.

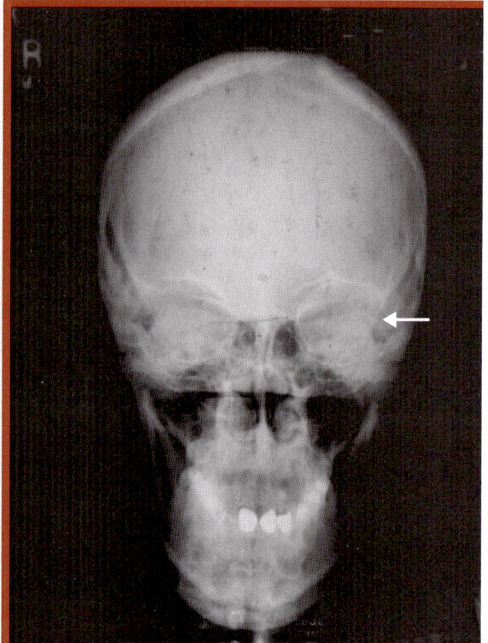

FIGURE 12-45

Caldwell skull view showing petrous ridges (arrow) in midorbits, equivalent to 12° of caudal angle by Figure 12-41. If a 15° caudal angle was used, the head must have been slightly overflexed (3°), cancelling out some of the angle.

Courtesy of Quinn B. Carroll

Figures 12-44, 12-45, 12-46, and 12-47 present a series of radiographs illustrating how the shift rule presented in Figure 12-41 can be used to great advantage. Figure 12-44 is an attempted PA skull in which the petrous ridges are seen about 1 centimeter *above* the orbits. To bring them back down, the chin must be raised at least 6° (or the x-ray beam must be angled *caudally* 6°). Figure 12-45 is an attempted Caldwell projection.

The ridges are seen right through the middle of the orbits. If a true 15° caudal angle was used, then for the ridges to be too high in the orbit, the patient's chin must have been *overflexed* downward by 3°. This would cancel out 3° of the 15° of angle, placing the ridges at midorbit for a net 12° as shown in Figure 12-41. The chin should be pulled back up slightly to correct the position.

On the other hand, if the head in Figure 12-45 had been perfectly positioned, then the CR angle must have been only 12° caudal, 3° short of what was needed.

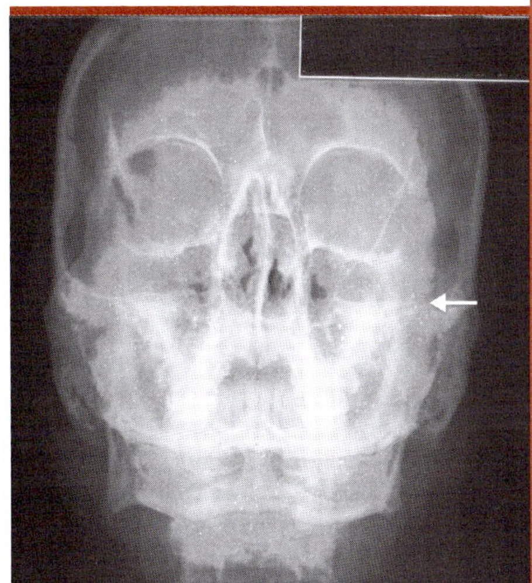

Courtesy of Quinn B. Carroll

FIGURE 12-46

Waters sinus view with the head only extended about 36° (see Figure 12-41), placing the petrous ridges through the middle of the maxillary sinuses. If the chin cannot be lifted further, a caudal angle of 17° should be added upon repeating the exposure for a total of 53°.

Figure 12-46 is a Waters projection with the petrous ridges projected right through the middle of the maxillary sinuses (the anatomy of interest). From the scale in Figure 12-41, we conclude that the patient's head was extended only 36°. The needed extension for a Waters position is 53°. If the chin cannot be lifted further, a *caudal* angle of 17° must be used to see the floor of the sinuses.

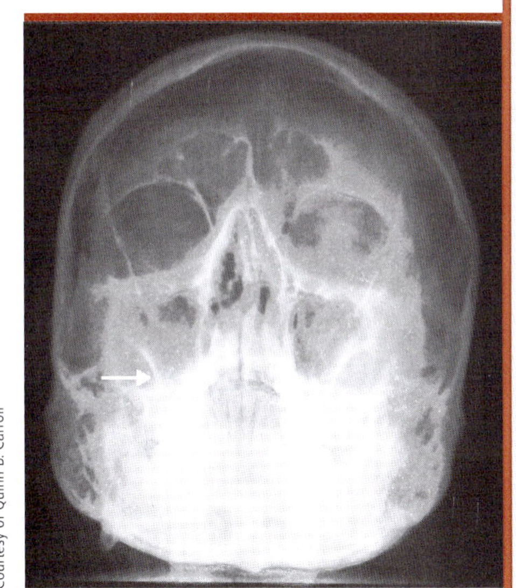

Courtesy of Quinn B. Carroll

FIGURE 12-47

A very common problem for the Waters sinus view: With the patient's chin as far up as he can stand, the petrous ridges (arrow) are still obscuring the floor of the sinuses. By Figure 12-41, this represents 47°–48° of head extension. A 4°–5° caudal angle will correct this *and still be close enough to horizontal to demonstrate fluid levels.*

Figure 12-47 is a very common situation for the Waters projection: With the patient's chin as far up as he can tolerate, the petrous ridges are still obscuring the floor of the sinuses. A 4°–5° caudal angle will correct this *and still be close enough to horizontal to demonstrate fluid levels.*

Lateral

For evaluating rotation on lateral views of the skull, sinuses, or facial bones, we strongly recommend observing the posterior edges of the two mandibular rami, as shown in Figures 11-9 and 11-13 in Chapter 11. These are also shown here by the large arrows in Figure 12-48. When the rami are difficult to see, or when they are not included in a "coned-down" view, the greater wings of the sphenoid bone are the next-best anatomy to use. These show up as reversed "C' shapes extending downward from the orbital plates about 1 inch

FIGURE 12-48

Use of the greater wings of the sphenoid bone (upper arrows) and the rami of the mandible (lower arrows) in determining rotation on a lateral skull view. The arrows indicate in **A**, the *downside* structures; in **B**, the *upside* structures; and **C** is presented as a clear view for practice identifying these structures. In **B**, both the greater wing and the mandibular ramus appear more blurry, although it is less obvious for the ramus. Therefore these are the *upside* structures. If the projection is a left lateral skull, then the upside is the patient's right side, which is shifted anteriorly here. The patient's head is rotated toward the *left*.

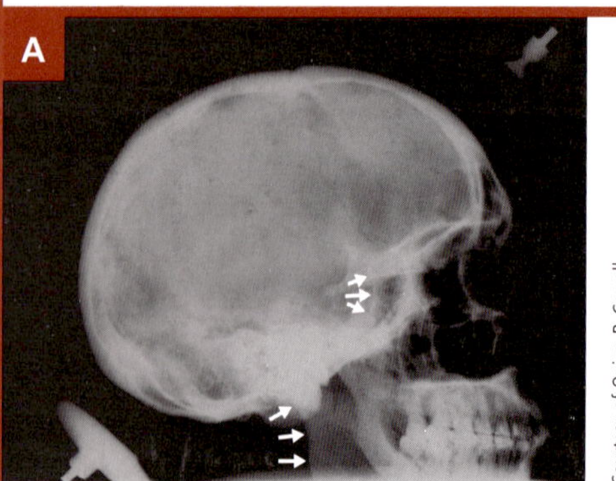

Courtesy of Quinn B. Carroll

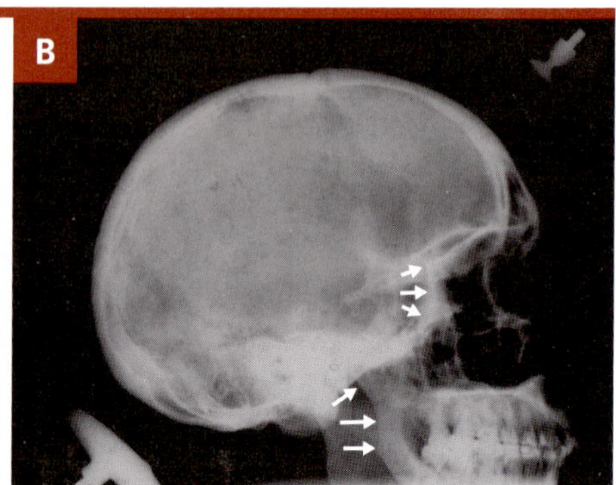

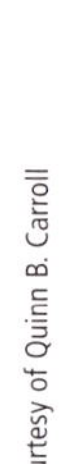

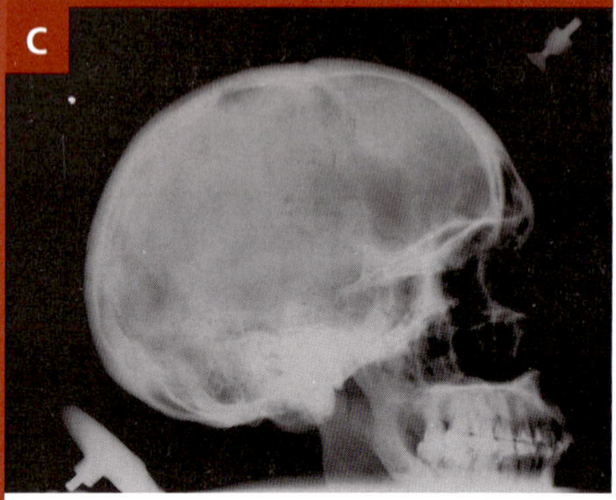

Courtesy of Quinn B. Carroll

anterior to the sella turcica. They are pointed out by the smaller arrows in Figure 12-48*A* and *B*.

To determine *which way* the skull is rotated, you must identify which of the mandibular rami or greater wings is the *upside* one. This can only be done by comparing the degree of magnification and blurriness present. In Figure 12-48, magnification of the mandibular rami, TMJs, and greater sphenoid wings is difficult to assess, but you can see the difference in *sharpness* with careful scrutiny. For clarity, three versions of this view are presented: In *A*, the *downside* greater wing and mandibular ramus are indicated with arrows; in **B**, the *upside* greater wing and ramus are indicated with arrows; and **C** is presented without arrows obscuring any anatomy so you can practice identifying these structures. Notice in *B* that the greater wing shifted anteriorly is visibly more blurred than the one in *A*. The same is true for the mandibular ramus in *B*, though it is less apparent. Therefore, these two structures shifted anteriorly in *B* are the *upside* structures. If the projection is a left lateral skull, then the upside is the patient's *right* side, which is shifting forward. Therefore, the patient's head is being turned toward the *left*.

For Figures 12-49 and 12-50, which demonstrate how to assess the *amount* of rotation and tilt in a lateral skull projection, a phantom skull was carefully positioned and a protractor was used to actually measure the degrees of rotation or tilt. This was done for precision.

Courtesy of Quinn B. Carroll

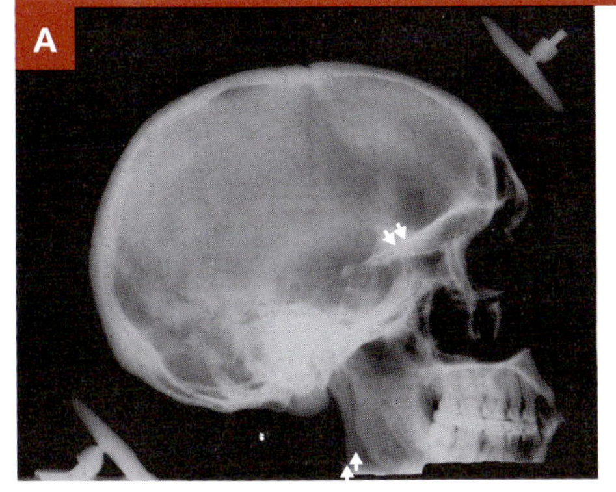

Courtesy of Quinn B. Carroll

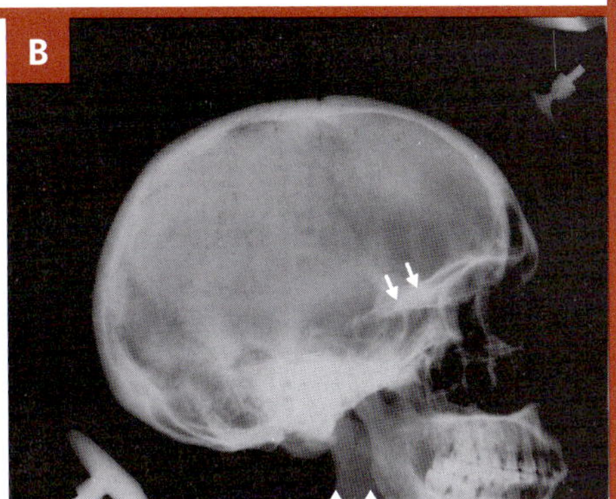

Courtesy of Quinn B. Carroll

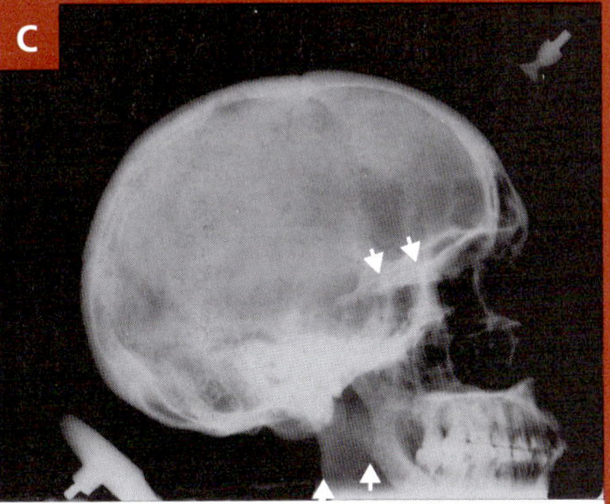

FIGURE 12-49

Lateral skull views showing the amount of horizontal shift caused by rotation: In Radiograph **A**, the rami of the mandible (large arrows at the very bottom) show only slight horizontal shift, indicating only slight rotation. The orbital plates (small arrows) show no vertical shift, indicating no tilt. Radiograph **A** is a nearly perfect lateral skull view. Radiograph **B** shows slightly more than 1 centimeter of horizontal shift in the mandibular rami as well as the greater wings—the skull was rotated 7°. Radiograph **C** demonstrates 2 centimeters of shift—the skull was rotated 12°.

Courtesy of Quinn B. Carroll

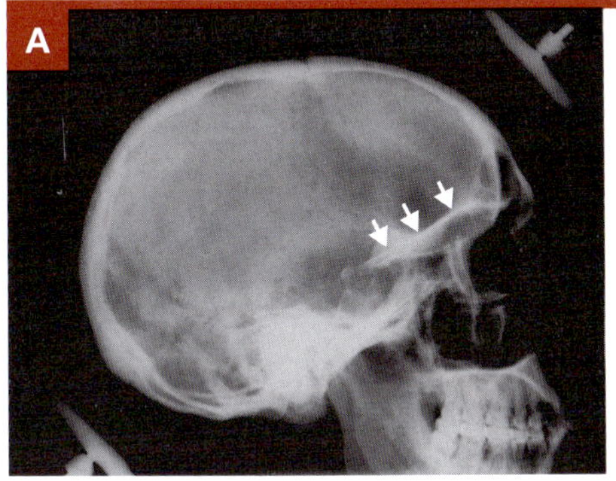

Courtesy of Quinn B. Carroll

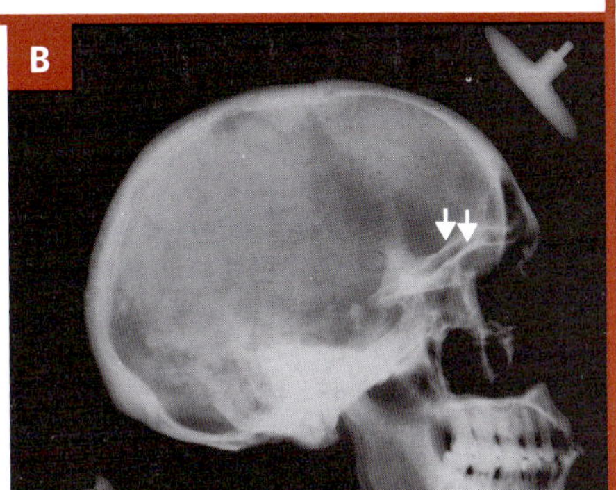

Courtesy of Quinn B. Carroll

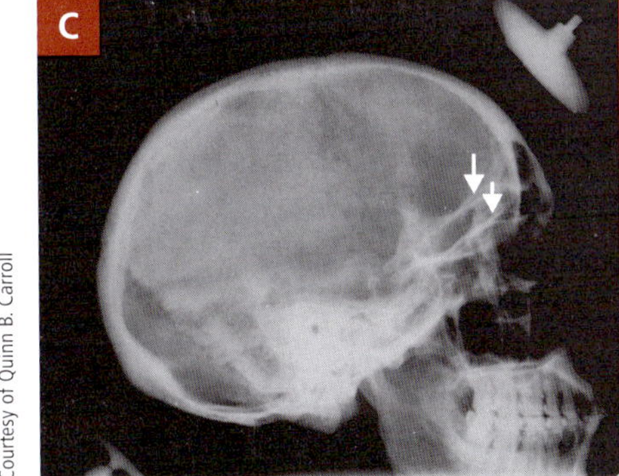

FIGURE 12-50

Lateral skull views demonstrating the amount of vertical shift caused by tilt. Radiograph **A** has no tilt present, and the orbital plates (arrows) are directly superimposed. Radiograph **B** shows 1 centimeter of vertical shift between the two orbital plates—the skull was tilted 6°. Radiograph **C** shows slightly less than 2 centimeters of shift in the orbital plates—the skull was tilted 10°.

You can use the general shift rule for rough estimation in skull positions, but for precision in the following examples, we will apply the specific rule for skulls presented in this chapter: *Each* ***centimeter*** *of side-to-side shift in the mandibular rami or greater wings represents 6° of rotation.*

Figure 12-49 is an exercise in determining the amount of rotation for a lateral skull view. In Figure 12-49***B***, both the mandibular rami and the greater wings show slightly more than 1 centimeter of horizontal shift—the skull was rotated about 7°. Radiograph **C** demonstrates 2 centimeters of shift between the two rami and the two greater wings—the skull was rotated 12°.

Tilt of the skull is best evaluated by examining the *orbital plates* of the frontal bone, as shown in Figure 12-50. Every centimeter of shift indicates 6° of tilt. The more blurry plate is the upside. Radiograph ***B*** shows 1 centimeter of vertical shift between the orbital plates—the skull was tilted 6°. Radiograph **C** shows slightly less than 2 centimeters of shift in the orbital plates—the skull was tilted 10°.

Townes (AP Axial)

When the proper CR angle is combined with correct flexion/extension of the head for the Townes projection of the skull, the sella turcica should be projected right into the foramen magnum behind it. The sella possesses low contrast and can be difficult to see, so Figure 12-51 includes a clear view, ***A***, and an identical view with an arrow pointing out the sella, ***B***. Note too, that three-quarters of the foramen magnum is visible above the junction of the petrous pyramids in the centerline. Insufficient angulation of the CR results in only a small portion of the foramen magnum appearing above this junction (Figure 12-52*A*), while excessive angulation causes the

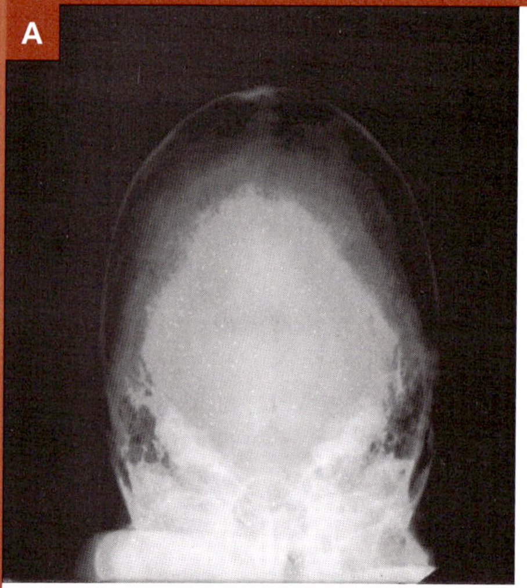

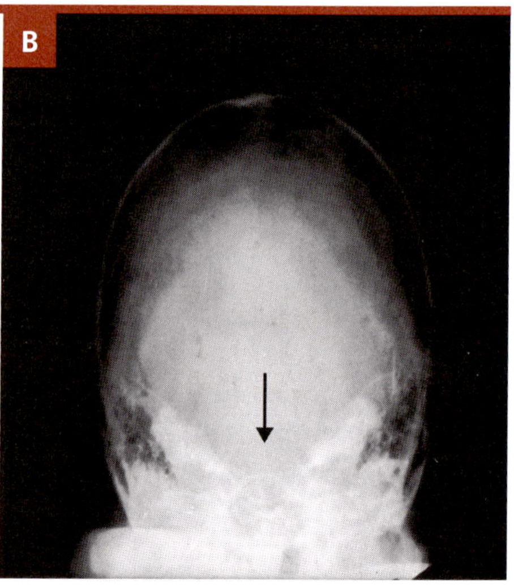

FIGURE 12-51

Proper Townes view of the skull, demonstrating three-fourths of the foramen magnum above the centerline junction of the petrous pyramids with the sella turcica (arrow in **B**) framed within the foramen. **A** is presented for a more clear view of this low-contrast structure.

Carroll, Q. Evaluating Radiographs, 1993, Figure 176, Courtesy of Charles C Thomas, Publisher, Ltd., Springfield, Illinois.

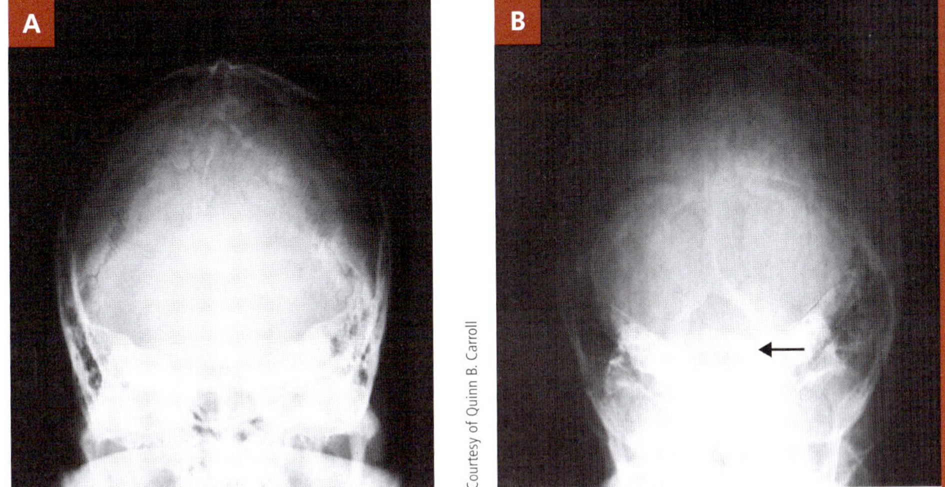

FIGURE 12-52

On the Townes view, underangulation of the CR (or extension of the skull) **A**, results in only a small portion of the foramen magnum rising above the centerline junction of the petrous pyramids, while overangulation of the CR results in the ring-shaped posterior arch of C1 appearing within the foramen **B**.

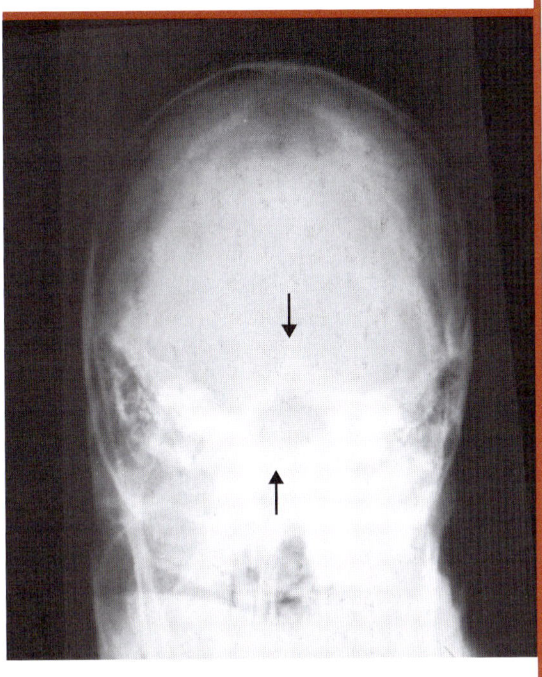

FIGURE 12-53

A Townes view demonstrating slight rotation of the skull. The right and left petrous pyramids are not symmetrical in appearance, and the centerline junction of the petrous pyramids (lower arrow) is shifted in the direction of rotation compared to the midline ridge of the occipital bone (upper arrow).

ring-shaped posterior arch of cervical vertebra #1 to appear within the foramen (Figure 12-52*B*).

A Townes view with rotation of the head is demonstrated in Figure 12-53. Rotation can be judged by the asymmetrical appearance of the petrous pyramids, as well as off-centering between the midline ridge of the occipital bone (upper arrow) and the midjunction of the petrous pyramids (lower arrow). The side toward which the junction of the petrous pyramids shifts relative to the foramen magnum and occipital bone is the direction in which the face has been rotated.

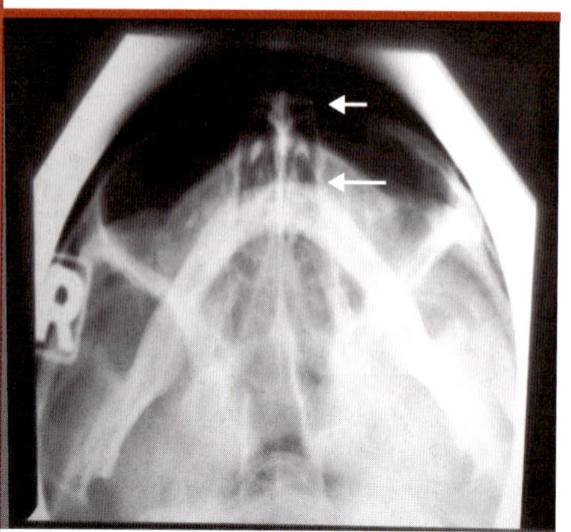

FIGURE 12-54

Basilar view of the skull showing insufficient extension of the head (10° for 1 inch of shift), as well as 5° tilt of the head (½ inch of shift).

Courtesy of Quinn B. Carroll

Basilar (SMV) Projections for Zygomatic Arches, Sinuses, Mandible, or Skull

Figure 12-54 demonstrates a basilar projection in which the skull is both tilted and insufficiently extended. The chin should superimpose the forehead, but it is more than 1 inch low, indicating that at least 10° more of head extension or cephalic angle is needed. (Since the axial measurement of the average head is 23 cm, you can use the general shift rule here.) The gonions of the mandible are seen to be shifted about ½ inch to the patient's right, indicating 5° of head tilt, the top of the head tilted toward the tabletop.

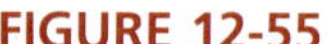

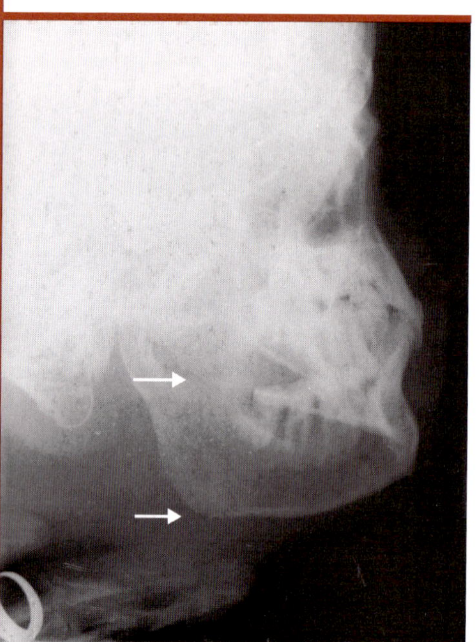

FIGURE 12-55

Lateral (oblique) mandible view showing only 2½ inches of vertical shift between the gonions. Using the general shift rule, this indicates 25° of angle and tilt, 10° short of what is needed.

Courtesy of Quinn B. Carroll

Mandible and Temporomandibular Joints

The oblique lateral mandible should show the upside gonion projected 3 to 3½ inches above the downside gonion, providing maximum desuperimposition of the downside body of the mandible. In Figure 12-55, insufficient cephalic beam angle or insufficient head tilt is evident, because there is only about 2½ inches of vertical shift between the two gonions. Using the general shift rule, this translates to about 25° of beam angle or head tilt, whereas 35° is ideal.

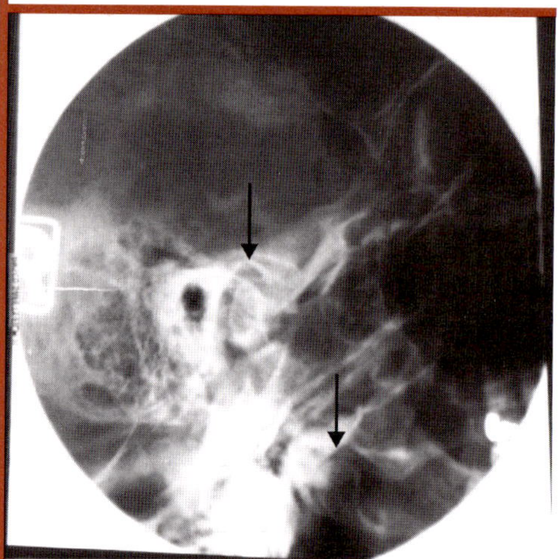

FIGURE 12-56

Laws view for the TMJ (or mastoids), showing proper 1½ inches of vertical shift corresponding to 15° of CR angle, but only 1 inch of lateral shift (arrows). Using the general shift rule, this indicates only 10° of head rotation. The head should be rotated another 5° toward the tabletop.

Carroll, Q. Evaluating Radiographs, 1993, Figure 200, Courtesy of Charles C Thomas, Publisher, Ltd., Springfield, Illinois.

Figure 12-56 is an attempted Laws projection for the TMJs. The blurry and magnified upside TMJ is seen about 1½ inches below the downside TMJ, and about 1 inch anterior. The vertical shift

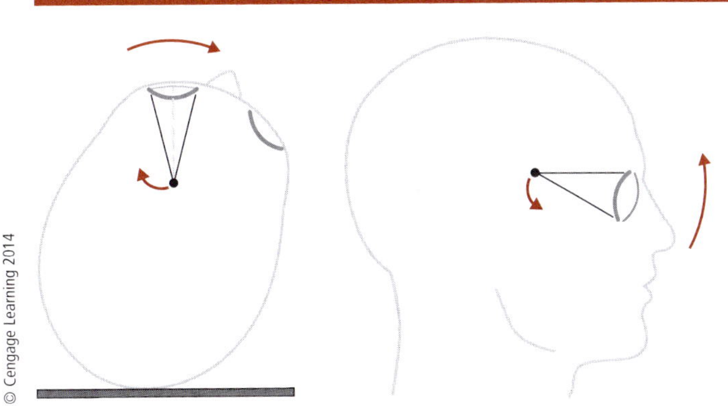

FIGURE 12-57
The optic foramen (shaded black) lies at the apex of the cone of the orbit almost midway from the front to the back of the head. This is well *posterior* to the orbital rim, so relative to the face, the optic foramen shifts *opposite,* that is, *left* when the face is turned to the right **A**, and *down* when the chin is lifted extending the head **B**.

of 1½ inches suggests a correct tube angle of 15° caudally. However, the patient's face should also be rotated toward the tabletop 15°. There is only 1 inch of side-to-side shift. Using the general shift rule, this indicates that the head was rotated only 10°. The head needs to be rotated another 5° toward the tabletop.

Orbits/Optic Foramina

The Rhese method for the orbit provides a perfect case study with which to summarize film critique skills. **Anterior surface anatomy always shifts with the rotation of the body part.** On a Rhese view, the *rim of the orbit* is at the front surface and moves to the patient's right as his head is turned to the right. The orbit also shifts upward as the chin is lifted. **Posterior anatomy always shifts against the rotation of the body part.** On the Rhese view, the *optic foramen* lies about midway through the skull, well posterior to the orbital rim, so turning the head to the patient's right shifts the small foramen to the *left*, and raising the chin shifts the foramen *downward* (Figure 12-57). The optic foramen always moves *opposite* of the direction the face is being turned. You can generally apply these principles to all radiographs, but in each case you must stop to consider which anatomical landmark is more posterior.

For the correctly positioned Rhese view, the optic foramen (which can be found at the end of the curving white line of the lesser sphenoid wing as best shown in Figure 12-60), should be projected into the middle of the lower-outer quadrant of the orbit (Figure 12-58). In Figure 12-59, the foramen is seen at the lateral rim of the right orbit, too lateral or too far to the patient's *right*. This indicates rotation of the head too far toward the *left*. To demonstrate

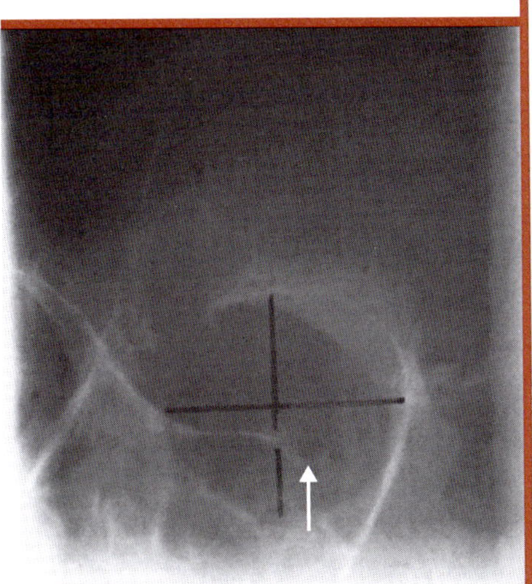

FIGURE 12-58
Rhese view for the orbit, showing the optic foramen (arrow) properly projected into the middle of the lower-outer quadrant of the orbit designated by the black lines.
Carroll, Q. Evaluating Radiographs, 1993, Figure 192, Courtesy of Charles C Thomas, Publisher, Ltd., Springfield, Illinois.

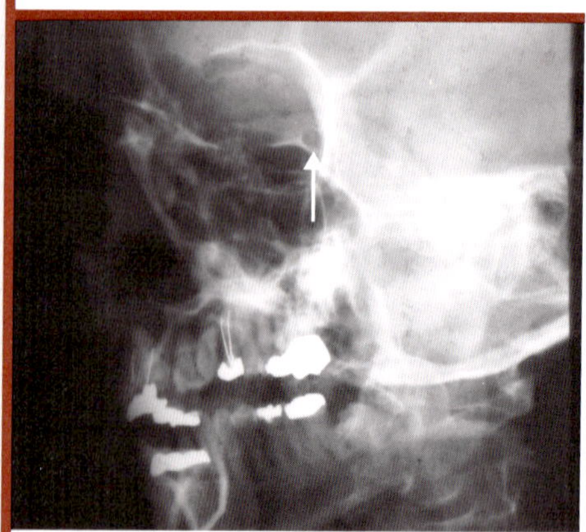

FIGURE 12-59

Rhese view for the orbit, showing the optic foramen right at the lateral orbital rim. This is too far laterally, and indicates that the head was overrotated toward the table, that is, too shallow. The off-shift is about one-quarter orbit or 1 centimeter, indicating 5° or 6° of overrotation.

Carroll, Q. Evaluating Radiographs, 1993, Figure 193, Courtesy of Charles C Thomas, Publisher, Ltd., Springfield, Illinois.

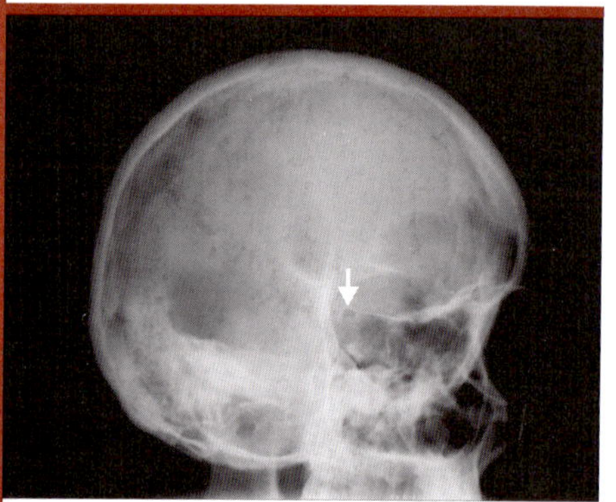

FIGURE 12-60

Rhese view for the orbit, showing the optic foramen too high within the orbit. This indicates underextension of the chin.

Courtesy of Quinn B. Carroll

the right orbit, the head is supposed to be turned toward the left. But, the head was turned *too far*, placing it shallower than the recommended 53°, or too *lateral*. Note that it is shifted about one quarter orbit or 1 centimeter from where it should be. Using the skull shift rule, this indicates 5° or 6° of overrotation.

For the Rhese view, when the optic foramen is too lateral, the *head* is too lateral. When the foramen is too medial, the head is too *steep*.

In Figure 12-60, the head rotation is correct, but the optic foramen is projected too *high* within the orbit. This indicates that the chin is not *extended* enough. It is one quarter orbit or 1 centimeter too high. Using the skull shift rule, to correct this position, the head must be *extended* another 6°–7°.

SUMMARY

1. Compared to downside anatomy, you must identify upside anatomy by its increased blur or magnification. Some anatomy will include tubercles or other details that help identify right from left. Along with the methods to quantify errors in positioning presented in the previous chapter, this allows us to identify the *direction* of the body movement.

2. Specific recommendations for each body part are made throughout this chapter. You can use the general shift rule (½ inch of shift equals 5° of movement or angle) for most of the body.

3. The specific shift rule for skull radiographs is that each quarter of the orbit (or each centimeter of shift) represents 6° of rotation, tilt, flexion, extension, or beam angle.

CORRECTIONS ON AN OPEN-MOUTH ODONTOID VIEW

CRITICAL THINKING CHALLENGE 12.1

Observe the radiograph of an attempted open-mouth (George) position in Figure 12-61 for the odontoid and upper two cervical vertebrae.

Analyze the flexion or extension of the head. Is the head overflexed or overextended and, if so, by how many degrees? State the specific correction, how many degrees and in which direction the chin should be moved, for the repeat exposure. If the head cannot be moved, state the degrees and direction of the compensating tube angle that should be used.

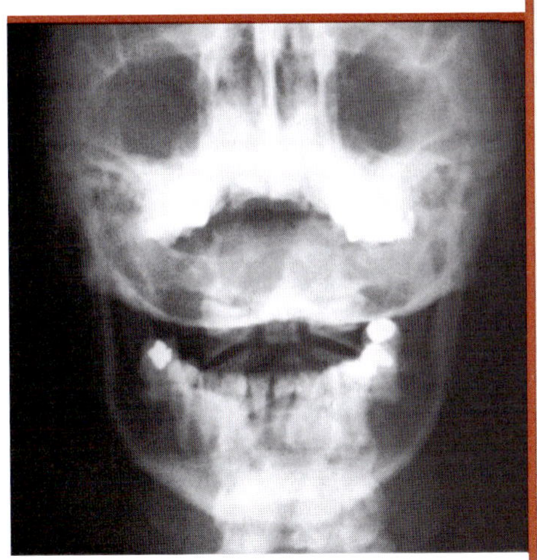

Courtesy of Quinn B. Carroll

FIGURE 12-61
For an attempted open-mouth (George) method view of the upper two cervical vertebrae and the odontoid, analyze the specific correction (including the amount in degrees) needed.

CORRECTION FOR FLEXION/EXTENSION ON A WATERS VIEW

CRITICAL THINKING CHALLENGE 12.2

Observe the radiograph of an attempted Waters position in Figure 12-62.

Based upon where the petrous ridges are projected, how many degrees was this head extended? If the patient cannot extend her chin any further, how many degrees of CR angle is needed,

and in which direction, to correct this view and project the ridges just below the maxillary sinuses? ■

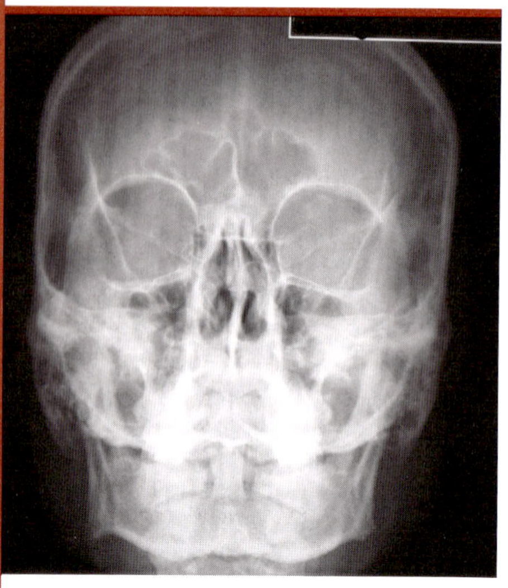

Courtesy of Quinn B. Carroll

FIGURE 12-62
For an attempted Waters position, analyze the specific correction needed based upon where the petrous ridges are projected.

CRITICAL THINKING CHALLENGE 12.3

CORRECTIONS ON A RHESE VIEW

Observe the radiograph of an attempted Rhese position in Figure 12-63 for the optic foramen (arrow).

Analyze both the rotation and the extension of the head. Is the head overflexed or overextended? If so, by how many degrees? Which way (too medial or too lateral) is the head off-rotated and by how many degrees? State the specific corrections to be made on the repeat exposure. ■

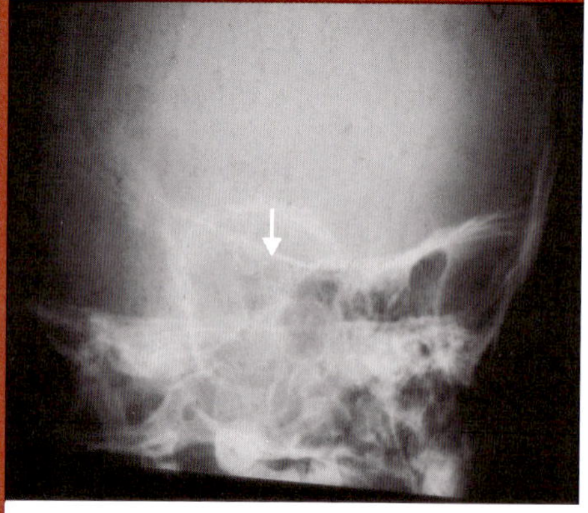

Courtesy of Quinn B. Carroll

FIGURE 12-63
For an attempted Rhese position, for the optic foramen (arrow), analyze both the rotation and the extension of the head.

(Answers to Critical Thinking Challenges are found in the Appendix.)

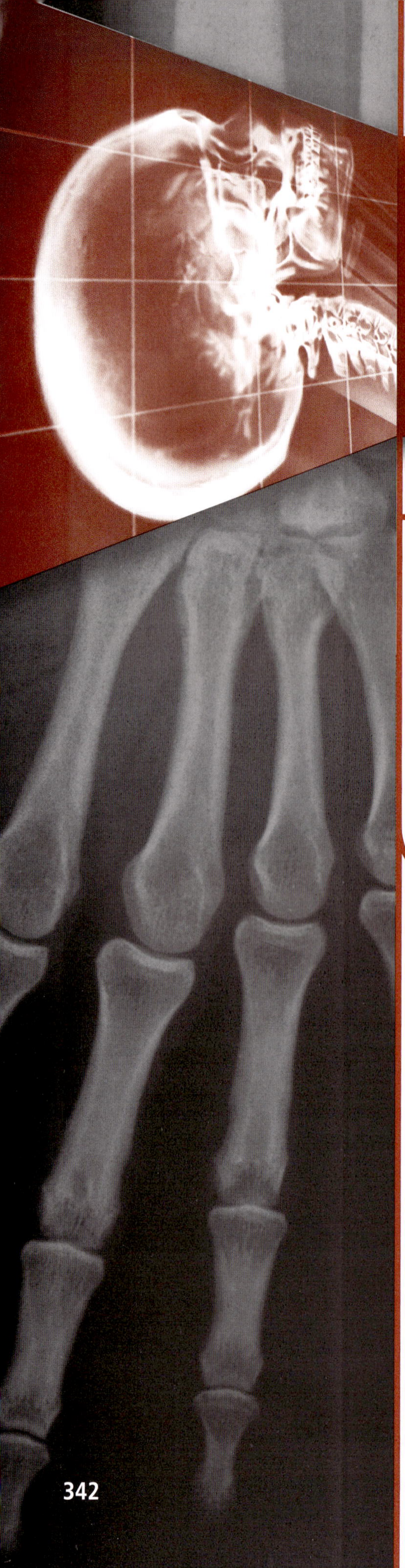

CHAPTER 13

Helpful Rules for Adapting Technique

OUTLINE

OBJECTIVES

Upon completion of this chapter, you should be able to:

1. Appreciate the need for continuing radiographic technique skills ("manual" and AEC) with digital imaging equipment.
2. Memorize technique adjustments for changes in SID.
3. Memorize the rule for adjusting overall technique for different body part thicknesses.
4. Describe the appropriate technique adjustments for different casts, soft-tissue technique, postmortem radiography, and various common additive diseases and destructive diseases.
5. Explain the appropriate radiographic techniques for breathing autotomography and for the air-gap method.
6. Describe the different magnitudes of technique adjustments for infants and small children from radiographic view to the next, as compared to adults.

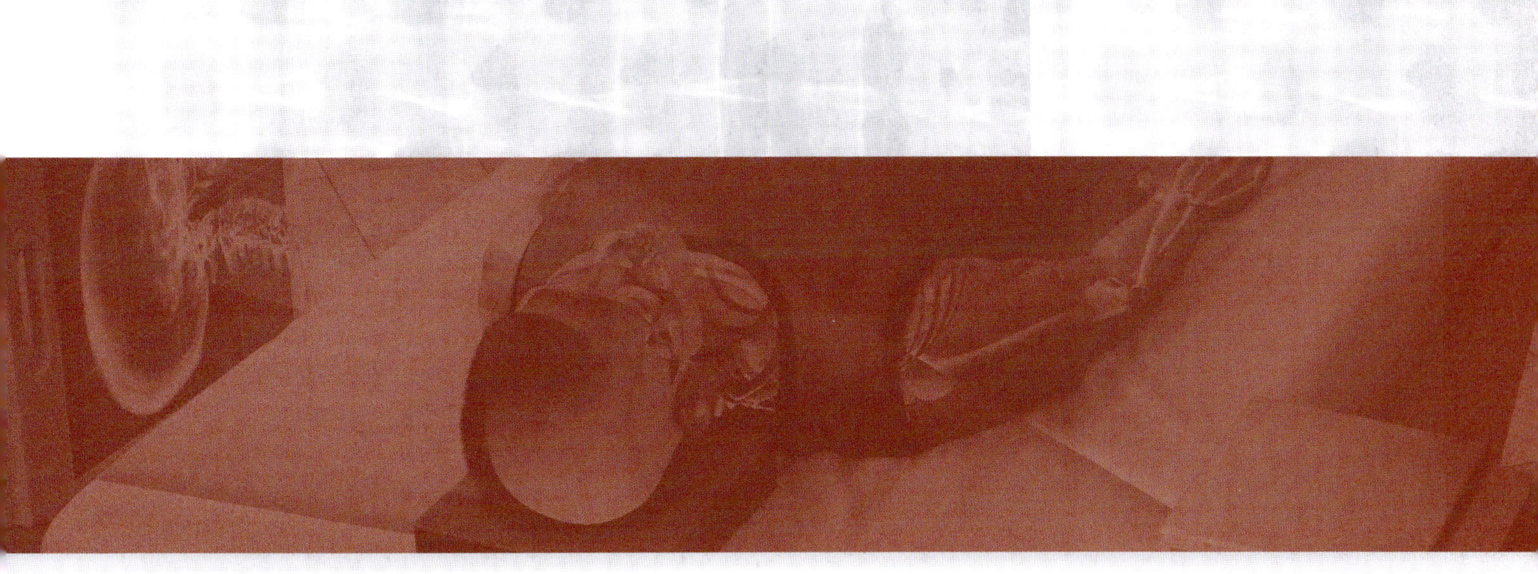

INTRODUCTION

Many special techniques such as soft-tissue technique and the use of wedge filters, were conventionally designed to maximize the visibility of particular radiographic details that were otherwise obscured. With the advent of digital radiography and its powerful postprocessing options to adjust the image, these are no longer strictly necessary.

However, breathing techniques are still required for some procedures, and the air-gap technique may be necessary on very large patients to minimize scatter radiation reaching the detectors or imaging plate. Also, the proper adjustment of technique for different patient conditions and thicknesses, and for variable distances, is absolutely required for the following two important reasons:

1. *Too little technique, **especially insufficient kVp**, results in an inadequate amount of useful signal (x-rays) reaching the detector elements or imaging plate. With all their postprocessing power in adjusting the image, digital systems are not (and* never *will be) capable of manipulating information that simply is not there in the first place. A sufficient quantity of exposure must penetrate through the patient and reach the detectors.*
2. *Too much technique, **especially too much mAs**, overexposes the patient to unnecessary and harmful radiation. This is not immediately obvious in the quality of the resulting digital image, which has only exacerbated the problem. The result has been an upward trend in patient exposure, dubbed as "dose creep," which is very real and has become a public health issue. Every radiographer* must *be conscientious to avoid overexposure to patients.*

For these reasons, we will present a short discussion of some very practical technique adjustments.

ADJUSTMENTS FOR DISTANCE

Table 13-1 presents rules for distance changes using a 40-inch SID as a starting point for comparison. These are based upon the inverse square law, but have been rounded out for practical application. That is, by memorizing these few numbers, everyday adjustments can be made without having to do calculations, something eminently useful for mobile and trauma radiography.

Note the bolded value for the 72-inch SID, a technique adjustment that is ever-present in daily practice: When adapting a 40-inch technique to a 72-inch distance, simply triple the mAs. This can be seen in a typical cervical spine series, in which the mAs for the lateral and oblique views taken at the chest board is usually three times the mAs used for the AP view on the table. A typical technique for the AP might be 5–6 mAs, but 15–18 mAs for the lateral and obliques. This is entirely due to the change in SID from 40 to 72 inches.

When changing SID from 40 to 72 inches, or from 72 to 40 inches, adjust the mAs by a factor of 3 (three times when increasing the distance, one-third when decreasing it).

The following two case studies provide other common examples.

BEST PRACTICE TIP

When changing SID from 40 to 72 inches, or from 72 to 40 inches, adjust the mAs by a factor of 3 (three times when increasing the distance, one-third when decreasing it).

CASE STUDY

Case Study #1: Upright Abdomen Following an Upright Chest

You have just shot a chest series at the chest board with the x-ray tube at 72-inch SID.

An upright abdomen has also been ordered on the patient. There is no need to go to the trouble of moving the x-ray tube closer to 40 inches (the longer SID actually provides better sharpness and less magnification, both *advantages*). All you need is a *technique* for an upright abdomen at the chest board. For this average patient, the technique chart indicates 80 kVp and 20 mAs for a routine supine abdomen at the table, but there is no technique for a 72-inch abdomen. What should you use?

ANSWER: *Simply triple the 40-inch technique from the chart. Use 60 mAs at the same 80 kVp.* ■

Case Study #2: Trauma Chest Supine on Gurney

You have a trauma patient supine on a gurney (stretcher) who cannot sit or stand. For this average patient, the technique chart indicates 2.4 mAs at 110 kVp for a routine PA chest at 72-inch SID, but there is no technique for a 40-inch chest. What should you use?

ANSWER: *Take one-third of the 72-inch technique—0.8 mAs—and use the same 110 kVp.* ■

TABLE 13-1

RULES OF THUMB FOR ADJUSTING TECHNIQUE FOR CHANGES IN SID FROM 40 INCHES

NEW DISTANCE	TECHNIQUE CHANGE COMPUTED BY THE SQUARE LAW	RULE-OF-THUMB TECHNIQUE CHANGE
30 inches (76 cm)	0.56	½
40 inches (100 cm)	1 (standard)	1
50 inches (127 cm)	1.56	1.5 X (50% incr.)
60 inches (152 cm)	2.25	2 X
72 inches (180 cm)	3.24	3 X
80 inches (200 cm)	4	4 X

ADJUSTING FOR PATIENT THICKNESS

From a trusted technique for the average thickness of a particular body part, adjust the overall technique according to the *4-centimeter rule* for variations in thickness. This rule is presented in the Best Practice Tip.

Change overall technique by a factor of 2 for every 4-centimeter difference in body part thickness.

Note that the rule adjusts for "overall" technique. This is to accommodate both the variable mAs and the variable kVp approaches to technique. To apply the rule to variable kVp, the 15% rule is used in conjunction with the 4-centimeter rule—that is, a 15% change in kVp is applied wherever a factor of 2 is indicated. Or, some combination of changes in mAs and kVp may be used as long as the *total, overall* change is equivalent to a net factor of 2.

For example, if a patient is 4 centimeters larger than average, the mAs may be doubled without adjusting the kVp, the kVp may be increased 15% without adjusting the mAs, or a combination of the two can be used in which the mAs is increased *halfway* to double and the kVp is increased halfway to 15%. The following case studies provide some practice in fully understanding the application of this concept.

BEST PRACTICE TIP

Change overall technique by a factor of 2 for every 4-centimeter difference in body part thickness.

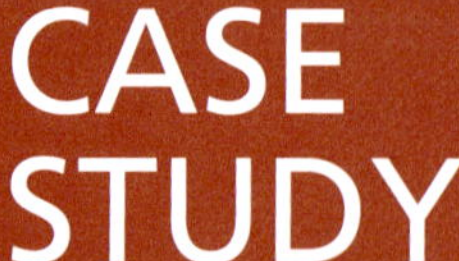

CASE STUDY

Case Study #3: Adjusting Technique for a Thin Patient

A trusted technique chart lists a technique for the average PA chest of 110 kVp and 2.4 mAs. The average chest measures 22 centimeters in PA projection. You have a thin patient measuring only 18 centimeters in the chest. What technique should you use?

ANSWER: *Cut the mAs in half to 1.2 mAs, OR bring the kVp down to 94.*

Case Study #4: Adjusting Technique in Increments for a Thick Patient

A trusted technique chart lists a technique for the average AP abdomen of 80 kVp and 20 mAs. The average abdomen measures 22 centimeters in AP projection. You have a thick patient measuring 28 centimeters in the abdomen. What new mAs should you use?

ANSWER: *Increase the mAs in steps as follows: From 22 centimeters to 26 centimeters, double the mAs to 40. From 26 centimeters to 28 centimeters is one-half of a 4-centimeter increase, so increase the mAs again one-half way to doubling, that is halfway from 40 to 80. The result is 60 mAs.*

In situations where the part thickness changes substantially from one end of the field to the other, such as the AP thoracic spine, a *wedge* filter can be placed on the collimator, or saline bags can be laid across the thinner part of the anatomy (upper chest for the AP T-spine) to effectively *equalize* the thickness of the part. However, with digital image processing, these types of measures are necessary only in fairly extreme cases.

ADJUSTING FOR PATIENT CONDITION

For extremity casts made of mixed fiberglass and plaster, also for most wood or plastic splints, and for plaster half-casts, increase the mAs by 50% (*or* the kVp by 8%). Casts made of pure plaster require double the technique, and if still wet or especially thick such as a femoral cast, can require up to three times the normal technique. Note that *pure fiberglass* casts do not attenuate the x-ray beam and require no adjustment in the normal technique. Nor do "air splints."

For most additive diseases, if you know the patient's condition in advance, increase the usual mAs by 50% (or kVp by 8%) as a general rule. Additive diseases include ascites, cardiomegaly, cirrhosis, pulmonary edema, hydrocephalus, hydrothorax or hemothorax, osteochondroma, osteopetrosis, Paget's disease, pneumoconiosis, pneumonia, syphilis, and pulmonary tuberculosis. The expiration chest projection also requires an increase in technique of at least 35%.

Destructive diseases include emphysema, severe pneumothorax, aseptic necrosis, blastomycosis, bowel obstruction (which creates trapped gas), osteolytic cancers, Ewing's tumor, exostosis, gout, Hodgkin's disease, hyperparathyroidism, osteomyelitis, and osteoporosis. These require a decrease in mAs by 30% (or in kVp by 5%).

Apply soft-tissue techniques to demonstrate small slivers or other subtle objects or anatomy by simply reducing the usual kVp by about 20% with no adjustment in mAs. However, with digital postprocessing of the image available, this is no longer strictly needed.

Immediately after death, all body fluids respond to gravity and pool to the lowest point throughout the body. Anticipate an increase in technique of 35%–50%. If the patient is supine, pooling of body fluids throughout the chest field makes this 35%–50% increase in technique absolutely mandatory to avoid a repeated exposure.

BREATHING TECHNIQUES

Breathing techniques are still useful with digital radiography in helping blur out overlying bony structures for views of the thoracic spine, the sternum, and the sternoclavicular joints. Unfortunately, many radiographers *underestimate* the amount of exposure time needed to achieve a good breathing technique. Consider the fact that the normal adult respiration rate is 12 breaths per minute or 5 seconds per breath. Radiographers often use a 2-second exposure time with 50 mA for a breathing technique. If one full inspiration and expiration requires 5 seconds, then at 2 seconds, the patient has not even completed a single *inspiration*, much less let that breath back out. It defeats the purpose of the procedure to attempt a "breathing technique," and then cut the exposure short of even a single breath being taken in!

Most modern x-ray units have available mA stations as low as 25, 12.5, and even 10 mA. By using these mA stations (instead of 50 mA), the exposure time can be doubled or extended even more. This is strongly recommended. *For breathing techniques, use exposure times of 4 to 6 seconds at the lowest mA station available.*

AIR-GAP TECHNIQUE

In the digital age, radiography of the abdomen and chest on extremely obese patients continues to present a particular technique challenge for radiographers. In these cases, even the use of a grid can prove insufficient to yield a satisfactory image. Although digital equipment can compensate for some scatter radiation by postprocessing contrast enhancement of the image, extremely obese patients can generate so much scatter radiation that it overwhelms the system and leads to errors in histogram analysis. When such excessive scatter is present, it is still imperative to eliminate as much of it as possible before the remnant x-ray beam reaches the digital detectors or plate.

This can be done by using the *air-gap technique* in combination with an appropriate grid. As with breathing techniques, the danger for radiographers in employing the air-gap technique lies in *underestimating* the adjustment needed. For example, frequently the patient is placed only 6 inches out in front of the plate. *Place the patient about 1 foot out in front of the imaging plate with a grid.* At 12 inches OID, randomly scattered radiation is allowed to spread out so much that its concentration at the plate itself is substantially reduced. Meanwhile, the geometry of the primary x-ray beam is not altered, so no primary radiation is lost at the plate. Some magnification and blurring result, but these are preferable to producing an image with digital processing errors that may not be diagnostic. With the patient placed 1 foot in front of the plate, use the usual mAs and kVp indicated for *that thickness of patient* (see the 4-centimeter rule described earlier).

Many radiographers have never attempted the air-gap technique due to unfamiliarity with it. It can pay great dividends to those willing to try it out.

PEDIATRIC TECHNIQUES

As described for NBICU infants in Chapter 8, the torso of a newborn is essentially round in shape, so that the same technique can be used for the lateral chest or abdomen projection as for the AP or PA. By the time a child is 6 months old, the torso is about 4 centimeters wider than it is thick, and technique must be approximately doubled when changing from the AP to the lateral projection. Many radiographers leave the same mAs and simply go up 10 or 12 kVp (which, in the range of 60–70 kVp, is equivalent). By the time a child is about 6 years old, the technique must be increased by three to four times when changing from the AP or PA to the lateral, just as with an adult patient.

There is surprising reliability in comparing the thickness of a child's various body parts with equivalent portions of the adult body when estimating technique. An adult knee technique can be used for a child's skull of comparable or slightly greater thickness. An adult hand technique can be used for the child's arms or legs, and so on.

SUMMARY

1. With digital equipment, technique skills are still essential. Too little technique results in a poor image, and too much technique overexposes the patient.
2. For a change in SID from 40 inches to 72 inches, triple the mAs, and vice versa for a change from 72 inches to 40 inches. We recommend that you memorize the technique adjustments in Table 13-1 for daily use.
3. Change overall technique by a factor of 2 for every 4-centimeter difference in body part thickness.
4. Generally, for most casts, additive diseases, and postmortem radiography, increase technique by 35%–50%. For destructive diseases, reduce it by 30%. For soft tissue, reduce it by 20%.
5. For breathing techniques, use the lowest mA station possible to achieve exposure times of 4–6 seconds. For air-gap techniques, use at least 12 inches of OID gap between the patient and the plate.
6. For infants and very small children, there is much less difference in the technique needed between the frontal and the lateral projections.

ADJUSTING TECHNIQUE FOR AN UNUSUAL SID

CRITICAL THINKING CHALLENGE 13.1

For the mobile unit, you have a trusted technique of 74 kVp and 2 mAs for a 40-inch supine chest. You are in a patient's room with another radiographer who insists on taking the lead. He has placed the patient in a semisitting position, and pulled the x-ray tube up and out to a distance you estimate to be 55 inches SID.

Using the rule for distance changes during mobile radiography, state the ideal new kVp and mAs you would use, adjusting from your 40-inch technique.

CRITICAL THINKING CHALLENGE 13.2

ADJUSTING KVP FOR A THICKER PATIENT

You face the same situation described in Case Study #4, but prefer a variable kVp approach to technique. A trusted technique chart lists a technique for the average AP abdomen of 80 kVp and 20 mAs. The average abdomen measures 22 centimeters in AP projection. You have a thick patient measuring 28 centimeters in the abdomen.

Leaving the mAs at 20, what new kVp would be indicated for this patient who is 6 centimeters thicker than average?

CRITICAL THINKING CHALLENGE 13.3

USING THE 15% RULE TO PREVENT MOTION FROM BREATHING

A large patient in the ICU needs a portable abdomen radiograph taken. The previous day the same image was properly exposed using 80 kVp at 60 mAs. At that time, the patient was cognizant and able to follow the breathing instruction to hold his breath (he was not intubated). Today, the patient is unable to understand the breathing command. At a typical built-in 100-mA station for a mobile unit, the previous exposure time would have been 0.6 seconds.

If the same exposure time is used on the patient who is now unable to hold his breath, is there a substantial risk of breathing motion blurring the image? If so, what new technique could be used to cut the exposure time in to half?

(Answers to Critical Thinking Challenges are found in the Appendix.)

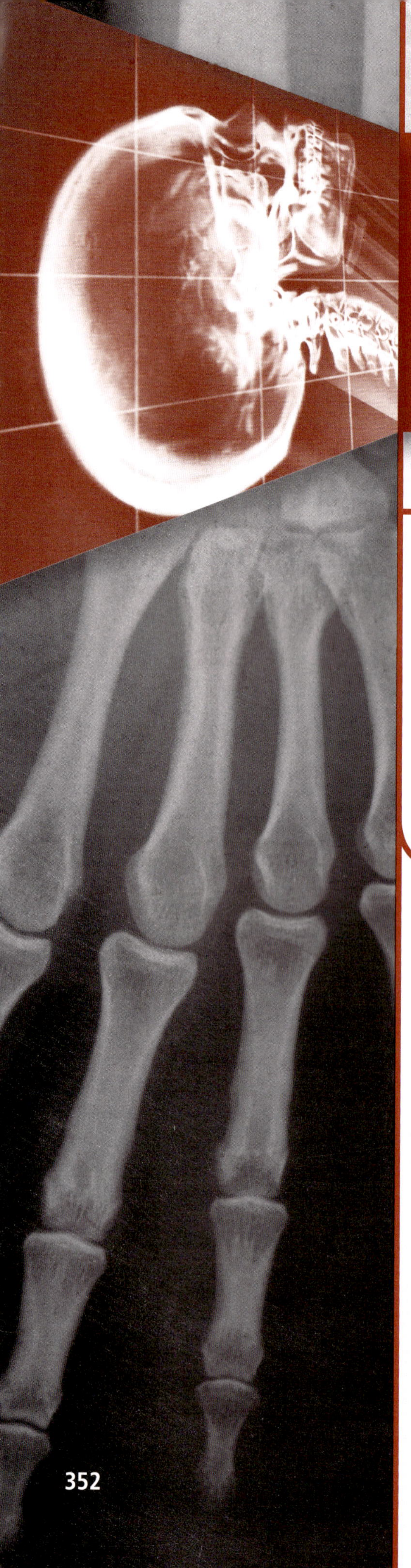

CHAPTER 14

Elements of Critical Thinking: Clinical Application

OUTLINE

Introduction
Sequencing Exams
Essential Intellectual Traits
Proactive Critical Thinking: Criteria for Grading
Summary
Critical Thinking Challenges 14.1, 14.2, 14.3, 14.4, & 14.5
Great Student Form
Great Student Evaluation

OBJECTIVES

Upon completion of this chapter, you should be able to:

1. Appreciate how critical thinking skills improve our safety, effectiveness, and efficiency in clinical practice.
2. List the three steps in the *process* of critical thinking.
3. Describe the eight *elements* of critical thinking, and for each, its antithesis.
4. Define the 10 *universal intellectual standards,* and for each, the questions that can be applied to use it as a grading criterion.

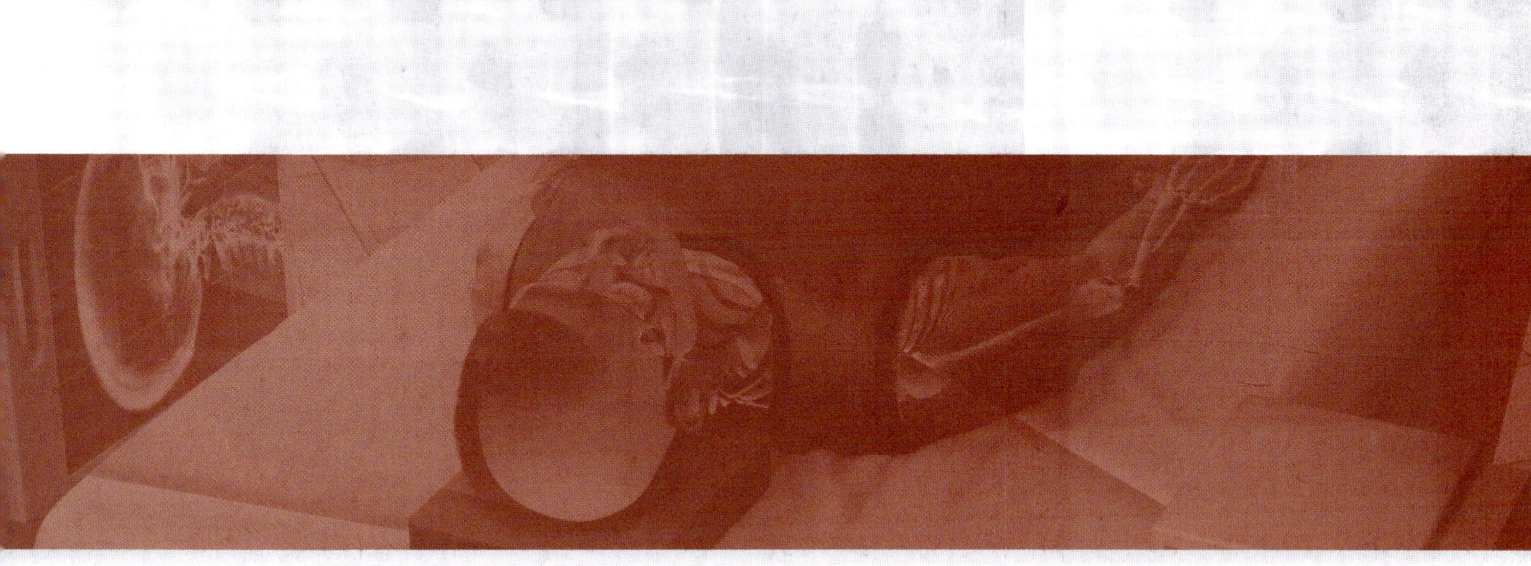

INTRODUCTION

The ability to think critically has an immediate, direct, and profound impact on the quality of our work, and even the quality of our personal daily life. When our thinking is uninformed, biased, or distorted, it can be costly to the patients we are responsible for, to us, and to our employer. In the practice of radiography, this cost can be more than monetary in nature, more than a matter of wasted time or resources—it can affect the amount of radiation exposure, physical discomfort, or injury to the patient, all serious issues of legal liability.

The notion of "being critical" often has a negative connotation when describing our social skills, but this is in a *behavioral* context that is not at all what we are describing here. Rather, the ability to *think* critically about something you have just read or heard is one of the most positive and desirable traits we can possibly have. By nurturing our critical thinking skills, we actually communicate *more effectively* with others, we are able to bring focus and precision to the discussion of problems, and we arrive at well-considered conclusions, with safer, quicker, and better solutions to problems. We become more effective and more efficient in our jobs.

But, the ability to read, listen, and consider issues critically does not come naturally to us—these are skills that we must develop by practice. The *process* of thinking critically about a problem or issue is fairly straightforward, and consists of three steps:

1. Focus on the desired outcome.
2. Develop a mental or written list of *all* possible approaches to reaching this outcome. Be creative, using the skill of "thinking out of the box."
3. Accurately and fully identify the consequences, positive and negative, of each option in making a final choice.

What does *not* come as intuitively to us is an appreciation for the *elements* of critical thinking—that which makes it "critical." These have been well-defined by the *Foundation for Critical Thinking,* and will be the focus of this chapter as "essential intellectual traits."

SEQUENCING EXAMS

A perfect example of clinical application for critical thinking skills is the proper sequencing of multiple radiographic studies ordered by a physician. Without first giving thorough consideration to *Step 1* described earlier, *focusing on the desired outcome(s),* Steps 2 and 3 cannot be effectual. The results are likely to include additional problems for the radiographer, unnecessary discomfort or even injury to the patient, and extended exam time.

So, what are the desired outcomes for sequencing the various radiographic positions to be taken, and how should these be prioritized? We suggest the following:

Priority #1: Avoid injury to the patient and unsafe conditions generally.

Priority #2: For patients in or from the ED, CCU, ICU, NBICU, or in other urgent situations, expeditiously provide to the physicians and other primary caregivers those images needed to *stabilize* the patient.

Priority #3: Minimize movement of the patient from projection to projection. This saves both time and discomfort for the patient.

The following case study will provide practice in applying these concepts.

CASE STUDY

Case Study #1: Sequencing Exams

The following series are ordered on a patient from the emergency department, using two separate requisitions. The patient has suffered multiple trauma from an automobile accident. Once in the x-ray department, the patient can be rolled as needed, or sat up, but not stood up due to administered drugs.

Requisition #1:
Right ankle three-view
Right lower leg
Right hip
Pelvis
Skull two-view
Cervical spine three-view
Upright chest two-view

Requisition #2:
Portable (mobile) AP chest
Portable (mobile) "cross-table" C-spine

List the order in which each specific projection should be taken.

CASE STUDY

ANSWER: *First, assume that, no matter what order the requisitions were received in, the portable procedures are intended for screening purposes to stabilize the patient. They not only take priority, but should be screened by a radiologist before proceeding with anything on requisition #1.*

Because the procedures requested imply the possibility of both pelvis and cervical spine injuries, do not sit this patient up for the portable AP chest, rather, perform the radiograph with the patient supine.

Having screened these views, permission is given to sit, move, and roll the patient as needed to obtain the exams on requisition #1. However, the patient has been given a heavy dose of "painkillers" and should not be stood up.

It would be wise to get the lateral projection of the C-spine while the patient is sitting and you can employ a long SID of 72 inches (180 cm). You might elect to do the two views of the chest (and the lateral C-spine) last in the sequence, such that all the other views have been obtained prior to sitting up the patient, which carries some risk.

To minimize movement, first take all AP projections:

AP skull

AP C-spine

Odontoid

AP pelvis

AP hip to include the upper length of the femur

AP leg

AP ankle

The oblique ankle might be taken next, because no other views will use an internal oblique position and it involves minimal movement from the AP projection. Next, take the right laterals:

R lateral ankle

R lateral leg

R lateral hip

R lateral skull, rolling the patient the rest of the way over into a prone obliqued body position

Finally, since the patient can be sat up, the lateral projection of the C-spine could be done with a proper long SID, at the end of the series, along with the two upright chest projections. ■

With this many projections to do, there is rarely a *single* correct answer for the best sequencing. Often, the entire sequence could be reversed without higher risk to the patient. But, the important thing is that there is a logical *rationale* developed for the sequence you choose, and that this rationale follows the three general priorities we have listed.

ESSENTIAL INTELLECTUAL TRAITS

The following eight mental habits are traits identified by the *Foundation for Critical Thinking* as essential components of critical thinking. Applied with honesty and consistency, they can profoundly affect our clinical practice, our legal liability, our academic performance, and even our personal lives.

Intellectual Humility versus Intellectual Arrogance

Having a consciousness of the limits of one's own knowledge, including a sensitivity to circumstances in which one's native egocentrism is likely to function self-deceptively; sensitivity to bias, prejudice, and limitations of one's viewpoint, intellectual humility depends on recognizing that one should not claim more than one actually knows. It does not imply spinelessness or submissiveness. It implies the lack of intellectual pretentiousness, boastfulness, or conceit, combined with insight into the logical foundations, or lack of such foundations, of one's own beliefs.

Intellectual Courage versus Intellectual Cowardice

Having a consciousness of the need to face and fairly address ideas, beliefs, or viewpoints toward which we have strong negative emotions and to which we have not given a serious hearing. This courage is connected with the recognition that ideas considered dangerous or absurd are sometimes rationally justified and that conclusions and beliefs inculcated in us are sometimes false or misleading. To determine for ourselves which is which, we must not passively and uncritically "accept" what we have "learned." Intellectual courage comes into play here, because inevitably we will come to see some truth in some ideas considered dangerous and absurd, and distortion or falsity in some ideas strongly held in our social group. We need courage to be true to our own thinking in such circumstances. The penalties for nonconformity can be severe.

Intellectual Empathy versus Intellectual Closed-Mindedness

Having a consciousness of the need to imaginatively put oneself in the place of others in order to genuinely understand them, which requires the consciousness of our egocentric tendency to identify truth with our immediate perceptions of long-standing thought or belief. This trait correlates with the ability to reconstruct accurately the viewpoints and reasoning of others and to reason from premises, assumptions, and ideas other than our own. This trait also correlates with the willingness to remember occasions when we were wrong in the past despite an intense conviction that we were right, and with the ability to imagine our being similarly deceived in a case at hand.

Intellectual Autonomy versus Intellectual Conformity

Having rational control of one's belief's, values, and inferences. The ideal of critical thinking is to learn to think for oneself, to gain command over one's thought processes. It entails a commitment to analyzing and evaluating beliefs on the basis of reason and evidence, to question when it is rational to question, to believe when it is rational to believe, and to conform when it is rational to conform.

Intellectual Integrity versus Intellectual Hypocrisy

Recognition of the need to be true to one's own thinking; to be consistent in the intellectual standards one applies; to hold one's self to the same rigorous standards of evidence and proof to which one holds one's antagonists; to practice what one advocates for others; and to honestly admit discrepancies and inconsistencies in one's own thought and action.

Intellectual Perseverance versus Intellectual Laziness

Having a consciousness of the need to use intellectual insights and truths in spite of difficulties, obstacles, and frustrations; firm adherence to rational principles despite the irrational opposition of others; a sense of the need to struggle with confusion and unsettled questions over an extended period of time to achieve deeper understanding or insight.

Confidence in Reason versus Distrust of Reason and Evidence

Confidence that, in the long run, one's own higher interests and those of humankind at large will be best served by giving the freest play to reason, by encouraging people to come to their own conclusions by developing their own rational faculties; faith that, with proper encouragement and cultivation, people can learn to think for themselves, to form rational viewpoints, draw reasonable conclusions, think coherently and logically, persuade each other by reason and become reasonable persons, despite the deep-seated obstacles in the native character of the human mind and in society as we know it.

Fair-Mindedness versus Intellectual Unfairness

Having a consciousness of the need to treat all viewpoints alike, without reference to one's own feelings or vested interests, or the feelings or vested interests of one's friends, community, or nation; implies adherence to intellectual standards without reference to one's own advantage or the advantage of one's group.

Source: Paul, Richard and Elder, Linda. *The Miniature Guide to Critical Thinking: Concepts and Tools,* 2007, Dillon Beach, CA: Foundation for Critical Thinking Press. www.criticalthinking.org. Reprinted with permission.

The Essential Intellectual Traits shown in the box are the *attitudes* that must become *habits* if we wish to hone our critical thinking skills. Based on these philosophical concepts, the *Foundation for Critical Thinking* has published a list of "universal intellectual standards," which you can directly apply to every conceivable problem-solving situation. These are *clarity, accuracy, precision, relevance, depth, breadth, logic, significance,* and *fairness*. They can be directly applied as *grading* criteria for student reports, extra-credit assignments, or clinical case studies. An example is presented in the next section, adding the criterion of *completeness,* with two or three key questions to answer for each criterion to determine if it has been met.

PROACTIVE CRITICAL THINKING

Criteria for Grading

1. **CLARITY**
   Could you elaborate further?
   Could you give me an example?
   Could you illustrate what you mean?
2. **ACCURACY**
   How could we check on that?
   How could we find out if that is true?
   How could we verify or test that?
3. **PRECISION**
   Could you be more specific?
   Could you give me more details?
   Could you be more exact?
4. **RELEVANCE**
   How does that relate to the problem?
   How does that bear on the question?
   How does that help us with the issue?
5. **DEPTH**
   What factors make this a difficult problem?
   What are some of the complexities of this question?
   What are some of the difficulties we need to deal with?
6. **BREADTH**
   Do we need to look at this from another perspective?
   Do we need to consider another point of view?
   Do we need to look at this in another way?
7. **LOGIC**
   Does all this make sense together?
   Do your early statements fit with your later statements?
   Does what you say follow from the evidence?
8. **SIGNIFICANCE**
   Is this one of the most important points to consider?
   Is this the central issue to focus on?
   Which of these facts are most important?
9. **FAIRNESS**
   Do I have any vested interest in this issue?
   Am I sympathetically representing the viewpoints of others?
10. **COMPLETENESS**
    Have I fully explained all relevant issues?
    Have I fully explained any terms or concepts I used that may not be familiar to my reader?

Source: Paul, Richard and Elder, Linda. *The Miniature Guide to Critical Thinking: Concepts and Tools,* 2007, Dillon Beach, CA: Foundation for Critical Thinking Press. www.criticalthinking.org. Reprinted with permission.

For clinical application, two generic forms are included at the end of this chapter, which the instructor or clinical instructor is given permission to copy and use. The first is a generic form that students can use to submit critical thinking challenges, the second an evaluation form for the instructor to use based on the preceding criteria. The criteria can be attached or printed on the back of the student form, and we strongly recommend conducting a full classroom discussion of the *Essential Intellectual Traits* when introducing any educational program to develop critical thinking skills.

SUMMARY

1. The ability to think critically improves our safety, effectiveness, and efficiency in clinical practice. Poor critical thinking skills can be costly. Critical thinking has a deep impact not only on our professional career, but also on our personal daily life.
2. The three basic steps in the *process* of critical thinking are to 1) focus on the desired outcome, 2) develop a list of *all* options to reach it, and 3) accurately identify the consequences, of each option in making a final choice.
3. The eight *elements* of critical thinking are *intellectual humility, intellectual courage, intellectual empathy, intellectual autonomy, intellectual integrity, intellectual perseverance, confidence in reason, and fair-mindedness.*
4. The ten *universal intellectual standards* are *clarity, accuracy, precision, relevance, depth, breadth, logic, significance, fairness,* and *completeness*. Using these standards, instructors can develop grading forms that measure critical thinking skills.

CRITICAL THINKING CHALLENGE 14.1

SERIES SEQUENCE FOR MULTIPLE TRAUMA #1

The following series are ordered on a patient suffering multiple trauma, including a puncture wound to the chest from a car accident. The patient is not to be moved from his supine position.

Left lower leg
Right shoulder
Chest one-view
Pelvis
Abdomen
Lumbar spine three-view

List the order in which each specific projection should be taken to minimize discomfort to the patient and expedite the procedure.

CRITICAL THINKING CHALLENGE 14.2

SERIES SEQUENCE FOR MULTIPLE TRAUMA #2

The following series are ordered on a patient experiencing multiple trauma from a car accident. The patient is not to be moved from her supine position. Rib injuries are on the left side of the patient's back, and include puncture wounds.

Skull two-view
Left ribs
Chest one-view
Sternum

List the order in which each specific projection should be taken to minimize discomfort to the patient and expedite the procedure.

CRITICAL THINKING CHALLENGE 14.3

SERIES SEQUENCE FOR MULTIPLE TRAUMA #3

The following series are ordered on a patient suffering multiple trauma from a skiing accident. After screening the lateral C-spine and lateral skull, approval is given to move the patient as needed, so the patient can be rolled onto his side (but not stood up, due to administered drugs).

Skull two-view
Cervical spine five-view
Chest one-view
Thoracic spine two-view
Lumbar spine five-view

List the order in which each specific projection should be taken to minimize discomfort to the patient and expedite the procedure.

CRITICAL THINKING CHALLENGE 14.4

SERIES SEQUENCE FOR MULTIPLE TRAUMA #4

The following series are ordered on a patient suffering multiple trauma, from a sporting accident. The patient is not to be moved from her supine position.

Right shoulder, one-view
Right humerus, two-view

Right elbow, two view
Right wrist, three-view
Right forearm, two-view
Right hand, three-view

List the order in which each specific projection should be taken to minimize discomfort to the patient and expedite the procedure.

SERIES SEQUENCE FOR MULTIPLE TRAUMA #5

CRITICAL THINKING CHALLENGE 14.5

The following series are ordered on a patient suffering multiple trauma from a boating accident. The patient can be rolled as needed (but not stood up due to administered drugs).

Skull two-view
Facial bones two-view
Mandible two-view
Zygomatic arches one-view
Cervical spine three-view

List the order in which each specific projection should be taken to minimize discomfort to the patient and expedite the procedure.

(Answers to Critical Thinking Challenges are found in the Appendix.)

GREAT STUDENT FORM

Great Student Form

Date *and* Time Submitted: ____________________ **Instructor's Signature** ________________________

Proactive Critical Thinking

Radiographic Position: ________________________ Name: ______________________________________

RANK (For submitting this concept): _____________________ Score: ______________________________________

Use back of form or attached pages as needed.

Sample Questions:

1. **Describe any centering or positioning method you thought was emphasized in class, lab, or clinical, or from a textbook:**

2. **Describe a different centering or positioning method you heard at a clinical site or from any other source, that you tried out and thought was most useful:**

3. **Concisely argue how or why, in your opinion, #1 works better than #2 OR #2 works better than #1, taking into consideration the *Criteria for Critical Thinking*:**

Topics (Must be relevant to the course for which they are submitted):

Centering points and collimation
Angles and distance
Flexion/extension, rotation, tilt, abduction/adduction of the part
Radiographic technique used
Patient care and safety issues
Criteria for image critique

(Particularly good topics are recommendations from a textbook that local radiographers do *not* practice, or that local radiographers practice that are *not* in the textbook.)

Based on: Paul, Richard and Elder, Linda. *The Miniature Guide to Critical Thinking: Concepts and Tools, 2007,* Dillon Beach, CA: Foundation for Critical Thinking Press. www.criticalthinking.org.

GREAT STUDENT EVALUATION

Great Student Evaluation

Proactive Critical Thinking

Radiographic Position: ______________________ Name: ______________________

RANK (For submitting this concept): ______________________ Score: ______________________

Comments:

1. **CLARITY:**

2. **ACCURACY:**

3. **PRECISION:**

4. **RELEVANCE:**

5. **DEPTH:**

6. **BREADTH:**

7. **LOGIC:**

8. **SIGNIFICANCE:**

9. **FAIRNESS:**

10. **COMPLETENESS:**

Based on: Paul, Richard and Elder, Linda. *The Miniature Guide to Critical Thinking: Concepts and Tools*, 2007, Dillon Beach, CA: Foundation for Critical Thinking Press. www.criticalthinking.org.

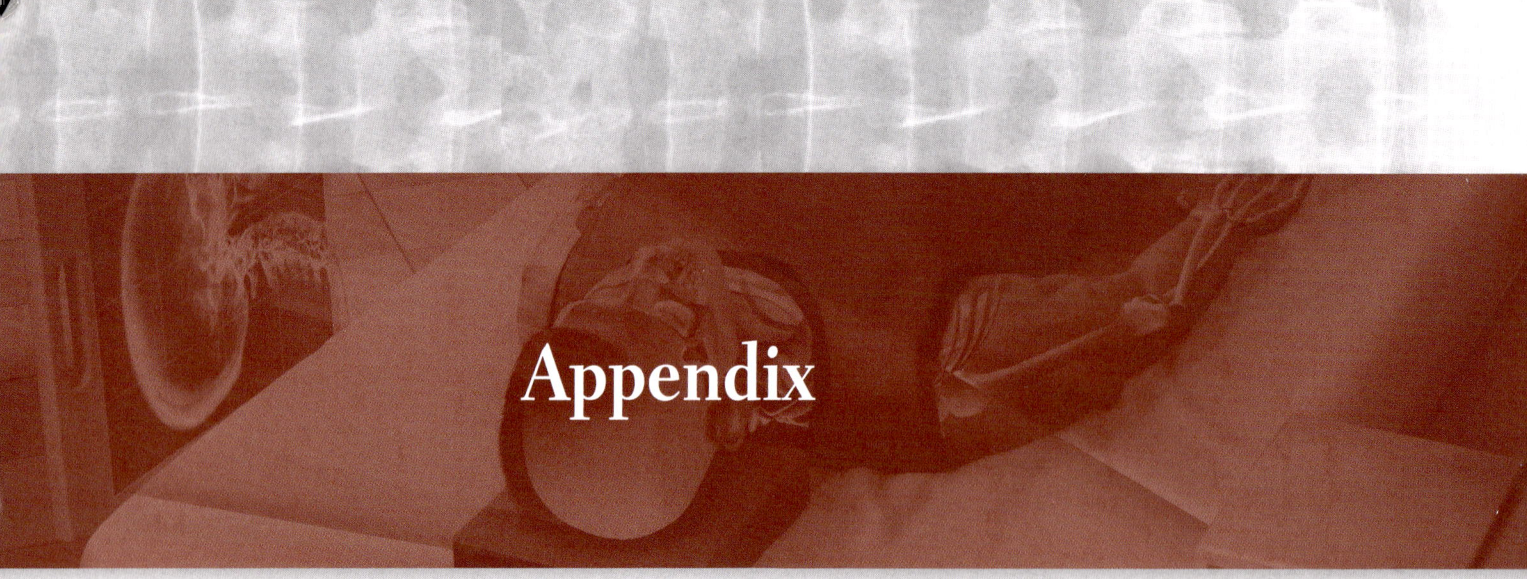

Appendix

ANSWERS TO CRITICAL THINKING CHALLENGES

1.1: Centering a Portable Chest

It is impossible to tell from that angle. The person evaluating any positioning line or plane must himself be positioned directly end-on to that plane in some cases, or at right angles (90°) to it in other cases. In this case, the CR itself could only be properly evaluated from a position directly behind the x-ray tube and squatting beneath it (or directly behind and above the patient, not likely in this scenario). If the x-ray tube is directly above the foot of a patient's bed, from a viewpoint at 90° directly to the side of the x-ray tube, the radiographer can see if the face of the collimator is parallel with the plane of the foot board of the bed. In both cases, standing as far back as possible improves the viewpoint.

1.2: Routine Chest Exam on a Kyphotic Patient

Reverse the position of the patient for an AP projection, allowing the patient's back to be placed in direct contact with the image receptor. If the chin obscures anatomy of interest, ask the referring physician or radiologist if an additional AP projection with a cephalic angle is desired, but a routine AP should be taken first to demonstrate the bases of the lungs.

1.3: Head Position for the Oblique Cervical Spine

An oblique C-spine radiograph taken with the head aligned to the oblique body will place the gonion and ramus portions of the mandible over the upper cervical vertebrae, obscuring the anatomy of interest. To prevent superimposition of the jaw over the cervical vertebrae, the head must be rotated somewhat (though not necessarily all the way) toward the lateral position. This is true whether performing a posterior oblique or an anterior oblique. Many radiographers routinely do this even though it is not generally recommended in textbooks.

Furthermore, one of the main purposes of the oblique view is to see, nicely opened, the intervertebral foramina. These do not all open precisely at 45°; rather, they gradually transition more laterally in the upper vertebrae. The intervertebral foramina between C2/C3 and C3/C4 are actually opened better with some rotation of the head toward the lateral (approaching parallel to the tabletop).

2.1: Centering for Different Cervical Spine Views

These are different because the AP and the AP oblique (posterior oblique) projections involve a *cephalic angle* on the beam that enters the anterior neck, whereas the spine itself lies posterior. In order to *exit* through the same vertebra, the surface centering point of an upward-angled beam must be shifted downward to compensate. (This is discussed in Chapter 2.)

The CR should always *exit* through C4, which is in the center of the seven cervical vertebrae with three above and three below. (The books state that it should enter *at the level* of C5, not that it should *pass through* the actual vertebra C5.)

This relates to the "1 inch for every 10° rule" because by this rule, a cephalic angle of 15° would be centered 1½ inches lower, and centering to the *bottom* of the thyroid cartilage rather than to the top of it approximates this point 1½ inches lower.

2.2: Centering for the PA Oblique Cervical Spine

The cervical spine lies *posterior* in the neck. The shift rule must be applied to centering points on the *front surface* of the neck because of the depth from there to the back of the neck. However, on the PA oblique, the CR enters the *back* of the neck where the C-spine can even be directly palpated. The CR can be directed right through C4 as it enters the neck. No shifting is needed, because the anatomy of interest is *close to the entrance surface* of the CR. The shift rule does not strictly apply in this case.

2.3: Centering for a Trauma AP Oblique Cervical Spine

Using the shift rule, "1 inch for every 10°," the correct centering point will lie 4½ inches off to the side of the midline (midsagittal plane), and 1½ inches inferior to the top of the thyroid cartilage.

3.1: Placement of a Lead Marker on a Patient

At a 40-inch (100-cm) SID, *each edge* of the light field will expand by about 2 inches (5 cm). The radiographer adjusted the field to a 14-inch (35-cm) width *on the surface of the patient,* with the marker placed near the edge. By the time this field reaches the IR below, the marker will have been projected off to the side of the IR. (This field will also run past the edges of the IR by 2 inches on every side, creating unnecessary amounts of scatter radiation.)

First, the field should be collimated so that it is 14 inches (35 cm) wide *at the image receptor* (as indicated by the collimator settings), not on the patient's surface. Second, the marker needs to be moved in accordingly, within the properly collimated field.

3.2: Rotation on a Lateral Chest Position

The only "straight" ray in the x-ray beam is the CR that, on a lateral chest, is passing through the midcoronal plane, *not the back* of the patient. Because of the fan-shaped divergence of the x-ray beam, the ray that skims the patient's back is diverging or *angled* toward the left.

Unfortunately, there is no symmetrical, bilateral bony anatomy in the midcoronal plane that can be used to evaluate rotation on a lateral chest. So we resort to the superimposition of the right and left posterior ribs or the posterior costophrenic angles.

If the patient's back surface is *perfectly perpendicular* to the plate, it is not in line with the diverging, angled ray that is projecting it. To get it in line, the patient's right shoulder must be slightly rotated *forward*. The angled beam will then project the right ribs and costophrenic angles directly on top of the left ones, and the view comes out appearing nonrotated.

3.3: Problems with the Tube on a Groin Lateral Hip

The problem is that the x-ray tube was angled to the *right* into horizontal position in the first place. If it is simply angled to the *left* into horizontal position, all these problems are avoided. It will be swiveled *clockwise* instead of counterclockwise. When it is brought vertically down, the yoke and handles will be positioned away from the table so they do not get in the way. The tube can be brought down until the collimator rests on the tabletop, placing the CR close to the midthigh. A 40-inch SID can be achieved while maintaining the proper 45° cephalic angle into the groin area.

If the tube yoke and handles are left in the improper position described, the best option between settling for an improper angle and an improper distance is to accept the improper *distance*, because an increase in technique is all that is required to correct for it. (The geometrical effects of increased distance are all *beneficial*: improved sharpness and reduced magnification. So there is no geometrical contraindication for allowing an increased SID.) On the other hand, using an improper angle distorts and superimposes the neck of the femur, producing an improper view.

4.1: Identifying the Upside Iliac Crest

In Figure 4-11, a lateral view of the lumbar spine, the iliac crest marked **B** is the right crest, and is upside.

For the lateral lumbar spine position, the central ray should be centered 1½ inches *above* the iliac crest to pass through L3. In *this* radiograph the CR is centered higher still, passing through L2. As long as the centering is *above* the level of the crests, then the beams passing through the crests are *diverging caudally*. This projects the upper crest *below* the downside crest. The lower of the two iliac crests must be the right side.

Extreme body habitus or pathology such as severe scoliosis, which tilts the pelvis, could reverse the iliac crest that is projected higher or lower and render this conclusion wrong, but such cases would be rare, because these two crests are usually projected an inch or more apart.

Note that in this radiograph the crest that is projected higher may subjectively appear more blurry, yet it is geometrically impossible for this to be true, because it is the downside crest right against the tabletop. The reason it may seem blurrier is that is has relatively low contrast. The upside crest, projected lower, is brighter because it is superimposed over the other crest, so you are seeing the contrast effect of the two bones stacked together. This high contrast makes the edge more visible, and this can fool the human eye into thinking the edge is actually sharper.

Judging the sharpness of specific anatomy on radiographs can be very tricky, and you must beware of high-contrast bones subjectively appearing "sharper" and low-contrast anatomy appearing "blurry." It takes great familiarity with the anatomy and practice to judge image sharpness.

4.2: Spatial Relations Applied to a Lateral Knee View

In Figure 4-12, a lateral knee view, the knee is *not* significantly rotated. (If it were, the subpatellar joint space would be completely closed off.) Begin by observing the *bottom edges* of the two femoral condyles and it becomes clear that they are shifted *vertically* one above the other. Vertical shift of horizontal lines indicates that the object is *tilted*, that the CR is *off-angled cephalically or caudally*, or that the CR is *off-centered cephalically or caudally*. In this particular radiograph, it was a combination of centering an inch too high and neglecting to angle the CR 5° cephalically.

In some portions of this image, most notably the upper anterior condyles above the patella, you can make out anatomical lines that appear at a glance to be shifted side to side. This would indicate rotation; however, it is an illusion. It is caused by the fact that two *circular* objects were shifted vertically, which will result in *different parts* of the circles desuperimposing in a side-to-side dimension. But for correct film critique, you must compare the exact *same* points on each condyle. When this is done, you again conclude that they are shifted *vertically*.

4.3: Sag on the Lateral Lumbar Spine

If the lumbar spine is built up until it lies parallel to the tabletop, all of the joints will open vertically and parallel to each other. But, this does not match the shape of the x-ray beam (see Figure 4-1 in Chapter 4). The x-rays are not emitted parallel to each other and vertically (except for the CR); rather, they diverge outward from the focal spot in a fan shape. By *allowing* the lumbar spine to "sag" moderately, the joints and vertebrae actually line up with the x-ray beam (see Figure 4-4 in Chapter 4), for a near-perfect view.

It is possible to have too much sagging of the lumbar spine for the lateral view, but it is also possible to *not have enough*.

5.1: Building Up an AP Odontoid View

For the "coned" AP projection of the odontoid, when the occipital bone comes down underneath the odontoid process, either the patient's head is *extended* too far, or the CR is *angled cephalic* too much (or a combination of these). By building the patient's head up on a sponge, the chin is tucked and the back of the head comes up. This is a correct adjustment, in and of itself. However, when the CR is then angled cephalically, it *cancels out this effect*, projecting the odontoid process back up over the occipital bone behind it. This is flawed thinking. If the sponge forces the head into 5° of flexion, and the CR is angled 5° cephalically, the *identical problem* will result in the repeated image. Another repeat *is* likely.

Let's take the analysis a step further: If these two corrections have cancelling effects on each other, then why does this "work," as claimed by the radiographer? Undoubtedly, this is because the *amount* of flexion caused by the sponge is different than the *amount* of the angle—most likely the flexion from the sponge is greater than 5°. Let us assume that the flexion caused by the sponge is 10°. Five of these degrees are cancelled out by the cephalic angle. This leaves 5° of effective flexion of the head. The radiographer's method may be working because the *net* result is 5° of head flexion, changed from the original position.

Is there a way that is simpler, quicker, and easier on the patient? Yes, there is. Note that, with the patient supine, 5° of head flexion is equivalent to 5° of *caudal* angle. *All that was needed to be done in the first place was to angle the CR 5° caudally.* This adjustment can be made without bothering to slide a sponge under the patient's head.

5.2: Reversed Lateral "Spot" View of L5–S1

Reversing the patient's position from left lateral to right lateral *will* improve the view. Since the joint was closed with a straight beam, and angling caudally made the projection of the joint space worse, the joint must be tilted *opposite* to the caudal angle. Turning the patient into the opposite lateral position will reverse the tilt of the joint so that at least it aligns with the *general direction* of the caudal angle, if not by the precise degree.

However, there *is* certainly a way to achieve the same thing without as much trouble to the patient. Keeping the patient in the original left lateral recumbent position on the table, simply *angle the CR cephalically*. Reversing the tube angle is equivalent to reversing the position, and just as effective. There is no compelling reason to have the patient stand up or even roll over.

Now, the *degree* of angulation can only be estimated, but given the fact that the straight projection had the joint completely closed, it is likely that more than 5° will be needed. A good estimation would be at least 7°–8° cephalic for the first attempt.

An important flaw in this reasoning is that when the patient stands up, the whole weight load dynamic of the spine is changed, which will likely alter the angle at which the joint lies. The "sagging" effect of the patient lying on his side is removed, and at the same time the lumbar spine is now weight-bearing for all of body weight above that level. The net result is unpredictable, so for all practical purposes you are starting all over again.

By keeping the patient recumbent on his left side and simply using a cephalic angle, you are correcting for a known situation, even though you must estimate the degrees. This is the most efficient course of action.

5.3: Determining the Angle for a Lateral "Spot" View of L5–S1

This type of measurement is *irrelevant* to the lateral projection of the L5–S1 joint space, because it is being taken on an *AP view with the patient supine*. Such a measurement will show any tilt of the joint space due to scoliosis or other pathology, and these may have *some* effect on the lateral position. But, it just fails to take into account the entirely different weight load dynamic when a patient lies on his side versus lying on his back. When a patient rolls up onto his side, it typically makes the spine sag to one degree or another. Furthermore, different breadths of the hips, waist, and shoulders all affect the way the spine lies in lateral position. None of these factors are taken into account on the AP view. Too many variables change between the AP and the lateral positions. This measurement is flawed thinking and amounts to "comparing apples to oranges."

6.1: Cross-Table Lateral Hip Pin with a Fixed DR Detector

Minimize OID by keeping the body part as close to the IR as possible, and use the longest feasible SID, which will minimize magnification of the pin.

6.2: Walker Shoulder Projection on a Large Patient with a Fixed DR Detector

Use a cephalic angle of 40°, and center the CR 1 inch (2.5 cm) lower than average.

6.3: Use of a Step Sponge for an Oblique Hand

First, for this particular design of sponge, the step for the fourth finger raises this finger off of the image receptor by approximately ½ inch, creating an OID gap. Indeed, an additional ½ inch is added to the OID for *all* fingers and the thumb, resulting in unnecessary magnification and blur in the projected image. Note that the entire bottom ½ inch of this sponge could be chopped off, and the patient instructed how to use the modified sponge by placing the fourth finger (fifth digit) directly on the image receptor, with the other fingers all supported by the sponge.

Second, a laboratory demonstration of this very sponge reveals that if the patient rests the wrist on the film, which the patient normally will, the sponge forces the entire palm up such that the metacarpals are now tilted in relation to the IR. This causes distortion of these bones, with the knuckles improperly bent to bring the fingers back down onto the steps of the sponge.

Experimentation shows that this sponge, as it is, can still be used by simply sliding all digits down one step so that the fifth digit is directly on the IR, with the thumb on the step marked for "finger #1," but take care not to overlap the soft tissue of the thumb with that of the second digit.

6.4: Oblique Projection on a Patient Who Must Remain on the Side

Yes. By backing the patient against the upright Bucky, you can place *vertical* angles on the x-ray beam without crossing grid lines. A 45° caudal angle will project the equivalent of a right posterior oblique position, and a cephalic angle will be equivalent to an LPO. For an illustration of this concept, see Figure 7-12 at the end of the next chapter relative to the discussion for Case Study #1.

7.1: Trauma External Oblique Elbow

The CR should be angled 45° mediolaterally.

7.2: Head Position for a Caldwell Skull Projection

The head needs to be extended more. As the face and orbits move up, the petrous pyramids move down posteriorly.

7.3: Series Modification for Tangential Foreign Body

You should take the "profile" view in a steep posterior oblique (AP oblique) position such that the wound is placed tangentially in the central ray. The CR should nearly "skim" the wound surface, but be directed about 1 inch into the tissue of the body.

You should not use AEC because a tangential projection leaves so much "raw" field past the patient's surface, and the center detector cell may not be fully covered with tissue, such that the exposure shuts off early. Placement of lead sheets over this "raw" field area may cause the opposite effect if it lies over any portion of the energized detector cell, causing the exposure to shut off much too late. You should use manual technique, at approximately one-third of the mAs normally used for an AP abdomen, because the thickness of tissue through the path of the CR is much less.

8.1: Alleged Effect of SID on CR Angle

The assisting radiographer is incorrect, and this would be a misapplication of the rules learned in this chapter, which apply to *recentering* the CR to some point that was *previously* in a diverging beam with different centering, not to the *original* centering point recommended for any particular routine position.

As described in this chapter, it is true that the longer 72-inch (180-cm) SID will reduce beam divergence, so there will be less *change* in the angle above and below the central ray as these beams pass through different intervertebral foramina. This will affect how well-opened these foramina *above and below the CR* will be projected. But, the original angle recommended for the oblique projection is the *average* angle needed for seven vertebrae, determined by the shape of the *middle* vertebra, which is C4. The central ray is passing directly through the IV foramen of C4. Any reduction in this angle, regardless of the SID, will begin to close off the space of the foramen by superimposing the bone of the pedicle above it, as well as those of the other vertebrae.

If we were to *recenter* the central ray to C2 or C7, adjustments would be necessary, but changing only the SID does not alter the *average* angle needed for all seven vertebrae.

8.2: Magnification on the Open-Mouth View of C1/C2

It is not accurate to state that magnification of C1/C2 and of the open mouth effectively cancels each other out at different SIDs, because *the OID to the open mouth is approximately double the OID to the odontoid process.* Object-to-image receptor distance (OID) has a profound effect on magnification. In fact, when the OID is close to 0, it renders the SID negligible insofar as magnification is concerned. In this case, both the odontoid and the open mouth are at very significant OIDs, and both undergo measurable magnification. From the tabletop, the OID to the odontoid is about 10 centimeters, while the OID to the mouth is about 20 centimeters.

It is not untrue to say that both are magnified as the SID is shortened. However, the *degree* of magnification is much greater for the open mouth because of the doubled OID. If the odontoid is magnified by 10%, but the open mouth is magnified by 20%, then the net effect will be equivalent to a wider opening of the mouth and less superimposition of the teeth over the upper vertebrae.

The open-mouth projection of C1 and C2 should *not* be done at a 72-inch SID. The shorter the distance, the better is the view of the upper vertebrae.

8.3: Standing Thoracic Spine Lateral

The radiographer is incorrect. Since the spine is a midline structure (side-to-side) and is equidistant from the IR from either the right or the left side, either lateral can be performed with an equal amount of magnification present in the image.

9.1: Adapting a Reversed Caldwell (#1)

The vertical lies above the orbitomeatal line (OML), so the head is flexed. The vertical is midway between the OML and the glabellomeatal line (GBL). The GBL lies at 10°, so a line midway to it represents 5° of flexion. Normally, a reversed Caldwell would use a 15° *cephalic* (reversed) angle. Flexion of the head tends to *cancel that angle out*, so the 5° must be added. *The answer is 20° cephalic.*

9.2: Adapting a Reversed Caldwell (#2)

The infraorbitomeatal line (IOML) is at 7°. The acanthiomeatal line (AML) is at 27°. The difference between them is 20°. Two-thirds of 20 is about 14, so the head is 7° (for the IOML) + 14° = 21° extended. Normally, a reversed Caldwell would use a 15° *cephalic* (reversed) angle. Extension of the head is *equivalent to the desired cephalic angle*, but it has gone too far, 6° *past* the 15° needed. To cancel out the extra 6°, the CR must be angled *caudally*.

Mathematically stated, extension of the head *contributes to a cephalic angle*, so the 21° must be subtracted from the normal angle. 15 − 21 = −6. The minus sign indicates that the angle is *opposite to cephalic, that is, caudal. The answer is 6° caudal.*

9.3: Adapting a Reversed Waters

The acanthiomeatal line (AML) is at 27°. The mentomeatal line (MML) is at 53°. The difference between them is 53 − 27 = 26. One-third of 26 is about 9, so the head is 27° (for the AML) + 9° = 36° extended. Normally, a reversed Waters would use a 53° *cephalic* (reversed) angle. Extension of the head is *equivalent to the desired cephalic angle*, so the 36° will be subtracted from the normal angle. 53 − 36 = 17. *The answer is 17° cephalic.*

9.4: Modified Waters for Infant

The usual amount of head extension used for an adult must be reduced by approximately one-third for an infant. *Beware, however, that the normal head extension is* ***53°****, not 37° (37° is the angle from the OML to the IR plate).* One-third of 53° is about 18°. Reducing it by that amount, 53 − 18 = 37. The child's head should be extended 37°.

Now, to obtain the angle from the OML to the IR plate, the 37° of head extension must be subtracted from 90° (the angle of the plate from the CR): 90 − 37 = 53. *The answer is that the angle between the OML and the IR plate should measure 53°.*

(You will note that this answer is *increased* from 37° which may seem backward when we are trying to *reduce* head extension. As explained in this chapter, for the Waters projection, head extension is measured from the position of the CR, not from the IR plate, so its angle moves *opposite* from the angle to the plate. As the child's chin is brought back down a bit, reducing extension, the angle between the OML and the plate goes *up*. This is the correct answer.)

9.5: Modified Townes

With the orbitomeatal line at 0°, the glabellomeatal line (GML) is at 10°. Two-thirds of 10 is about 7, so the head is 7° flexed. If the chin could be flexed enough to place the OML vertical, a Townes projection would use a 30° caudal angle. Flexion of the head is *equivalent to the desired cephalic angle*, so the 7° will be subtracted from the normal angle: 30 − 7 = 23. *The answer is 23° caudal.*

10.1: Centering Rule for PA Chest

This rule meets criteria 2 through 5. It is self-correcting and automatically compensates for patient size because larger patients have larger scapulae, bringing the centering point down from the shoulders more as the entire chest expands. It is independent of the radiographer's own body size. It is simple and requires no special equipment. And, it is quick and easy on the patient.

The rule does not (at least fully) meet criterion #1. Whether the scapula is directly related to the lung size is at best debatable, but more importantly, *the scapulae move when the patient shrugs his shoulders forward for the PA projection, and more so when he raises his arms for the lateral position.* The rule assumes that the shoulders are shrugged forward when the centering is checked. If the patient cannot or has not pulled the shoulders forward, the result will be slightly low centering. For the lateral, raising the arms pulls the scapulae up by an inch or more, so the rule cannot be directly applied to the lateral, but lateral centering can be derived from the PA centering.

All in all, the rule meets four of the first five criteria, and is especially good at compensating for differences in patient size. It is therefore good enough for adoption by those who prefer it, but it is helpful to double-check it against *other* rules. (It is always wise to use more than one rule, and learn to split the differences when they do not precisely agree.) Criterion #6 provides the final analysis, whether over a period of time and given ample data, the rule can be shown to *reduce repeat rates*.

10.2: Head Position for the Lateral (Oblique) Mandible

You will find by experimentation that when the face is rotated 15° toward the tabletop, the gonion and ramus of the *downside* mandible, the anatomy of interest, shifts posteriorly enough to run into the cervical spine. That is, the cervical spine is projected over the ramus, preventing a clear view of the very anatomy the position is supposedly designed to demonstrate.

An unobstructed view can be obtained using 35° of head *tilt*, cephalic angulation, or a combination of the two, while leaving the head lateral or rotating it toward the table no more than 5°.

10.3: Correcting Head Rotation for the Rhese Position

First, in a prone position with a PA projection, rotating the face toward the left is equivalent to angling the CR toward the patient's *right*. (Both result in the *left* side of the face coming into view from behind.) The correct degree of angle is 37°, not 53° (as stated in some books). The 53° angle is the *position* angle as measured from the tabletop, or from the *horizontal*, to the midsagittal plane. What is needed is the *projection* angle from the usual central ray, or from the *vertical*. You must subtract the position angle from 90° to obtain the projection angle.

Second, since this is a transverse angle, you will need to swivel the x-ray tube for a typical fixed unit 90° so that you can use the normal angle lock to angle across the table.

You cannot use a transverse angle with the plate in the Bucky tray. There are two options: 1) Just shoot the projection *nongrid* with a plate placed on the tabletop, or 2) use a wafer grid with the plate or a gridded cassette, but be sure to place it on the tabletop such that the grid lines run *transversely across the table* aligned with the angulation of the beam.

10.4: Angulation Adjustment for Normal Lateral L5–S1 "Spot"

For a normal patient, if the L5–S1 joint space is "locked" into place within the pelvic girdle, then any determined tilt of the joint space would also imply that the entire pelvis was tilted by the same amount. This would then raise the upper crest toward the head such that a line drawn between the two iliac crests would parallel the joint space itself. With this being the case, any normal centering based on the upper iliac crest (such as "1½ inches below the crest") would correctly apply *without recentering* relative to the crest. The angle of the CR would simply parallel the pelvic tilt and pass through the L5–S1 joint space.

11.1: Correction for an AP Cervical Spine Projection

The patient's head (chin) was overflexed. The chin must be lifted and the base of the skull will move downward accordingly. Since the distance between them on the image was 1½ inches, but *both* move in opposite directions, the chin must be extended by just ¾ inch from its original position.

11.2: Precise Cassette Critique for TMJs/Mastoids

The sharper of the two mandibular rami is at the upper arrow. The upper ramus and surrounding anatomy is the *downside* anatomy on the patient.

(Note that when observing the TMJs themselves, the lower one is more *visible*. It is not superimposed by the parietal portion of the skull as is the upper one. Therefore, it is presented with better contrast and is more visible. It is easy to visually mistake this improved visibility for higher *sharpness*. By also comparing other anatomy, such as the rami, you can reaffirm a better conclusion. Note that where the arrows are placed, we are comparing two similar points on the mandible, but with *both of them* in identical circumstances. That is, at the arrows, neither ramus is superimposed by skull bones. Both have soft tissue behind them. We can expect the contrast of the two to be equal, and therefore any differences observed are more certainly due to sharpness. This is not true for the two TMJs, in which the superimposition of skull bones over the upper one changes the background contrast and therefore makes it more difficult to determine differences in sharpness.)

The distance between the two TMJs (or EAMs) is 3 to 3½ inches, with the one almost in a straight line directly below the other. Using the "1 inch for every 10°" rule, this translates to 30°–35° of tube angle (or of head tilt), and almost no rotation of the head. Having determined that the upper TMJ is the *downside*, we conclude that the *upside TMJ is being projected straight downward by a 30°–35°* caudal *angle of the CR*.

At first glance, you may conclude that there is substantial rotation, but *most of the shift in the image is up-down shift*. You must use identical anatomical points from each side. Comparing the two TMJs (similar points on the mandible), there is slight side-to-side shift of the lower one behind the upper one. This only amounts to about ½ centimeter, representing only 2° or 3° of rotation, and is not repeatable for a lateral skull position. Slight rotation is present.

This view has the traditional name of the *Schuller method*, in which the head is in a true lateral position and a 35° caudal angle is used to project the upside TMJ and mastoids well down below the downside. In this way, the only bones superimposing the downside TMJ is the flat parietal portion of the skull, rather than the opposite petrous portions, mastoids, TMJ, and ramus.

11.3: Correcting Head Extension for the Rhese Position

First, recall from this chapter that the acanthiomeatal line (AML) lies at 27°. To place it perpendicular for the Rhese position, then, means that the head should be *extended* 27°. You have estimated that her head is extended about 20°, so another 7° is needed, and you must achieve this with tube angulation. For the routine Rhese method with the patient prone and the head in PA projection, *caudal* angulation is equivalent to raising the chin. (Both result in looking *downward* more on the head from behind.) *The answer is 7° caudal.*

12.1: Corrections on an Open-Mouth Odontoid View

In the radiograph, the base of the occipital bone is projected not quite 1½ inches (3 cm) below the bottom edge of the upper incisor teeth. The general shift rule is "1 inch for every 10°," but remember that for the skull, this rule is somewhat *under*stated. For 1½ inches of shift, we conclude that the head is extended *at least* 15°. (Using the more precise rule for the skull, "1 centimeter for every 6°," we conclude that the head is extended 18°.) There is no rotation in the view. *On the repeat exposure, the chin must be tucked 15°–18°, which will likely require a thick sponge.*

In AP projection, flexing the head is equivalent to *caudal* angulation (both result in looking *down* on the face from front). *The angle needed to correct this view is 15°–18° caudal.*

12.2: Correction for Flexion/Extension on a Waters View

In the radiograph, the petrous ridges are projected 1 centimeter or slightly more below the floors of the orbits. By Figure 12-41 in this chapter, this is 6°–8° below the orbital floors, which are themselves 24° below the zero point for a PA projection. This patient's orbitomeatal line (OML) has been extended 30°–32°.

For the Waters projection, 53° of head extension is needed. Subtracting the actual extension from that needed, the head extension here is 21°–23°. In PA projection, head extension is equivalent to *caudal* angulation (both result in looking *down* on the head from behind). *The angle needed to correct this view is 21°–23° caudal.*

12.3: Corrections on a Rhese View

For the Rhese view, you should project the optic foramen in the center of the lower-outer quadrant of the orbit. Here it is both much too high in the orbit and much too medial. The orbit can be divided into four equal levels, each about 1 centimeter apart and represent 6° each (see Figure 12-41 in chapter 12). You can apply the same measurement system to approximate side-to-side shift for rotation. The foramen is posterior to the orbital rim, so flexing the head moves it *up* within the orbit, and rotating the head *shallower* toward lateral moves it medially.

Here, the foramen is at the upper quarter rather than the lower quarter, about 2 centimeters too high. This means the chin was lifted 12° *short* of the head extension needed (it is 12° overflexed).

Side to side, the foramen is a bit past the midline of the orbit moving medially. This is a little more than 1 centimeter more medial than it should be. This translates to about 8° of overrotation shallower toward lateral.

To correct this projection, first you must extend the head another 12° *or use a 12° caudal angle* on the CR. Then, you must rotate the head *steeper* by 8°.

13.1: Adjusting Technique for an Unusual SID

Refer to the "at least one step in mAs (at least 35%) for every 10 inches" rule, but with adaptations as follows: From your 40-inch technique to a 50-inch SID, increase by one step in mAs. Now, from 50 inches to 60 inches would be another step, but the actual increase in SID is halfway from 50 inches to 60 inches, so the equivalent of a half-step additional increase is needed.

This will not be available on the mAs settings, but an equivalent increase in kVp could be used, by applying the 15% rule in proportions. For the mobile unit, if every two steps in mAs is usually a doubling or a 100% increase, then each step will be approximately halfway to double or a 50% increase. We need roughly half of that, or a 25% increase. This is *one-quarter* of the way to a doubling. The 15% rule states that this amount of increase in kVp is equivalent to a doubling of the mAs. We need one-fourth of that, or one-quarter of the way to 15%. This would be about 4%. Four percent of 74 is 3 kVp.

The most precise answer for this situation is to increase the mAs by one step and also add 3 or 4 kVp.

13.2: Adjusting kVp for a Thicker Patient

Use the rule "For each 4-centimeter change in part thickness, adjust technique by a factor of 2," but adapted for the 15% rule for kVp as follows: For the first 4-centimeter increase, from the average 22 centimeters to 26 centimeters, a doubling is needed. Employing kVp, this will be a one-step increase of 15%. Now, 15% of 80 is 12, so this brings the kVp from 80 up to 92.

From here, we need another increase equivalent to *halfway to a doubling*. If the patient were 30 centimeters thick, another doubling would be needed. The actual patient thickness, 28 centimeters, falls halfway from 26 to 30. An increase in kVp equal to *one-half of 15%* will accomplish this, but this increase must be based on the *adjusted* kVp of 92 rather than the original 80 kVp. Fifteen percent of 92 is 14. Half of this is 7: 92 + 7 = 99 kVp. *The answer is to change the kVp from 80 to 99 or 100 kVp.*

13.3: Using the 15% Rule to Prevent Motion from Breathing

Yes, an exposure time of 0.6 seconds could result in a blurred image due to breathing motion. Using a 15% increase in kVp, the new technique should be 92 kVp at 30 mAs.

14.1: Series Sequence for Multiple Trauma #1

1. Chest one-view
2. Pelvis
3. Abdomen
4. AP L-spine
5. AP shoulders (internal and external rotation)
6. AP leg
7. Cross-table lateral leg
8. Cross-table lateral L-spine
9. Cross-table lateral L-spine spot

14.2: Series Sequence for Multiple Trauma #2

1. Chest one-view
2. AP left ribs
3. AP left ribs below the diaphragm
4. Modified oblique left ribs (using angle)
5. Modified oblique AP sternum (using angle)
6. Cross-table lateral sternum
7. Cross-table lateral skull
8. AP skull

14.3: Series Sequence for Multiple Trauma #3

1. Cross-table lateral C-spine
2. Cross-table lateral skull
3. AP skull
4. AP C-spine
5. AP odontoid
6. AP chest
7. AP T-spine
8. AP L-spine
9. Right oblique L-spine
10. Right oblique C-spine
11. Left oblique C-spine
12. Left oblique L-spine
13. Left lateral L-spine
14. Left lateral L-spine spot
15. Left lateral T-spine

14.4: Series Sequence for Multiple Trauma #4

1. AP right shoulder
2. AP right humerus
3. AP right elbow
4. AP right forearm
5. AP right wrist
6. AP right hand
7. Cross-table lateral right hand
8. Cross-table lateral right wrist
9. Cross-table lateral right forearm
10. Cross-table lateral right elbow
11. Cross-table lateral right humerus
12. Cross-table oblique hand
13. Cross-table oblique wrist

14.5: Series Sequence for Multiple Trauma #5

1. Cross-table lateral C-spine (for long SID)
2. Lateral skull
3. Lateral facial bones
4. Oblique lateral mandible
5. Zygomatic arches
6. AP C-spine
7. AP odontoid
8. PA mandible
9. PA facial bones
10. PA skull

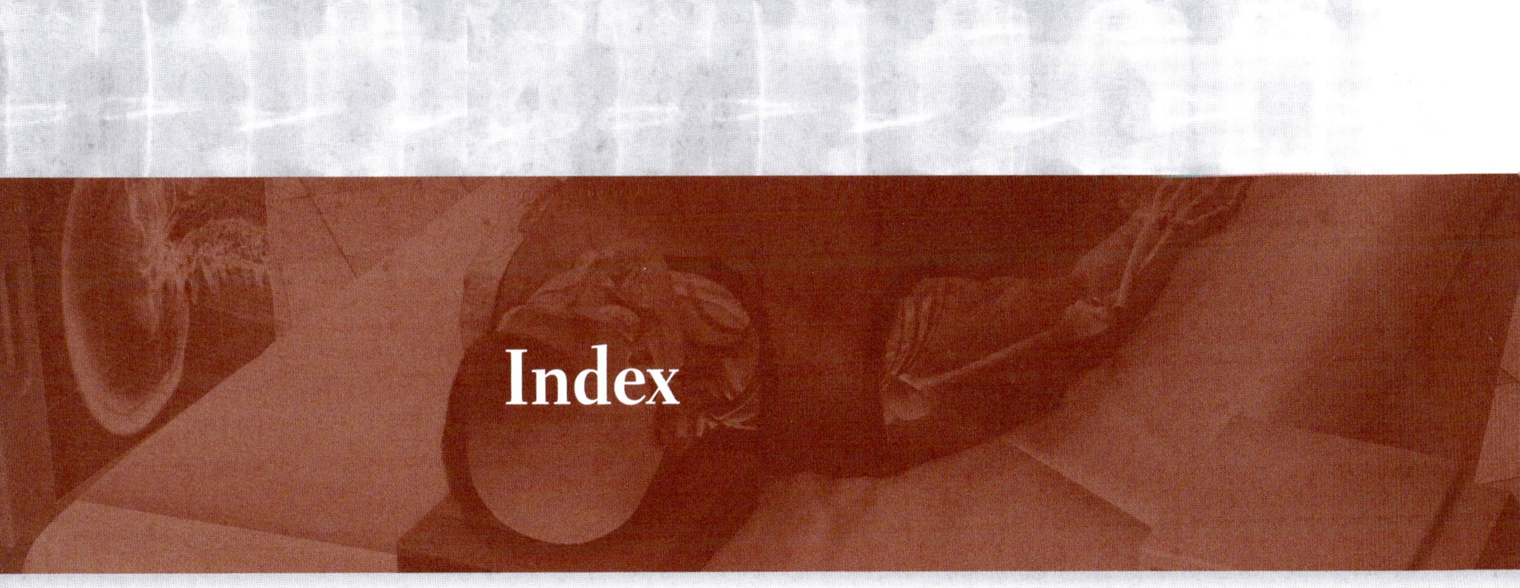

Index

A

B

C

D

H

I

J

K

L

T

U

V

W

X

Z

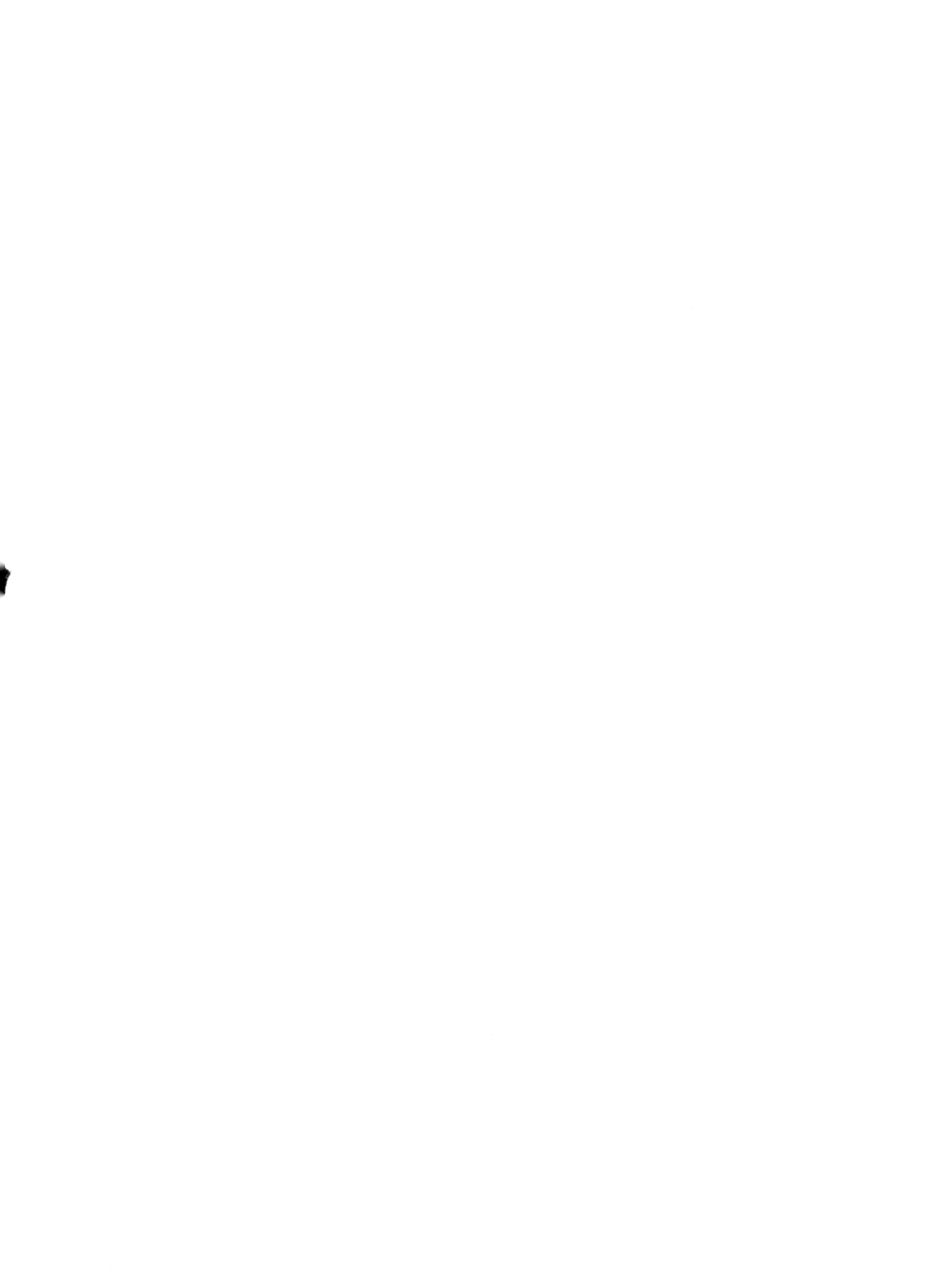